Biomechanical Basis of Human Movement

SECOND EDITION

Biomechanical Basis of Human Movement

SECOND EDITION

Joseph Hamill, PhD
Professor,
Department of Exercise Science
University of Massachusetts at Amherst
Amherst, Massachusetts

Kathleen M. Knutzen, PhD
Professor, Department of Physical Education,
    Health and Recreation
Western Washington University
Bellingham, Washington

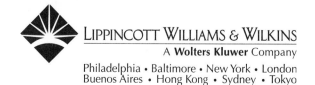

LIPPINCOTT WILLIAMS & WILKINS
A **Wolters Kluwer** Company
Philadelphia • Baltimore • New York • London
Buenos Aires • Hong Kong • Sydney • Tokyo

Editor: Peter J. Darcy
Managing Editor: Linda S. Napora
Marketing Manager: Christen DeMarco
Production Editor: Jennifer Ajello
Designer: Doug Smock
Compositor: Techbooks
Printer: Quebecor World-Versailles

Printed in the United States of America

First Edition, 1995

Library of Congress Cataloging-in-Publication Data

Hamill, Joseph, 1946–
    Biomechanical basis of human movement / Joseph Hamill, Kathleen M. Knutzen.—2nd ed.
        p. cm.
    Includes bibliographical references and index.
    ISBN 0-7817-3405-3
    1. Human mechanics.   I. Knutzen, Kathleen.   II. Title.

    QP303 .H354 2003
    612.7′6—dc21   2002034025

The publishers have made every effort to trace the copyright holders for borrowed material. If they have inadvertently overlooked any, will be pleased to make the necessary arrangements at the first opportunity.

Dedication

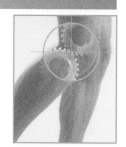

To my mother, Ruth; father, David; brothers, David and Matthew; and sister, Adelaide; to my wife, Donna; and to my numerous graduate and undergraduate students who have made the journey well worth it.

J. H.

With love to my mother, Pauline, and daughter, Amanda, and with great respect for the many students over the years.

K. K.

Acknowledgments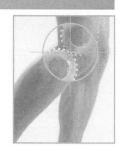

To those who reviewed this edition of the book and who made a substantial contribution to its development, we express our sincere appreciation. We also thank Pete Darcy, Linda Napora, and Jennifer Ajello of Lippincott Williams & Wilkins and Tim Hengst and Joyce Lavery, medical illustrators, for their expertise throughout the publishing process. A special thanks also to Collan Clark for the photography used throughout.

Preface

Biomechanics can be taught from either a quantitative or qualitative perspective within the disciplines of movement sciences. Biomechanical Basis of Human Movement is an introductory textbook that stresses the quantitative rather than qualitative nature of biomechanics. Although this approach stresses the quantification of human movement, the text is also accessible to those with a limited background in mathematics. The quantitative examples are presented in a detailed, logical manner that highlights topics of interest. Our goal is to provide an introductory text in biomechanics that integrates basic anatomy, physics, calculus, and physiology for the study of human movement. We chose this approach because numerical examples are meaningful and easily clear up misconceptions concerning the mechanics of human movement.

This text is organized in three sections: Part I, Foundations of Human Movement (Chapters 1 to 4); Part II, Functional Anatomy (Chapters 5 to 7); and Part III, Mechanical Analysis of Human Motion (Chapters 8 to 11). The chapters are ordered to provide a logical progression of material essential for understanding the biomechanics of human movement.

Part I, Foundations of Human Movement, Chapter 1, Basic Movement Terminology, presents some of the terminology and nomenclature generally used in biomechanics. Chapter 2, Skeletal Considerations for Movement, covers the skeletal system with particular emphasis on joint articulation. Chapter 3, Muscular Considerations for Movement, discusses the organization of the muscular system. Chapter 4, Neurological Considerations for Movement, presents the control and activation systems for human movement.

Part II, Functional Anatomy, Chapters 5 to 7, deals with specific regions of the body: the upper extremity, lower extremity, and trunk, respectively. Each chapter integrates the general information presented in Part I relative to each region.

Part III, Mechanical Analysis of Human Motion, Chapters 8 to 11, covers the quantitative mechanical techniques for the analysis of human movement. Chapter 8 and 9 provide the concepts of linear and angular kinematics.

These chapters include the equations used to describe the motion of projectiles and the conventions for the study of angular motion in the analysis of human movement. Chapters 10 and 11 present the concepts of linear and angular kinetics, including discussions of the forces and torques that act on the human body during daily activities. These chapters also discuss the inertial characteristics of the segments of the body. A portion of each chapter is devoted to a review of the research literature on human locomotion, wheelchair propulsion, and golf, with applications related to the section being studied. Mechanical analysis methods are incorporated into the kinematic and kinetic chapters. A walking data set has been created to provide students with a hands-on approach to computing a wide range of biomechanical parameters. All four chapters have numerous references to the data set, with relevant assignments in relation to the content being studied.

The book is organized to enable instructors to delete or de-emphasize certain sections. Although the chapters follow a progressive order, the major sections are generally self-contained. Parts I and II, Foundations of Human Movement and Functional Anatomy, for example, could be used in a more traditional kinesiology course; Part III, Mechanical Analysis of Human Motion, could be used for a biomechanics course.

Several features of this text serve as effective means for students to comprehend biomechanics as a field of study:

Objectives and Outline: To reinforce the principles, each chapter begins with objectives to enable the student to focus on key points in the material and an outline to guide the reader through the chapter. Each chapter is accompanied by a series of problems that highlight the concepts in the chapter. A key element of this textbook is its examples of human movement. Whereas illustrations of the principles of human movement are easily seen in most sports examples, applications from ergonomics, orthopaedics, and exercise are presented too, with references from the current biomechanics literature. In this way, the full continuum of human movement potential is covered by actual examples.

Chapter Summary: A summary at the end of each chapter outlines the major concepts.

Glossary: The glossary on the last page or pages of each chapter defines the terms found in each chapter, as a source of reinforcement and reference.

References and Additional Reading: Both an up-to-date reference list of the research literature cited in the chapter and a list of additional readings for students who wish to study the material in more depth are included.

Review Questions: Each chapter contains a series of review questions (both true–false and multiple choice) to challenge students and to help them digest and integrate the material.

Appendices: The appendices present information on bony landmarks, ligaments, muscles, units of measurement, trigonometric functions, and the kinematic data on a walking stride.

It is our hope that readers will find the second edition of Biomechanical Basis of Human Movement a helpful guide for studying the basic anatomy, physics, calculus, and physiology of human movement.

Joseph Hamill
Kathleen M. Knutzen

Contents

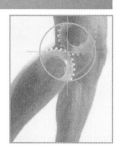

Foundations of Human Movement

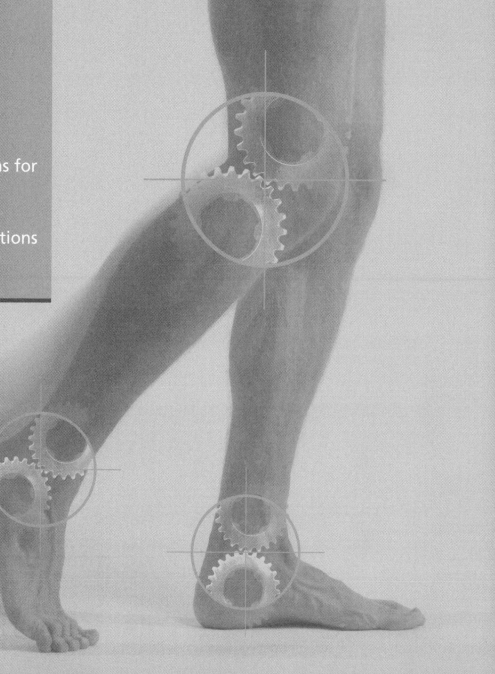

Basic Terminology

OBJECTIVES

After reading this chapter, the student will be able to:

1. Define mechanics, biomechanics, and kinesiology and differentiate among their uses in the analysis of human movement.
2. Define and provide examples of linear and angular motion.
3. Define kinematics and kinetics.
4. Explain the difference between relative and absolute reference systems.
5. Define how the mechanical properties of a structure can be expressed in terms of its stress–strain relationship.
6. Define stress, strain, elastic region, plastic region, yield point, failure point, and elastic modulus.
7. Describe the difference between an elastic and a viscoelastic material.
8. Differentiate between brittle, stiff, and compliant materials.
9. Define sagittal, frontal, and transverse planes along with corresponding frontal, sagittal, and longitudinal axes. Provide examples of human movements that occur in each plane.
10. Explain *degree of freedom* and provide examples of degrees of freedom associated with numerous joints in the body.
11. Describe the location of segments or landmarks using correct anatomical terms, such as medial, lateral, proximal, and distal.
12. Identify segments by their correct name, define all segmental movement descriptors, and provide specific examples in the body.

Introduction

To begin or renew the study of kinesiology and biomechanics using this textbook requires a fresh mind. Remember that human movement is the theme and the focus of study in both biomechanics and kinesiology. A thorough understanding of various aspects of human movement may facilitate better teaching, successful coaching, more observant therapy, knowledgeable exercise prescription, or new research ideas. Movement is the means by which we interact with our environment, whether it be simply to take a walk in a park, to strengthen muscles in a bench press, to compete in the high jump at a collegiate track meet, or to stretch or rehabilitate an injured joint. Movement, or motion, involves a change in place, position, or posture relative to some point in the environment.

This textbook focuses on developing knowledge in the area of human movement in such a manner that you will feel comfortable observing human movement and solving movement problems. There are many approaches to the study of movement, such as observing movement using only the human eye and collecting data on movement parameters using laboratory equipment. Observers of activities also have different concerns: a coach may be interested in the final outcome of a tennis serve, while a therapist may be interested in identifying where in the serve the athlete is placing the stress on the elbow with tendinitis. Some applications of biomechanics and kinesiology will require only a cursory view of a movement, such as visual inspection of the forearm position in the jump shot. Other applications, such as evaluating the forces applied by the hand on the basketball during the shot, will require some advanced knowledge and the use of sophisticated equipment and techniques.

Elaborate equipment is not needed to apply the material in this text, but it will be necessary to understand and interpret numerical examples collected using such intricate instruments. Qualitative examples in this text describe the characteristics of movement. A **qualitative analysis** is a nonnumeric evaluation of motion based on direct observation. These examples can be applied directly to a particular movement situation using visual observation or video.

This text also presents quantitative information. A **quantitative analysis** is a numeric evaluation of the motion based on data collected during the performance. For example, movement characteristics can be presented to describe the forces or the temporal and spatial components of the activity. The application of this material to a practical setting, such as teaching a sport skill, is more difficult, since it is more abstract and often cannot be visually observed. However, quantitative information is very important, since it substantiates what is seen visually in a qualitative analysis. It also directs the instructional technique, because a quantitative analysis will identify the source of a movement. For example, a front handspring

can be qualitatively evaluated through visual observation by focusing on such things as whether the legs are together and straight, the back arched, the landing solid and whether it was too fast or slow. But it is through the quantitative analysis that the source of the movement, the magnitude of the forces generated, can be identified. A force cannot be observed qualitatively, but knowing it is the source of the movement will help with qualitative assessment of its effects, that is, the success of the handspring.

This chapter introduces terminology that will be used throughout the text. The chapter begins by defining and introducing the various areas of study for movement analysis. This will be the first exposure to the areas presented in much greater depth later in the text. Next, it discusses methods and terminology describing how we arrive at the basic mechanical properties of various structures. Finally, this chapter establishes a working vocabulary for movement description at both structural and whole-body levels.

 Core Areas of Study

BIOMECHANICS VS KINESIOLOGY

Those who study human movement often disagree over the use of the terms *kinesiology* and *biomechanics*. *Kinesiology* can be used in two ways. First, **kinesiology** as the scientific study of human movement can be an umbrella term used to describe any form of anatomical, physiological, psychological, or mechanical human movement evaluation. Kinesiology also describes the content of a class in which human movement is evaluated by examination of its source and characteristics. Consequently, kinesiology has been used by several disciplines to describe many different content areas. Some departments of physical education and movement science have gone so far as to adopt kinesiology as their department name. However, a class in kinesiology may consist primarily of functional anatomy at one university and strictly biomechanics at another.

Historically, a kinesiology course has been part of college curricula as long as there have been physical education and movement science programs. The course originally focused on the musculoskeletal system, movement efficiency from the anatomical standpoint, and joint and muscular actions during simple and complex movements. A typical student activity in the kinesiology course was to identify discrete phases in an activity, describe the segmental movements occurring in each phase, and identify the major muscular contributors to each joint movement. Thus, if one were completing a kinesiological analysis of the act of rising from a chair, the movements would be hip extension, knee extension, and plantarflexion via the hamstrings, quadriceps femoris, and triceps surae muscle groups, respectively. Most kinesiological analyses are considered qualitative because they involve observing a

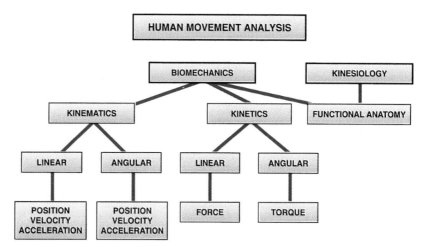

FIGURE 1-1 Types of movement analysis. Movement can be analyzed by assessing the anatomical contributions to the movement (functional anatomy), describing the motion characteristics (kinematics), or determining the cause of the motion (kinetics).

movement and providing a breakdown of the skills and identification of the muscular contributions to the movement.

The content of the study of kinesiology is incorporated into many biomechanics courses and is used as a precursor to the introduction of the more quantitative biomechanical content. In this text, biomechanics will be used as an umbrella term to describe content previously covered in courses in kinesiology, as well as content developed as a result of growth of the area of biomechanics.

In the 1960s and 1970s, biomechanics was developed as an area of study in the undergraduate and graduate curricula across North America. The content of biomechanics was extracted from mechanics, an area of physics that consists of the study of motion and the effect of forces on an object. Mechanics is used by engineers to design and build structures such as bridges and machines such as airplanes, since it provides the tools for analyzing the strength of structures and ways of predicting and measuring the movement of a machine. It was a natural transition to take the tools of mechanics and apply them to living organisms. Thus evolved **biomechanics**, the study of the application of mechanics to biological systems.

A biomechanical analysis evaluates the motion of a living organism and the effect of forces on the living organism. The biomechanical approach to movement analysis can be qualitative, with movement observed and described, or quantitative, meaning that some aspect of the movement will be measured. The use of the term *biomechanics* in this text incorporates qualitative components with a more specific quantitative approach. In such an approach, the motion characteristics of a human or an object are described using such parameters as speed and direction, how the motion is created through application of forces both inside and outside the body, and the optimal body positions and actions for efficient, effective motion. For example, to biomechanically evaluate the motion of rising from a chair, one attempts to measure and identify joint forces acting at the hip, knee, and ankle along with the

force between the foot and the floor, all of which act together to produce the movement up out of the chair. The components of a biomechanical and kinesiologic movement analysis are presented in Figure 1-1. We now examine some of these components individually.

ANATOMY VS FUNCTIONAL ANATOMY

Anatomy, the science of the structure of the body, is the base of the pyramid from which expertise about human movement is developed. It is helpful to develop a strong understanding of regional anatomy so that for a specific region such as the shoulder, the bones, arrangement of muscles, nerve innervation of those muscles, blood supply to those muscles, and other significant structures, such as ligaments, can be identified. A knowledge of anatomy can be put to good use if, for example, one is trying to assess an injury. Assume a patient has a pain on the inside of the elbow. One's knowledge of anatomy allows one to recognize the medial epicondyle of the humerus as the prominent bony structure of the medial elbow. It also indicates that the muscles that pull the hand and fingers toward the forearm into flexion attach to the epicondyle. Thus, familiarity with anatomy may lead to a diagnosis of medial epicondylitis, possibly caused by overuse of the hand flexor muscles.

Functional anatomy is the study of the body components needed to achieve or perform a human movement or function. Functional anatomy, used to analyze a dumbbell lateral raise of the arm, identifies the deltoid, trapezius, levator scapulae, rhomboid, and supraspinatus muscles as contributors to upward rotation and elevation of the shoulder girdle and abduction of the arm. Knowledge of functional anatomy will be useful in a variety of situations, for example to set up an exercise or weight training program and to assess the injury potential in a movement or sport or when establishing training techniques and drills for athletes. The prime consideration of functional anatomy is not the muscle's location but the movement produced by the muscle or muscle group.

LINEAR VS ANGULAR MOTION

Two types of motion are present in a human movement or an object propelled by a human. First is **linear motion,** often termed translation or translational motion. Linear motion is movement along a straight or curved pathway in which all points on a body or an object move the same distance in the same amount of time. Examples are the path of a sprinter, the trajectory of a baseball, the bar movement in a bench press, and the movement of the foot during a football punt. The focus in these activities is on the direction, path, and speed of the movement of the body or object. Figure 1-2 illustrates two focal points for linear movement analysis.

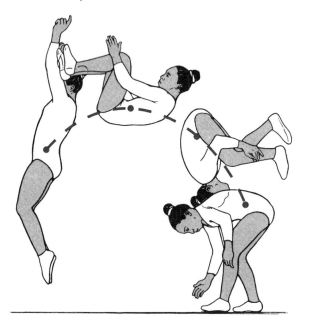

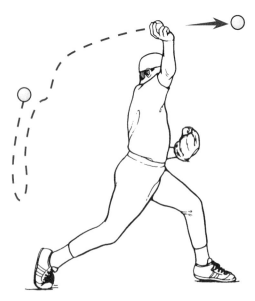

FIGURE 1-2 Examples of linear motion. Ways to apply linear motion analysis include examination of the motion of the center of gravity or the path of a projected object.

The center of mass of the body, of a segment, or of an object is usually the point monitored in a linear analysis (Fig. 1-2). The center of mass is the point at which the mass of the object appears to be concentrated, and it represents the point at which the total effect of gravity acts on the object. However, any point can be selected and evaluated for linear motion. In skill analysis, for example, it is often helpful to monitor the motion of the top of the head to gain an indication of certain trunk motions. An examination of the head in running is a prime example. Does the head move up and down? Side to side? If so, it is an indication that the central mass of the body is also moving in those directions. The path of the hand or racket is important in throwing and racket sports, so visually monitoring the linear movement of the hand or racket throughout the execution of the motion is beneficial. In an activity such as sprinting, the linear movement of the whole body is the most important component to analyze, since the object of the sprint is to move the body quickly from one point to another.

The second type of motion is **angular motion,** which is motion around some point so that different regions of the same body segment or object do not move through the same distance in a given amount of time. As illustrated in Figure 1-3, swinging around a high bar represents angular motion because the whole body rotates around the contact point with the bar. To make one full revolution around the bar, the feet travel through a much greater distance than the arms because they are farther from the point of turning. It is typical in biomechanics to examine the linear motion characteristics of an activity and then follow up with a closer look at the angular motions that create and contribute to the linear motion.

All linear movements of the human and objects propelled by humans occur as a consequence of angular contributions. The only exceptions to this rule are movements such as skydiving or free falling, in which the body is held in a position to let gravity create the linear movement downward, and when an external pull or push moves the body or an object. It is important to identify the angular motions and their sequence that make up a skill or human movement, because the angular motions will determine the success or failure of the linear movement.

Angular motions occur about an imaginary line called the axis of rotation. Angular motion of a segment, such as the arm, occurs about an axis running through the joint. For example, lowering the body into a deep squat entails angular motion of the thigh about the hip joint, angular motion of the leg about the knee joint and angular motion of the foot about the ankle joint. Angular motion can also occur about an axis through the center of mass. Examples of this type of angular motion are a somersault in the air and a figure skater's vertical spin. Finally, angular motion can occur about a fixed external axis. For example, the body follows an angular motion path when swinging

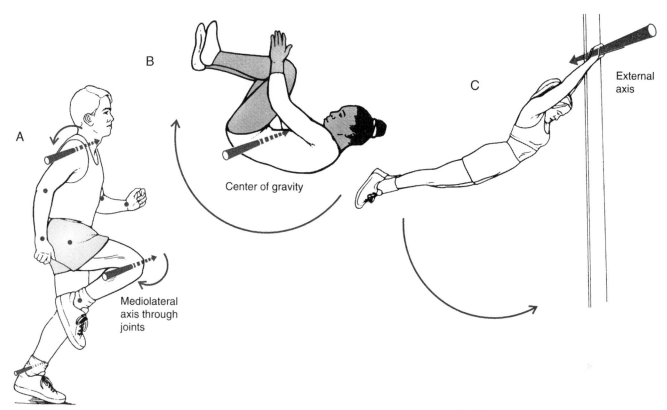

FIGURE 1-3 Examples of angular motion. Angular motion of the body, an object, or segment can take place around an axis running through a joint **(A)**, through the center of gravity **(B)**, or about an external axis **(C)**.

around a high bar, with the high bar acting as the axis of rotation.

For proficiency in human movement analysis, it is necessary to identify the angular motion contributions to the linear motion of the body or an object. This is apparent in a simple activity such as kicking a ball for maximum distance. The intent of the kick is to make solid contact between a foot traveling at a high linear speed and moving in the proper direction to send the ball in the desired direction. The linear motion of interest is the path and velocity of the ball after it leaves the foot. To create the high speeds and the correct path, the angular motions in the kicking leg are sequential, drawing speed from each other so that the velocity of the foot is determined by the summation of the individual velocities of the connecting segments. The kicking leg moves into a preparatory phase, drawing back through angular motions of the thigh, leg, and foot. The leg whips back underneath the thigh very quickly as the thigh starts to move forward to initiate the kick. In the power phase of the kick, the thigh moves vigorously forward and rapidly extends the leg and foot forward at very fast angular speeds. As contact is made with the ball, the foot is moving very fast because the velocities of the thigh and leg have been transferred to the foot. Skilled observation of human movement allows the relationship between angular and linear motion shown in this kicking example to serve as a foundation for techniques used to correct or facilitate a movement pattern or skill.

KINEMATICS VS KINETICS

A biomechanical analysis can be conducted from either of two perspectives. The first, **kinematics**, is concerned with motion characteristics and examines motion from a spatial and temporal perspective without reference to the forces causing the motion. A kinematic analysis involves the description of movement to determine how fast an object is moving, how high it goes, or how far it travels. Thus, position, velocity, and acceleration are the components of interest in a kinematic analysis. Examples of linear kinematic analysis are the examination of the projectile characteristics of a high jumper and a study of the performance of elite swimmers. Examples of angular kinematic analysis are an observation of the joint movement sequence for a tennis serve and an examination of the segmental velocities and accelerations in a vertical jump. Figure 1-4 presents both an angular (*top*) and linear (*bottom*) example of the kinematics of the golf swing. By examining an angular or linear movement kinematically, we can identify segments of a movement that require improvement or obtain ideas and technique enhancements from elite performers or break a skill down into identifiable parts. By each of these, we can further our understanding of human movement.

Pushing on a table may or may not move the table, depending upon the direction and strength of the push. A push or pull between two objects that may or may not result in motion is termed a force. **Kinetics** is the area of because forces cannot be seen (Fig. 1-5). Only the effects of forces can be observed. Watch someone lift a 200-lb barbell in a squat. How much force has been applied? Since the force cannot be seen, there is no way of accurately evaluating the force unless it can be measured with recording instruments. A likely estimate of the force is at least 200 lb, since that is the weight of the bar. The estimate may be off

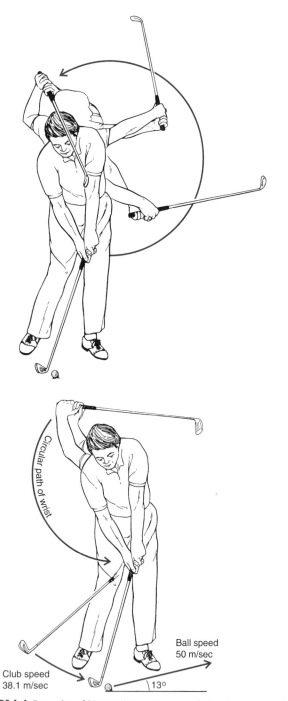

FIGURE 1-4 Examples of kinematic movement analysis. Kinematic analysis focuses on the amount and type of movement, the direction of the movement, and the speed or change in speed of the body or an object. The golf shot is presented from two of these perspectives: the angular components of the golf swing **(top)** and the direction and speed of the club and ball **(bottom)**.

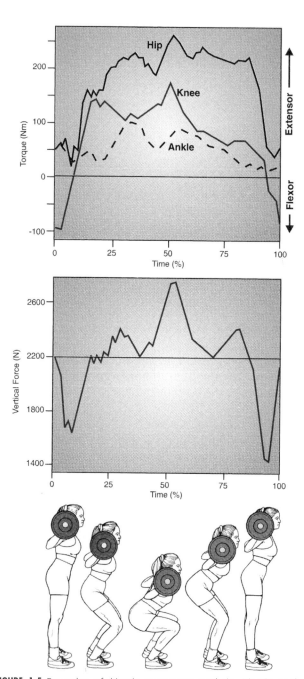

FIGURE 1-5 Examples of kinetic movement analysis. Kinetic analysis focuses on the cause of movement. The weight lifter demonstrates how lifting can be analyzed by looking at the vertical forces on the ground that produce the lift (linear) and the torques produced at the three lower extremity joints that generate the muscular force required for the lift (Redrawn from Lander, J. et al. [1986]. Biomechanics of the squat exercise using a modified center of mass bar. *Medicine and Science in Sports and Exercise,* 18:469–478).

study that examines the forces acting on a system, such as the human body, or any object. A kinetic movement analysis attempts to define the forces causing a movement. A kinetic movement analysis is more difficult than a kinematic analysis both to comprehend and to evaluate, by a significant amount if the weight of the body lifted and the speed of the bar were not considered.

The forces produced during human movement are very important, since they are responsible for creating all of our movements and for maintaining positions or postures having no movement. The assessment of these forces represents the greatest technical challenge in this field, since it requires sophisticated equipment and significant expertise. Thus, for the novice movement analyst, concepts relating to maximizing or minimizing force production in the body will be more important than evaluating the actual forces themselves.

A kinetic analysis can provide the teacher, therapist, coach, or researcher with valuable information about how the movement is produced or how a position is maintained. This information can direct conditioning and training for a sport or movement. For example, kinetic analyses performed by researchers have identified weak and strong positions in various joint movements. Thus, we know that the weakest position for starting an arm curl is with the weights hanging down and the forearm straight. If the same exercise is started with the elbow slightly bent, more weight can be lifted.

Kinetics also identifies the important parts of a skill in terms of movement production. For example, what is the best technique for maximizing a vertical jump? After measuring the forces produced against the ground that are used to propel the body upward, researchers have concluded that the vertical jump incorporating a very quick drop downward and stop-and-pop upward action (often called a countermovement action) produces more effective forces at the ground than the slow, deep gather jump.

Last, kinetics has played a crucial role in identifying aspects of a skill or movement that make the performer prone to injury. Why do 43% of participants and 76% of instructors of high-impact aerobics incur an injury (4)? The answer was clearly identified through a kinetic analysis that found forces in typical high-impact aerobic exercises to be in the magnitude of 4 to 5 times body weight (5). For an individual weighing 667.5 N (newtons) or 150 lb, repeated exposure to forces in the range of 2670 to 3337.5 N (600–750 lb) partially contributes to injury of the musculoskeletal system.

Examination of both the kinematic and kinetic components are essential to full understanding of all aspects of a movement. It is also important to study the kinematic and kinetic relationships, since any acceleration of a limb, of an object, or of the human body is a result of a force applied at some point, at a particular time, of a given magnitude, and for a particular duration. While it is of some use merely to describe the motion characteristics kinematically, one must also explore the kinetic sources before a thorough comprehension of a movement or skill is possible.

STATICS VS DYNAMICS

Examine the posture used to sit at a desk and work at a computer. Are forces being exerted? Yes, even though there is no movement, there are forces between the back and the chair and the foot and the ground. In addition, muscular forces are acting throughout the body to counteract gravity and keep the head and trunk erect. Forces are present without motion and are produced continuously to maintain positions and postures that do not involve movement. Principles of statics are used to evaluate the sitting posture. **Statics** is a branch of mechanics that examines systems that are not moving or are moving at a constant speed. Static systems are considered to be in equilibrium. Equilibrium is a balanced state in which there is no acceleration because the forces causing a person or object to begin moving, to speed up, or to slow down are neutralized by opposite forces that cancel them out.

Statics is also useful for determining stresses on anatomical structures in the body, identifying the magnitude of muscular forces, and identifying the magnitude of force that would result in the loss of equilibrium. How much force generated by the deltoid muscle is required to hold the arm out to the side? Why is it easier to hold an arm at the side if you lower the arm so that it is no longer perpendicular to the body? What is the effect of an increased curvature, or swayback, on forces coming through the lumbar vertebrae? These are the types of questions static analysis may answer. Since the static case involves no change in the kinematics of the system, a static analysis is usually performed using kinetic techniques to identify the forces and the site of the force applications responsible for maintaining a posture, position, or constant speed. However, kinematic analyses can be applied in statics to substantiate whether there is equilibrium through the absence of acceleration.

To leave the computer workstation and get up out of the chair, it is necessary to produce forces in the lower extremity and on the ground. **Dynamics** is the branch of mechanics used to evaluate this type of movement, since it examines systems that are being accelerated. Dynamics uses a kinematic or kinetic approach or both to analyze movement. An analysis of the dynamics of an activity such as running may incorporate a kinematic analysis in which the linear motion of the total body and the angular motion of the segments are described. The kinematic analysis may be related to a kinetic analysis that describes forces applied to the ground and across the joints as the person runs. Since this textbook deals with numerous examples involving motion of the human or a human-propelled object, dynamics is addressed in detail in specific chapters on linear and angular kinematics and kinetics.

 ## Basic Structural Analysis

Section 1 of this book discusses the basic structures that make up the human body. These structures include bone, tendon, ligament, and muscle. Of great interest to biomechanists are the mechanical properties of these tissues. Generally, when analyzing the mechanical properties of such structures, we discern the external forces that are applied to the structure and relate these to the resulting deformation of the structure. The ability of a structure to resist deformation is dependent on its material organization and overall shape. Therefore, this type of analysis is important because it gives us information on the mechanical properties of the structure that may ultimately influence its function.

STRESS–STRAIN

The force applied to deform a structure and the resulting deformation are referred to as stress and strain, respectively. To enable comparison of structures of different sizes, stress and strain are scaled quantities of the force applied and the deformation of the structure, respectively. The values of stress and strain are measured on a machine that can place either tension (pulling stress) or compression (pushing stress) on the structure (Fig. 1-6). In this figure, the load cell measures the tension, or pulling force, applied to the tendon, and the extensiometer measures the length to which the tendon is stretched. The actuator is a motor that initiates the pull on the tendon. Figure 1-7 shows a similar setup to determine the compression stress on an amputated foot. The graph relating stress to strain is the **stress–strain curve** of a structure. A stress–strain analysis can be used in such ways as to discern how a material changes with age, how materials react to different force applications, and how a material reacts to lack of everyday

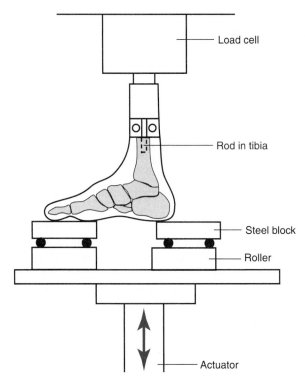

FIGURE 1-7 A testing machine that determines the stress–strain properties of an amputated foot. (Reprinted with permission from Alexander, R. McN. (1992). *The Human Machine*. New York: Columbia University Press.)

stress. Figure 1-8 illustrates the stress–strain relationships of bone vertebrae of normal rhesus monkeys versus those that have been immobilized. A stress–strain analysis can be performed with either pulling force (tension), pushing force (compression) or shear force (a push or pull along the surface of the material). This book deals only with tension and compression stress–strain relationships.

In this type of test, **stress** is defined as the force per unit area and is designated with the Greek letter sigma (σ). Stress is calculated thus:

$$\sigma = \frac{F}{A}$$

where F is the applied force and A is the unit area over which the force is applied. The force is applied perpendicular to the surface of the structure over a predetermined area. The unit in which a force is measured is the newton (N). The unit of area is the square meter (m^2). Thus, the unit of stress is newtons per square meter (N/m^2), or the pascal (Pa).

Deformation or strain is also scaled to the initial length of the structure being tested. That is, the deformation caused by the applied stress is compared to the initial, or resting, length of the material, when no force is applied. Strain, designated by the Greek letter epsilon (ϵ), is therefore defined as the ratio of the change in length to the resting length. Thus:

$$\varepsilon = \frac{\Delta L}{L}$$

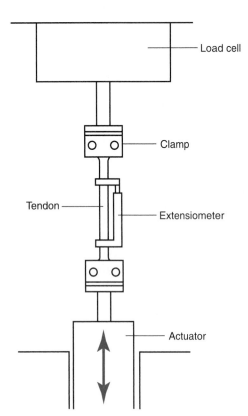

FIGURE 1-6 A testing machine that determines the stress–strain properties of a tendon. The actuator stretches the tendon, which is then allowed to recoil. (Reprinted with permission from Alexander, R. McN. (1992). *The Human Machine*. New York: Columbia University Press.)

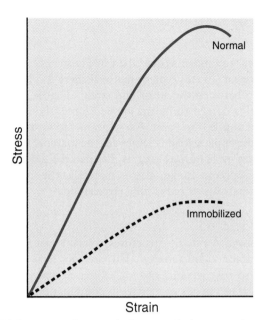

FIGURE 1-8 Stress–strain curves for bone vertebral segments from a normal and immobilized rhesus monkey (Adapted from Kazarian, L. E., Von Gierke, H. E. [1969]. Bone loss as a result of immobilization and chelation. Preliminary results in *Macaca mulatta. Clinical Orthopaedics,* 65:67–75.).

where ΔL is the change in length of the structure and L is the initial length. Because we are dividing a length by a length, there are no units and so strain is a dimensionless number.

A stress–strain curve is presented in Figure 1-9. A number of key points on this curve are important to the ultimate function of the structure. In this curve, the slope of the linear portion of the curve is the **elastic modulus,** or stiffness of the material. Stiffness is thus calculated as:

$$k = \frac{Stress}{Strain} = \frac{\sigma}{\varepsilon}$$

As greater force is applied to the structure, the slope of the curve will eventually decrease. At this point, the structure is said to yield or reach its **yield** point. Up to the yield

point, the structure is said to be in the **elastic region.** If the stress is removed while the material is in this region, the material will return to its original length with no structural damage. After the yield point, the molecular components of the material are permanently displaced with respect to each other, and if the applied force is removed, the material will not return to its original length (Fig. 1-10). The difference between the original length of the material and the (resting) length resulting from stress into the plastic region is the **residual strain**.

The region after the yield point is the **plastic region**. For rigid materials, such as bone, the yield or plastic region is relatively small, while for other materials it can be relatively large. If the applied force continues beyond the plastic region, the structure will eventually reach **failure**, at which point the stress quickly falls to zero. The maximal stress reached when failure occurs determines the failure strength and failure strain of the material.

In normal functional activities, the stress applied will not cause a strain that reaches the yield point. When structures are designed by an engineer, the engineer considers a **safety factor** when determining the stress–strain relationship of the structure. This safety factor is generally in the range of 5 to 10 times the stress that would normally be placed on the structure. That is, the applied force to reach the yield point is significantly greater than the force generally applied in everyday activities. It is obvious and has been suggested that biological materials and biological structures must have a significantly large safety factor. Needless to say, the stresses placed on a biological structure in everyday activities are much less than the structure can handle. Figure 1-11 illustrates a stress–strain curve for a human adult tibia and the actual stress–strain relationship during jogging.

When a structure is deformed by an applied force, the strain developed in the material relates to the mechanical

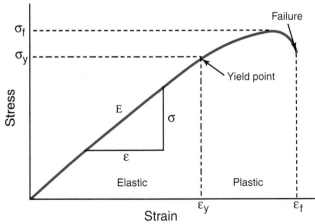

FIGURE 1-9 An idealized stress–strain curve showing the elastic and plastic regions and the elastic modulus.

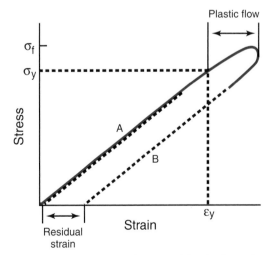

FIGURE 1-10 A stress–strain curve of a material that has been elongated into the plastic region. *A,* The period of the applied load. *B,* The period when the applied load is removed. The residual strain results because of the reorganization of the material at the molecular level.

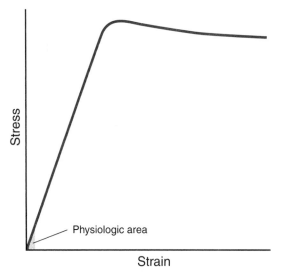

FIGURE 1-11 The shaded area represents the tension stress–strain values of an adult human tibia during jogging while the solid line represents bone samples tested to failure (Adapted with permission from Nordin, M., Frankel, V. H. [1989]. *Basic Biomechanics of the Musculoskeletal System*. Philadelphia: Lea and Febiger.).

energy absorbed by the material. The amount of mechanical energy stored is proportional to the area under the stress–strain curve (Fig. 1-12). That is, the stored mechanical energy is:

$$ME = \frac{1}{2}\,\sigma\varepsilon$$

When the applied force is removed, the stored energy is released. For example, a rubber band can be stretched by pulling on both ends. When one end is released, the rubber band rebounds back to its original length but in doing so releases the energy stored during stretching. For practical purposes, this is the same concept as a trampoline. The weight of the person bouncing on it deforms the bed and stores energy. The trampoline rebounds and releases the stored energy to the person.

TYPES OF MATERIALS

Elastic

The idealized material described in Figure 1-9 is an **elastic material**. In this type of material there is a linear relationship between the stress and strain. That is, when the material is deformed by the applied force, the amount of deformation is the same for a given amount of stress. When the applied load is removed, the material will return to its resting length as long as the material did not reach its yield point. In an elastic material, the mechanical energy that was stored is fully recovered.

Viscoelastic

As opposed to elastic structures, certain materials show stress–strain characteristics that are not strictly linear; these are **viscoelastic** materials. These structures have nonlinear or viscous properties in combination with linear elastic properties. The combination of these properties results in the magnitude of the stress being dependent on the rate of loading, or how fast the load is applied. Nearly all biological materials, such as tendon and ligament, show some level of viscoelasticity.

Figure 1-13 illustrates a viscoelastic material. On a stress– strain curve of a viscoleastic material, the terms stiffness, yield point, and failure point also apply. The elastic and plastic regions are defined similarly as in an elastic material. However, in contrast to an elastic structure, stiffness has several values that can be determined by where it was calculated on the curve. In Figure 1-13, the stiffness designated by E_1 is less than that of E_2. However, E_3 is certainly less than E_2. In addition, in a viscoelastic material, the stored mechanical energy is not completely returned when the applied load is removed. Thus, the energy returned is not equal to the energy stored. The energy that is lost is **hysteresis** (Fig. 1-14).

Materials, whether they are elastic or viscoelastic, are often referred to as stiff, compliant, or brittle, depending on

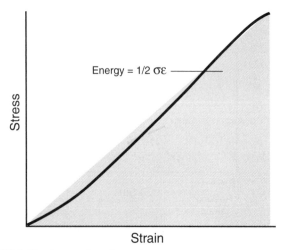

FIGURE 1-12 The stored mechanical energy (*shaded area*) is equal to the area under the stress–strain curve.

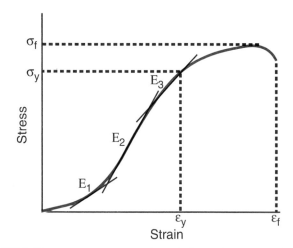

FIGURE 1-13 A stress–strain curve of a typical viscoelastic material. The elastic modulus (slope of the curve) varies according to the portion of the curve on which it is calculated.

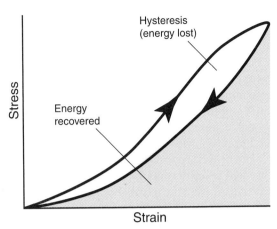

FIGURE 1-14 A stress–strain curve of a typical viscoelastic material showing the energy recovered when the material is allowed to return to its resting length. The hysteresis or energy lost is equal to the energy stored when the material is deformed minus the energy recovered.

the elastic modulus. Stress–strain curves of these materials are presented in Figure 1-15. A compliant material will have an elastic modulus less than that of a stiff material. The compliant material will store considerably more energy than a stiff material. On the other hand, a brittle material will have a greater elastic modulus and will store less energy than a stiff material. Nonetheless, all of these terms are relative. Depending on the materials being tested, a brittle material may be considered stiff relative to one material and compliant relative to another. For example, bone is brittle relative to tendon but compliant relative to glass.

 Anatomical Movement Descriptors

SEGMENT NAMES

To flex the arm, does one lift at the elbow with weights in the hand or raise the whole arm in front? Whatever interpretation is placed on the segment name, the term *arm* will determine the type of movement performed. It is important to identify segment names correctly and use

them consistently when analyzing movement. The correct interpretation of flexing the arm is to raise the whole arm, since the arm is the segment between the shoulder and the elbow, not the segment between the elbow and the wrist or the hand segment. A review of segment names is worthwhile preparation for more extensive use of them in the study of biomechanics.

The head, neck, and trunk are segments composing the main part of the body and the **axial** portion of the skeleton. This portion of the body is large, accounting for more than 50% of a person's weight, and it usually moves much more slowly than the other parts of the body. Because of its large size and slow speed, the trunk is a good segment to observe visually when one is learning to analyze movement or following the total body activity.

The upper and lower extremities are termed the **appendicular** portion of the skeleton. Generally speaking, as one moves away from the trunk, the segments become smaller, move faster, and are more difficult to observe because of their size and speed. Thus, arm flexion is raising the upper extremity in front, while forearm flexion describes a movement at the elbow. The movements of the arm will typically be described as they occur in the shoulder joint; the forearm movements will be described in relation to elbow joint activity; and hand movements will be described relative to wrist joint activity. Figure 1-16 illustrates the axial and appendicular regions of the body with the correct segment names.

In the lower extremity, the thigh is the region between the hip and knee joints; the leg is the region between the knee and ankle joints; and the foot is the region distal to the ankle joint. The movement of the thigh will typically

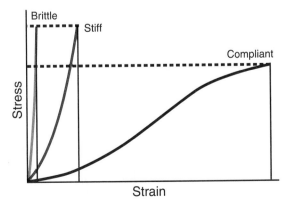

FIGURE 1-15 Stress–strain curves of compliant, stiff and brittle materials. The elastic modulus is significantly different in the three materials.

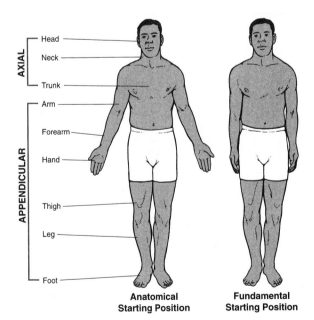

FIGURE 1-16 Anatomical vs fundamental starting position. The anatomical and fundamental starting positions serve as a reference point for the description of joint movements.

be described as it occurs at the hip joint; leg movement, described by actions at the knee joint; and the foot movements, determined by ankle joint activity.

ANATOMICAL TERMS

The description of a segmental position or joint movement is typically expressed relative to a designated starting position. This reference position, the **anatomical position,** has been a standard reference point used for many years by anatomists, biomechanists, and the medical profession. In this position, the body is in an erect stance with the head facing forward, arms at the side of the trunk with palms facing forward, and the legs together with the feet pointing forward. Some biomechanists prefer to use what is called the **fundamental position** as the reference position. This reference position is similar to the anatomical position except that the arms are in a more relaxed posture at the sides with the palms facing in toward the trunk. Whatever starting position is used, all segmental movement descriptions are made relative to some reference position. Both of these reference positions are illustrated in Figure 1-16.

To discuss joint position, we must define the joint angle, or more correctly, the relative angle between two segments. A relative angle is the included angle between the two segments (Fig. 1-17). The calculation of the relative angle will be illustrated in a later section of this book.

The starting position is also called the zero position, or origin, for description of most joint movements. For example, when a person is standing, there is zero movement at the hip joint. If the thigh is lifted or rotated in or out, the amount of movement is described relative to the fundamental or anatomical starting position. Most zero

positions appear to be quite obvious, since there is usually a straight line between the two segments so that no relative angle is formed between them. Zero position in the trunk occurs when the trunk is vertical and lined up with the lower extremity. The zero position at the knee is found in the standing posture when there is no angle between the thigh and the leg. One not so obvious zero position is at the ankle joint. For this joint, the zero position is assumed in stance with the foot at a right angle to the leg.

Movement description or anatomical location can best be presented using terminology universally accepted and understood. Movement terms should become a part of a working vocabulary, regardless of the level of application of kinesiology required. Development of solid knowledge of the movement characteristics of the various phases of a human movement or sport skill can improve the effectiveness of teaching a skill, assist in correcting flaws in a performance, identify important movements and segments for emphasis in conditioning, and identify aspects of the skill that may be associated with injury. The experienced coach or teacher can determine the most relevant movements in a skill and will use a specific vocabulary of terms to instruct students or athletes. A standardized set of terms is most helpful in this situation.

The anatomical terms describing the relative position or direction are illustrated in Figure 1-18. The term **medial** refers to a position relatively close to the midline of the body or object or a movement that moves toward the midline. In the anatomical position, the little finger and the big toe are on the medial side of the extremity, since they are on the side of the limb closest to the midline of the body. Also, pointing the toes toward the midline of the body is considered a medial movement. The opposite of medial is **lateral,** that is, a position relatively far from the midline or a movement away from the midline. The thumb and the little toe are on the lateral side of the hand and foot, respectively, since they are farther from midline. Likewise, pointing the toes out is a lateral movement. Landmarks are also commonly designated as medial or lateral based on their relative position to the midline, such as medial and lateral condyles, epicondyles, and malleoli.

Proximal and **distal** are used to describe the relative position with respect to a designated reference point, with proximal representing a position closer to the reference point and distal being a point farther from the reference. The elbow joint is proximal and the wrist joint is distal relative to the shoulder joint. The ankle joint is proximal and the knee joint is distal relative to the point of heel contact with the ground. Both proximal and distal must be expressed relative to some reference point.

A segment or anatomical landmark may lie on the **superior** aspect of the body, placing it above a particular reference point or closer to the top of the head. It may lie on an **inferior** aspect, that is, lower than a reference segment or landmark. For example, the head is positioned superior to the trunk, the trunk is superior to the thigh, and so on. The greater trochanter is located on the

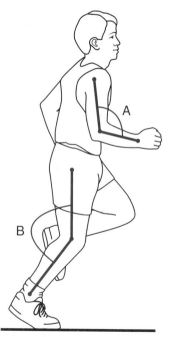

FIGURE 1-17 Relative angles of the elbow **(A)** and the knee **(B)**.

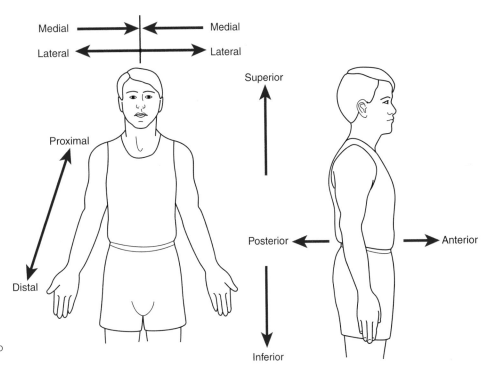

FIGURE 1-18 Anatomical terms used to describe relative position or direction.

superior aspect of the femur, and the medial epicondyle of the humerus is located on the inferior end of the humerus.

The location of an object or a movement relative to the front or back is **anterior** or **posterior**, respectively. Thus, the quadriceps muscle group is located on the anterior aspect of the thigh, while the hamstrings muscle group is located on the posterior aspect of the thigh. Anterior is also synonymous with **ventral** for a location on the human body, while posterior refers to the **dorsal** surface or position on the human.

The term **ipsilateral** describes activity or location of a segment or landmark positioned on the same side as a particular reference point. Actions, positions, and landmark locations on the opposite side can be designated as **contralateral**. Thus, when a person lifts the right leg forward, there is extensive muscular activity in the iliopsoas muscle of that leg, the ipsilateral leg, and extensive activity in the gluteus medius of the contralateral leg to maintain balance and support. In walking, as the ipsilateral lower limb is swinging forward, the other limb, the contralateral limb, is pushing on the ground to propel the walker forward.

MOVEMENT DESCRIPTION

Basic Movements

Six basic movements occur in varying combinations in the joints of the body. The first two movements, flexion and extension, are movements found in almost all of the freely movable joints in the body, including the toe, ankle, knee, hip, trunk, shoulder, elbow, wrist, and finger. **Flexion** is a bending movement in which the relative angle of the joint between two adjacent segments decreases. **Extension** is a straightening movement in which the relative angle of the joint between two adjacent segments increases as the joint returns to the zero or reference position. Numerous examples of both flexion and extension are provided in Figure 1-19. A person can also perform **hyperflexion** if the flexion movement goes beyond the normal range of flexion. For example, this can happen at the shoulder only when the arm moves forward and up in flexion through 180° until it is at the side of the head, and then hyperflexes as it continues to move past the head toward the back. **Hyperextension** can occur in many joints as the extension movement continues past the original zero position. It is common to see hyperextension movements in the trunk, arm, thigh, and hand.

A toe-touch movement entails flexion at the vertebral, shoulder, and hip joints. The return to the standing position involves the opposite movements: of vertebral extension, hip extension, and shoulder extension. The power phase of the jump shot is produced via smooth timing of lower extremity hip extension, knee extension, and ankle extension coordinated with shoulder flexion, elbow extension, and wrist flexion in the shooting limb. This example illustrates the importance of the lower extremity extension movements to the production of power. Lower extremity extension often serves to produce upward propulsion working against the pull of gravity. It is opposite in the shoulder joint, where flexion movements are primarily used to develop propulsion upward against gravity to raise the limb.

The second pair of movements, abduction and adduction, are not as common as flexion and extension, occurring only in the metatarsophalangeal (foot), hip, shoulder, wrist, and metacarpophalangeal (hand) joints.

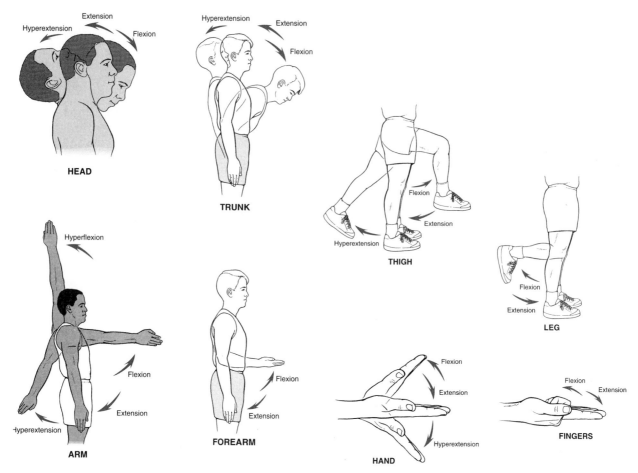

FIGURE 1-19 Flexion and extension. These movements occur in many joints in the body, including vertebra, shoulder, elbow, wrist, metacarpophalanx, interphalanx, hip, knee, and metatarsophalanx.

Many of these movements are presented in Figure 1-20. **Abduction** is a movement away from the midline of the body or the segment. Raising an arm or leg out to the side or the spreading of the fingers or toes is an example of abduction. **Hyperabduction** can occur in the shoulder joint as the arm moves more than 180° from the side all the way up past the head. **Adduction** is the return movement of the segment back toward the midline of the body or segment; bringing the arms back to the trunk, bringing the legs together, and closing the toes or fingers are examples of adduction. **Hyperadduction** occurs frequently in the arm and thigh as the adduction continues past the zero position so that the limb crosses the body. These side-to-side movements are commonly used to maintain balance and stability during the performance of both upper and lower extremity sport skills. Controlling or preventing abduction and adduction movements of the thigh is especially crucial to the maintenance of pelvic and limb stability during walking and running.

The last two basic movements are segment rotations, illustrated in Figure 1-21. A **rotation** can be either medial (also known as internal) or lateral (also known as external). Rotations are designated as right and left for the head and trunk only. When in the fundamental starting position, medial or internal rotation refers to the movement of a segment about a vertical axis running through the segment so that the anterior surface of the segment moves toward the midline of the body while the posterior surface moves away from the midline. Lateral or external rotation is the opposite movement in which the anterior surface moves away from the midline and the posterior surface of the segment moves toward the midline. Since the midline runs through the trunk and head segments, the rotations in these segments are described as left or right from the perspective of the performer. Right rotation is the movement of the anterior surface of the trunk so that it faces right while the posterior surface faces left, and left rotation is the opposite movement so that the anterior trunk faces left and the posterior trunk faces right. Rotations occur in the vertebrae, shoulder, hip, and knee joints. Rotation movements are very important in the power phase of sport skills involving the trunk, arm, or thigh. For throwing, the throwing arm laterally rotates in the preparatory phase and medially rotates in the power and follow-through phases. The trunk complements the arm action with right rotation in the preparatory phase (right-handed thrower) and left rotation in the power and follow-through phase. Likewise, the right thigh laterally rotates in the preparatory phase

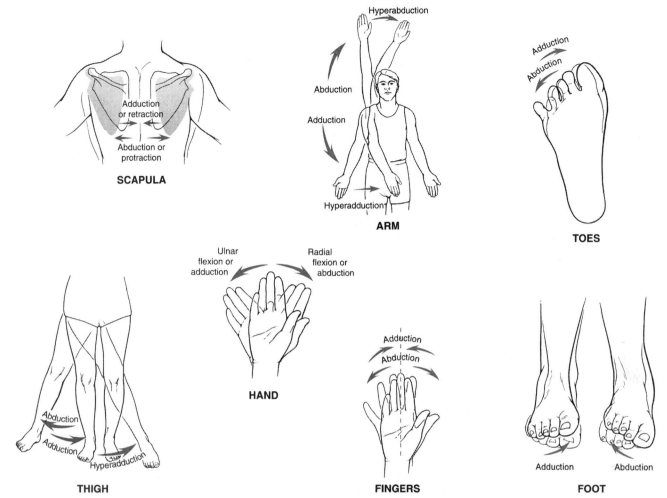

FIGURE 1-20 Abduction and adduction. These movements occur in the sternoclavicular, shoulder, wrist, metacarpophalangeal, hip, intertarsal, and metatarsophalangeal joints.

and medially rotates until the lower extremity comes off the ground in the power phase.

Specialized Movement Descriptors

Specialized movement names are assigned to a variety of segmental movements (Fig. 1-22). While most of these segmental movements are technically among the six basic movements, the specialized movement name is the terminology commonly used by movement professionals. Right and left **lateral flexion** applies only to movement of the head or trunk. When the trunk or head tilts sideways, the movement is termed lateral flexion. If the right side of the trunk or head moves so that it faces down, the movement is termed right lateral flexion and vice versa.

The shoulder girdle has specialized movement names that can best be described by observing the movements of the scapula. The raising of the scapula, as in a shoulder shrug, is termed **elevation**, while the opposite lowering movement is **depression**. If the two scapulae move apart, as in rounding the shoulders, the movement is termed **protraction**. The return movement, in which the scapulae move toward each other with the shoulders back, is called **retraction**. Finally, the scapulae can swing out so that the

bottom of the scapula moves away from the trunk and the top of the scapula moves toward the trunk. This movement is termed **upward rotation**; the return movement, when the scapula swings back down into the resting position, is **downward rotation**.

In the arm and the thigh, a combination of flexion and adduction is termed **horizontal adduction** and a combination of extension and abduction is called **horizontal abduction**. Horizontal adduction, sometimes called horizontal flexion, is the movement of the arm or thigh across the body, toward the midline, using a movement horizontal to the ground. Horizontal abduction, or horizontal extension, is a horizontal movement of the arm or thigh away from the midline of the body. These movements are used in a wide variety of sport skills. The arm action of the discus throw is a good example of the use of horizontal abduction in the preparatory phase and horizontal adduction in the power and follow-through phase. Many soccer skills use horizontal adduction of the thigh to bring the leg up and across the body for a shot or pass.

In the forearm, pronation and supination occur as the distal end of the radius rotates over and back on the ulna

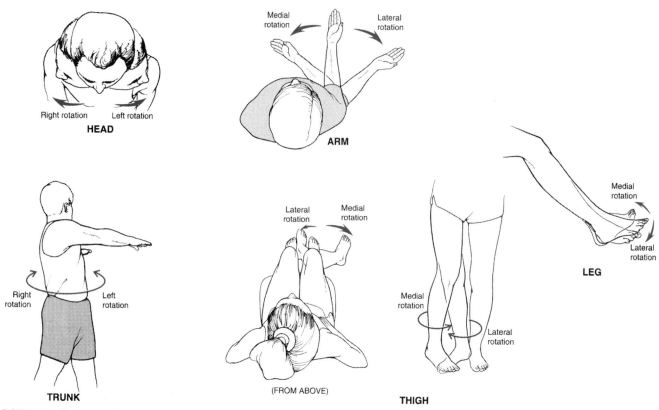

FIGURE 1-21 Rotation. Rotation occurs in the vertebral, shoulder, hip, and knee joints.

at the radioulnar joints. **Supination** is the movement of the forearm in which the palm rotates to face forward from the fundamental starting position. **Pronation** is the movement in which the palms face backward. Supination and pronation joint movements have also been referred to as external and internal rotation, respectively. As the forearm moves from a supinated position to a pronated position, the forearm passes through the semiprone position, in which the palms face the midline of the body with the thumbs forward. The actions of forearm pronation and supination are used with arm rotation movements to increase the range of motion, add spin, enhance power, and change direction during the force application phases in racket sports, volleyball, and throwing.

At the wrist joint, the movement of the hand toward the thumb is called **radial flexion**, while the opposite movement of the hand toward the little finger is called **ulnar flexion**. These specialized movement names are easier to remember because they do not depend on forearm or arm position, as do the interpretation of abduction and adduction, and they can easily be interpreted if the location of the radius (thumb side) and the ulna (little finger side) is known. Ulnar and radial flexion are important in racket sports for control and stabilization of the racket. Also, in volleyball, ulnar flexion is a valuable component of the forearm pass, as it helps to maintain the extended arm position and increases the contact area of the forearms.

In the foot, plantarflexion and dorsiflexion are specialized names for foot extension and flexion, respectively. **Plantarflexion** is the movement in which the bottom of the foot moves down and the angle formed between the foot and the leg increases. This movement can be created by raising the heel so the weight is shifted up on the toes or by placing the foot flat on the ground in front and moving the leg backward so that the body weight is behind the foot. **Dorsiflexion** is the movement of the foot up toward the leg that decreases the relative angle between the leg and the foot. This movement may be created by putting weight on the heels and raising the toes or by keeping the feet flat on the floor and lowering with weight centered over the foot. Any foot–leg angle greater than 90° is termed a plantarflexed position, while any foot–leg angle less than 90° is termed dorsiflexion.

The foot has another set of specialized movements, called inversion and eversion, that occur in the intertarsal and metatarsal articulations. **Inversion** of the foot takes place when the medial border of the foot lifts so that the sole of the foot faces in toward the other foot. **Eversion** is the opposite movement of the foot: the lateral aspect of the foot lifts so that the sole of the foot faces away from the other foot.

Often there is confusion over the use of the terms inversion and eversion and the popularized use of pronation and

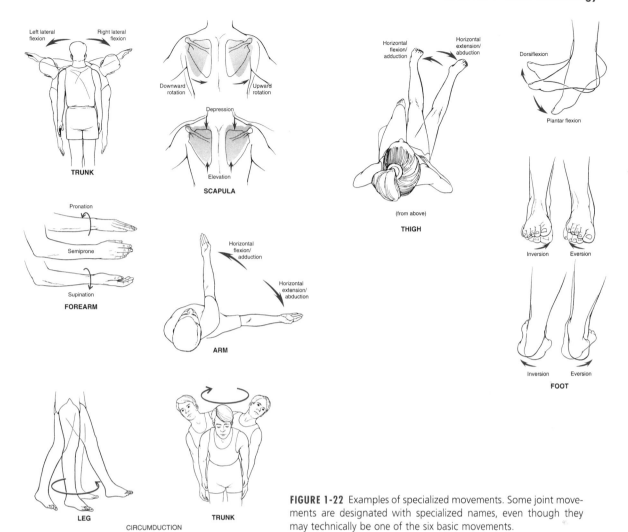

FIGURE 1-22 Examples of specialized movements. Some joint movements are designated with specialized names, even though they may technically be one of the six basic movements.

supination as descriptors of foot motion. Inversion and eversion are not the same as pronation and supination; in fact, they are only a part of pronation and supination. Pronation of the foot is actually a set of movements consisting of dorsiflexion at the ankle joint, eversion in the tarsals, and abduction of the forefoot. Supination is created through ankle plantarflexion, tarsal inversion, and forefoot adduction. Pronation and supination are dynamic movements of the foot and ankle occurring when the foot is on the ground during a run or walk. These two movements are determined by structure and laxity of the foot, body weight, playing surfaces, and footwear.

The final specialized movement, **circumduction**, can be created in any joint or segment that has the potential to move in two directions, so that the segment can be moved in a conic fashion as the end of the segment moves in a circular path. An example of circumduction is placing the arm out in front and drawing an imaginary O in the air. Circumduction is not a simple rotation but four movements in sequence. The movement of the arm in the creation of the imaginary O is actually a combination of flexion, adduction, extension, and abduction.

Circumduction movements are also possible in the foot, thigh, trunk, head, and hand. The movements of all of the major segments are reviewed in Table 1-1.

Reference Systems

RELATIVE VS ABSOLUTE

A reference system is necessary for accurate observation and description of any type of motion. The use of joint movements relative to the fundamental or anatomical starting position is an example of a simple reference system. This system was previously used in this chapter to describe movement of the segments. To improve upon the precision of a movement analysis, a movement can be evaluated with respect to a different starting point or position.

A **reference system** is necessary to specify position of the body, segment, or object so as to describe motion or identify whether any motion has occurred. The reference frame or system is arbitrary and may be within or outside of the body. The reference frame is placed at a designated spot and

🌐 TABLE 1-1 Movement Review

Segment	Joint	Df	Movements
Head	Intervertebral	3	Flexion, extension, hyperextension, R/L lateral flexion, R/L rotation, circumduction
	Atlantoaxial (3 jts)	1 each	R/L rotation
Trunk	Intervertebral	3	Flexion, extension, hyperextension, R/L rotation, R/L lateral flexion, circumduction
Arm	Shoulder	3	Flexion, extension, hyperextension, abduction, adduction, hyperabduction, hyperadduction, horizontal abduction, horizontal adduction, med/lat rotation, circumduction
Arm/shoulder	Sternoclavicular	3	Elevation, depression
Girdle	Acromioclavicular	3	Abduction, adduction (protraction, retraction), upward/downward rotation
Forearm	Elbow	1	Flexion, extension, hyperextension
	Radioulnar	1	Pronation, supination
Hand	Wrist	2	Flexion, extension, hyperextension, radial flexion, ulnar flexion, circumduction
Fingers	Metacarpophalangeal	2	Flexion, extension, hyperextension, abduction, adduction, circumduction
	Interphalangeal	1	Flexion, extension, hyperextension
Thumb	Carpometacarpal	2	Flexion, extension, abduction, adduction, opposition, circumduction
	Metacarpophalangeal	1	Flexion, extension
	Interphalangeal	1	
Thigh	Hip	3	Flexion, extension, hyperextension, abduction, adduction, hyperadduction, horizontal adduction, horizontal abduction, med/lat rotation, circumduction
Leg	Knee	2	Flexion, extension, hyperextension, med/lat rotation
Foot	Ankle	1	Plantarflexion, dorsiflexion
	Intertarsal	3	Inversion, eversion
Toes	Metatarsophalangeal	2	Flexion, extension, abduction, adduction, circumduction
	Interphalangeal	1	Flexion, extension

R/L, right–left; med/lat, medial–lateral.

usually consists of imaginary lines called **axes** that intersect at right angles at a common point termed the **origin**. The axes are generally given letter representations to differentiate the direction in which they are pointing. Any position can be described by identifying the distance of the object from each of the three axes. It is important to identify the frame of reference used in the description of motion.

An example of a reference system placed outside the body is the starting line in a race. The center of an anatomical joint, such as the shoulder, can be used as a reference system within the body. The arm can be described as moving through a 90° angle if abducted until perpendicular to the trunk. However, if the ground is used as a frame of reference, the same arm abduction movement can be described with respect to the ground, such as movement to a height of 1.6 m from the ground.

When angular motion is described, the joint positions, velocities, and accelerations can be described using either an absolute or a relative frame of reference. An **absolute** reference frame is one in which the axes intersect in the center of the joint and movement of a segment is described with respect to that joint. The axes are generally oriented horizontally (X-axis) and vertically (Y-axis), and the segment angle is measured from the right horizontal axes (Fig. 1-23A). The absolute positioning of an abducted arm perpendicular to the trunk is 0° or 360° when described relative to the axes running through the shoulder joint. A **relative reference frame** is one in which the movement of a segment is described relative to the adjacent segment. This type of reference frame is often used to describe a joint angle. The axes in this reference frame are not horizontal and vertical. Figure 1-23B shows the Y-axis placed along one segment, the leg, and the X-axis perpendicular to the Y-axis. The knee angle can then be determined from the lower portion of the Y-axis to the dotted line describing the thigh segment.

In the previously described example of the arm, with abduction perpendicular to the trunk, the relative

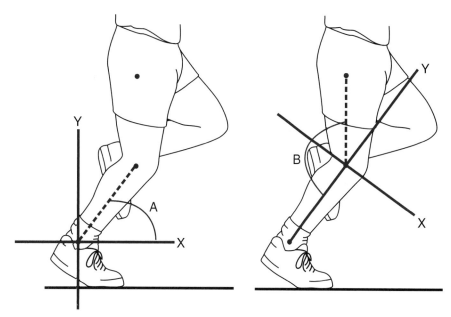

FIGURE 1-23 Absolute vs relative reference frame. **Left,** An absolute reference frame measures the segment angle (A) with respect to the distal joint. **Right,** A relative reference frame measures the relative angle (B) formed by the two segments. It is important to designate the reference frame in movement description.

positioning of the arm with respect to the trunk is 90°. The reference frame should be clearly identified so that the results can be interpreted accordingly, and since reference systems vary among researchers, the reference system and reference point must be identified before comparing and contrasting results between studies. For example, some researchers label a fully extended forearm as a 180° position, and others label the position 0°. After 30° of flexion at the elbow joint, the final position is 150° or 30°, respectively, for the two systems described above. There can be considerable confusion when trying to interpret an article using a different reference system from that of the authors.

PLANES AND AXES

The universally used method of describing human movements is based on a system of planes and axes. A **plane** is a flat two-dimensional surface. Three imaginary planes are positioned through the body at right angles to each other so they intersect at the center of mass of the body. These are the **cardinal planes** of the body. Movement is said to occur in a specific plane if it is actually along the plane or parallel to it. Movement in a plane always occurs about an **axis of rotation** perpendicular to the plane (Fig. 1-24). Stick a pin through a piece of cardboard and spin the paper around the pin. The movement of the cardboard takes place in the plane and the pin represents the axis of rotation. The cardboard can spin around the pin while the pin is front-to-back horizontal, vertical, or sideways, for movement of the cardboard in all three of the planes. This example can be applied to describe imaginary lines running through the total body center of mass in the same three pin directions. These planes allow full description of a motion and contrast of an arm movement straight out in front of the body with one straight

out to the side of the body. The planes and axes of the human body for motion description are presented in Figure 1-25.

The **sagittal plane** bisects the body into right and left halves. Movements in the sagittal plane occur about a **mediolateral axis** running side to side through the center of mass of the body. Sagittal plane movements involving the whole body rotating around the center of mass include somersaults, backward and forward handsprings, and flexing to a pike position in a dive. The **frontal** or **coronal plane** bisects the body to create front and back halves. The axis about which frontal plane movements occur is the **anteroposterior axis** that runs anterior and posterior from the plane. Frontal plane motions of the whole body

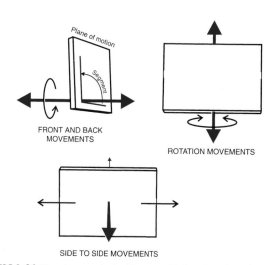

FIGURE 1-24 The plane and axis. Movement takes place in a plane about an axis perpendicular to the plane.

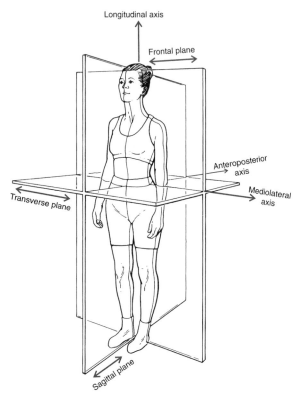

FIGURE 1-25 Planes and axes on the human body. The three cardinal planes that originate at the center of gravity are the sagittal plane, which divides the body into right and left; the frontal plane, dividing the body into front and back; and the transverse plane, dividing the body into top and bottom. Movement takes place in or parallel to the planes about a mediolateral axis (sagittal plane), an anteroposterior axis (frontal plane), or a longitudinal axis (transverse plane).

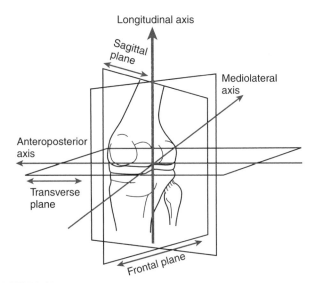

FIGURE 1-26 Planes and axes for the knee.

about the center of mass are not as common as movements in the other planes. The **transverse** or **horizontal plane** bisects the body to create upper and lower halves. Movements occurring in this plane are primarily rotations about a **longitudinal axis**. An example of transverse plane movement about the body's center of mass is spinning vertically around the body while in the air.

Although we have described the sagittal, transverse, and frontal cardinal planes, actually any number of other planes can pass through the body. For example, we can define many sagittal planes that do not pass through the center of mass of the body. The only requirement for defining such a plane is that it is parallel to the cardinal sagittal plane. Likewise we can have multiple transverse or frontal planes. Defining these noncardinal planes is useful for describing joint or limb movements. The intersection of the three planes is placed at the joint center so that joint actions can be described in a sagittal, transverse, or frontal plane (Fig. 1-26). Noncardinal planes can also be used in examining movements that take place about an external axis.

Most planar or two-dimensional analyses in biomechanics are concerned with motion in the sagittal plane through

a joint center. Examples of sagittal plane movements at a joint can be demonstrated by performing flexion and extension movements, such as raising the arm in front, bending the trunk forward and back, lifting and lowering the leg in front, and rising on the toes. Examples of sagittal plane movements of the body about an external support point include rotating the body over the planted foot running and rotating the body over the hands in a vault. The most accurate view of any motion in a plane is obtained from a position perpendicular to the plane of movement to allow viewing along the axis of rotation. Therefore, sagittal plane movements are best viewed from the side of the body to allow focus on a frontal axis of rotation (Fig. 1-27).

Like sagittal plane movements, frontal plane movements can occur about a joint. Characteristic joint movements in the frontal plane include thigh abduction and adduction, finger and hand abduction and adduction, lateral flexion of the head and trunk, and inversion and eversion of the foot. Frontal plane motion about an external point of contact can be seen often in dance and ballet especially, as the dancers move laterally from a pivot point, and in gymnastics with the body rotating sideways over the hands, such as in the cartwheel. The best position to view frontal plane movements is in front or in back of the body to focus on the joint or the point about which the whole body is going to rotate (Fig. 1-28).

Examples of movements in the transverse plane about longitudinal joint axes are rotations at the vertebrae, shoulder, and hip joints. Pronation and supination of the forearm at the radioulnar joints is also a transverse plane movement. The axis for all of these movements is an imaginary line running vertically through the vertebrae, the shoulder, the radioulnar or the hip joints. This is a very common movement in gymnastics, dance, and ice skating.

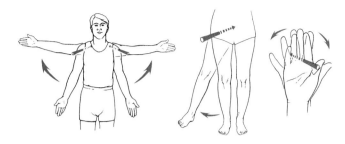

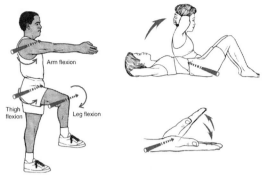

SAGITTAL PLANE MOVEMENTS ABOUT AXIS JOINTS

FRONTAL PLANE MOVEMENTS ABOUT JOINT AXES

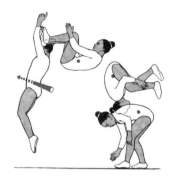

SAGITTAL PLANE MOVEMENTS ABOUT THE CENTER OF GRAVITY

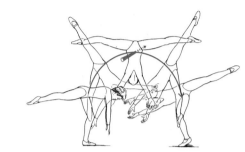

FRONTAL PLANE MOVEMENT ABOUT THE CENTER OF GRAVITY

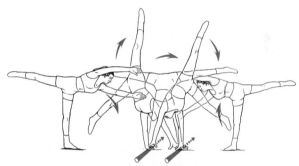

FRONTAL PLANE MOVEMENT ABOUT EXTERNAL AXIS

FIGURE 1-28 Movements in the frontal plane. Segmental movements in the frontal plane about anteroposterior joint axes are abduction and adduction or some specialized side-to-side movement. Frontal plane movements about the center of gravity or an external point involve sideways movement of the body, which is more difficult than movement to the front or back.

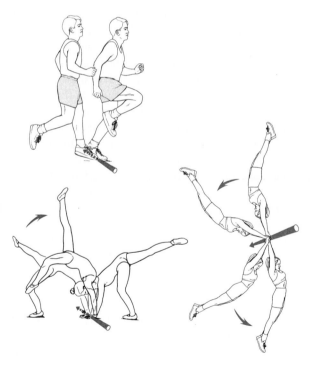

SAGITTAL PLANE MOVEMENTS ABOUT AN EXTERNAL AXIS

FIGURE 1-27 Movements in the sagittal plane. Sagittal plane movements are typically flexions and extensions or some forward or backward turning exercise. The movements can take place about a joint axis, the center of gravity, or an external axis.

There are also numerous examples from dance, skating, and gymnastics in which the athlete performs transverse plane movements about an external axis running through a pivot point between the foot and the ground. All spinning movements that have the whole body turning about the ground or the ice are examples. While transverse plane motions are vital aspects of most successful sport skills, these movements are difficult to follow visually, since the best viewing position is either above or below the movement, perpendicular to the plane of motion. Consequently, rotation motions are evaluated by following the linear movement of some point on the body if vertical positioning cannot be achieved. Examples of movements in the transverse plane are presented in Figure 1-29.

Most human movements take place in multiple planes at the various joints. In running, for example, the lower extremity appears to move predominantly in the sagittal

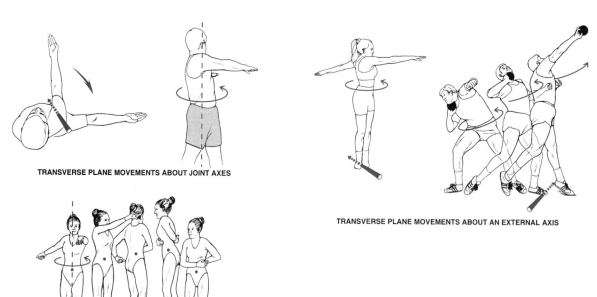

TRANSVERSE PLANE MOVEMENTS ABOUT JOINT AXES

TRANSVERSE PLANE MOVEMENTS ABOUT AN EXTERNAL AXIS

TRANSVERSE PLANE MOVEMENTS ABOUT THE CENTER OF GRAVITY

FIGURE 1-29 Movements in the transverse plane. Most transverse plane movements are rotations about a longitudinal axis running through a joint, the center of gravity, or an external contact point.

plane as the limbs swing forward and back through the gait cycle. Upon closer examination of the limbs and joints, one will find movements in all of the planes. At the hip joint, for example, the thigh will perform flexion and extension in the sagittal plane, abduction and adduction in the frontal plane, and internal and external rotation in the transverse plane. If human movements were confined to single-plane motion, we would look like robots as we performed our skills or joint motions. Examine the three-dimensional motion for an overhand throw presented in Figure 1-30. Note the positioning for viewing motion in each of the three planes.

The movement in a plane can also be described as a single **degree of freedom** (df). This terminology is commonly used to describe the type and amount of motion structurally allowed by the anatomical joints. A joint with 1 df indicates that the joint allows the segment to move through one plane of motion. A joint with 1 df is also termed uniaxial, since there is one axis perpendicular to the plane of motion about which movement occurs. A 1-df joint, the elbow, allows only flexion and extension in the sagittal plane.

Conventionally, most joints are considered to have 1, 2, or 3 df offering movement potential that is uniaxial, biaxial, or triaxial, respectively. The shoulder is an example of a 3-df, or triaxial, joint because it allows the arm to move in the frontal plane via abduction and adduction, in the sagittal plane via flexion and extension, and in the transverse plane via rotation.

Joints with 3 df include the vertebrae, shoulder, and hip; 2-df joints include the knee, metacarpophalangeal (hand), wrist, and thumb carpometacarpal joints; 1-df

joints include the atlantoaxial (neck), interphalangeal (hand and foot), radioulnar (elbow), and ankle joints. Three degrees of freedom does not always imply great mobility, but it does indicate that the joint allows movement in all three planes of motion. The shoulder is much more mobile than the hip, even though they both are triaxial joints and are capable of performing the same movements. The trunk movements, although classified as having 3 df, are quite restricted if one evaluates movement at a single vertebral level. For example, the lumbar and cervical areas of the vertebrae allow the trunk to flex and extend, but this plane of movement is limited in the middle thoracic portion of the vertebrae. Likewise, the rotation actions of the trunk occur primarily in the thoracic and cervical regions, since the lumbar region has limited movement potential in the horizontal plane. It is only the combination of all of the vertebral segments that allows the 3-df motion produced by the spine.

Also, gliding movements occur across the joint surfaces. Gliding movements may be interpreted as adding more degrees of freedom to those defined in the literature. For example, the knee joint is considered to have 2 df for flexion and extension in the sagittal plane and rotation in the transverse plane. However, the knee joint also demonstrates linear translation and it is well known that there is movement in the joint in the frontal plane as the joint surfaces glide over one another to create side-to-side translation movements. While these movements have been measured and are relatively significant, they have not been established as an additional degree of freedom for the joint. The degrees of freedom for most of the joints in the body are shown in Table 1-1.

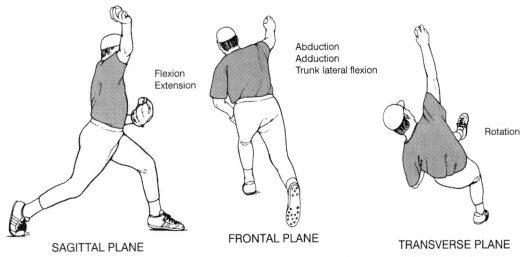

FIGURE 1-30 Movements in all three planes. Most human movements employ movement in all three planes. The release phase of the overhand throw illustrates movements in all three planes. The sagittal plane movements are viewed from the side; the frontal plane movements, from the rear; and the transverse plane movements, from above.

A kinematic chain is derived from combining degrees of freedom at various joints to produce a skill or movement. The chain is the summation of the degrees of freedom in adjacent joints that identifies the total degrees of freedom available or necessary for the performance of a movement. For example, kicking a ball might involve an 11-df system relative to the trunk. This would include perhaps 3 df at the hip, 2 df at the knee, 1 df at the ankle, 3 df in the tarsals (foot), and 2 df in the toes.

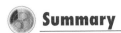 **Summary**

Biomechanics, the application of the laws of physics to the study of motion, is a useful tool for studying human movement. Human motion can be qualitatively or quantitatively assessed biomechanically. A qualitative analysis is a nonnumeric assessment of the movement. A quantitative analysis uses kinematic or kinetic applications that analyze a skill or movement by identifying its components or by assessing the forces creating the motion, respectively.

Individual structures of the human body may be analyzed mechanically using a stress–strain curve to help determine its basic properties. Stress–strain curves illustrate the elastic and plastic regions and the elastic modulus of the structure. Structures and materials can be differentiated as elastic or viscoelastic based on their stress–strain curves. These basic mechanical properties may give insight into how a movement may take place.

To provide a specific description of a movement, it is helpful to define movements with respect to a starting point or to one of the three planes of motion: sagittal, frontal, or transverse.

Anatomical movement descriptors should be used to describe segmental movements. This requires acknowledgment of the starting position (fundamental or anatomical), standardized use of segment names (arm, forearm, hand, thigh, leg, foot), and the correct use of movement descriptors (flexion, extension, abduction, adduction, rotation).

REVIEW QUESTIONS

True or False

1. ____ Biomechanics is the application of the laws of physics to human motion.

2. ____ A biomechanical analysis can be accomplished only qualitatively.

3. ____ Kinesiology is essentially the same as biomechanics.

4. ____ The appendicular skeleton includes the head, trunk, and upper extremities.

5. ____ For each rotation, an axis of rotation can be defined.

6. ____ A relative angle measures the position of a segment in space.

7. ____ When the relative angle between two segments increases, flexion is said to take place.

8. ____ Pronation and supination describe motions of the forearm and can be used for motions of the foot.

9. ____ The right leg is ipsilateral to the left leg.

10. ____ When a material reaches its failure point, the applied force immediately drops to zero.

11. ____ Hysteresis is the energy stored in a stress–strain test.

12. ____ Both the anatomical and fundamental reference positions are used by biomechanists.

13. ___ The foot is distal to the leg relative to the thigh.

14. ___ Lower extremity motion in running can be studied as if it occurred only in the sagittal plane.

15. ___ A viscoelastic material has no elastic properties at all.

16. ___ The foot is inferior to the thigh relative to the head.

17. ___ A mediolateral axis runs from the medial side of the body to the distal side.

18. ___ When a material remains in its elastic region during a stress–strain test, it exhibits no residual strain.

19. ___ Statics is a branch of mechanics that studies systems that do not move.

20. ___ Angular motion occurs about an axis of rotation.

21. ___ A biomechanist must have a sound knowledge of anatomy.

22. ___ The stiffness of a material can be determined by calculating the slope of the linear portion of the stress–strain curve.

23. ___ A joint that has only 1° of freedom can also be called a uniaxial joint.

24. ___ All joints in the human body have at least 3° of freedom.

25. ___ All analyses in biomechanics must be quantitative.

Multiple Choice

1. Which of the following are not essential areas of study for a biomechanist?
   a. Anatomy
   b. Physics
   c. Philanthropy
   d. Mathematics

2. Which of the following is not an example of a qualitative analysis?
   a. A coach correcting a free throw
   b. A force profile of a weight lifter
   c. A physical therapist watching a patient exercise
   d. All of the above

3. Which of the following are examples of linear motion?
   a. The arm of a pitcher throwing a ball
   b. A parachutist in free-fall
   c. A runner's leg motion during a 100-m race
   d. None of the above

4. Which of the following are examples of angular motion?
   a. The ball after being thrown by the pitcher
   b. A parachutist in free fall
   c. A runner's leg motion during a 100-m race
   d. None of the above

5. Which of the following could be a kinetics study?
   a. The position of a runner during each segment of a race
   b. The velocity of a runner during portion of a race
   c. The angular motion of a runner's leg during a race
   d. None of the above

6. An example of a kinematic study is ___.
   a. The force acting on a runner during a race
   b. The velocity of a runner during portion of a race
   c. The force applied to a ball being kicked
   d. None of the above

7. Which of the following are examples of a static analysis?
   a. A weight-lifter holding a barbell over his head
   b. An isometric exercise
   c. The path of a spaceship in flight in space
   d. All of the above

8. The unit of force is ___.
   a. Gram
   b. Centimeter
   c. Newton
   d. All of the above

9. A dynamic analysis of human movement could use ___.
   a. Both a kinematic and kinetic approach
   b. Neither a kinematic nor a kinetic approach
   c. A kinematic but not a kinetic approach
   d. A kinetic but not a kinematic approach

10. The force applied to a structure will cause a ___.
    a. Strain
    b. Stress
    c. Both A and B
    d. Neither A nor B

11. To compare the stress–strain properties of two different materials, the applied force must be applied to ___.
    a. Both materials at the same time
    b. The same side of each material
    c. The same volume
    d. The same area

12. When stressed in its elastic region, a material will exhibit ___.
    a. Structural reorganization
    b. Failure
    c. No effect
    d. Residual strain

13. A viscoelastic material ___.
    a. Has elastic and viscous properties
    b. Exhibits non-linear behavior
    c. Has multiple stiffnesses
    d. All of the above

14. The difference between the anatomical and fundamental positions is ___.
    a. The position of the hands relative to the trunk
    b. The position of the head
    c. Both A and B
    d. There is no difference

15. The elbow joint in relation to to the wrist relative to the trunk is ___.
    a. Proximal
    b. Medial
    c. Inferior
    d. Anterior

16. The hip joint relative to the head is ___.
    a. Proximal
    b. Medial
    c. Inferior
    d. Anterior

17. The right knee relative to the left knee is ___.
    a. Proximal
    b. Contralateral
    c. Inferior
    d. Ipsilateral

18. A joint in which the relative angle continues past its zero position undergoes ___.
   a. Hyperextension
   b. Hyperflexion
   c. Hyperadduction
   d. Hyperabduction

19. Which of the following are not movements of the scapula?
   a. Depression
   b. Lateral flexion
   c. Upward rotation
   d. Retraction

20. Radial flexion takes place on ___.
   a. The thumb side of the hand
   b. The little finger side of the hand
   c. The big toe side of the foot
   d. The little toe side of the foot

21. A reference system has ___.
   a. Planes
   b. Axes
   c. An origin
   d. All of the above

22. Motion in the coronal plane take place about which axis?
   a. Longitudinal
   b. Mediolateral
   c. Transverse
   d. Anteroposterior

23. Most human movements take place in ___.
   a. The sagittal plane
   b. The frontal plane
   c. The transverse plane
   d. Multiple planes

24. A degree of freedom is ___.
   a. The type of movement structurally allowed by a joint
   b. The number of movements possible at a joint
   c. Both A and B
   d. Neither A nor B

25. A uniaxial joint has how many degrees of freedom?
   a. 3
   b. 1
   c. 2
   d. Multiple

REFERENCES

1. Richie, D. H., et al. (1985). Aerobic dance injuries: A retrospective study of instructors and participants. *Physician and Sports Medicine*, 13:130–140.
2. Ulibarri, V. D., et al. (1987). Ground reaction forces in selected aerobics movements. *Biomechanics in Sport*. New York: Bioengineering Division of the American Society of Mechanical Engineering, 19–21.
3. Lander, J., et al. (1986). Biomechanics of the squat exercise using a modified center of mass bar. *Medicine and Science in Sports and Exercise*, 18:469–478.
4. Kazarian, L. E., Von Gierke, H. E. (1969). Bone loss as a result of immobilization and chelation. Preliminary results in *Macaca mulatta*. *Clinical Orthopaedics*, 65:67–75.
5. Nordin, M., Frankel, V. H. (1989). *Basic Biomechanics of the Musculoskeletal System*. Philadelphia: Lea and Febiger.

ADDITIONAL READING

Alexander, R. McN. (1992). *The Human Machine*. New York: Columbia University Press.

Marieb, E. N., Mallatt, J. (2001). *Human Anatomy* (3rd ed.). San Francisco: Benjamin Cummings.

Roozbazar, A. (1974). Biomechanics of lifting. In R.C. Nelson and C.A. Morehouse (Eds.), *Biomechanics IV*. Baltimore: University Park Press, 37–43.

Vetter, W. L., et al. (1985). Aerobic dance injuries. *Physician and Sports Medicine*, 13:114–120.

GLOSSARY

Abduction: A movement away from the midline of the body.

Absolute Reference Frame: A reference frame in which the origin is at the joint center.

Adduction: A movement toward the midline of the body.

Anatomy: The science of the structure of the body.

Anatomical Position: The standardized reference position used in the medical profession.

Angular Motion: Motion around an axis of rotation in which different regions of the same object do not move through the same distance.

Anterior: A position in front of a designated reference point.

Anteroposterior Axis: The axis through the center of mass of the body running from posterior to anterior.

Appendicular Skeleton: The bones of the extremities.

Axes: The imaginary lines of a reference system along which position is measured.

Axial Skeleton: The bones of the head, neck, and trunk.

Axis of Rotation: The imaginary line about which an object rotates.

Biomechanics: The study of motion and the effect of forces on biological systems.

Cardinal Planes: The planes of the body that intersect at the total body center of mass.

Circumduction: A movement that is a combination of flexion, adduction, extension, and abduction.

Contralateral: On the opposite side.

Degree of Freedom: The movement of a joint in a plane.

Depression: The lowering movement of the scapula.

Distal: A position relatively far from a designated reference point.

Dorsal: See Posterior.

Dorsiflexion: The motion in which the relative angle between the foot and the leg decreases.

Downward Rotation: The action whereby the scapula swings toward the midline of the body.

Dynamics: The branch of mechanics in which the system being studied undergoes an acceleration.

Elastic Material: A material that exhibits only elastic properties on a stress–strain curve.

Elastic Modulus: The linear portion of a stress–strain curve.

Elastic Region: The area of a stress–strain curve before the yield point. The area in which the material will return to its resting length when the applied force is removed.

Elevation: The raising of the scapula.

Eversion: The movement in which the lateral border of the foot lifts so that the sole of the foot faces away from the midline of the body.

Extension: The action in which the relative angle between two adjacent segments gets larger.

Failure Point: The point on a stress–strain curve when the applied force causes a complete rupture of the material.

Flexion: The action in which the relative angle between two adjacent segments becomes smaller.

Frontal (Coronal) Plane: The plane that bisects the body into front and back halves.

Fundamental Position: A standardized reference position similar to the anatomical position.

Functional Anatomy: The study of the body components needed to achieve a human movement or function.

Horizontal Abduction: A combination of extension and abduction of the arm or thigh.

Horizontal Adduction: A combination of flexion and adduction of the arm or thigh.

Hysteresis: The mechanical energy lost by a material that has been deformed.

Inferior: A position below a designated reference point.

Inversion: The movement in which the medial border of the foot lifts so that the sole of the foot faces away from the midline of the body.

Ipsilateral: On the same side.

Kinematics: Area of study that examines the spatial and temporal components of motion (position, velocity, acceleration).

Kinesiology: Study of human movement.

Kinetics: Study of the forces that act on a system.

Lateral: A position relatively far from the midline of the body.

Lateral Flexion: A flexion movement of the head or trunk.

Linear Motion: Motion in a straight or curved line in which different regions of the same object move the same distance.

Longitudinal Axis: The axis through the center of mass of the body running from top to bottom.

Medial: A position relatively closer to the midline of the body.

Mediolateral Axis: The axis through the center of mass of the body running from right to left.

Movement: A change in place, position, or posture occurring over time and relative to some point in the environment.

Origin: The intersection of the axes of a reference system and the reference point from which measures are taken.

Plane of Motion: A two-dimensional flat surface running through an object. Motion occurs in the plane or parallel to the plane.

Plantarflexion: The motion in which the relative angle between the foot and the leg increases.

Plastic Region: The region between the yield point and the failure point on a stress–strain curve. The region in which the material will not return to its initial length after it is deformed.

Posterior: A position behind a designated reference point.

Pronation: Movement in which the forearm rotates to a palms down position relative to anatomical position.

Protraction: The motion describing the separating action of the scapula.

Proximal: A position relatively closer to a designated reference point.

Qualitative Analysis: A nonnumeric description or evaluation of movement based on direct observation.

Quantitative Analysis: A numeric description or evaluation of movement based on data collected during the performance of the movement.

Radial Flexion: The flexion movement of the hand toward the forearm on the thumb side of the hand.

Reference System: A system to locate a point in space.

Relative Angle: The included angle between two adjacent segments.

Relative Reference Frame: A reference frame in which the origin is at the joint center and one of the axes is placed along one of the segments.

Retraction: The motion describing the coming together action of the scapula.

Residual Strain: The difference between the initial length of a material and the length when the material has gone beyond its yield point.

Rotation: A movement about an axis of rotation in which not every point of the segment or body covers the same distance in the same time.

Safety Factor: The ratio of the stress to reach the yield point to the stress of everyday activity.

Sagittal Plane: The plane that bisects the body into right and left sides.

Statics: A branch of mechanics in which the system being studied undergoes no acceleration.

Stress: Force per unit area.

Stress–strain Curve: A plot of the stress placed on a material against the strain imposed by the stress.

Transverse (Horizontal) Plane: The plane that bisects the body into top and bottom halves.

Superior: A position above a designated reference point.

Supination: The movement in the forearm in which the forearm rotates to a palms-up position relative to anatomical position.

Ulnar Flexion: The flexion movement of the hand toward the forearm on the little finger side of the hand.

Upward Rotation: The action whereby the scapula swings out from the midline of the body.

Ventral: See Anterior.

Viscoelastic Material: A material that exhibits nonlinear properties on a stress–strain curve.

Yield Point: The point on a stress–strain curve at which the material reaches the plastic region.

Skeletal Considerations for Movement

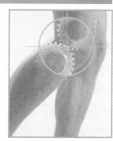

OBJECTIVES

After reading this chapter, the student will be able to:

1. List the functions of the skeletal system and the types of bones found in the skeletal system and describe the role each type of bone plays in human movement or support.

2. Describe the characteristics of compact and spongy bone and the mechanical properties of bone under load.

3. Identify the elastic region, yield point, plastic region, and failure point on a stress–strain curve.

4. Define the following types of loads that bone must absorb and provide an example to illustrate each load on the skeletal system: compression, tension, shear, bending, and torsion.

5. Describe some common injuries to the skeletal system and explain the load causing the injury.

6. Describe the types of cartilage and their function in the skeletal system.

7. Describe the function of ligaments in the skeletal system.

8. Describe all of the components of the diarthrodial joint, factors that contribute to joint stability, and examples of injury to the diarthrodial joint.

9. List the seven different types of diarthrodial joints, providing examples for each one.

10. Describe the characteristics of the synarthrodial and amphiarthrodial joint and provide an example of each.

I. Introduction
  A. Functions of the Skeletal System
    1. Levers
    2. Support
    3. Other Functions
  B. Architecture of Bone
    1. Cortical Bone
    2. Cancellous Bone
  C. Types of Bones
    1. Long Bones
    2. Short Bones
    3. Flat Bones
    4. Irregular Bones
    5. Sesamoid Bones

II. Biomechanical Characteristics of Bone
  A. Bone Tissue
    1. Constitution
    2. Resorption and Deposit of Bone
    3. Physical Activity vs Bone Remodeling
    4. Lack of Activity vs Bone Remodeling
    5. Bone Deposit in Soft Tissue
    6. Osteoporosis
  B. Strength and Stiffness of Bone
    1. Anisotropic Characteristics
    2. Viscoelastic Characteristics
    3. Elastic Response

Introduction

The skeletal system consists of the bones, cartilage, ligaments, and joints of the body. Bones constitute the majority of the structures in the skeletal system. Joints, or articulations, are the intersections between bones, while ligaments connect bones at the articulations, thus reinforcing the joints. The skeleton consists of approximately 20% of total body weight. The skeletal system is generally broken down into axial and appendicular skeletons. The major bones of the body are presented in Figure 2-1.

The skeletal framework determines shape and body size. While one can roughly predict adult height by doubling the height of a 2-year-old, the skeletal system and frame can be greatly influenced by nutrition, activity level, and postural habits. Although the general size and shape of the bones are inherited, structural adaptations in shape, size, and landmarks can be induced by weight bearing and the forces exerted by tendons, ligaments, and muscles (31). In the developing or immature skeleton, the influence of weight bearing and muscular forces will have a more substantial effect on the formation of the size and shape of the bones than the same forces will have on a mature skeleton. For this reason, it is important to pay careful attention to the types of activities and habitual postures of a preadolescent child.

A common example of skeletal alteration in the immature skeleton is idiopathic scoliosis, a lateral curvature in the spine, present in approximately 15 to 20% of girls aged 10 to 12. It is termed idiopathic because the forces causing the lateral curve have not been identified. Is it because young girls spend too much time weight bearing on one limb? Is it related to posture that includes hyperextended knees and swayback? It is easy to speculate on possible causes, but the scientific substantiation of this disorder still evades us. We do know that the skeletal system is a malleable system that can be shaped and formed through activity. It is important to understand how the skeletal system responds in order to institute programs that will promote skeletal health and prevent skeletal injury.

FUNCTIONS OF THE SKELETAL SYSTEM

The skeletal system performs many functions: leverage, support, protection, storage, and blood cell formation. Two of these functions, leverage and support, are critically important for human movement.

Levers

The skeletal system provides the levers and axes of rotation about which the muscular system generates the movements. A **lever** is a simple machine that magnifies the force and/or speed of movement. The levers are primarily the long bones of the body, and the axes are the joints where the bones meet. Chapter 9 provides an in-depth discussion of levers.

The morphology of the bones determines the manner in which the skeleton contributes to movement. **Morphology** is the shape and structural arrangement of the bones and the characteristics of the articulations connecting the bones. For example, if the forearm moves into a position of maximum flexion so that it is up against the arm and then is extended until it stops, hyperextension is

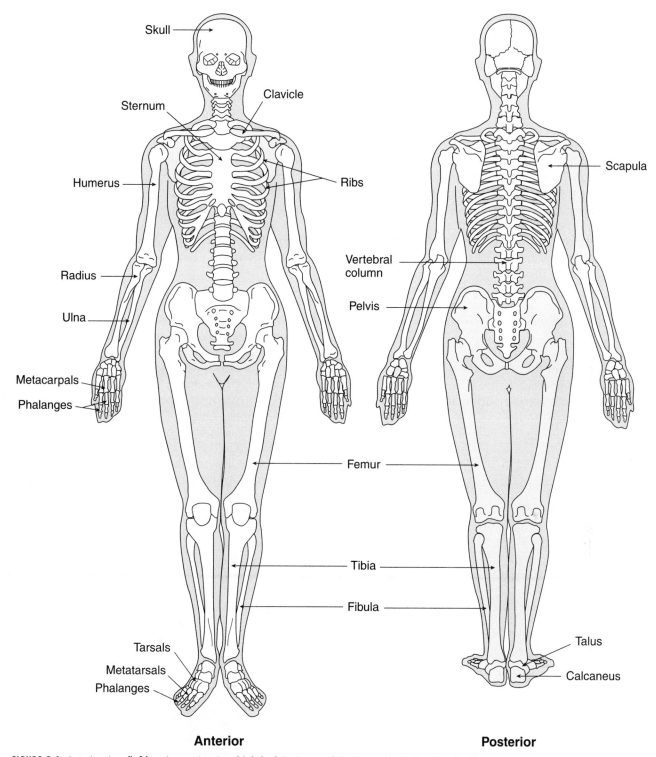

Anterior   **Posterior**

FIGURE 2-1 Anterior view **(left)** and posterior view **(right)** of the bones of the human body. (Reprinted with permission from Willis, M. C. [1996]. *Medical Terminology: The Language of Health Care*. Baltimore: Williams & Wilkins.)

limited because of the shape of the bones forming the elbow joint. Conversely, if the arm moves by shoulder flexion so that it is pointed straight above the head, followed by shoulder extension back to anatomical position, the arm will continue into a hyperextended position because the structure of the shoulder joint will allow the movement.

The skeleton also restricts motion in other areas of the body, as shown in Figure 2-2. A movement up on the toes will wedge the talus against the calcaneus and restrict the amount of plantar flexion. Dancers consider this a serious limitation, since they desire maximum plantar flexion for many maneuvers. Some dancers even undergo surgery that involves shaving the posterior portion of the talus to allow greater freedom of movement in plantar flexion. Dancers have been known to have this operation two or three times during their careers. Understanding skeletal structure and shape provides information on the movement potential in each joint that can be used to work within the limits of the system.

Support

A second important function of the skeletal system is the provision of a support structure. The skeleton can maintain a posture while accommodating large external forces,

such as those involved in jumping. The bones increase in size from top to bottom in proportion to the amount of body weight they bear; thus, the bones of the lower extremity and the lower vertebrae and pelvic bones are larger than their upper extremity and upper torso counterparts. A visual comparison of the humerus and femur or the cervical vertebrae and lumbar vertebrae demonstrates these size relationships.

Other Functions

There are three additional bone functions not specifically related to movement: protection, storage, and blood cell formation. The bones protect the brain and internal organs. Bone also stores fat and minerals. Finally, blood cell formation, called hematopoiesis, takes place within the cavities of bone.

ARCHITECTURE OF BONE

Bone is composed of a matrix of inorganic salts and connective tissue referred to as **collagen** fibers. Bone cells are referred to as **osteocytes**. The two types of these cells are referred to as **osteoblasts** and **osteoclasts**. These cells are responsible for remodeling bone. Bone is composed of two types of **osseous**, or bone tissue: **cortical** bone and **cancellous** bone. The hard outer layer is compact bone; internal to this is spongy bone. A section of the femoral head presented in Figure 2-3 illustrates the architecture of the long bone. The architectural arrangement of bony tissue is remarkably well suited for the mechanical demands imposed upon the skeletal system during physical activity.

Cortical Bone

Cortical bone is often referred to as compact bone. Cortical bone looks solid, but closer examination reveals many passageways for blood vessels and nerves. The

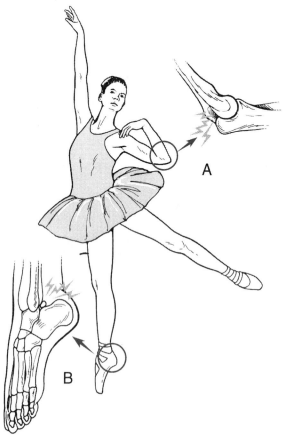

FIGURE 2-2 Skeletal obstructions limit joint movement in many areas of the body. **A.** In the elbow joint, the olecranon process and the olecranon fossa meet to restrict the amount of forearm hyperextension. **B.** In the foot, the talus and calcaneus make contact to restrict plantar flexion.

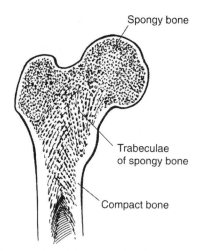

FIGURE 2-3 This midsection of the proximal end of the femur shows both compact and spongy bone. The dense compact bone lines the outside of the bone, continuing down to form the shaft of the bone. Spongy bone is found in the ends and is distinguishable by its latticelike appearance. Note the curvature in the trabeculae, which forms to withstand the stresses.

exterior layer of bone is very dense and has a porosity less than 15% (32).

Cortical bone consists of a system of hollow tubes called **lamellae** that are placed inside one another. Lamellae are composed of collagen fibers, all running in a single direction. The collagen fibers of adjacent lamellae always run in different directions. A series of lamellae form an **osteon** or **haversian** system. Osteons are pillarlike structures that are oriented parallel to the stresses that are placed on the bone. The arrangement of these weight-bearing pillars and the density of the compact bone provide strength and stiffness to the skeletal system. Cortical bone can withstand high levels of weight bearing or muscle tension in the longitudinal direction before it will fail and fracture (31).

Cortical bone is especially capable of absorbing tensile loads if the collagen fibers are parallel to the load. Typically, the collagen is arranged in layers running in longitudinal, circumferential, and oblique configurations. This offers resistance to tensile forces in different directions, because the more layers there are, the greater the strength and stiffness the bone will have. Also, where muscles, ligaments, and tendons attach to the skeleton, the collagen fibers are arranged parallel to the insertion of the soft tissue, thereby offering greater tensile strength for these attachments.

A thick layer of compact bone is found in the shafts of long bones, where strength is necessary to respond to the high loads imposed down the length of the bone during weight bearing or in response to muscular tension. Thin layers of compact bone are found on the ends of the long bones, the epiphyses, and also covering the short or irregular bones.

Cancellous Bone

The bone tissue interior to cortical bone is referred to as cancellous or spongy bone. This bone has a latticelike structure with a porosity greater than 70% (32). Cancellous bone structure, although quite rigid, is weaker and less stiff than the compact bone. The small, flat pieces of bone making up the spongy bone are called **trabeculae** (Fig. 2-3). The trabeculae adapt to the direction of the imposed stress on the bone, providing strength without adding much weight (5). Collagen runs along the axis of the trabeculae, providing cancellous bone with both tensile and compressive resistance.

The high porosity gives spongy bone high-energy storage capacity, so that this type of bone becomes a crucial element in energy absorption and stress distribution when loads are applied to the skeletal structure (28). Cancellous

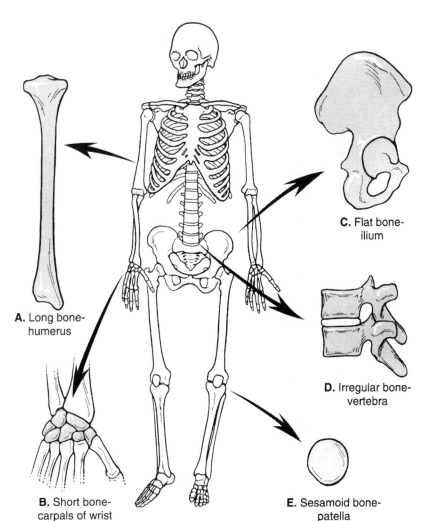

C. Flat bone-ilium

D. Irregular bone-vertebra

E. Sesamoid bone-patella

A. Long bone-humerus

B. Short bone-carpals of wrist

FIGURE 2-4 Various types of bones serve specific functions. **A.** Long bones serve as levers. **B.** Short bones offer support and shock absorption. **C.** Flat bones protect and offer large muscular attachment sites. **D.** Irregular bones have specialized functions. **E.** Sesamoid bones alter the angle of muscular insertion.

bone is not as strong as compact bone, and there is a high incidence of fracture in the cancellous bone of the elderly. This is believed to be caused by loss of compressive strength due to mineral loss (osteoporosis).

TYPES OF BONES

The skeletal system consists of types of bones categorized according to shape, function, and the proportion of spongy and compact bone tissue. Five types of bones are illustrated in Figure 2-4. These include bones designated as long, short, flat, irregular, and sesamoid.

Long Bones

The long bones are longer than they are wide. The long bones in the body are the clavicle, humerus, radius, ulna, femur, tibia, fibula, metatarsals, metacarpals, and phalanges. The long bone has a shaft, the **diaphysis**, a thick layer of compact bone surrounding the bone marrow cavity (Fig. 2-5). The shaft widens toward the end into the section called the **metaphysis**. In the immature skeleton the end of the long bone, the **epiphysis**, is separated from the diaphysis by a cartilaginous disc. The epiphyses consist of a thin outer layer of compact bone covering spongy inner bone. A thin white membrane, the **periosteum**, covers the outside of the bone with the exception of the parts covered by cartilage.

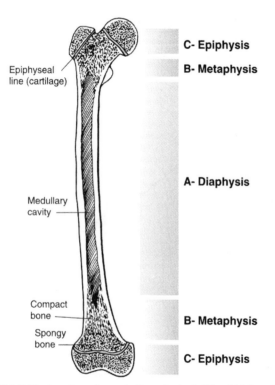

FIGURE 2-5 The long bone has a shaft, or diaphysis **(A),** which broadens out into the metaphysis **(B)** and the epiphysis **(C).** Layers of compact bone make up the diaphysis. The metaphysis and epiphysis are made up of spongy bone inside a thin layer of compact bone.

Long bones offer the body support and provide the interconnected set of levers and linkages that allow us to move. A long bone is strongest when it is stressed by forces acting along the long axis of the bone. Muscle attachment sites and protuberances are formed by tensile forces of muscles pulling on the bones. Most long bones are beam-shaped to handle and minimize the bending loads imposed upon them.

Short Bones

The short bones, such as the carpals of the hand and tarsals of the foot, consist primarily of spongy bone covered with a thin layer of compact bone. These bones play an important role in shock absorption and the transmission of forces.

Flat Bones

A third type of bone, the flat bone, is represented by the ribs, ilium, sternum, and scapula. These bones consist of two layers of compact bone, with spongy bone and marrow in between. Flat bones protect internal structures and offer broad surfaces for muscular attachment.

Irregular Bones

Irregular bones, such as those found in the skull, pelvis, and vertebrae, consist of spongy bone with a thin exterior of compact bone. These bones are termed irregular because of their specialized shapes and functions. The irregular bones perform a variety of functions, including supporting weight, dissipating loads, protecting the spinal cord, contributing to movement, and providing sites for muscular attachment.

Sesamoid Bones

The last type of bone, the sesamoid bone, is a short bone embedded in a tendon or joint capsule. The patella is a sesamoid bone at the knee joint: it is embedded in the tendon of the quadriceps. Other sesamoid bones can be found at the base of the first metatarsal in the foot, where the bones are embedded in the distal tendon of the flexor hallucis brevis muscle, and at the thumb, where the bones are embedded in the tendon of the flexor pollicis brevis muscle. The role of the sesamoid bone is to alter the angle of insertion of the muscle.

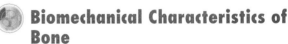 Biomechanical Characteristics of Bone

BONE TISSUE

Constitution

Osseous tissue is strong and one of the body's hardest structures because of its combination of inorganic and organic elements. The minerals, calcium and phosphate, along with collagen, constitute the organic element in bone and make up approximately 60 to 70% of bone tissue. Water constitutes approximately 25 to 30% of the weight of bone tissue (28).

Bone tissue is a viscoelastic material whose mechanical properties are affected by its deformation rate. The ductile properties of bone are provided by the collagenous material in bone. The collagen content gives bone the ability to withstand tensile loads. Bone is also brittle, and its strength depends on the loading mechanism. The brittleness of bone is provided by the mineral constituents that provide bone with the ability to withstand compressive loads. These properties are discussed later in the chapter.

Resorption and Deposit of Bone

Bone is a highly adaptive material that is very sensitive to disuse, immobilization, or vigorous activity and high levels of loading. Bone tissue is self-repairing and can alter its properties and configuration in response to mechanical demand. This was first determined by the German anatomist Julius Wolff, who provided the theory of bone development, termed Wolff's law. This law states: "Every change in the form and function of a bone or of their function alone is followed by certain definitive changes in their internal architecture and equally definite secondary alteration in their external conformation, in accordance with mathematical laws" (21).

During growth and in life, the bones are subjected to externally applied loads and muscular forces to which the bone responds. Bone is remodeled and repaired throughout life. It is a dynamic and active tissue in which large volumes of bone are removed through bone **resorption** or reabsorption and replaced through bone **deposition**. Bone resorption is accomplished by osteocytes called osteoclasts and depostion by osteoblasts. This process is not the same in all bones or even in a single bone. For example, the bone in the distal part of the femur is replaced every 5 to 6 months, whereas the bone in the shaft is replaced much more slowly. In young adults, bone deposits equal bone resorption, and the total bone mass is relatively constant. However, through exercise, the bone mass can be increased even up through young adulthood. This is one of the major benefits of physical activity.

Bone deposits will exceed bone resorption when greater strength is required or when there is an injury. Thus, weight lifters develop thickenings at the insertion of very active muscles, and bones are densest where stresses are greatest. The dominant arm of professional tennis players have cortical thicknesses that are 35% greater than the contralateral arm (21). The shape of bone also changes during fracture healing.

Physical Activity vs Bone Remodeling

Bones require mechanical stress to grow and strengthen. Thus physical activity is an important component of the development and maintenance of skeletal integrity and strength. Bone tissue must have a daily stimulus to maintain health. The daily applied loading history, comprising the number of loading cycles and the stress magnitude, influences the density of the bone. Intermittent loading for 100 cycles a day has been shown to produce a significant increase in the bone cross-section (36). Body weight and activity level are examples of factors that regulate density in the weight-bearing bones. Increases in the activity level produce a moderate increase in bone mass.

Lack of Activity vs Bone Remodeling

Bone loss following a decrease in the activity level may be significant (36). In microgravity, astronauts, subjected to reduced activity and the loss of body weight influences, lose significant bone mass in relatively short periods. Some of the changes occurring to bone as a result of space travel include loss of rigidity, increased bending displacement, a decrease in bone length and cortical cross-section, and slowing of bone formation (37).

Bone Deposit in Soft Tissue

A condition known as myositis ossificans occurs when bone deposits are laid down in soft tissue near bone as a safety response to repeated trauma or a hematoma (bruise) to an area. The body first responds to the repeated bruising by developing fibrous tissue that eventually develops into cartilage and then into bone. The anterior portion of the thigh and the hip joint are regions where this condition is common. Football players who are repeatedly hit in the thigh are susceptible to this type of injury. It has also been seen in the hip region of soccer players who repeatedly fall on the hip (1). Recognizing that the body will develop a fibrous, cartilaginous, and osseus proliferation at the specific site of repeated trauma, some performers in the martial arts deliberately attempt to obtain this response in the hands and feet.

Osteoporosis

Bone resorption exceeds bone deposits in osteoporosis. The symptoms of osteoporosis often begin to appear in the elderly, especially postmenopausal women. However, osteoporosis may begin earlier in life, when bone mineral density decreases. When bone deposition cannot keep up with bone resorption, bone mineral mass decreases, resulting in reduced bone density accompanied by loss of trabecular integrity. The loss of bone mineral density means loss of the stiffness in bone, and the loss of trabecular integrity weakens the structure. Both of these losses create the potential for a much greater incidence of fracture (6), ranging from 2 to 3.7% in nonosteoporotic individuals and almost doubling to 5 to 7% in osteoporotic individuals (19).

The exact causes of osteoporosis are not fully understood, but the condition has been shown to be related to hormonal factors, nutritional imbalances, and lack of exercise. Normal bone volume is 1.5 to 2 L, and the cortical diameter of bone is at its maximum between ages 30 and 40 for both men and women (12, 29). After age 30, there is a

0.2 to 0.5% yearly loss in the mineral weight of bone (36), accelerating after menopause in women to bone loss that is 50% greater than in men of similar age (29). It is speculated that a substantial proportion of this bone loss may be related to the accompanying reduction in activity level (36).

Mild or moderate exercise can increase bone mineral content in the elderly (3). In one study, bone mineral content in runners aged 50 to 72 was shown to be greater than in subjects who did not run. There was also a decreased rate of age-related bone loss: 4% over 2 years for the runners and 6 to 7% over 2 years for the nonrunner group (23). However, when the runners stopped running or moved to walking as an alternative exercise, bone loss increased substantially, to 10 to 13% (23). Therefore, it is suggested that a substitute activity for running is one that provides high-intensity loads and low repetitions, such as weight lifting.

Lifestyle and activity habits seem to play an important role in the maintenance of bone health. In one study, the incidence of osteoporosis was 47% in a sedentary population, compared to only 23% in a population whose occupations included hard physical labor (3). It is clear that the elderly may benefit from some form of weight-bearing exercise even though the exercise intensity and durations have not been determined.

Estrogen levels in anorexic women and amenorrheic female athletes have also been related to the presence of osteoporosis in this population. There is speculation that stress fractures in the femoral neck of female runners may be related to a noted loss of bone mineral density due to osteoporosis (6). Elite female athletes in a variety of sports have had bone loss, usually associated with bouts of heavy training and associated menstrual irregularity. Some of these athletes have lost so much bone mass that their skeletal characteristics resemble those of elderly women.

STRENGTH AND STIFFNESS OF BONE

The behavior of any material under loading conditions is determined by its strength and stiffness. When an external force is applied to a bone or any other material, there is an internal reaction. The strength can be evaluated by examining the relationship between the load imposed (external force) and the amount of deformation (internal reaction) occurring in the material. The methods and terminology of this type of evaluation were presented in Chapter 1.

Anisotropic Characteristics

Bone tissue is an anisotropic material, which means that the behavior of bone will vary with the direction of the load application (Fig. 2-6). In general, tissue of long bones can handle the greatest loads in the longitudinal direction and the least amount of load across the surface of the bone (31). Long bones are stronger withstanding longitudinal loads because they are habitually loaded in that direction.

Viscoelastic Characteristics

Bone is also viscoelastic, meaning that its response depends on the rate at which the load is applied and the duration of the load. At a higher speed of loading, bone can handle greater loads before it fails, or fractures. As shown in Figure 2-7, the bone loaded slowly fractures at a load that is approximately half of the load handled by bone at a fast rate of loading.

Elastic Response

At the onset of loading, bone exhibits a linearly elastic response. When a load is first applied, a bone will deform through a change in length or angular shape. Bone deforms no more than approximately 3% (34). This is considered in the elastic region of the stress–strain curve because when the load is removed, the bone will recover and return to its original shape or length.

Plastic Response

With continued loading the bone tissue reaches its yield point, after which its outer fibers begin to yield, with microtears and debonding of the material in the bone. This is termed the plastic region of the stress–strain curve. The bone tissue begins to deform permanently and eventually fractures if loading continues in the plastic region. Thus, when the load is removed, the bone tissue does not return to its original length but stays permanently elongated.

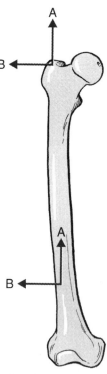

FIGURE 2-6 Bone is considered anisotrophic because it responds differently if forces are applied in different directions. **A.** Bone can handle large forces applied in the longitudinal direction. **B.** Bone is not as strong in handling forces applied transversely across its surface.

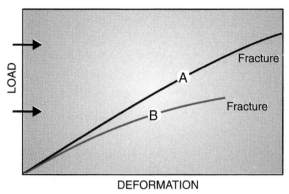

FIGURE 2-7 Bone is considered viscoelastic because it responds differently when loaded at different rates. **A.** When loaded quickly, bone responds with more stiffness and can handle a greater load before fracturing. **B.** When loaded slowly, bone is not as stiff or strong, fracturing under lower loads.

Although bone can exhibit a plastic response, normal loading remains well within the elastic region.

Strength

The strength of bone or any other material is defined by the failure point or the load sustained before failure. The failure of bone depends on the type of load imposed (Fig. 2-8). Failure of bone involves either a single traumatic event or the accumulation of microfractures. Thus, both fracture and fatigue behaviors of bone are important. Strength is assessed in terms of energy storage or the area under a stress–strain curve.

Stiffness

Stiffness, or the modulus of elasticity, is determined by the slope of the load deformation curve in the elastic response range and is representative of the material's resistance to load as the structure deforms. The stress–strain curve for ductile, brittle, and bone material is shown in Figure 2-9. Bone is not as stiff as glass or metal, and unlike these materials, it does not respond in a linear fashion because it yields and deforms nonuniformly during the loading phase (28).

The greater the load imposed upon the bone, the greater the deformation. Furthermore, if the load exceeds the material's elastic limits, permanent deformation and failure of the material result. If a material continues to elongate and deform a great deal in the plastic phase, it is termed a ductile material. Skin is an example of material that will deform a considerable amount before failure. Bone has properties that respond in both a brittle and ductile manner.

Figure 2-10 plots a variety of materials according to strength and stiffness. Examples of material considered stiff and weak are glass and copper; stiff and strong materials include steel and iron; flexible and strong materials include fiberglass and silk; and flexible and weak materials include oak, lead, and a spiderweb. Bone is considered flexible and weak (33).

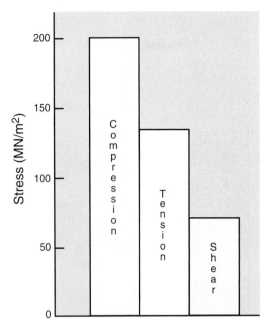

FIGURE 2-8 Ultimate stress for human adult cortical bone specimens. (Adapted with permission from Nordin, M. & Frankel, V.H. [Eds.] [1989]. *Basic Biomechanics of the Musculoskeletal System*. Philadelphia: Lea & Febiger.)

Normal and Shear Stress

Stress can be perpendicular to the plane of a cross-section of the loaded object. This is termed **normal stress**. If stress is applied parallel to the plane of the cross-section, it is termed **shear stress**. Each type of stress produces a strain. For example, normal strain involves a change in the length of an object, whereas shear strain is characterized by a change in the original angle of the object. An example of both normal strain and shear strain is the response of the femur to weight bearing. The femur shortens in response to normal strain and bends anteriorly in response

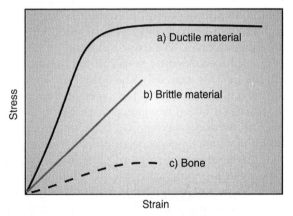

FIGURE 2-9 These stress–strain curves illustrate the differences in the behavior between ductile material **(A)**, brittle material **(B)**, and bone **(C)**, which has both brittle and ductile properties. When a load is applied, a brittle material responds linearly and fails or fractures before undergoing any permanent deformation. The ductile material enters the plastic region and deforms considerably before failure or fracture. Bone deforms slightly before failure.

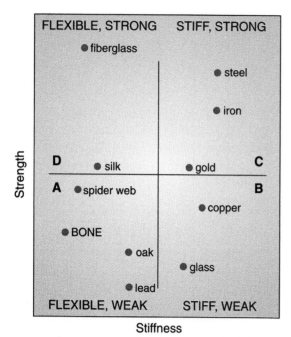

FIGURE 2-10 The strength and stiffness of a variety of materials are plotted in four quadrants representing material that is flexible and weak **(A)**; stiff and weak **(B)**; stiff and strong **(C)**; and flexible and strong **(D)**. Bone is categorized as being flexible and weak, along with other materials, such as spider web and oak wood. (Adapted with permission from Shipman, P., Walker, A., and Bichell, D. [1985]. *The Human Skeleton.* Cambridge, MA: Harvard University Press.)

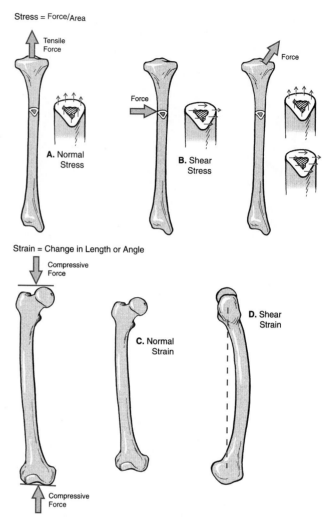

FIGURE 2-11 Stress, or force per unit area, can be perpendicular to the plane (normal stress) **(A)** or parallel to the plane (shear stress) **(B)**. Strain, or deformation of the material, is normal **(C)**, in which the length varies, or shear **(D)**, in which the angle changes.

to shear strain imposed by the body weight (31). Normal stress and shear stress, developed in response to tension applied to the tibia, are presented in Figure 2-11. Normal and shear strain, developed in response to compression of the femur, are also illustrated.

TYPES OF LOAD

The skeletal system is subject to a variety of applied forces as bone is loaded in various directions. Loads are produced by weight bearing, by gravity, by muscular forces, and by external forces. The stress and strain produced by forces applied to bones are responsible for facilitating the deposit of osseous material. The loads are applied in various directions, producing five types of forces: compression, tension, shear, bending, and torsion.

Injury to the skeletal system can be produced by a single high-magnitude application of one of these types of loads or by repeated application of a low-magnitude load over time. The former injury is referred to as a **traumatic fracture**. The latter type is a **stress fracture**, **fatigue fracture**, or **bone strain**. Figure 2-12 shows a radiograph of a stress fracture to the metatarsal. These fractures occur as a consequence of cumulative **microtrauma** imposed upon the skeletal system when loading of the system is so frequent that bone repair cannot keep up with the breakdown of bone tissue. The development of a stress fracture is discussed in greater detail at the end of this section.

Compression Forces

A **compression force** presses the ends of the bones together and is produced by muscles, weight bearing, gravity, or some external loading along the length of the bone. The compressive stress and strain inside the bone shorten and widen the bone. The bone absorbs maximal stress on a plane perpendicular to the compressive load. Figure 2-13 shows the effects of compressive force. Compressive forces are necessary for development and growth in the bone.

If a large compressive force is applied and if the load surpasses the stress limits of the structure, a compression fracture will occur. Numerous sites in the body are susceptible to compressive fractures. Compressive forces are responsible for patellar pain and softening and destruction of the cartilage underneath the patella. This injury is known as chondromalacia patellae. As the knee joint moves through a range of motion, the patella moves up and down in the femoral groove. The load between the

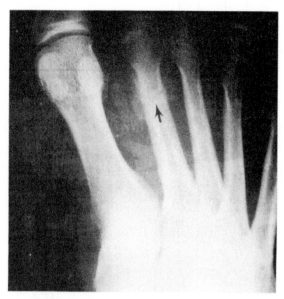

FIGURE 2-12 Stress fractures occur in response to overloading of the skeletal system so that cumulative microtraumas occur in the bone. A stress fracture to the second metatarsal, as shown in this radiograph, is caused by running on hard surfaces or in stiff shoes. It is also associated with persons with high arches and can be created by fatigue of the surrounding muscles. (Reprinted with permission from Fu, H. F., and Stone, D.A. [1994]. *Sports Injuries*. Baltimore: Williams & Wilkins.)

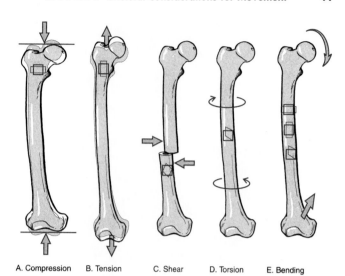

A. Compression   B. Tension   C. Shear   D. Torsion   E. Bending

FIGURE 2-13 The skeletal system is subjected to a variety of loads that alter the stresses in the bone. The square in the femur indicates the original state of the bone tissue. The colored area illustrates the effect of the force applied to the bone. **A.** Compressive force causes shortening and widening. **B.** Tensile force causes narrowing and lengthening. **C** and **D.** Shear force and torsion create angular distortion. **E.** Bending force includes all of the changes seen in compression, tension, and shear.

patella and the femur increases and decreases to a point at which the compressive patellofemoral force is greatest at approximately 50° of flexion and least at full extension or hyperextension of the knee joint. The high-compressive force in flexion, primarily on the lateral patellofemoral surface, is the source of the destructive process that breaks down the cartilage and underlying surface of the patella (10).

Compression is also the source of fractures to the vertebrae (11). Fractures to the cervical area have been reported in activities such as water sports, gymnastics, wrestling, rugby, ice hockey and football. Normally the cervical spine is slightly extended with a curve anteriorly convex. If the head is lowered, the cervical spine will flatten out to approximately 30° of flexion. If a force is applied against the top of the head when it is in this position, the cervical vertebrae are loaded along the length of the cervical vertebrae by a compressive force, creating a dislocation or fracture–dislocation of the facets of the vertebrae. When spearing or butting during tackling with the head in flexion was outlawed in football, the number of cervical spine injuries was dramatically reduced (11).

Compression fractures in the lumbar vertebrae of weight lifters, football linemen, and gymnasts who load the vertebrae while the spine is held in hyperlordotic or swayback position have also been reported (13). Figure 2-14 is a radiograph of a fracture to the lumbar vertebrae, demonstrating the shortening and widening effect of the compressive force. Finally, compression fractures are common in individuals with osteoporosis.

Specific lifts in weight training result in spondylolysis, a stress fracture of the pars interarticularis section of the vertebra. Lifts that have a high incidence of this fracture are the clean and jerk and the snatch from the Olympic lifts and the squat and dead lift from power lifting (13, 14). In gymnasts it is associated with extreme extension positions in the lumbar vertebrae. This injury will be discussed in greater detail in Chapter 7, when the trunk is reviewed.

A compressive force at the hip joint can increase or decrease the injury potential of the femoral neck. The hip joint must absorb compressive forces of approximately 3 to 7 times body weight during walking (28, 31). Compressive forces are up to 15 to 20 times body weight in jumping (31). In a normal standing posture, the hip joint assumes approximately a third of the body weight if both limbs are on the ground (28). This creates large compressive forces on the inferior portion of the femoral neck and a large pulling, or tensile, force on the superior portion of the neck. Figure 2-15 shows how this happens as the body pushes down on the femoral head, pushing the bottom of the femoral neck together and pulling the top of the femoral neck apart as it creates bending.

The hip abductors, specifically the gluteus medius, contract to counteract the body weight during stance. As shown in Figure 2-15, they also produce a compressive load on the superior aspect of the femoral neck that reduces the tensile forces and injury potential in the femoral neck, since bone usually fractures sooner with a tensile force (28). It is proposed that runners develop femoral neck fractures because the gluteus medius fatigues and cannot maintain its reduction of the high tensile force producing the fracture (20, 31). A femoral neck fracture

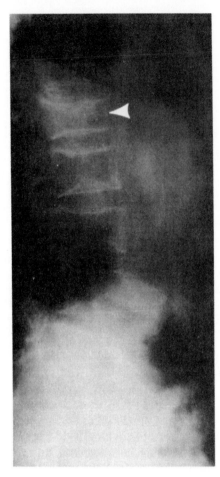

FIGURE 2-14 The lumbar vertebrae can incur compressive fracture, in which the body of the vertebra is shortened and widened. This type of fracture has been associated with loading of the vertebrae while maintaining a hyperlordotic position. (Reprinted with permission from Nordin, M., and Frankel, V.H. [1989]. *Basic Biomechanics of the Musculoskeletal System*. [2nd Ed.]. Philadelphia: Lea & Febiger.)

can also be produced by a strong cocontraction of the hip muscles, specifically the abductors and adductors, creating excessive compressive forces on the superior neck.

Tension Forces

Tension force is usually applied to the bony surface and pulls or stretches the bone apart so that it tends to lengthen and narrow (Fig. 2-13). The maximum stress, as with compression, is perpendicular to the plane of the applied load. The source of the tensile force is usually the pull of a contracting muscle tendon. When muscle applies a tensile force to the system through the tendon, the collagen in the bone tissue arranges itself in line with the tensile force of the tendon. Figure 2-16 shows an example of collagen alignment at the tibial tuberosity. This figure also illustrates the influence of tensile forces on the development of apophyses. An **apophysis** is bony outgrowth, such as a process, tubercle, or tuberosity. Figure 2-16 illustrates how an apophysis, the tibial tuberosity, is formed by tensile forces.

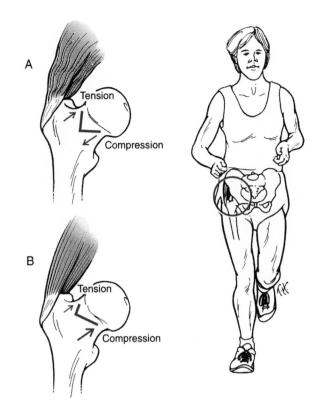

FIGURE 2-15 **A.** During standing or in the stance phase of walking and running, bending force applied to the femoral neck creates a large compressive force on the inferior neck and tensile force on the superior neck. **B.** If the gluteus medius contracts, the compressive force increases and the tensile force decreases. This reduces the injury potential, since injury is more likely to occur in tension.

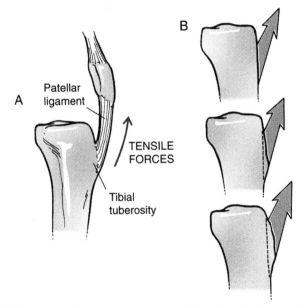

FIGURE 2-16 **A.** When tensile forces are applied to the skeletal system, the bone strengthens in the direction of the pull as collagen fibers align with the pull of the tendon or ligament. **B.** Tensile forces are also responsible for the development of apophyses, bony outgrowths such as processes, tubercles, and tuberosities.

Failure of the bone usually occurs at the site of muscle insertion. Tensile forces can also create ligament avulsions. A ligament avulsion, or an **avulsion fracture**, occurs when a portion of the bone at the insertion of the ligament is torn away. This occurs more frequently in children than in adults. Avulsion fractures occur when the tensile strength of the bone is not sufficient to prevent the fracture. This is typical of some of the injuries occurring in the high-velocity throwing motion of a Little Leaguer's pitching arm. The avulsion fracture in this case is commonly on the medial epicondyle as a result of tension generated in the wrist flexors.

Two other common tension-produced fractures are at the fifth metatarsal, caused by the tensile forces generated by the peroneal muscle group, and at the calcaneus, where the forces are generated by the triceps surae muscle group. The tensile force on the calcaneus can also be produced in the stance phase of gait as the arch is depressed and the plantar fascia covering the plantar surface of the foot tightens, exerting tensile force on the calcaneus. Some sites of avulsion fractures for the pelvic region, presented in Figure 2-17, include the anterior superior and inferior spines, the lesser trochanter, the ischial tuberosity, and the pubic bone.

Tension forces are generally responsible for sprains and strains. For example, the typical ankle inversion sprain occurs when the foot is oversupinated. That is, the foot rolls over its lateral border, stretching the ligaments on the lateral side of the ankle. Tensile forces are also identified with shin splints. This injury occurs when the tibialis anterior pulls on its attachment site on the tibia and on the interosseous membrane between the tibia and the fibula.

Another site exposed to high-tensile forces is the tibial tuberosity, which transmits very high tensile forces when the quadriceps femoris muscle group is active. This tensile force, if sufficient in magnitude and duration, may cause tendinitis or inflammation of the tendon in the older participant. In the younger participant, however, the damage usually occurs at the site of tendon–bone attachment and can result in inflammation, bony deposits, or an avulsion fracture of the tibial tuberosity. Osgood-Schlatter disease is the name of the condition characterized by inflammation and formation of bony deposits at the tendon–bone junction.

Bone responds to the demands placed upon it as described by Wolff's law (21). Therefore, different bones and different sections in a bone will respond to tension and compressive forces differently. For example, the tibia and femur participate in weight bearing in the lower extremity and are strongest when loaded with a compressive force. The fibula, which does not participate significantly in weight bearing but is a site for muscle attachment, is strongest when tensile forces are applied (31). An evaluation of the differences found in the femur uncovered greater tensile strength capabilities in the middle third of the shaft, which is loaded through a bending force in weight bearing. In the femoral neck, the bone can withstand large compressive forces, and the attachment sites of the muscles have great tensile strength (31).

Shear Forces

A **shear force** is applied parallel to the surface of an object, creating deformation internally in an angular direction (Fig. 2-13). Maximum shear stress acts on the surface parallel to the plane of the applied force. Shear stresses are created when a bone is subjected to compressive forces, tension forces, or both. Figure 2-18 shows how shear stress can develop with the application of a compressive or tensile force. Note the change in shape of the diamond. As the diamond undergoes distortion through compression or tension, shear force is applied across the surface of the bone. Bone fails more rapidly when exposed to shear force than tensile or compressive

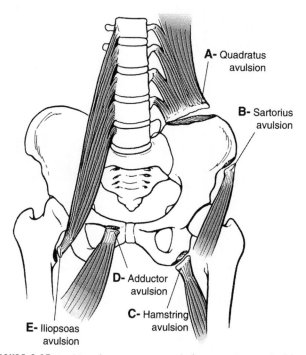

FIGURE 2-17 Avulsion fractures can result from tension applied by a tendon or a ligament. Sites of avulsion fractures in the pelvic region include the anterior superior spine **(A)**; anterior inferior spine **(B)**; ischial tuberosity **(C)**; pubic bone **(D)**; and lesser trochanter **(E)**.

A- Quadratus avulsion

B- Sartorius avulsion

D- Adductor avulsion

C- Hamstring avulsion

E- Iliopsoas avulsion

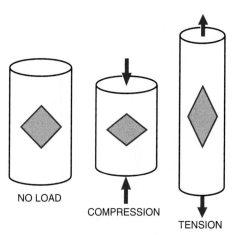

NO LOAD

COMPRESSION

TENSION

FIGURE 2-18 Shear stress and strain accompany both compression and tension loads.

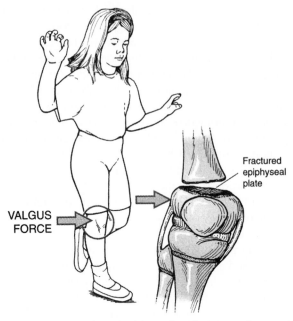

VALGUS
FORCE

Fractured
epiphyseal
plate

FIGURE 2-19 Fracture of the distal femoral epiphysis is usually created by shear force. This is commonly produced by a valgus force applied to the thigh or shank with the foot fixed and the knee hyperextended.

shear force increases with increased swayback, or hyperlordosis (14). The pull of the psoas muscle on the lumbar vertebrae also increases shear force on the vertebrae. This injury will be discussed in greater detail in Chapter 7.

Examples of fractures due to shear forces are commonly found in the femoral condyles and the tibial plateau. The mechanism of injury for both is usually hyperextension in the knee through some fixation of the foot and valgus or medial force to the thigh or shank. In the adult, this shear force can fracture a bone as well as injure the collateral or cruciate ligaments (25). In the developing child, this shear force can create epiphyseal fractures, such as in the distal femoral epiphysis. The mechanism of injury and the resulting epiphyseal damage are presented in Figure 2-19. The effects of such a fracture in the developing child can be significant, since this epiphysis accounts for approximately 37% of the bone growth in length (8).

It is common for bone to be loaded with more than one type of force at a time. Figures 2-20 and 2-21 show the multiple loads absorbed by the tibia in walking and running, respectively (28). In walking, a compressive

force. This is because bone is anisotropic and responds differently when loaded from different directions.

Shear forces are responsible for some vertebral disc problems, for example spondylolisthesis, in which the vertebrae slip anteriorly over one another. In the lumbar vertebrae,

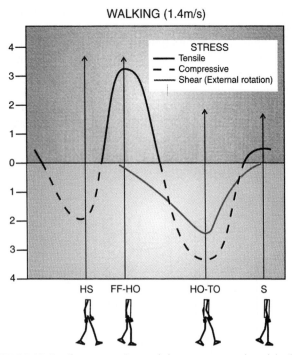

WALKING (1.4m/s)

STRESS
Tensile
Compressive
Shear (External rotation)

HS FF-HO HO-TO S

FIGURE 2-20 Tensile, compressive, and shear stresses on the adult tibia during walking. HS, heel strike; FF, foot flat; HO, heel off; TO, toe off; S, swing. (Reprinted with permission from Nordin, M., and Frankel, V.H. [1989]. *Basic Biomechanics of the Musculoskeletal System*. [2nd Ed.]. Philadelphia: Lea & Febiger.)

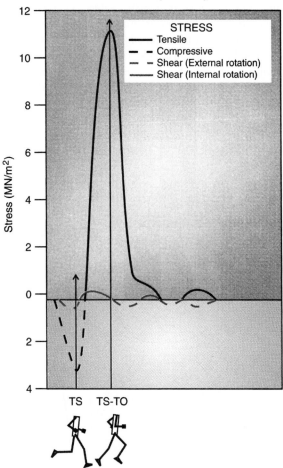

JOGGING (2.2 m/s)

STRESS
Tensile
Compressive
Shear (External rotation)
Shear (Internal rotation)

Stress (MN/m^2)

TS TS-TO

FIGURE 2-21 Tensile, compressive, and shear stresses on the adult tibia during running. TS, toe strike; TO, toe off. (Reprinted with permission from Slaby, F., and Jacobs, E.R. [1990]. *Radiographic Anatomy*. Philadelphia: Harwal.)

stress at heel strike is created by body weight, contact with the ground, and muscular contraction. Tensile stress dominates in mid support as a result of muscular contraction. Compressive stress develops in preparation for propulsion as the force on the ground and the muscular contractions increase. Shear force occurs in the propulsive phase of support and is believed to be related to torsion created through external rotation of the tibia.

In running, the stress increases substantially and the patterns of stress are different from those seen in walking. There are similarities in the foot strike phase, as a compressive stress is created by contact with the ground, body weight, and muscular contraction. This is followed by large tensile stress continuing on through the toe-off phase and into the swing phase. The pattern of shear stress is also different, representative of torsion created in response to internal and external rotation of the tibia (28).

Compressive, tensile, and shear forces applied simultaneously to the bone are important in development of strength of the bones. Figure 2-22 illustrates both compressive and tensile stress lines in the tibia and femur during running. Bone strength develops along these lines of stress.

Bending Forces

A **bending force** is applied to an area having no direct support offered by the structure. When a bone is subjected to a bending force and deformation occurs, one side of the bone will form a convexity where tensile forces are present and the other side of the bone will form a concavity where compressive forces are present (Fig. 2-13). Typically, the bone will fail and fracture on the convex side in response to the high tensile forces, since bone can withstand greater compressive forces than tensile forces (28). The magnitude of the compressive and tensile forces produced by bending increases with distance from the axis of the bone. Thus, the force magnitudes are greater on the outer portions of the bone.

During normal stance, both the femur and the tibia bend. The femur bends both anteriorly and laterally

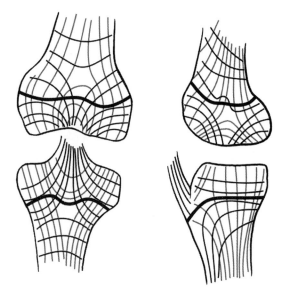

FIGURE 2-22 The lines of compressive stress (*bold black lines*) and tension stress (*lighter black and red lines*) for the distal femur and proximal tibia during the stance phase of running.

because of its shape and the manner of the force transmission caused by weight bearing. Weight bearing produces an anterior bend in the tibia. Although these bending forces are not injury producing, the bone is strongest in the regions where the bending force is greatest (31).

Injury-producing bending loads are caused by multiple forces applied at different points on the bone. Generally these situations are called three- or four-point force applications. Usually a force is applied perpendicular to the bone at both ends of the bone and a force applied in the opposite direction at some point between the other two forces. The bone will break at the point of the middle force application, as is the case in a ski boot fracture shown in Figure 2-23. This fracture is produced as the skier falls over the top of the boot with the ski and boot pushing in the other direction. The bone will usually fracture on the posterior side, since that is where the convexity and the tensile forces are applied.

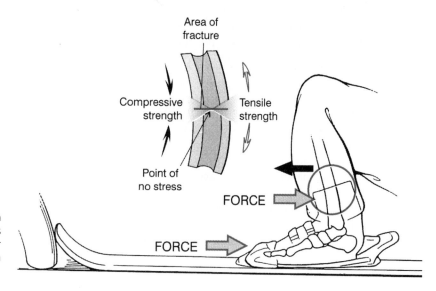

FIGURE 2-23 The ski boot fracture, created by a three-point bending load, occurs when the ski stops abruptly. Compressive force is created on the anterior tibia and tensile force on the posterior tibia. The tibia usually fractures on the posterior side.

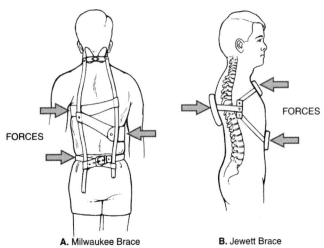

A. Milwaukee Brace   **B. Jewett Brace**

FIGURE 2-24 Three-point bending loads are used in many braces. **A.** The Milwaukee brace, used for correction of lateral curvature of the spine, applies three-point bending force to the spine. **B.** The Jewett brace applies three-point bending force to the thoracic spine to create spinal extension in that region.

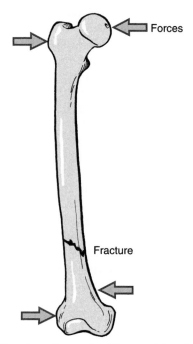

FIGURE 2-25 Hypothetical example of four-point bending load applied to the femur, creating a fracture or failure at the weakest point.

Ski boot fractures have been significantly reduced because of improvements in bindings, skis that turn more easily, well-groomed slopes, and the change in skiing technique that puts the weight forward on the skis. However, the reduction of tibial fractures through the improvement of equipment and technique has led to an increase in the number of knee injuries for the same reasons (7).

The three-point bending force is also responsible for injuries to a finger that is jammed and forced into hyperextension and to the knee or lower extremity when the foot is fixed in the ground and the lower body bends. Just eliminating the long cleats in the shoes of football players, and playing on good resurfaced fields, reduce this type of injury by half (14). Three-point bending force applications are also used in bracing. Figure 2-24 presents two brace applications using the three-point force application to correct a postural deviation or stabilize a region.

A four-point bending load is two equal and opposite pairs of forces at each end of the bone. In the case of four-point bending, the bone will break at its weakest point. This is illustrated in Figure 2-25 with the application of a four-point bending force to the femur.

Torsional Forces

A **torsional force** applied to a bone is a twisting force creating a shear stress over the entire material (Fig. 2-13). The magnitude of the stress increases with distance from the axis of rotation, and maximum shear stress acts both perpendicular and parallel to the axis of the bone. Torsional loading also produces both tensile and compressive forces at an angle across the structure.

Fractures resulting from torsional force can occur in the humerus when poor throwing technique creates a twist on the arm (31) and in the lower extremity when the foot is planted and the body changes direction. A spiral fracture

is a result of torsional force. An example of the mechanism of spiral fracture to the humerus in a pitcher is shown in Figure 2-26. Spiral fractures usually begin on the outside of the bone parallel to the middle of the bone. Torsional loading of the lower extremity is also responsible for knee cartilage and ligament injuries (14).

Injury vs Loading

Whether or not a bone incurs an injury as a result of an applied force is determined by the critical strength limits of the material and the loading history of the bone. These limits are primarily influenced by the loading on the bone. The loading of the bone can be increased or decreased by physical activity and conditioning, immobilization, and skeletal maturity of the individual. The rate of loading is also important because the response and tolerance of bone is rate sensitive. At high rates of loading, when bone tissue cannot deform fast enough, an injury can occur.

Muscular Activity vs Loading

Muscular activity can also influence the loads that bone can manage. Muscles alter the forces applied to the bone by creating compressive and tensile forces. These muscular forces may reduce tensile forces or redistribute the forces on the bone. Since most bones can handle greater compressive forces, the total amount of load can increase with the muscular contribution. However, if muscles fatigue during an exercise bout, their ability to alleviate the load on the bone diminishes. The altered stress distribution or increase in tensile forces leaves the athlete or performer susceptible to injury.

TABLE 2-1 Injuries to the Skeletal System

Injury to Bone Type of Injury	Activity Examples	Load Causing Injury	Mechanism of Injury
Tibial stress fracture	Dancing Running Basketball	Compression	Poor conditioning, stiff footwear, unyielding surfaces, hypermobile foot (overpronation)
Medial epicondyle	Gymnastics	Tension compression	Too much work on floor exercise and tumbling
Stress fracture of big toe	Sprinting Fencing Rugby	Tension	Toe extensors create bowstring effect on big toe when up on toes; primarily in individuals with hallux valgus
Stress fracture of femoral neck	Running Gymnastics	Compression	Muscle fatigue, high-arched foot
Stress fracture in calcaneus	Running Basketball Volleyball	Compression	Hard surface, stiff footwear
Stress fracture in lumbar vertebrae	Weight lifting Gymnastics Football	Compression Tension	High loads with hyperlordotic low-back posture
Tibial plateau fractures	Skiing	Compression	Hyperextension and valgus of the knee, as in turning, with the force on the inside edge of the downhill ski, abruptly halted with heavy snow
Stress fracture to medial malleolus	Running	Compression	Ankle sprain to outside causing compression between talus and medial malleolus or excessive pronation, since the medial malleolus rotates in with tibial rotation and pronation
Hamate fracture of hand	Baseball Golf Tennis Racquet sports	Compression	Relaxed grip in the swing that stops suddenly at the end of the swing as the club hits the ground, the bat is forcefully checked, or the racket is out of control
Fracture of tibia	Skiing	Bending Compression Tension	Three-point bending fall in which the body weight, boot, and ground bend the tibia posteriorly
Fracture of femoral condyles	Skiing Football	Shear	Hyperextension of knee with valgus force
Stress fracture in fibula	Running Aerobics Jumping	Tension	Jumping or deep-knee bends with a walk. Pull by soleus, tibialis posterior, peroneals, and toe flexors pulling tibia and fibula together
Meniscus tear of knee	Basketball Football Jumping Volleyball Soccer	Compression Torsion	Turning on a weight-bearing limb or valgus force to knee
Stress fracture in metatarsal	Running	Compression	Hard surfaces, stiff footwear, high-arched foot, fatigue
Stress fracture in femoral shaft	Running Triathlon	Tension	Excessive training and mileage. Created by pull of vastus medialis or adductor brevis

Stress Fractures

A **stress fracture** occurs when bone resorption weakens the bone too much and the bone deposit does not occur rapidly enough to strengthen the area. Stress fractures in the lower extremity can be attributed to muscle fatigue that reduces shock absorption and causes redistribution of forces to specific focal points in the bone. In the upper extremity, stress fractures result from repetitive muscular forces pulling on the bone. Stress fractures account for 10% of injuries to athletes (24).

The typical stress fracture injury occurs during a load application that produces shear or tensile strain and results in laceration, fracture, rupture, or avulsion. Bone tissue can also develop a stress fracture in response to compressive or

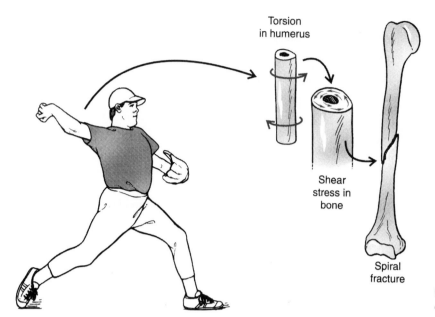

Torsion
in humerus

Shear
stress in
bone

Spiral
fracture

FIGURE 2-26 Example of torsion applied to the humerus, creating shear stress across the surface.

tensile loading that overloads the system, either through excessive force applied one or a few times or through too-frequent application of a low or moderate level of force (20, 22, 24). The relationship between the magnitude and frequency of applications of load on bone is presented in Figure 2-27. The tolerance of bone to injury is a function of the load and the cycles of loading.

Examples of injuries to the skeletal system are presented in Table 2-1. The activity associated with the injury, the type of load causing the injury, and the mechanism of injury are summarized.

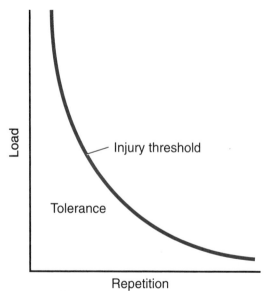

FIGURE 2-27 Injury can occur when a high load is applied a small number of times or when low loads are applied numerous times. It is important to remain within the injury tolerance range.

 Cartilage

Cartilage is a firm, flexible tissue made up of cells called **chondrocytes** surrounded by an extracellular matrix. There are two main types of cartilage that will be discussed in this chapter: articular or hyaline cartilage and fibrocartilage.

Articulating joints connect the different bones of the skeleton. In freely moving joints, the articulating ends of the bones are covered with a connective tissue referred to as articular cartilage.

ARTICULAR CARTILAGE

Articular or **hyaline cartilage** is an avascular substance consisting of 60 to 80% water and a solid matrix composed of collagen and proteoglycan. Collagen is a protein with the important mechanical properties of stiffness and strength. Proteoglycan is a highly hydrated gel. It is unclear how collagen and the proteoglycan gel interact during stress to the cartilage. However, the interaction between the two materials determines cartilage's mechanical properties. Cartilage has no blood supply and no nerves and is nourished by the fluid within the joint (26).

Articular cartilage is anisotropic, having different material properties for different orientations relative to the joint surface. The properties of cartilage make it well suited to resisting shear forces because it responds to load in a viscoelastic manner. It deforms instantaneously to a low or moderate load, and if rapidly loaded, it will become stiffer and deforms over a longer period. The force distribution across the area in the joint determines the stress in the cartilage, and the distribution of the force depends on the cartilage thickness.

Cartilage is important to the stability and function of a joint because it distributes loads over the surface and reduces the contact stresses by half (34). Collagen fibers are arranged to withstand load bearing. For example, in the knee, the medial meniscus transmits 50% of the compression load. Removal of just a small part of the cartilage has been shown to increase the contact stress by as much as 350% (16). Several years ago, a cartilage tear would have meant removal of the whole cartilage, but today orthopaedists trim the cartilage and remove only minimal amounts to maintain as much shock absorption and stability in the joint as possible.

Cartilage is 1 to 7 mm thick, depending on the stress and the incongruity of the joint surfaces (17). For example, in the ankle and the elbow joints, the cartilage is very thin, while at the hip and knee joints, it is thick. The cartilage is thin in the ankle because of the ankle's architecture. A substantial area of force distribution imposes less stress on the cartilage. Conversely, the knee joint is exposed to lower forces, but the area of force distribution is smaller, imposing more stress on the cartilage. Some of the thickest cartilage in the body, approximately 5 mm, lies on the underside of the patella (35).

Articular cartilage allows movement between two bones with minimal friction and wear. The joint surfaces have remarkably low coefficients of friction. Articular cartilage contributes significantly to this. The coefficient of friction in some joints has been reported to range from 0.01 to 0.04, whereas the coefficient of friction of ice at 0°C is about 0.1. These almost frictionless surfaces allow the surfaces to glide over each other smoothly.

FIBROCARTILAGE

Another type of cartilage is **fibrocartilage**, often found where articular cartilage meets a tendon or a ligament. Fibrocartilage acts as an intermediary between hyaline cartilage and the other connective tissues. Fibrocartilage is found where both tensile strength and the ability to withstand high pressures are necessary, for example in the intervertebral disks, the jaw, and the knee joint. A fibrocartilage structure is referred to as an articular disc, or **meniscus**. The menisci also improve the fit between articulating bones that have slightly different shapes. Meniscus tears usually occur during a sudden change of direction with the weight all on one limb. The resultant compression and tension on the meniscus tear the fibrocartilage. There is no pain associated with the actual tear; the peripheral attachment sites are the site of the irritation and resulting sensitivity.

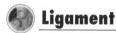 **Ligament**

A **ligament** connects bone to bone and consists of collagen, elastin, and reticulin fibers. Ligaments can be capsular, extracapsular, or intra-articular. **Capsular ligaments** are just thickenings in the wall of the capsule, much like the glenohumeral ligaments in the front of the shoulder capsule. **Extracapsular ligaments** lie outside the joint itself. The collateral ligaments found in numerous joints are extracapsular (i.e., fibular collateral ligament of knee). Finally, **intra-articular ligaments**, such as the cruciate ligaments of the knee and the capitate ligaments in the hip, are located inside a joint. The major ligaments of the body are presented in Appendix B.

The maximum stress that a ligament can endure is related to its cross-sectional area. Ligaments exhibit viscoelastic behavior. They respond to loads by becoming stronger and stiffer over time. The collagen fibers in a ligament are arranged so that it can handle both tensile loads and shear loads; however, it is best suited for tensile loading. An example of viscoelastic behavior is presented in Figure 2-28. The collagen fibers in ligament have a nearly parallel configuration. When unloaded, they have a wavy or crimped configuration. At low stresses, the crimp in the collagen fibers of the ligament disappears. At this point, ligament behaves almost linearly, with strains that are relatively small and within the physiological limit. At greater stresses, ligament tears, either partially or completely. Generally, when a tensile load is applied to a joint very quickly, the ligament is more likely to fail than the bone at the ligament attachment.

The strength of a ligament also diminishes rapidly with immobilization. A tensile injury to a ligament is termed a sprain. Sprains are rated 1, 2, or 3 in severity, depending on whether there is a partial tear of the fibers (rated 1), tear with some loss of stability (rated 2), or a complete tear with loss of joint stability (rated 3) (17).

At the end of the range of motion for every joint there is usually a ligament tightening up to terminate the motion.

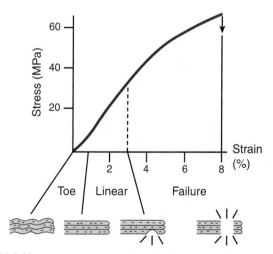

FIGURE 2-28 A stress–strain curve for a ligament. In the toe region, the collagen fibers of the ligament are wavy. The fibers straighten out in the linear region. In the plastic region, some of the collagen fibers tear. (Adapted with permission from Butler, D. L., Grood, E. S., Noyes, F. R., and Zernike, R. F. [1978]. Biomechanics of ligaments and tendons. *Exercise and Sports Science Reviews*, 6:125–181.)

Since the ligaments stabilize, control, and limit joint motion, any injury to a ligament will influence joint motion.

 Bony Articulations

THE DIARTHRODIAL OR SYNOVIAL JOINT

Movement potential of a segment is determined by the structure and function of the **diarthrodial** or **synovial joint**. The diarthrodial joint provides low-friction articulation capable of withstanding significant wear and tear. The characteristics of all diarthrodial joints are similar. For example, the knee has similar structures to the finger joints. Because of this similarity, it is worthwhile to look at the various components of the diarthrodial joint to gain general knowledge about joint function, support, and nourishment. Figure 2-29 shows the characteristics of the diarthrodial joint.

Characteristics of the Diarthrodial Joint

Covering the ends of the bones is the **articular end plate**, a thin layer of compact bone over spongy bone. On top of the end plate is articular cartilage. This cartilage in the joint offers additional load transmission, stability, improved fit of the surfaces, protection of the joint edges, and lubrication.

Another important characteristic of the diarthrodial joint is the **capsule**, a fibrous white connective tissue made primarily of collagen. It protects the joint. Thickenings in the capsule, known as ligaments, are common where additional support is needed. The capsule basically defines the

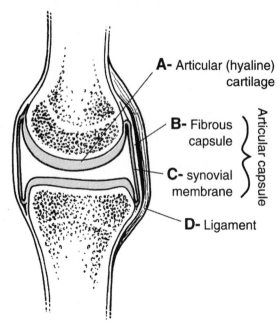

A- Articular (hyaline) cartilage

B- Fibrous capsule

C- synovial membrane

} Articular capsule

D- Ligament

FIGURE 2-29 The diarthrodial joints have similar characteristics. If you study the knee, interphalanges, elbow, or any other diarthrodial joint, you will find the same structures. These include **(A)** articular or hyaline cartilage, **(B)** capsule, **(C)** synovial membrane, and **(D)** ligaments.

joint, creating the interarticular portion, or inside, of the joint, which has a joint cavity and a reduced atmospheric pressure (34). Although soft tissue loads are difficult to compute, the capsule sustains some of the load imposed upon the joint (18).

Any immobilization of the capsule alters the mechanical properties of the capsular tissue and may result in joint stiffness. Likewise, injury to the capsule usually results in the development of a thick or fibrous section that can be externally palpable (9).

On the inner surface of the joint capsule is the **synovial membrane**, a loose, vascularized connective tissue that secretes **synovial fluid** into the joint to lubricate and provide nutrition to the joint. The fluid, having the consistency of an egg white, decreases in viscosity as shear rates increase. It is like catsup, hard to start but easy to move once it is going. When the joint moves slowly, the fluid is highly viscous and the support is high. Conversely, when the joint moves rapidly, the fluid is elastic in its response, decreasing the friction in the joint (34).

Any injury to the joint is noticeable in both a thickening in the membrane and a change in the consistency of the fluid. The fluid fills the capsular compartment and creates pain in the joint. Physicians will drain the joint to relieve the pressure, often finding that the fluid is blood-stained.

Stability of the Diarthrodial Joint

Stability in a diarthrodial joint is provided by the structure—the ligaments surrounding the joints, the capsule, and the tendons spanning the joint—gravity, and the vacuum in the joint produced by negative atmospheric pressure. The hip is one of the most stable joints in the body because it has good muscular, capsular, and ligamentous support. The hip joint has congruency between the surfaces, with a high degree of bone-to-bone contact. However, most of the stability in the hip is derived from the effects of gravity and the vacuum in the joint (17). The negative pressure in the joint is sufficient to hold the femur in the joint if all other structures, such as supporting ligaments and muscles, are removed.

In contrast, stability of the shoulder is supplied only by the capsule and the muscles surrounding the joint. Also, the congruency of the shoulder joint is limited, with only a small proportion of the head of the humerus making contact with the glenoid cavity.

Degeneration of the Diarthrodial Joint

Injury to the structures of the diarthrodial joint can occur during high load or through repetitive loading over an extended period. The articular cartilage in the joint is especially subject to wear during one's lifetime. Any trauma to or repeated wear on the joint causes a change in the articular substance to the point of enzymatic degradation, loss of proteoglycan, and removal of actual material by mechanical action. This results in diminished contact areas and erosion of the cartilage through development of rough

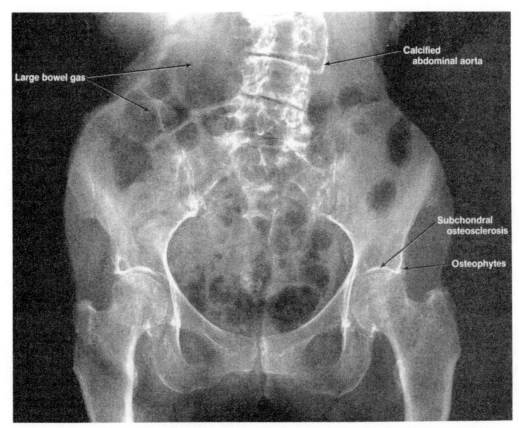

FIGURE 2-30 Osteoarthritis is characterized by physical changes in the joint consisting of cartilage erosion and formation of cysts and osteophytes. This radiograph shows osteoarthritis in the hip and vertebrae.

spots in the cartilage. The rough spots develop into fissures and eventually go deep enough that only subchondral bone is exposed. Osteophytes or cysts form in and around the joint, and this is the beginning of degenerative joint disease, or osteoarthritis. The radiographs in Figure 2-30 show the areas of joint degeneration associated with osteoarthritis in the hip and vertebrae.

It is theorized that osteoarthritis develops first in the subchondral, or cancellous, bone underlying the joint (30). The cartilage overlying the bone in the joint is thin; consequently, the underlying subchondral bone absorbs the shock of loading. Repetitive loading or unequal loading in the joint causes microfractures in the subchondral bone. When the microfractures heal, the subchondral bone is stiffer and less able to absorb shock, passing this role on to the cartilage. The cartilage deteriorates as a consequence of this overloading and the body lays down bone in the form of osteophytes to increase the contact area.

Osteoarthritis has been shown to have no relationship to hyperlaxity in the joint (2), to levels of osteoporosis (15), or to levels of physical activity (23). However, an injured joint deteriorates at a faster rate, making it more susceptible to the development of osteoarthritis.

Osteoarthritis can also be created by joint immobilization, because the joint and the cartilage require loading and compression to exchange nutrients and wastes (27).

After only 30 days of immobilization, the fluid in the cartilage is increased, and an early form of osteoarthritis develops. Fortunately, this process can be reversed with a return to activity.

Injury to other structures in the diarthrodial joint can also be serious. An injury to the joint capsule will result in formation of more fibrous tissue and possibly stretching of the capsule (9). Injury to the meniscus can create instability, loss of range of motion, and an increase in synovial effusion into the joint (swelling). Injury to the synovial membrane causes an increase in vascularity and produces gradual fibrosis of the tissue, eventually leading to chronic synovitis or inflammation of the membrane. Amazingly, many of these injury responses can also be reproduced through immobilization of the joint, which can produce adhesions, loss of range of motion, fibrosis, and synovitis.

Simple, Compound, and Complex Joints

The articulating surfaces in the joints vary in size and shape. There is typically a concave surface meeting a convex surface on the adjacent bone, termed female and male surfaces, respectively. Also, there can be more than two contact points or articulating surfaces. A joint with only two articulating surfaces is a **simple joint**, while a joint with three or more articulating surfaces is a **compound joint**. A joint with more than two articulating surfaces and with an articular disc or fibrocartilage is a **complex joint**. The hip and the ankle (talotibial) are simple joints; the wrist is a compound joint; and the knee is a complex joint.

Close-Packed vs Loose-Packed Positions

As movement through a range of motion occurs, the actual contact area varies between the articulating surfaces. When the joint position is such that the two adjacent bones fit together best and there is maximum contact between the two surfaces, the joint is considered to be in a **close-packed position**. This is the position of maximum compression of the joint, in which the ligaments and the capsule are tense and the forces travel through the joint as if it did not exist. Examples of close-packed positions are full extension for the knee, extension of the wrist, extension of the interphalangeal joints and maximum dorsiflexion of the foot (34). All other joint positions are termed **loose-packed positions** because there is less contact area between the two surfaces and the contact areas are frequently changing. There is more sliding and rolling of the bones over one another in a loose-packed position. This position allows for continuous movement, reducing the friction in the joint. Although the loose-packed joint position is less stable than the close-packed position, it is not as susceptible to injury because of its mobility. The close- and loose-packed positions of the knee joint are presented in Figure 2-31. Note the greater contact area in the close-packed position.

While in the close-packed position, the joint is very stable but vulnerable to injury, since the structures are taut and the joint surfaces are pressed together. The joint is especially susceptible to injury if hit by an external force, such as hitting the knee when it is fully extended.

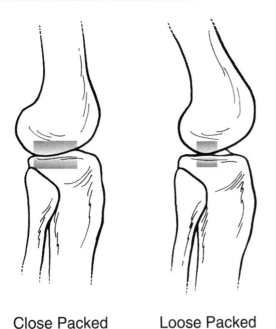

Close Packed   **Loose Packed**

FIGURE 2-31 In the close-packed position, contact between the two joint surfaces is maximal and mobility is minimal. In the loose-packed joint position, there is less contact between the surfaces in the joint and more mobility and movement between the two surfaces.

TYPES OF DIARTHRODIAL JOINTS

A classification system categorizes seven types of diarthrodial joints according to the differences in articulating surfaces, the degrees of freedom allowed by the joint and the type of movement occurring between the segments. Figure 2-32 offers a graphic representation of these seven joints.

Plane or Gliding Joint

The first type of joint is the **plane** or **gliding joint**, found in the foot among the tarsals and in the hand among the carpals. Movement at this type of joint is termed nonaxial, since it consists of two flat surfaces that slide over each other rather than around an axis.

In the hand, for example, the carpals slide over each other as the hand moves to positions of flexion, extension, radial deviation, and ulnar deviation. Likewise, in the foot, the tarsals shift during pronation and supination, sliding over each other in the process.

Hinge Joint

The **hinge joint** allows movement in one plane (flexion, extension); it is uniaxial. Examples of the hinge joint in the body are the interphalangeal joints in the foot and hand and the ulnohumeral articulation at the elbow.

Pivot Joint

The **pivot joint** also allows movement in one plane (rotation; pronation, supination) and is uniaxial. Pivot joints are found at the superior and inferior radioulnar joint and the atlantoaxial articulation at the base of the skull.

Condylar Joint

The **condylar joint** allows a primary movement in one plane (flexion and extension) with small amounts of movement in another plane (rotation). Examples are the knee and the temporomandibular joint.

Ellipsoid Joint

The **ellipsoid joint** allows movement in two planes (flexion and extension; abduction and adduction) and is biaxial. Examples of this joint are the radiocarpal articulation at the wrist and the metacarpophalangeal articulation in the phalanges.

Saddle Joint

The **saddle joint**, found only at the carpometacarpal articulation of the thumb, allows two planes of motion (flexion and extension; abduction and adduction) plus a small amount of rotation. It is similar to the ellipsoid joint in function.

Ball-and-Socket Joint

The last type of diarthrodial joint, the **ball-and-socket joint**, allows movement in three planes (flexion and extension; abduction and adduction; rotation) and is the most mobile of the diarthrodial joints. The hip and shoulder are examples of ball-and-socket joints. A summary of the major joints in the body is presented in Table 2-2.

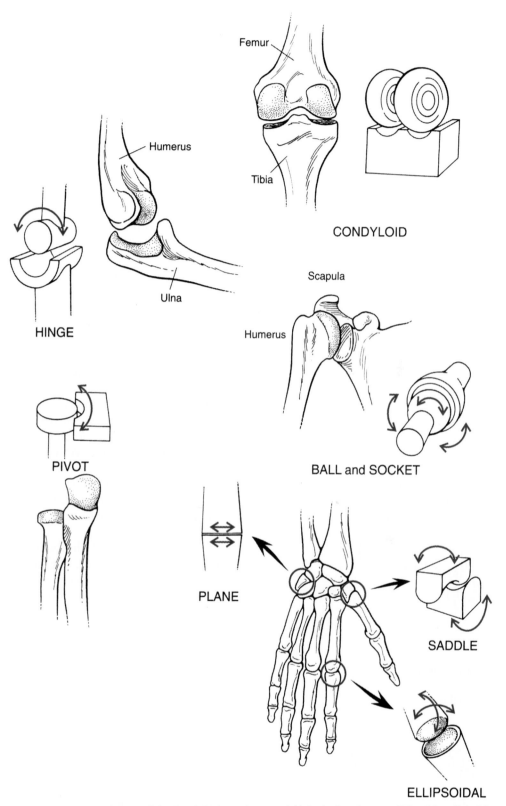

FIGURE 2-32 The seven types of diarthrodial joints. The nonaxial joint is the plane or gliding joint. Uniaxial joints include the hinge and pivot joints; biaxial joints are the condylar, ellipsoid, and saddle joint. The ball-and-socket joint is the only triaxial diarthrodial joint.

TABLE 2-2 Major Joints of the Body

Joint	Type	Degrees of Freedom
Vertebra	Amphiarthrodial	3
Hip	Ball-and-socket	3
Shoulder	Ball-and-socket	3
Knee	Condyloid	2
Wrist	Ellipsoid	2
Metacarpophalangeal (fingers)	Ellipsoid	2
Carpometacarpal (thumb)	Saddle	2
Elbow	Hinge	1
Radioulnar	Pivot	1
Atlantoaxial	Pivot	1
Ankle	Hinge	1
Interphalangeal	Hinge	1

A. Synarthrodial

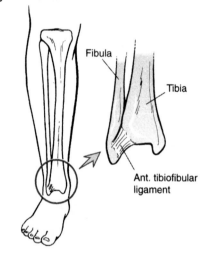

Fibula

Tibia

Ant. tibiofibular ligament

Distal Tibiofibular Joint

B. Amphiarthrodial

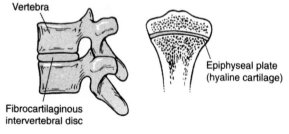

Vertebra

Epiphyseal plate (hyaline cartilage)

Fibrocartilaginous intervertebral disc

Intervertebral Disc

Epiphysis

FIGURE 2-33 A. An example of the synarthrodial joint is the fibrous articulation at the distal tibiofibular joint. **B.** The amphiarthrodial, or cartilaginous, joint can be found between the vertebrae or in the epiphyseal plate of a growing bone.

OTHER TYPES OF JOINTS

Synarthrodial or Fibrous Joints

Other articulations are limited in movement characteristics but nonetheless play an important role in stabilization of the skeletal system. Some bones are held together by fibrous articulations such as those found in the sutures of the skull. These articulations, referred to as **synarthrodial joints**, allow little or no movement between the bones and hold the bones firmly together (Fig. 2-33).

Amphiarthrodial or Cartilaginous Joints

Cartilaginous or **amphiarthrodial joints** hold bones together with either hyaline cartilage, such as is found at the epiphyseal plates, or fibrocartilage, as in the pubic symphysis and the intervertebral articulations (Fig. 2-32). The movement at these articulations is also limited, although not to the degree of the synarthrodial joints.

 Summary

The skeleton comprises bones, joints, cartilage, and ligaments. It provides a system of levers that allows a variety of movements at the joints, provides a support structure, protects the internal structures, stores fats and minerals, and participates in blood cell formation. Bone is an organ with blood vessels and nerves running through it. The types of bones that compose the skeletal system (long, short, flat, irregular, sesamoid) are shaped differently, perform different functions and are made up of different proportions of spongy and compact bone tissue.

Bone tissue is one of the body's hardest structures because of its organic and inorganic components. Bone tissue continuously remodels through deposition and resorption of tissue. Bone is also sensitive to disuse and loading. Bone tissue is deposited in response to stress on the bone and removed through resorption when not stressed. One of the ways of increasing the strength and density of bone is through a program of physical activity. Osteoporosis occurs when bone resorption exceeds bone deposit and the bone becomes weak.

The study of the architecture of bone tissue has identified two types of bone, compact and spongy. Compact bone, found on the exterior of bone and in the shaft of the long bones, is suited to handling high levels of compression and high tensile loads produced by the muscles. Spongy bone is suited for high-energy storage and facilitates stress distribution within the bone.

Bone is both anisotropic and viscoelastic in its response to loads and responds differently to variety in the direction of the load and to the rate at which the load is applied. When first loaded, bone responds by deforming through a change in length or shape, known as the elastic response. With continued loading, microtears occur in the bone as it yields during the plastic phase. Bone is considered to be a flexible and weak material compared to other materials such as glass and steel.

The skeletal system is subject to a variety of loads and can handle larger compressive loads than tensile or shear loads. Commonly, bone is loaded in more than one direction, as with bending, in which both compression and tension are applied, and in torsion loads, in which shear, compression, and tensile loads are all produced. Injury to bone occurs when the applied load exceeds the strength of the material.

Two types of cartilage are found in the skeletal system. Articular or hyaline cartilage covers the ends of the bones at synovial joints. This cartilage is composed of water and a solid matrix of collagen and proteoglycan. Articular cartilage functions to attenuate shock in the joint, to improve the fit of the joint, and to provide minimal friction in the joint. Cartilage has viscolelastic properties in its response to loads. A second type of cartilage, fibrocartilage, offers additional load transmission and stability in a joint. Fibrocartilage is often referred to as anarticular disc or meniscus.

Ligaments connect bone to bone and are categorized as capsular, intracapsular, or extracapsular, depending on their location relative to the joint capsule. Ligaments exhibit viscoleastic behavior. They respond to loads by becoming stiffer as the load increases.

The movements of the long bones occur at a synovial joint, a joint with common characteristics such as articular cartilage, a capsule, a synovial membrane, and ligaments. The synovial joint can be injured through a sprain, in which the ligaments are injured. Joints are also susceptible to degeneration characterized by breakdown in the cartilage and bone. This degeneration is known as osteoarthritis.

The amount of motion between two segments is largely influenced by the type of synovial joint. For example, the planar joint allows simple translation between the joint surfaces; the hinge joint allows flexion and extension; the pivot joint allows rotation; the condylar joint allows flexion and extension with some rotation; the ellipsoid and the saddle joints allow flexion, extension, abduction, and adduction; and the ball-and-socket joint allows flexion, extension, abduction, adduction, and rotation. Other types of joints, synarthrodial and amphiarthrodial, allow little or no movement.

REVIEW QUESTIONS

True or False

1. ___ The cause of idiopathic scoliosis is known to be related to posture.
2. ___ Idiopathic scoliosis is anterior curvature of the spine.
3. ___ A lever alters only the speed of a movement.
4. ___ A lever must have an axis.
5. ___ Bones decrease in size from top to bottom.
6. ___ Spongy bone is not very porous.
7. ___ Spongy bone transmits energy.
8. ___ The phalanges are short bones.
9. ___ The shaft of a long bone is called the epiphysis.
10. ___ The diaphysis is composed primarily of compact bone.
11. ___ The role of sesamoid bone is to protect internal structures.
12. ___ Bone is approximately10–15% inorganic.
13. ___ Bone tissue is a viscoelastic material whose mechanical properties are affected by its structure.
14. ___ The mineral constituents of bone allow it to withstand compressive loads.
15. ___ Bone adapts to both internal and external forces.
16. ___ Bones do not require mechanical stress to grow and function.
17. ___ Immobilization has little effect on bone.
18. ___ A condition in which bone resorption exceeds bone deposits is called osteopetrosis.
19. ___ The term that best describes the fact that the behavior of bone depends on the direction of loading is viscoelastic.
20. ___ Cartilage is approximately 70% water and has little blood supply.
21. ___ Some of the thickest cartilage in the body is found at the ankle joint.
22. ___ A ligament connects muscle to bone.
23. ___ The shoulder has substantial ligamentous support.
24. ___ It is theorized that osteoarthritis develops first in the cartilage.
25. ___ The knee is a complex joint.

Multiple Choice

1. A lever alters the ___ of a movement.
   a. Speed
   b. Force
   c. Change in direction
   d. Both a and b
2. A lever must have ___.
   a. Axis of rotation
   b. Muscles
   c. Spongy bone
   d. None of the above
3. The olecranon process and the olecranon fossa meet to prevent ___.
   a. Pronation
   b. Hyperflexion
   c. Internal rotation
   d. Hyperextension
4. Hematopoiesis is ___.
   a. Internal bleeding
   b. Inflammation of bone marrow
   c. Blood cell formation
   d. None of the above
5. Compact bone ___ is and ___.
   a. Flexible, strong
   b. Strong, stiff
   c. Stiff, weak
   d. Ductile, weak

6. The shaft of a long bone is called the___.
   a. Epiphysis
   b. Diaphysis
   c. Metaphysis
   d. Duraphysis

7. Bone tissue is a viscoelastic material whose mechanical properties are afflicted by its ___.
   a. Structure
   b. Deformation rate
   c. Percentage of compact bone
   d. Both a and b

8. The bone in the distal part of the femur is replaced every ___.
   a. 5–6 months
   b. 10–12 months
   c. 2 years
   d. 4 years

9. Myositis ossificans is ___.
   a. An irritation of muscle due to irregular bone growth
   b. Desirable by some martial artists
   c. A breakdown of bone tissue
   d. None of the above

10. After age 30 there is a ___ yearly loss in the mineral weight of bone.
   a. 0.1–0.3%
   b. 0.2–0.5%
   c. 0.3–0.6%
   d. 1–2%

11. Compact bone is less than ___ percent porous.
   a. 2
   b. 5
   c. 10
   d. 15

12. At muscle insertion sites collagen fibers are arranged ___, maximizing strength.
   a. Obliquely
   b. Circumferentially
   c. Longitudinally
   d. In series

13. The small, flat pieces of bone making up the spongy bone are called ___.
   a. Tolmetin
   b. Trabiculae
   c. Treponema
   d. Lacunae

14. The term that best describes the fact that the response of bone depends on the rate of loading is ___.
   a. Isotropic
   b. Anisotropic
   c. Anisotonic
   d. Viscoelastic

15. A stress fracture can be the result of ___.
   a. A single high-magnitude force
   b. A repeated low-magnitude force
   c. A repated high-magnitude force
   d. None of the above

16. A standing person has ___ forces on the inferior portion and ___ forces on the superior portion of the femoral neck.
   a. Torsion, tensile
   b. Tensile, compressive
   c. Compressive, tensile
   d. Tensile, torsion

17. When a bone is subjected to an excessive bending force it will fail on the ___ side because it is weaker under ___ forces.
   a. Concave, tensile
   b. Convex, tensile
   c. Convex, compressive
   d. None of the above

18. Cartilage reduces contact forces by ___.
   a. 50%
   b. 60%
   c. 70%
   d. None of the above

19. Cartilage ___.
   a. Improves the fit of the ends of the bones in a joint
   b. Decreases the friction in a joint
   c. Helps to attenuate shock
   d. All of the above

20. Cartilage exhibits ___ characteristics.
   a. Isotropic
   b. Anisotropic
   c. Both a and b
   d. Neither a nor b

21. With no tension on it, the collagen fibers in a ligament are ___.
   a. Perpendicular to the length
   b. Crimped
   c. Stretched
   d. No specific pattern

22. The strength of a ligament ___ with immobilization.
   a. Increases
   b. Is not affected
   c. Decreases
   d. None of the above

23. The knee is an example of a ___ joint.
   a. Ellipsoid
   b. Hinge
   c. Condylar
   d. Simple

24. Synarthrodial joints allow for ___ movements.
   a. Small
   b. Large
   c. No movement
   d. None of the above

25. Amphiarthrodial joints allow ___ movement compared with synarthrodial joints.
   a. More
   b. Less
   c. The same
   d. All of the above

REFERENCES

1. Antao, N.A. (1988). Myositis of the hip in a professional soccer player. *American Journal of Sports Medicine*, 16:82.
2. Bird, H.A. (1986). A clinical review of the hyperlaxity of joints with particular reference to osteoarthrosis. *Engineering in Medicine*, 15:81.
3. Brewer, V., et al. (1983). Role of exercise in prevention of involutional bone loss. *Medicine and Science in Sports and Exercise*, 15:445.
4. Butler, D. L., et al. (1978). Biomechanics of ligaments and tendons. *Exercise and Sports Science Reviews*, 6:125–181.
5. Choi, K., Goldstein, S.A. (1922). A comparison of the fatigue behavior of human trabecular and cortical bone tissue. *Journal of Biomechanics*, 25:1371.
6. Cook, S.D., et al. Trabecular bone density and menstrual function in women runners. *American Journal of Sports Medicine*, 15:503, 1987.
7. Dolinar, J. (1990). Keeping ski injuries on the down slope. *Physician and Sports Medicine.* 19(2):120–123.
8. Downing, J. F., et al. (Eds. 1991). Four complex joint injuries. *Physician and Sports Medicine.* Vol 19(10): 80–97.
9. Egan, J.M. A constitutive model for the mechanical behavior of soft connective tissues. *Journal of Biomechanics*, 20:681–692, 1987.
10. Eisele, S.A. (1991). A precise approach to anterior knee pain. *Physician and Sports Medicine*, 19(6): 126–130; 137–139.
11. Fine, K. M., et al. (1991). Prevention of cervical spine injuries in football. *Physician and Sports Medicine*, 19(10): 54–64.
12. Frost, H. M. (1985). The pathomechanics of osteoporoses. *Clinical Orthopaedics and Related Research*, 200:198.
13. Halpbern, B. C., Smith, A. D. (1991). Catching the cause of low back pain. *Physician and Sports Medicine*, 19(6): 71–79.
14. Halpbern, B., et al. (1987). High school football injuries: Identifying the risk factors. *American Journal of Sports Medicine*, 15:316.
15. Healey, J. H., et al. (1985). The coexistence and characteristics of osteoarthritis and osteoporosis. *Journal of Bone and Joint Surgery*, 67A:586–592.
16. Henning, C.E. (1988). Semilunar cartilage of the knee: Function and pathology. In K. N. Pandolf (Ed.). *Exercise and Sport Sciences Review*. New York: Macmillan, 205–214.
17. Hettinga, D. L. (1985). Inflammatory response of synovial joint structures. In J. Gould, G. J. Davies (Eds.). *Orthopaedics and Sports Physical Therapy*. St. Louis: Mosby, 87–117.
18. Hoffman, A. H., Grigg, P. (1989). Measurement of joint capsule tissue loading in the cat knee using calibrated mechanoreceptors. *Journal of Biomechanics*, 22:787–791.
19. Iskrant, A. P., Smith, R. W. (1969). Osteoporosis in women 45 years and related to subsequent fractures. *Public Health Reports*, 84:33–38.
20. Jackson, D. L. (1990). Stress fracture of the femur. *Physician and Sports Medicine*, 19(7):39–44.
21. Keller, T. S., Spengler, D. M. (1989). Regulation of bone stress and strain in the immature and mature rat femur. *Journal of Biomechanics*, 22:1115–1127.
22. Lakes, R. S., et al. (1990). Fracture mechanics of bone with short cracks. *Journal of Biomechanics*, 23:967–975.
23. Lane, N. E., et al. (1990). Running, osteoarthritis, and bone density: Initial 2-year longitudinal study. *American Journal of Medicine*, 88:452–459.
24. Matheson, G. O., et al. (1987). Stress fractures in athletes. *American Journal of Sports Medicine*, 15:46–58.
25. McConkey, J. P., Meeuwisse, W. (1988). Tibial plateau fractures in alpine skiing. *American Journal of Sports Medicine*, 16:159–164.
26. Mow, V. C., et al. (1989). Biomechanics of articular cartilage. In M. Nordin, V. H. Frankel (Eds.). *Basic Biomechanics of the Musculoskeletal System*. Philadelphia: Lea Febiger, 31–58.
27. Navarro, A. H., Sutton, J. D. (1985). Osteoarthritis IX: Biomechanical factors, prevention, and nonpharmacologic management. *Maryland Medical Journal*, 34:591–594.
28. Nordin, M., Frankel, V. H. (1989). Biomechanics of bone. In M. Nordin, V. H. Frankel (Eds.). *Basic Biomechanics of the Musculoskeletal System*. Philadelphia, Lea & Febiger, 3–30.
29. Oyster, N., et al. (1984). Physical activity and osteoporosis in post-menopausal women. *Medicine and Science in Sports and Exercise*, 16:44–50.
30. Radin, E. L., et al. (1972). Role of mechanical factors in the pathogenesis of primary osteoarthritis. *Lancet*, 1:519–522.
31. Riegger, C. L. (1985). Mechanical properties of bone. In J. A. Gould, G. J. Davies (Eds.). *Orthopaedic and Sports Physical Therapy*. St. Louis, Mosby, 3–49.
32. Schaffler, M. B., Burr, D. B. (1988). Stiffness of compact bone: Effects of porosity and density. *Journal of Biomechanics*, 21:13–16.
33. Shipman, P., et al. (1985). *The Human Skeleton*. Cambridge, MA: Harvard University.
34. Soderberg, G. L. (1986). *Kinesiology: Application to Pathological Motion*. Baltimore: Williams & Wilkins, 1986.
35. Wallace, L. A., et al. (1985). The knee. In J. A. Gould, G. J.Davies (Eds.). *Orthopaedic and Sports Physical Therapy*. St. Louis: Mosby, 342–364.
36. Whalen, R. T., et al. (1988). Influence of physical activity on the regulation of bone density. *Journal of Biomechanics*, 21:825–837.
37. Zernicke, R. F., et al. (1990). Biomechanical response of bone to weightlessness. In K. B. Pandolf, J. O. Holloszy (Eds.). *Exercise and Sport Sciences Reviews*. Baltimore: Williams & Wilkins, 167–192.

ADDITIONAL READING

An, K. N., et al. (1991). Pressure distribution on articular surfaces: Application to joint stability evaluation. *Journal of Biomechanics*, 23:1013.

Blank, S. (1987). Transverse tibial stress fractures. *American Journal of Sports Medicine*, 15:597.

Brown, T. D., et al. (1990). Toward an identification of mechanical parameters initiating periosteal remodeling: a combined experimental and analytic approach. *Journal of Biomechanics*, 23:893.

Currey, J. (1984). *The Mechanical Adaptations of Bones*. Princeton, NJ: Princeton University.

Keller, C. S., et al. (1987). The medical aspects of soccer injury epidemiology. *American Journal of Sports Medicine*, 15:230–237.

McAuley, E., et al. (1987). Injuries in womens gymnastics. *American Journal of Sports Medicine*, 15:558–565.

Nambu, T., et al. (1991). Deformation of the distal femur: A contribution towards the pathogenesis of osteochondrosis dissecans in the knee joint. *Journal of Biomechanics*, 24:421–433.

Nichols, J. N., Tehranzadeh, J. (1987). A review of tibial spine fractures in bicycle injury. *American Journal of Sports Medicine*, 15:172–174.

Nigg, B. M., Bobbert, M. (1990). On the potential of various approaches in load analysis to reduce the frequency of sports injuries. *Journal of Biomechanics*, 23:3–12.

Parker, R. D., et al. (1986). Hook of the hamate fractures in athletes. *American Journal of Sports Medicine*, 14:517–523.

Rohl, L., et al. (1991). Tensile and compressive properties of cancellous bone. *Journal of Biomechanics*, 24:1143–1149.

Shelbourne, K. D., et al. (1988). Stress fractures of the medial malleolus. *American Journal of Sports Medicine*, 16:60–63.

Thompson, N., et al. (1987). High school football injuries: Evaluation. *American Journal of Sports Medicine*, 15:117–124.

Tursz, A., Crost, M. (1986). Sports-related injuries in children. *American Journal of Sports Medicine*, 14:294–299.

Viano, D. C., et al. (1986). Injury biomechanics research: An essential element in the prevention of trauma. *Journal of Biomechanics*, 22:403–417.

Watson, M. D., DiMartino, P. P. (1987). Incidence of injuries in high school track and field athletes and its relation to performance ability. *American Journal of Sports Medicine*, 15:251–254.

Yokoe, K., Mannoji, T. (1986). Stress fracture of the proximal phalanx of the great toe. *American Journal of Sports Medicine*, 14:240–242.

GLOSSARY

Amphiarthrodial Joint: A type of joint whose bones are connected by cartilage; some movement may be allowed at these joints. Also called cartilaginous joint.

Anisotropic: Having different properties in different directions.

Apophysis: A bony outgrowth such as a process, tubercle, or tuberosity.

Articular Cartilage: Hyaline cartilage consisting of tough, fibrous connective tissue.

Avulsion Fracture: The tearing away of a part of bone when a tensile force is applied.

Ball-and-Socket Joint: A type of diarthrodial joint that allows motion through three planes.

Bending Force: A force causing a change in the angle of the bone, offsetting in the horizontal plane. The material bends in the region of no direct structural support.

Bone Strain: See stress fracture.

Cancellous Bone: See spongy bone.

Capsular Ligament: Ligaments within the wall of the capsule; thickening in the capsule wall.

Capsule: A fibrous connective tissue that encloses the diarthrodial joint.

Cartilaginous Joint: A type of joint whose bones are connected by cartilage. Some movement may be allowed at these joints. Also called amphiarthrodial joint.

Chondrocytes: Cartilage cells.

Close-Packed Position: The joint position with maximum contact between the two joint surfaces and in which the ligaments are taut, forcing the two bones to act as a single unit.

Collagen: A connective tissue that is the main protein of skin, tendon, ligament, bone, and cartilage.

Compact Bone: A dense, compact tissue on the exterior of bone that provides strength and stiffness to the skeletal system. Also called cortical bone.

Complex Joint: A joint in which two or more bones articulate and a disc or fibrocartilage is present.

Compound Joint: A joint in which three or more bones articulate.

Compression Force: A force pressing the ends of the bone together, shortening and widening the structure.

Condylar Joint: A type of diarthrodial joint that is biaxial, with one plane of movement that dominates the movement in the joint.

Cortical Bone: Dense, compact tissue on the exterior of bone that provides strength and stiffness to the skeletal system. Also called compact bone.

Deposition: A phase of bone remodeling during which bone is formed through osteoblastic activity.

Diaphysis: The shaft of a long bone.

Diarthrodial Joint: Freely movable joint; also called synovial joint.

Ellipsoid Joint: A type of diarthrodial joint with two degrees of freedom that resembles the ball-and-socket joint.

Epiphysis: The ends of a long bone.

Extracapsular Ligament: Ligament outside of the joint capsule.

Fibrocartilage: A type of cartilage having parallel thick, collagenous bundles.

Fibrous Joint: A type of joint whose bones are connected by fibrous material; little or no movement is allowed at these joints; also called synarthrodial joint.

Flat Bone: A thin bone consisting of thin layers of compact and spongy bone.

Gliding Joint: A type of diarthrodial joint with flat surfaces that allows translation between the two bones; also called plane joint.

Haversian System: See osteon.

Hinge Joint: A type of diarthrodial joint allowing one degree of freedom.

Hyaline Cartilage: See articular cartilage.

Intra-articular Ligament: Ligament inside the joint.

Irregular Bone: A bone having a specialized shape and function.

Lamellae: The concentric tubes of collagen that encircle an osteon.

Lever: A simple machine that magnifies force or speed of movement.

Ligament: A band of fibrous, collagenous tissue connecting bone or cartilage to each other; supports the joint.

Long Bone: A bone longer than it is wide, having a shaft, diaphysis, and wide ends, the epiphyses.

Loose-Packed Position: The joint position with less than maximum contact between the two joint surfaces and in which contact areas frequently change.

Metaphysis: The wide shaft toward the end of a long bone.

Meniscus: Crescent-shaped disc of fibrocartilage.

Microtrauma: A disturbance or abnormal condition that is initially too small to be seen.

Morphology: The study of shape and form.

Normal Stress: The amount of load per cross-sectional area applied perpendicular to the plane of a cross-section of the loaded object.

Normal Strain: Deformation in a material involving a change in the length of the object.

Osseous: Having the nature or quality of bone.

Osteoarthritis: Degenerative joint disease characterized by degeneration in the articular cartilage, osteophyte formation and reduction in the joint space.

Osteocyte: A bone cell.

Osteoblast: A type of bone cell responsible for bone deposition.

Osteoclast: A type of bone cell responsible for bone resorption.

Osteon: Long cylindrical structure in bone that serves as weight-bearing pillar.

Osteoporosis: A condition in which the rate of bone formation is decreased, demineralization occurs, and the bone softens.

Periosteum: A white membrane of connective tissue that covers the outer surface of a bone except over articular cartilage.

Pivot Joint: A type of diarthrodial joint that allows movement in one plane; pronation, supination, or rotation.

Plane Joint: A type of diarthrodial joint with flat surfaces that allows translation between the two bones; also called gliding joint.

Porosity: The ratio of pore space to the total volume.

Resorption: A phase of bone remodeling in which bone is lost through osteoclastic activity.

Saddle Joint: A type of diarthrodial joint having two saddle-shaped surfaces allowing two degrees of freedom.

Sesamoid Bone: A type of short bone embedded in a tendon or joint capsule.

Shear Force: A force applied parallel to the surface, creating deformation internally in an angular direction.

Shear Stress: The amount of load per cross-sectional area applied parallel to the plane of a cross-section of the loaded object.

Shear Strain: Deformation in a material involving a change in the original angle of the object.

Short Bone: A bone having dimensions that are approximately equal.

Simple Joint: A joint with only two articulating surfaces.

Spongy Bone: Bone tissue that is latticelike, with high porosity; capable of high energy storage. Also called cancellous bone.

Stress Fracture: A fracture created when loading of the skeletal system is so frequent that bone repair cannot keep up with the breakdown of bone tissue; also called fatigue fracture.

Synarthrodial Joint: A type of joint whose bones are connected by fibrous material; little or no movement is allowed at these joints; also called fibrous joint.

Synovial Fluid: Liquid secreted by the synovial membrane that reduces friction in the joint; the fluid changes viscosity in response to the speed of joint movement.

Synovial Joint: Freely movable joint; also called diarthrodial joint.

Synovial Membrane: Loose vascularized connective tissue that lines the joint capsule.

Tension Force: Force pulling the bone apart, lengthening and narrowing the bone.

Torsion Force: Twisting force that creates shear stress over the entire material.

Trabeculae: Strands within spongy bone that adapt to the direction of stress on the bone.

Traumatic Fracture: A break in a bone as a result of a single high-magnitude force application.

Muscular Considerations for Movement

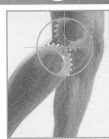

OBJECTIVES

After reading this chapter, the student will be able to:

1. Define the properties, functions, and roles of skeletal muscle.

2. Describe the gross and microscopic anatomical structure of the muscle.

3. Explain the differences in shape and function of muscles.

4. Describe the difference in the force output between the three muscle fiber types (Types I, IIa, IIb).

5. Describe the characteristics of the muscle attachment to the bone and explain the viscoelastic response of the tendon.

6. Compare isometric, concentric, and eccentric muscle actions.

7. Explain how muscles contract and how the angle of muscular attachment, the elastic component, the length–tension relationship, the force–velocity relationship, and the presence of a prestretch all influence tension development in the muscle.

8. Explain what electromyography is, the effect of increased muscle force on it, how to record it, and its limitations.

9. Explain the physical changes that occur in the muscle as a result of strength training and elaborate on how genetic predisposition, training specificity, intensity, and training volume influence strength training outcomes.

10. Describe types of resistance training and explain how training should be adjusted for the athlete or nonathlete.

11. Identify some of the major contributors to muscle injury, the location of common injuries, and means for prevention of injury to the muscle.

Muscles exert forces and thus are a major contributor to human movement. Muscles are used to hold a position, to raise or lower a body part, to slow down a fast-moving segment, and to generate great speed in the body or in an object that is propelled into the air. The tension developed by muscles applies compression to the joints, enhancing their stability. However, in some joint positions, the tension generated by the muscles can act to pull the segments apart and create instability.

Exercise programming for a young, healthy population usually uses exercises that push the muscular system to high levels of performance. Muscles can exert force and develop power. Many athletic training programs with the young and healthy are designed to achieve maximum performance. However, the same exercise principles used with young, active individuals can be scaled down for use by persons of limited ability. Using the elderly as an example, it is apparent that strength decrement is one of the major factors influencing efficiency in daily living activities. The loss of strength and efficiency in the muscular system can create a variety of problems, ranging from inability to reach overhead or open a jar lid to difficulty using stairs and getting up out of a chair. Another example is the overweight individual who has difficulty walking any distance because the muscular system cannot generate sufficient power and the person fatigues easily. These two examples are really no different from the power lifter trying to perform a maximum lift in the squat. In all three cases, the muscular system is overloaded, with only the magnitude of the load and output varying.

Muscles are either striated or smooth. Striated muscles include skeletal and cardiac muscle. Both cardiac and smooth muscles are under the control of the autonomic nervous system. That is, they are not under voluntary control. Skeletal muscle, on the other hand, is under direct voluntary control. Of primary interest in this chapter is skeletal muscle. All aspects of muscle structure and function related to human movement and efficiency of

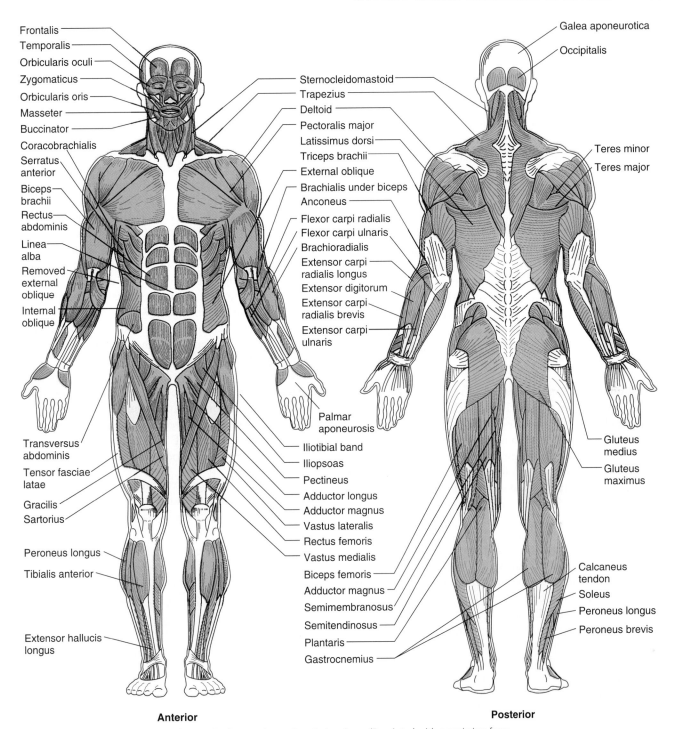

Frontalis
Temporalis
Orbicularis oculi
Zygomaticus
Orbicularis oris
Masseter
Buccinator
Coracobrachialis
Serratus anterior
Biceps brachii
Rectus abdominis
Linea alba
Removed external oblique
Internal oblique

Galea aponeurotica
Occipitalis

Sternocleidomastoid
Trapezius
Deltoid
Pectoralis major
Latissimus dorsi
Triceps brachii
External oblique
Brachialis under biceps
Anconeus
Flexor carpi radialis
Flexor carpi ulnaris
Brachioradialis
Extensor carpi radialis longus
Extensor digitorum
Extensor carpi radialis brevis
Extensor carpi ulnaris

Teres minor
Teres major

Transversus abdominis
Tensor fasciae latae
Gracilis
Sartorius
Peroneus longus
Tibialis anterior
Extensor hallucis longus

Palmar aponeurosis
Iliotibial band
Iliopsoas
Pectineus
Adductor longus
Adductor magnus
Vastus lateralis
Rectus femoris
Vastus medialis
Biceps femoris
Adductor magnus
Semimembranosus
Semitendinosus
Plantaris
Gastrocnemius

Gluteus medius
Gluteus maximus

Calcaneus tendon
Soleus
Peroneus longus
Peroneus brevis

Anterior

Posterior

FIGURE 3-1 Skeletal muscles of the human body: anterior and posterior views. (Reprinted with permission from Willis, M. C. [1986]. *Medical Terminology: The Language of Health Care.* Baltimore: Williams & Wilkins.)

muscular contribution are explored in this chapter. Since muscles are responsible for locomotion, limb movements, and posture and joint stability, a good understanding of the features and limitations of muscle action is necessary. While it is not the function of this chapter to teach you all of the muscles and their actions, it is necessary for you to have a good understanding of the location and action of the primary skeletal muscles. Figure 3-1 illustrates the surface skeletal muscles of the human body.

Characteristics of Muscle Tissue

Skeletal muscle is very resilient and can be stretched or shortened at fairly high speeds without major damage to the tissue. The performance of the muscle under varying loads and velocities is determined by the four properties of the skeletal muscle tissue: **irritability**, **contractility**, **extensibility**, and **elasticity**.

Irritability

Irritability is the ability to respond to stimulation. In a muscle, the stimulation is provided by a motor neuron releasing a chemical neurotransmitter. Skeletal muscle tissue is one of the most sensitive and responsive tissues in the body. Only nerve tissue is more sensitive than skeletal muscle. As an excitable tissue, skeletal muscle can be recruited quickly, with significant control over how many muscle fibers and which ones will be stimulated for a movement.

Contractility

Contractility is the ability of a muscle to shorten when it receives sufficient stimulation. Some muscles can shorten as much as 50 to 70% of their resting length. The average range is about 57% of resting length for all skeletal muscles. The distance through which a muscle shortens is usually limited by the physical confinement of the body. For example, the sartorius muscle can shorten more than half of its length if it is removed and stimulated in a laboratory, but in the body, the shortening distance is restrained by the hip joint and positioning of the trunk and thigh.

Extensibility

Extensibility is the muscle's ability to lengthen, or stretch beyond the resting length. The muscle itself cannot produce the elongation; another muscle or an external force is required. Taking a joint through a passive range of motion, that is, pushing another's limb past its resting length, is a good example of elongation in muscle tissue. The amount of extensibility in the muscle is determined by the connective tissue surrounding and within the muscle.

Elasticity

Elasticity is the ability of muscle fiber to return to its resting length once the stretch is removed. Elasticity in the muscle is determined by the connective tissue in the muscle rather than the fibrils themselves. The properties of elasticity and extensibility are protective mechanisms that maintain the integrity and basic length of the muscle. Elasticity is also a critical component in facilitating output in a shortening muscle action that is preceded by a stretch.

Using a ligament as a comparison makes it easy to see how elasticity benefits muscle tissue. The ligament, largely collagenous, has little elasticity, and if it is stretched beyond its resting length, it will not return to the original length but rather will remain extended. This can create laxity around the joint when the ligament is too long to exert much control over the joint motion. On the other hand, muscle tissue will always return to its original length. If the muscle is stretched too far, it will eventually tear.

 Gross Structure of the Muscle

PHYSICAL ORGANIZATION OF MUSCLE

Muscles and muscle groups are arranged so that they may contribute individually or collectively to produce a very small, fine movement or a very large, powerful movement.

Muscles rarely act individually but rather interact with other muscles in a multitude of roles. To understand muscle function, the structural organization of muscle from the macroscopic external anatomy all the way down to the microscopic level of muscular action must be examined. A good starting point is the gross anatomy and external arrangement of muscles and the microscopic view of the muscle fiber.

Groups of Muscles

Groups of muscles are contained within compartments that are defined by **fascia**, a sheet of fibrous tissue. The compartments divide the muscles into functional groups, and it is common for muscles in a compartment to be innervated by the same nerve. The thigh has three compartments: the anterior compartment, containing the quadriceps femoris; the posterior compartment, containing the hamstrings; and the medial compartment, containing the adductors. Compartments for the thigh and the leg are illustrated in Figure 3-2.

The compartments keep the muscles organized and contained in one region, but sometimes the compartment is not large enough to accommodate the muscle or muscle groups. In the anterior tibial region, the compartment is small, and problems arise if the muscles are overdeveloped for the amount of space defined by the compartment. This is known as anterior compartment syndrome, and it can be serious if the cramped compartment impinges on nerves or blood supply to the leg and foot.

Individual Muscle Organization

The anatomy of a skeletal muscle is presented in Figure 3-3. Each individual muscle usually has a thick central portion,

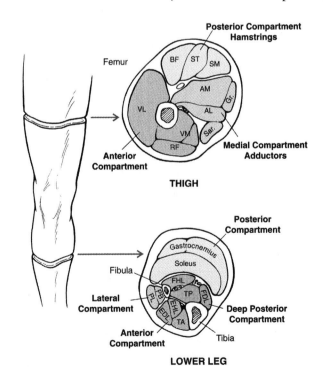

FIGURE 3-2 Muscles are grouped into compartments in each segment. Each compartment is maintained by fascial sheaths. The muscles in each compartment are functionally similar and define groups of muscles that we classify according to function, such as extensors and flexors.

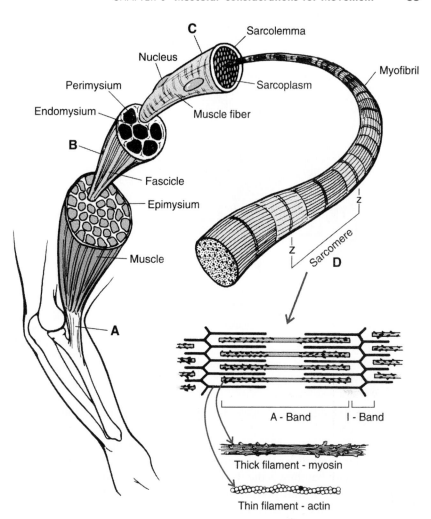

FIGURE 3-3 **A.** Each muscle connects to the bone via a tendon or aponeurosis. **B.** Within the muscle, the fibers are bundled into fascicles. **C.** Each fiber contains myofibril strands that run the length of the fiber. **D.** The actual contractile unit is the sarcomere. Many sarcomeres are connected in series down the length of each myofibril. Muscle shortening occurs in the sarcomere as the myofilaments in the sarcomere, actin and myosin, slide toward each other.

the **belly** of the muscle. Some muscles, like the biceps brachii, have very pronounced bellies, while other muscles, such as the wrist flexors and extensors, have bellies that are not as apparent.

Covering the outside of the muscle is another fibrous tissue, the **epimysium**. This structure plays a vital role in the transfer of muscular tension to the bone. Tension in the muscle is generated at various sites, and the epimysium transfers the various tensions to the tendon, providing a smooth application of the muscular force to the bone.

Each muscle may contain thousands of muscle fibers that are carefully organized into compartments within the muscle itself. Bundles of muscle fibers are called **fascicles**. Each fascicle may contain as many as 200 muscle fibers. A fascicle is covered with a dense connective sheath called the **perimysium** that protects the muscle fibers and provides pathways for the nerves and blood vessels. The connective tissue in the perimysium and the epimysium give muscle much of its ability to stretch and return to a normal resting length. The perimysium is also the focus of flexibility training because the connective tissue in the muscle can be stretched, allowing the muscle to elongate.

The fascicles run parallel to each other. Each fascicle contains the long, cylindrical muscle **fibers**, the cells of skeletal muscles, where the force is generated. Muscle

fibers can be as large as 50 μm wide and 10 cm long (8). Fibers also run parallel to each other and are covered with a membrane, the **endomysium**. The endomysium is a very fine sheath carrying the capillaries and nerves that nourish and innervate each muscle fiber. The vessels and the nerves usually enter in the middle of the muscle and are distributed throughout the muscle by a path through the endomysium. The endomysium also serves as an insulator for the neurological activity within the muscle.

Directly underneath the endomysium is the **sarcolemma**. This is a thin plasma membrane surface that branches into the muscle. The neurological innervation of the muscle travels through the sarcolemma and eventually reaches each individual contractile unit by means of a chemical neurotransmission.

At the microscopic level, a fiber can be further broken down into numerous **myofibrils**. These delicate rodlike strands run the total length of the muscle. There can be hundreds or thousands of myofibrils in each muscle fiber, and each fiber is filled with 80% myofibrils (8). The remainder of the fiber consists of the usual organelles, such as the mitochondria, the **sarcoplasm**, **sarcoplasmic reticulum** and the **t-tubules**, or **transverse tubules**. Myofibrils are 1 to 2 μm in diameter (about a 4-millionth of an inch wide) and run the length of the muscle fiber

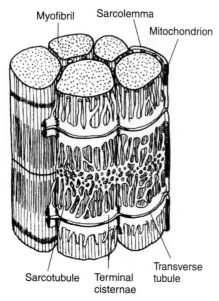

FIGURE 3-4 A portion of a skeletal muscle fiber illustrating the sarcoplasmic reticulum that surrounds the myofibril. (Adapted with permission from Pittman, M. I., Peterson, L. (1989). Biomechanics of Skeletal Muscle. In M. Nordin, V. H. Frankel (Eds.). *Basic Biomechanics of the Musculoskeletal System* (2nd ed.). Philadelphia: Lea & Febiger, 89–111.

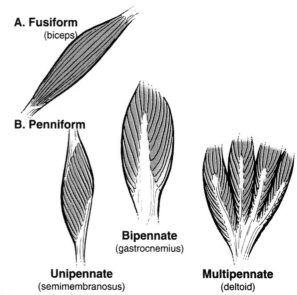

FIGURE 3-5 **A.** The fusiform muscles are spindle shaped, and the fibers run so that they pull in the same direction as the whole muscle. **B.** Penniform muscles have fibers that run diagonally to a central tendon through the muscle. The muscle fibers of a penniform muscle do not pull in the same direction as the whole muscle.

(8). Figure 3-4 illustrates muscle myofibrils and some of these organelles.

The myofibrils are cross-striated by light and dark filaments placed in an order that forms repeating patterns of bands. The dark banding is the thick protein **myosin**, and the light band is a thin polypeptide, **actin**. One unit of these bands is called a **sarcomere**. This structure is the actual contractile unit of the muscle that develops tension. Sarcomeres are in series along a myofibril. That is, sarcomeres form units along the length of the myofibril much like the links in a chain.

FIBER ORGANIZATION

The shape and arrangement of the fibers in the muscle will determine whether the muscle can generate large amounts of force and whether it can change its length significantly. In the case of the latter, the shortening ability of a muscle is reflected by both change in length and speed, depending on the situation. Two basic types of fiber arrangements are found in the muscle: **fusiform** and **penniform** (Fig. 3-5).

Fusiform Muscles

The fusiform fiber arrangement has parallel muscle fibers and fascicles that run the length of the muscle. The fibers in a fusiform muscle run parallel to the line of pull of the muscle so that the fiber force is in the same direction as the musculature (26). This spindle-shaped fiber arrangement is known for offering the potential for large amounts of shortening and high velocity movements in the body. This is basically because the fusiform muscles are typically longer than other types of muscles and the muscle fiber is

longer than the tendon. Fiber lengths of the fusiform muscle are shown in Figure 3-6.

A muscle having a greater ratio of muscle length to tendon length has the potential to shorten over a greater distance. Consequently, muscles attaching to the bone with a short tendon (for example, the rectus abdominus) can move through a greater shortening distance than muscles with longer tendons (for example, the gastrocnemius) (20). Great amounts of shortening also occur because skeletal muscle can shorten up to approximately 30 to 50% of its resting length. Examples of fusiform muscles are the sartorius, the biceps brachii, and the brachialis.

Penniform Muscles

In the second type of fiber arrangement, penniform, the fibers run diagonally with respect to a central tendon running the length of the muscle. The general shape of the penniform muscle is featherlike, as the fascicles are short and run at an angle to the length of the muscle. Because the fibers of the penniform muscle run at an angle relative to the line of pull of the muscle, the force generated by each fiber is in a different direction than the muscle force (26). The fibers are shorter than the muscle, and the change in the individual fiber length is not equal to the change in the muscle length (26). The fibers can run diagonally off one side of the tendon, termed **unipennate**, off both sides of the tendon, termed **bipennate**, or both, termed **multipennate**.

Since the muscle fibers are shorter and run diagonally into the tendon, the penniform fibers create slower movements through a smaller range of motion than a fusiform muscle. The trade-off is that a penniform muscle has a much greater physiological cross-section that can generally produce more strength than can a fusiform muscle.

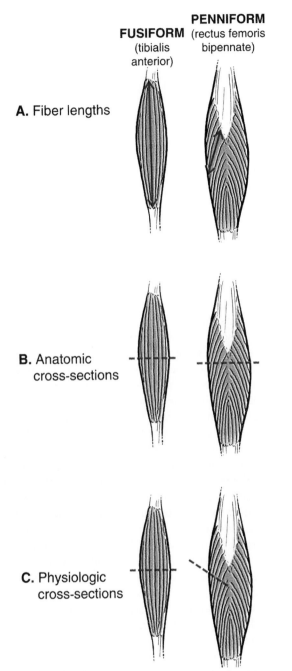

PENNIFORM
FUSIFORM (rectus femoris
(tibialis bipennate)
anterior)

A. Fiber lengths

B. Anatomic
cross-sections

C. Physiologic
cross-sections

FIGURE 3-6 A. Fusiform muscle fiber arrangements usually have longer fibers than penniform fiber arrangements. **B** and **C.** The anatomical cross-sections of the fusiform and penniform fiber arrangements may or may not be similar, but the physiological cross-section of the fusiform fiber arrangement is usually smaller. Thus, fusiform muscles are typically weaker but can move through greater distances than penniform muscles.

The physiological cross-section is the sum total of all of the cross-sections of fibers in the muscle in the plane perpendicular to the direction of the fibers. The anatomical cross-section is the cross-section perpendicular to the longitudinal axis of the muscle. Examine the anatomical and physiological cross-sections of the two types of muscles in Figure 3-6. In the fusiform muscle, the physiological and anatomical cross-sections are equal. In the penniform muscle, the physiological cross-section is greater than the

anatomical cross-section (20). Thus, a penniform muscle having the same anatomical cross-section as a fusiform muscle will be capable of generating greater force because it has a greater physiological cross-section (greater number of fibers). The penniform muscles are the high-force and power-producing muscles. Examples of unipennate muscles are flexor pollicis longus, tibialis posterior, semimembranosus, and extensor digitorum longus. Bipennate muscles include the gastrocnemius, soleus, vastus medialis, vastus lateralis, and rectus femoris. Examples of multipennate muscles are the deltoid and the gluteus maximus.

The mechanical actions of broad pennate muscles that have fibers attaching directly into bone over a large attachment site, such as the pectoralis major and trapezius, are difficult to describe using one movement for the whole muscle (61). For example, the lower trapezius attaches to the scapula at an angle opposite that of the upper trapezius; thus, these sections of the same muscle are functionally independent. When the shoulder girdle is elevated and abducted as the arm is moved up in front of the body, the lower portion of the trapezius may be inactive. This presents a complicated problem when studying the function of the muscle as a whole and requires multiple lines of action and effect (61).

FIBER TYPE

Each muscle contains a combination of fiber types that are categorized as **slow-twitch fibers** (Type I) or **fast-twitch fibers** (Type II). Fast-twitch fibers are further broken down into Type IIa and Type IIb. Fiber type is an important consideration in muscle metabolism and energy consumption, and muscle fiber type is thoroughly studied in exercise physiology. There are also mechanical differences in the response of slow- and fast-twitch muscle fibers warranting an examination of fiber type.

Slow-Twitch Fiber Types
Slow-twitch, or Type I, fibers are oxidative. The fibers are red because of the high content of myoglobin in the muscle. A stained cross-section of the slow-twitch fiber is presented in Figure 3-7. These fibers have slow contraction times and are well-suited for prolonged, low-intensity work. Endurance athletes usually have a high quantity of slow-twitch fibers.

Intermediate and Fast-Twitch Fiber Types
Fast-twitch, or Type II, fibers are further broken down into Type IIa, oxidative–glycolytic, and Type IIb, glycolytic. The Type IIa fiber is a red muscle fiber known as the intermediate fast-twitch fiber because it can sustain activity for long periods or contract with a burst of force and then fatigue (Fig. 3-7). The white Type IIb fiber provides us with rapid force production and then fatigues quickly.

Most muscles, if not all, contain both fiber types. An example is the vastus lateralis, typically half fast-twitch and half slow-twitch fibers (34). The fiber type will influence how the muscle is trained and developed and what techniques will

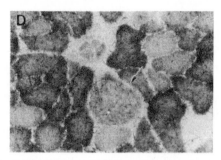

FIGURE 3-7 A histological stained cross-section of the three muscle types. The arrow points to a Type IIb fast-twitch glycolytic fiber. A slow-twitch oxidative fiber contacts the Type IIb fiber on the underside and an intermediate fast-twitch fiber (oxidative glycolytic) is making contact directly above and to the right of the Type IIb fiber. (Lieber, R. L. (1992). *Skeletal Muscle Structure and Function*. Baltimore: Williams & Wilkins.)

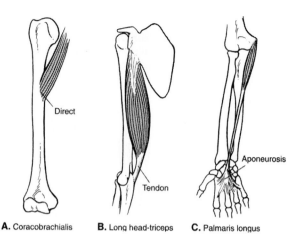

A. Coracobrachialis   **B.** Long head-triceps   **C.** Palmaris longus

FIGURE 3-8 A muscle can attach directly into the bone **(A)** or indirectly via a tendon **(B)** or aponeurosis **(C)**.

best suit individuals with specific fiber types. For example, sprinters and jumpers usually have great concentrations of fast-twitch fibers. These fiber types are also found in high concentrations in muscles on which these athletes rely, such as the gastrocnemius. On the other hand, distance runners usually have greater concentrations of slow-twitch fibers.

MUSCLE ATTACHMENT

Tendon vs Aponeurosis

A muscle attaches to bone in one of three ways: (*a*) directly into the bone, (*b*) via a **tendon**, or (*c*) via an **aponeurosis**. These three types of attachments are presented in Figure 3-8. Muscle can attach directly to the periosteum of the bone through fusion between the epimysium and the surface of the bone, such as the attachment of the trapezius (61). Muscle can attach via a tendon that is fused with the muscle fascia, such as in the hamstrings, biceps brachii, and flexor carpi radialis. Last, muscle can attach to a bone via a sheath of fibrous tissue known as an aponeurosis seen in the abdominals and the trunk attachment of the latissimus dorsi.

Characteristics of the Tendon

The most common form of attachment, the tendon, transmits the force of the associated muscle to bone. Tendon is an inelastic bundle of collagen fibers arranged parallel to the direction of the force application of the muscle. Even though the fibers are inelastic, the tendon can respond in an elastic fashion through recoiling and the elasticity of connective tissue. Tendons can withstand high tensile forces produced by the muscles, and they exhibit viscoelastic behavior in response to loading. The Achilles tendon has been reported to resist tensile loads to a degree equal to or greater than that of steel of similar dimensions.

The stress–strain response of a tendon is viscoelastic. That is, the tendon will show a nonlinear response and exhibit hysteresis. Tendons are relatively stiff and much stronger than other structures. Tendons will respond very stiffly when exposed to a high rate of loading. This stiff behavior of tendon is thought to be related to the relatively high collagen content. However, tendon is also very

resilient, showing relatively little hysteresis or energy loss. These characteristics are necessary to the function of tendons. Tendons must be stiff and strong enough to transmit force to bone without deforming much. Also, because of the low hysteresis of tendons, they are capable of storing and releasing elastic strain energy. The differences in the strength and performance characteristics of the tendon versus muscle or bone is presented in Figure 3-9.

Tendon and muscle join at the **myotendinous junction**, where the actual myofibrils of the muscle fiber join the collagen fibers of the tendon to produce a multilayered interface (66). The tendon connection to the bone consists of fibrocartilage that joins to mineralized fibrocartilage and then to the lamellar bone. This interface blends with the periosteum and the subchondral bone.

Tendons and muscles work together to absorb or generate tension in the system. Tendons are arranged in series, or in line with the muscles; consequently, the tendon bears the same tension as the muscle (51). The mechanical interaction between the muscle and tendon depends on the amount of force that is being applied or generated, the speed of the muscle action, and the slack in the tendon.

If tension is generated in the muscle fibers while the tendon is slack, it will begin to recoil, or spring back to its initial length. As the slack in the tendon is taken up by the recoiling action, the time taken to stretch the tendon causes a delay in the achievement of the required level of tension in the muscle fibers (51).

Recoiling of the tendon also reduces the speed at which a muscle may shorten, which in turn increases the load a muscle can support (51). If the tendon is stiff and has no recoil, the tension will be transmitted directly to the muscle fibers, creating higher velocities and decreasing the load the muscle can support. The stiff response in a tendon allows for the development of rapid tensions in the muscle, and results in brisk, accurate movements.

The tendon and the muscle are very susceptible to injury if the muscle is contracting as it is being stretched. An example is the follow-through phase of throwing. Here, the posterior rotator cuff stretches as it contracts to slow the

MUSCLE

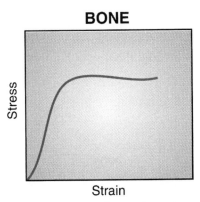

TENDON

BONE

FIGURE 3-9 The stress–strain curves for muscle, tendon, and bone tissue. Top. Muscle is viscoelastic and thus deforms under low load and then responds stiffly. **Middle.** Tendon is capable of handling high loads. The end of the elastic limits of the tendon is also the ultimate strength level (no plastic phase). **Bottom.** Bone is a brittle material that responds stiffly and then undergoes minimal deformation before failure.

movement. Another example is the lengthening and contraction of the quadriceps femoris muscle group during the support phase of running as the center of mass is lowered via knee flexion. The tendon picks up the initial stretch of the relaxed muscle, and if the muscle contracts as it is stretched, the tension rises steeply in both muscle and tendon (51).

When tension is generated in a tendon at a slow rate, injury is more likely to occur at the tendon–bone junction

than other regions. At a faster rate of tension development, the actual tendon is the more common site of failure (59). For the total muscle–tendon unit, the likely site of injury is the belly of the muscle or the myotendinous junction.

Many tendons travel over bony protuberances that reduce some of the tension on the tendon by changing the angle of pull of the muscle and reducing the tension generated in the muscle. Examples of this can be found with the quadriceps femoris muscles and the patella and with the tendons of the hamstrings and the gastrocnemius as they travel over condyles on the femur.

The tension in the tendons also produces the actual ridges and protuberances on bone. The apophyses found on a bone are developed by tension forces applied to the bone through the tendon (see Chapter 2). This is of interest to physical anthropologists because they can study skeletal remains and make sound predictions about lifestyle and occupations of a civilization by evaluating prominent ridges, size of the trochanters and tuberosities, and basic size of the specimen.

Origin vs Insertion

A muscle typically attaches to a bone at both ends. The attachment closest to the middle of the body, or more proximal, is termed the **origin**. The attachment farther from the midline, or more distal, is called the **insertion**. Traditional anatomy classes usually incorporate a study of the origins and insertions of the muscles. It is a common mistake to view the origin as the bony attachment that does not move when the muscle contracts. It is important to remember that muscles pull equally on both ends, so that both attachment sites receive equal forces. The reason that both bones do not move when a muscle contracts is the stabilizing force of adjacent muscles or the difference in the mass of the two segments or bones to which the muscle is attached.

There are numerous examples of a muscle shifting between moving one end of its attachment and the other, depending upon the activity. One example is the psoas muscle, which crosses the hip joint. This muscle flexes the thigh, as in leg raises, or raises the trunk, as in a curl-up or sit-up (Fig. 3-10). Another example is the gluteus medius, which moves the pelvis when the foot is on the ground and the leg when the foot is off the ground. The effect of tension in a muscle should be evaluated at all attachment sites even if no movement is resulting from the force. Evaluating all attachment sites allows assessment of the magnitude of the required stabilizing forces and the actual forces applied at the bony insertion.

 Functional Characteristics of Muscle

FUNCTIONS OF MUSCLE

Skeletal muscle performs a variety of different functions, all of which are important to efficient performance of the human body. The three functions relating specifically to human movement are (*a*) contributing to the production

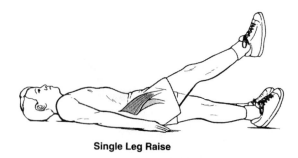

Single Leg Raise

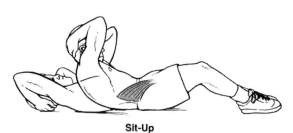

Sit-Up

FIGURE 3-10 The origin of the psoas muscle is on the bodies of the last thoracic and all of the lumbar vertebrae, and the insertion is on the lesser trochanter of the femur. It is incorrect to assume that the origin remains stable in a movement. Here the psoas pulls on both the vertebrae and the femur. With the trunk stabilized, the femur moves (leg raise), and with the legs stabilized, the trunk moves (sit-up).

of skeletal movement; (*b*) assisting in joint stability; and (*c*) maintaining posture and body positioning.

Produce Movement
Skeletal movement is created as muscle actions generate tensions that are transferred to the bone. The resulting movements are necessary for locomotion or other segmental manipulations.

Maintain Postures and Positions
Muscle actions of a lesser magnitude are used to maintain postures. This muscle activity is continuous and results in small adjustments as the head is maintained in position and the body weight is balanced over the feet.

Stabilize Joints
Muscle actions also contribute significantly to stability of the joints. Muscle tensions are generated and applied across the joints via the tendons, providing stability where they cross the joint. In most joints, especially the shoulder and the knee, the muscles spanning the joint via the tendons are among the primary stabilizers.

Other Functions
The skeletal muscles also provide four other functions that are not directly related to human movement. First, muscles support and protect the visceral organs and protect the internal tissues from injury. Second, tension in the muscle tissue can alter and control pressures within the cavities. Third, skeletal muscle contributes to the maintenance of body temperature by producing heat. Fourth, the muscles

control the entrances and exits to the body through voluntary control over swallowing, defecation, and urination.

ROLE OF MUSCLE

In the performance of a motor skill, only a very small portion of the potential movement capability of the musculoskeletal system is used. There may be 20 to 30 degrees of freedom available to raise your arm above your head and comb your hair (37). However, many of the available movements may be inefficient in terms of the desired movement, combing the hair. To eliminate the undesirable movements and create the skill or desired movement, muscles or groups of muscles will have to play a variety of roles. To perform a motor skill at a given time, only a small percentage of the potential movement capability of the motor system will be used.

Prime Mover vs Assistant Mover
The muscle or muscles primarily responsible for producing a given movement are called **prime movers**, and if more force is required, other muscles will contribute as **assistant movers**. For example, the latissimus dorsi and the pectoralis major are prime movers as they shorten to produce extension of the arm. If more force is required in the movement of extension, the teres major and triceps brachii may assist.

Agonists and Antagonists
The various roles of selected muscles in a simple arm abduction exercise are presented in Figure 3-11. Muscles creating the same joint movement are termed **agonists**. Conversely, muscles opposing or producing the opposite joint movement are called **antagonists**. It is the antagonists that must relax to allow a movement to occur or contract concurrently with the agonists to control or slow a joint movement. Thus, when the thigh swings forward and upward,

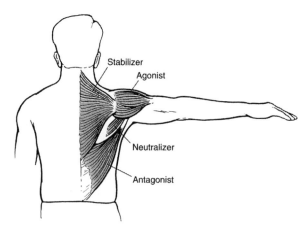

FIGURE 3-11 Muscles perform a variety of roles in movement. In arm abduction, the deltoid is the agonist, since it is responsible for the abduction movement. The latissimus dorsi is the antagonistic muscle, since it resists abduction. There are also muscles stabilizing in the region so the movement can occur. Here, the trapezius is shown stabilizing and holding the scapula in place. Last, there may be some neutralizing action: the teres minor may neutralize via external rotation any internal rotation produced by the latissimus dorsi.

the agonists producing the movement are the hip flexors, that is, the iliopsoas, rectus femoris, pectineus, sartorius, and gracilis muscles. The antagonists, or the muscles opposing the motion of hip flexion, are the hip extensors, hamstrings, and gluteus maximus. It is the antagonists combined with the effect of gravity that slow down the movement of hip flexion and terminate the joint action.

When a muscle is playing the role of an antagonist, it is more susceptible to injury at the site of muscle attachment or in the muscle fiber itself. This is because the muscle is contracting to slow the limb while being stretched.

Stabilizers and Neutralizers

Muscles are also used as **stabilizers**, acting in one segment so that a specific movement in an adjacent joint can occur. Stabilization is important, for example, in the shoulder girdle, which must be supported so that arm movements can occur smoothly and efficiently. It is also important in the pelvic girdle and hip region during gait. When one foot is on the ground in walking or running, the gluteus medius contracts to maintain the stability of the pelvis so it does not drop to one side.

The last role muscles are required to play is that of **synergist**, or **neutralizer**, in which a muscle will contract to eliminate an undesired joint action of another muscle. For example, the gluteus maximus is contracted at the hip joint to produce thigh extension, but the gluteus maximus will also attempt to rotate the thigh externally. If external rotation is an undesired action, the gluteus minimus and the tensor fascia latae will contract to produce a neutralizing internal rotation action that cancels out the external rotation action of the gluteus maximus, leaving the desired extension movement.

NET MUSCLE ACTIONS

Isometric Muscle Action

Muscle tension is generated against resistance to maintain position, raise a segment or object, or lower or control a segment. If the muscle is active and develops tension with no visible or external change in joint position, the muscle action is termed **isometric** (34). Examples of isometric muscle actions are illustrated in Figure 3-12. To bend over into 30° of trunk flexion and hold that position, the muscle action used to hold the position would be termed isometric since there is no movement. The muscles contracting isometrically to hold the trunk in a position of flexion are the back muscles since they are resisting the force of gravity that tends to flex the trunk further.

To take the opposite perspective, consider the movement in which the trunk is curled up to 30° and that position held. To hold this position of trunk flexion, an isometric muscle action using the trunk flexors is produced. This muscle action resists the action of gravity that is forcing the trunk to extend.

Concentric Muscle Action

If a muscle visibly shortens while generating tension actively, the muscle action is termed **concentric** (34). In concentric joint action, the net muscle forces producing movement are in the same direction as the change in joint angle, meaning that the agonists are the controlling muscles (Fig. 3-12). Also, the limb movement produced in a concentric muscle action is termed positive, since the joint actions are usually against gravity or are the initiating source of movement of a mass.

Many joint movements are created by a concentric muscle action. For example, flexion of the arm or forearm from

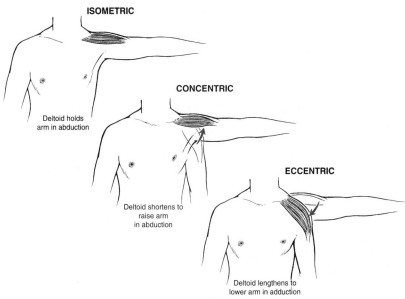

FIGURE 3-12 A muscle action is isometric when the tension creates no change in joint position. A concentric muscle action occurs when the tension shortens the muscle. An eccentric muscle action is generated by an external force when the muscle lengthens.

the standing position will be produced by a concentric muscle action from the respective agonists or flexor muscles. Additionally, to initiate a movement of the arm across the body in a horizontal adduction movement, the horizontal adductors will initiate the movement via a concentric muscle action. Concentric muscle actions are used to generate forces against external resistances, such as raising a weight, pushing off the ground or throwing an implement.

Eccentric Muscle Action

When a muscle is subjected to an external torque that is greater than the torque generated by the muscle, the muscle lengthens, and the action is known as **eccentric** (34). The source of the external force developing the external torque that produces an eccentric muscle action is usually gravity or the muscle action of an antagonistic muscle group (8).

In eccentric joint action, the net muscular forces producing the rotation are in the opposite direction of the change in joint angle, meaning that the antagonists are the controlling muscles (Fig. 3-12). Also, the limb movement produced in eccentric muscle action is termed negative, since the joint actions are usually moving down with gravity or are controlling rather than initiating the movement of a mass.

Most movements downward, unless they are very fast, are controlled by an eccentric action of the antagonistic muscle groups. To reverse the example shown in Figure 3-12, during extension of the arm or forearm from flexed position, the muscle action is eccentrically produced by the flexors or antagonistic muscle group. Likewise, lowering into a squat position, which involves hip and knee flexion, requires an eccentric movement controlled by the hip and knee extensors. Conversely, the reverse thigh and shank extension movements up against gravity are produced concentrically by the extensors.

From these examples, the potential sites of muscular imbalances in the body can be identified, since the extensors in the trunk and the lower extremity are used to both lower and raise the segments. In the upper extremity, the flexors both raise the segments concentrically and lower the segments eccentrically, thereby obtaining more use.

Eccentric actions are also used to slow a movement. When the thigh flexes rapidly, as in a kicking action, the antagonists (extensors) will eccentrically control and slow the joint action near the end of the range of motion.

Comparison of Isometric, Concentric, and Eccentric

Isometric, concentric, and eccentric muscle actions are not used in isolation but rather in combination. Typically, isometric actions are used to stabilize a body part, and eccentric and concentric muscle actions are used sequentially to maximize energy storage and muscle performance. This natural sequence of muscle function during which an eccentric action precedes a concentric action is known as the stretch–shortening cycle.

These three muscle actions are very different in terms of their energy cost and force output. The eccentric muscle action can develop the same force output as the other

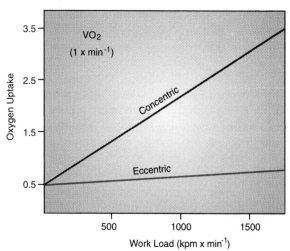

FIGURE 3-13 It has been illustrated that eccentric muscle action can produce high work loads at lower oxygen uptake levels than the same loads produced with concentric muscle action. (Adapted with permission from Asmussen, E. (1952). Positive and negative muscular work. *Acta Physiologica Scandinavica*, 28:364–382.)

two types of muscle actions with fewer muscle fibers activated. Consequently, eccentric action is more efficient and can produce the same force output with less oxygen consumption than the others (3) (Fig. 3-13).

In addition, the eccentric muscle action is capable of greater force output than isometric or concentric actions (Fig. 3-14). This occurs at the level of the sarcomere, where the force increases beyond the maximum isometric force if the myofibril is stretched and stimulated (14,15).

Concentric muscle actions generate the lowest force output of the three types. Force is related to the number of cross-bridges formed in the myofibril. In isometric muscle action, the number of bridges attached remains constant. As the muscle shortens, the number of attached bridges is reduced with increased velocity (15). This reduces the level of force output generated by tension in

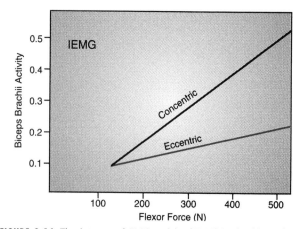

FIGURE 3-14 The integrated EMG activity (IEMG) in the biceps brachii muscle was higher as the same forces were generated using concentric muscle action as compared to eccentric muscle action (Adapted with permission from Komi, P. V. (1986). The stretch–shortening cycle and human power output. In N. L. Jones et al. (Eds.). *Human Muscle Power*. Champaign, IL: Human Kinetics, 27–40.)

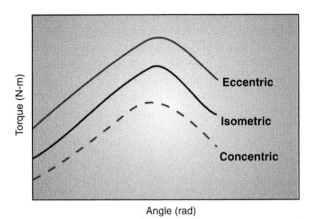

FIGURE 3-15 Eccentric muscle action can generate the greatest amount of torque through a given range of motion. Isometric muscle action can generate the next highest level of torque, and concentric muscle action generates the least torque (Adapted with permission from Enoka, R. M. (1988). *Neuromuscular Basis of Kinesiology.* Champaign, IL: Human Kinetics.)

the muscle fibers. A hypothetical torque output curve for the three muscle actions is presented in Figure 3-15.

An additional factor contributing to noticeable force output differences between eccentric and concentric muscle actions is present when the actions are producing vertical movements. In this case, the force output in both concentric and eccentric actions is influenced by torques created by gravity. The gravitational force creates torque that contributes to the force output in an eccentric action as the muscles generate torque that controls the lowering of the limb or body. The total force output in a lowering action is the result of both muscular torques and gravitational torques.

The force of gravity inhibits the movement of a limb upward, and before any movement can occur, the concentric muscle action must develop a force output that is greater than the force of gravity acting on the limb or body (weight). The total force output in a raising action is predominantly muscle force. This is another reason concentric muscle action is more demanding than the eccentric or isometric action.

This information is useful when one is considering exercise programs for unconditioned individuals or rehabilitation programs. Even the weakest individual may be able to perform a controlled lowering of a body part or a small weight but may not be able to hold or raise the weight. A program that starts with eccentric exercises and then leads into isometric followed by concentric exercises may prove to be beneficial in the progression of strength or in rehabilitation of a body part. Thus, a person unable to do a push-up should start at the extended position and lower into the push-up, then receiving assistance on the up phase until enough strength is developed for the concentric portion of the skill. Factors to consider in the use of eccentric exercises are the control of the speed at which the limb or weight is lowered and control over the magnitude of the load imposed eccentrically, since muscle injury and soreness can occur more readily with eccentric muscle action in high-load and high-speed conditions.

STRETCH–SHORTENING CYCLE

Elastic Component Contributions

If concentric, or shortening, muscle action is preceded by eccentric, or prestretch, muscle action, the resulting concentric action is capable of generating greater force. This is because a stretch on the muscle increases its tension through storage of potential elastic energy in the series elastic component of the muscle (35) (Fig. 3-16). When a muscle is stretched, there is a small change in the muscle and tendon length (36) and maximum accumulation of stored energy. Thus, when a concentric muscle action follows, an enhanced recoil effect adds to the force output through the muscle tendon complex (27).

A concentric muscle action beginning at the end of a prestretch will also be enhanced by the stored elastic energy in the connective tissue around the muscle fibers. This contributes to a high-force output at the initial portion of the concentric muscle action as these tissues return to their normal length.

If the shortening contraction of the muscle occurs within a reasonable time after the stretch (up to 0.9 second), the stored energy is recovered and used. If the stretch is held too long before the shortening occurs, the stored elastic energy is lost through conversion to heat (34).

Neural Contributions

The stretch preceding the concentric muscle action also initiates a stimulation of the muscle group through reflex potentiation. This activation accounts for only approximately 30% of the increase in the concentric muscle action

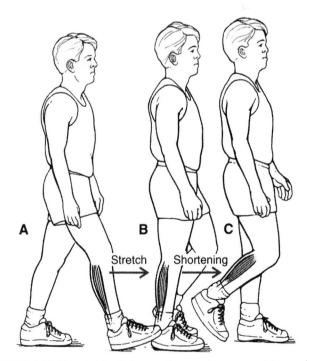

FIGURE 3-16 If a stretch of the muscle precedes a concentric muscle action, the resulting force output is greater. The increased force output is due to contributions from stored elastic energy in the muscle, tendon and connective tissue, and through some neural facilitation.

(34). The remaining increase is attributed to stored energy. The actual process of proprioceptive activation through the reflex loop is presented in the next chapter.

Use of the Prestretch

A short-range or low-amplitude prestretch occurring over a short time is the best technique to improve significantly the output of concentric muscle action through return of elastic energy and increased activation of the muscle (4,34). To get the greatest return of energy absorbed in the negative or eccentric action, go into the stretch quickly but not too far. Also, do not pause at the end of the stretch but move immediately into the concentric muscle action. In jumping, for example, a quick counterjump from the

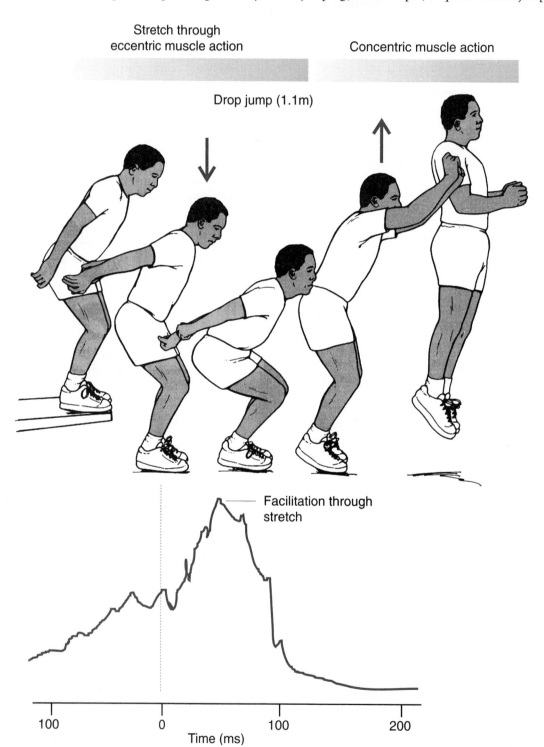

FIGURE 3-17 Neural facilitation in the gastrocnemius. In trained jumpers, the prestretch is used to facilitate the neural activity of the lower extremity muscles. Neural facilitation coupled with the recoil effect of the elastic components adds to the jump if it is performed with the correct timing and amplitude. (Adapted with permission from Sale, D. G. (1986). Neural adaptation in strength and power training. In N. L. Jones et al. (Eds.). *Human Muscle Power*. Champaign, Ill: Human Kinetics, 289–308.)

anatomical position, featuring a drop–stop–pop action, lowering only through 8 to 12 inches, is much more effective than a jump from a squat position or a jump from a height that forces the limbs into more flexion (4). The influence of this type of jumping technique on the gastrocnemius is presented in Figure 3-17.

The stretch–shortening cycle is also evident in gait when the body is subjected to impact forces and lowered by gravity (35). The muscles lengthen eccentrically at contact, at which point the velocity of the stretch is high and large muscle forces are present at the end of the eccentric muscle action. The extensors and the plantarflexors eccentrically lengthen and absorb energy returned in the propulsive stage, when the foot and lower limb push off the ground.

Fiber Type and the Prestretch
There is a difference in the way slow- and fast-twitch fibers handle a prestretch. Muscles with predominantly fast-twitch fibers benefit from a very high velocity prestretch over a small distance because they can store more elastic energy (34). The fast-twitch fibers can handle a fast stretch because myosin cross-bridging occurs quickly, whereas in slow-twitch fibers, the cross-bridging is slower (18).

In the slow-twitch fiber, the small-amplitude prestretch is not advantageous, since the energy cannot be stored fast enough and the cross-bridging is slower (18,34). Therefore, slow-twitch fibers will benefit from a prestretch that is slower and advances through a greater range of motion. Some athletes with predominantly slow-twitch fibers should be encouraged to use longer prestretches of the muscle to gain the benefits of the stretch. For most athletes, however, the quick prestretch through a small range of motion is the preferred method.

Plyometrics
This principle should be incorporated into both drills and conditioning for a sport or physical activity. The use of a quick prestretch is part of a conditioning protocol known as **plyometrics**. In this protocol, the muscle is put on a rapid stretch and a concentric muscle action is initiated at the end of the stretch. Single-leg bounding, depth jumps,

and stair hopping are all plyometric activities for the lower extremity. Surgical tubing or elastic bands are also used to produce a rapid stretch on muscles in the upper extremity. Plyometrics is covered in greater detail in Chapter 4.

ONE- AND TWO-JOINTED MUSCLES
As stated earlier, one cannot determine the function or contribution of a muscle to a joint movement by just locating the attachment sites. A muscle action can move a segment at one end of its attachment or two segments at both ends of its attachment. In fact, a muscle can accelerate and create movement at all joints, whether the muscle spans the joint or not. For example, the soleus is a plantarflexor of the ankle, but it can also force the knee into extension even though it does not cross the knee joint (65). This can occur in the standing posture. The soleus contracts and creates plantarflexion at the ankle. Since the foot is on the ground, the plantarflexion movement necessitates extension of the knee joint. In this manner, the soleus accelerates the knee joint twice as much as it accelerates the ankle, even though the soleus does not even span the knee.

Most muscles cross only one joint, so the dominating action of the one-joint muscle is at the joint it crosses. The two-joint muscle is a special case in which the muscle crosses two joints, creating a multitude of movements that often occur in opposite sequences to each other. For example, the rectus femoris is a two-joint muscle creating both hip flexion and knee extension. Take the example of jumping. Hip extension and knee extension propel the body upward. Does the rectus femoris, a hip flexor and knee extensor, contribute to the extension of the knee, does it resist the movement of hip extension, or does it do both?

The action of a two-joint, or biarticulate, muscle depends on the position of the body and the muscle's interaction with external objects such as the ground (65). In the case of the rectus femoris, the muscle will contribute primarily to the extension of the knee because of the hip joint position. This position results in the force of the rectus femoris acting close to the hip, thereby limiting the action of the muscle and its effectiveness in producing hip flexion (Fig. 3-18).

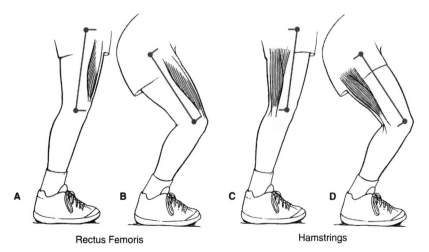

FIGURE 3-18 The rectus femoris moment arms at the hip and knee while standing **(A)** and in a squat **(B)** demonstrate why this muscle is more effective as an extender of the knee than as a flexor at the hip. Likewise, the hamstring moment arm while standing **(C)** and in a squat **(D)** demonstrates why the hamstrings are more effective as hip extensors than as knee flexors.

Rectus Femoris   Hamstrings

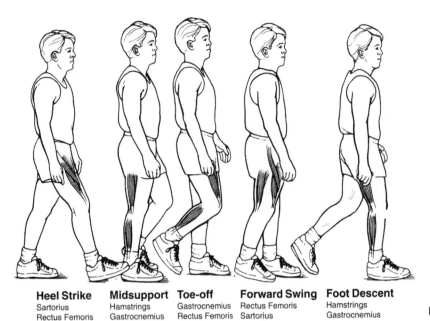

Heel Strike	**Midsupport**	**Toe-off**	**Forward Swing**	**Foot Descent**
Sartorius	Hamstrings	Gastrocnemius	Rectus Femoris	Hamstrings
Rectus Femoris	Gastrocnemius	Rectus Femoris	Sartorius	Gastrocnemius
			Hamstrings	

FIGURE 3-19 Two-joint muscles work synergistically to optimize performance, shown here for walking.

The perpendicular distance from the action line of the force of the muscle over to the hip joint is termed the moment arm, and the product of the force and the moment arm is the muscle torque. If the moment arm increases, torque at the joint increases even if the applied muscle force is the same. Thus, in the case of a two-joint muscle, the muscle will primarily act on the joint where it has the largest moment arm or where it is farther from the joint. The hamstring group will primarily create hip extension rather than knee flexion because of the greater moment arm at the hip (Fig. 3-18). The gastrocnemius will produce plantarflexion at the ankle rather than flexion at the knee joint because the moment arm is greater at the ankle.

For example, in vertical jumping, maximum height is achieved by extending the proximal joints first and then moving distally to where extension (plantarflexion) occurs in the ankle joint. By the time the ankle joint is involved in the sequence, very high joint moments and extension velocities are required (62). The role of the two-joint muscle becomes very important. The biarticular gastrocnemius muscle crosses both the knee and ankle joints. Its contribution to jumping is influenced by the knee joint. In jumping, the knee joint extends and effectively optimizes the length of the gastrocnemius (9). This keeps the contraction velocity in the gastrocnemius muscle low even when the ankle is plantarflexing very quickly. With the velocity lowered, the gastrocnemius is able to produce greater force in the jumping action.

The most important contribution of the two-joint muscle in the lower extremity is the reduction of the work required from the single-joint muscles. Two joint muscles initiate a mechanical coupling of the joints that allows for a rapid release of stored elastic energy in the system (65).

Two-joint muscles save energy by allowing positive work at one joint and negative work at the adjacent joint.

Thus, while the muscles acting at the ankle are producing a concentric action and positive work, the knee muscles can be eccentrically storing elastic energy through negative work (65).

The two-joint muscle actions for walking are presented in Figure 3-19. Two-joint muscles that work together in walking are the sartorius and rectus femoris at heel strike; the hamstrings and gastrocnemius at midsupport; the gastrocnemius and rectus femoris at toe-off; the rectus femoris, sartorius, and hamstrings at forward swing; and the hamstrings and gastrocnemius at foot descent (64). At heel strike, the sartorius, a hip flexor and a knee flexor, works with the rectus femoris, a hip flexor and knee extensor. As the heel strikes the surface, the rectus femoris performs negative work, absorbing energy at the knee as it moves into flexion. The sartorius, on the other hand, performs positive work as the knee and the hip both flex with gravity (64).

 Force Generation

MOTOR UNIT

Skeletal muscle is organized into functional groups called motor units. A **motor unit** consists of a group of muscle fibers that are innervated by the same motor neuron. Motor units are discussed in more detail in Chapter 5, but it is important to discuss some aspects in this chapter. Motor units can consist of only a few muscle fibers (for example, the optic muscles) or may have up to 2000 muscle fibers (for example, the gastrocnemius). The signal to contract that is transmitted from the motor neuron to the muscle is called an **action potential**. When a motor neuron is stimulated enough to cause a contraction, all muscle fibers innervated by that motor neuron contract.

MUSCLE CONTRACTION

The action potential from a motor neuron reaches a muscle fiber at a **neuromuscular junction** or **motor end plate** that lies near the center of the fiber. At this point there is a synapse, or space, between the motor neuron and the fiber membrane. When the action potential reaches the synapse, a series of chemical reactions take place and acetylcholine (ACH) is released. ACH diffuses across the synapse and causes an increase in permeability of the membrane of the fiber. The ACH rapidly breaks down to prevent continuous stimulation of the muscle fiber. The velocity at which the action potential is propagated along the membrane is the **conduction velocity**.

The muscle membrane potential is -70 mV. At the threshold level of the membrane potential, a change in potential of the fiber membrane or sarcolemma occurs. The action potential is characterized by a **depolarization** from the **resting potential** of the membrane so that the potential becomes positive and is said to overshoot. This is followed by a **repolarization**, or a return to the polarized state. Actually, there is a hyperpolarized state (**hyperpolarization**) before returning to the resting potential.

The changes in the membrane potential are brought about by alterations in the sodium (Na^+) and potassium (K^+) conductances. Both Na^+ and K^+ are positive, and their movements across the membrane do not alter the membrane potential. However, the movement of Na^+ into the muscle cell occurs before the movement of K^+ out of the muscle cell. In addition, Na^+ conductance has a much shorter term than K^+ conductance. As a result, the membrane depolarizes and repolarizes. The membrane potential reflects the imbalance in Na^+ and K^+ conductances. The hyperpolarization is the result of the Na^+ conductance returning to a resting level before the K^+ conductance. Gradually, Na^+ is returned to the

extra-cellular fluid and K^+ to inside the cell and the membrane potential returns to its steady state.

When the action potential reaches the muscle fibers, calcium ions (Ca^{2+}) are released into the area surrounding the myofibrils. These Ca^{2+} ions promote cross-bridge formation that results in an interaction between the actin and myosin filaments (see Sliding Filament Theory, discussed next). When the stimulation stops, ions are actively removed from the area surrounding the myofibrils, releasing the cross-bridges. This process is **excitation–contraction coupling**.

Muscle force production is achieved in two ways. First, muscle force can be increased by recruiting increasingly larger motor units. Initially, during a muscle contraction, smaller motor units are activated. As muscle force increases, more and larger motor units are engaged. This is the size principle (22). Second, a motor unit may be activated at any of several frequencies. A single action potential that activates a fiber will cause the force to rise and fall. This is referred to as a **twitch**. If a second stimulus occurs before the initial twitch has subsided, another twitch builds upon the first. With subsequent high frequency of stimulations, the force continues to build and forms a state called unfused **tetanus**. Finally, the force builds to a level in which there is no increase in muscle force. At this point, the force level has reached **tetanus**. This scenario is illustrated in Figure 3-20. In a muscle contraction, both size recruitment and frequency of stimulation are used simultaneously to increase muscle force.

SLIDING FILAMENT THEORY

How a muscle generates tension has been an area of much research. An explanation of the shortening of the sarcomere has been presented via the **sliding filament theory** presented by A. F. Huxley (28). This theory is the most widely accepted explanation of muscular contraction but certainly is not the only one. In the past, muscle contraction was thought, for example, to be similar to (*a*) the principle of blood clotting, (*b*) the behavior of India rubber, (*c*) a chain of circular elastic rings, and (*d*) a sliding movement caused by opposite electric charges in the different filaments (46).

For Huxley's sliding filament theory, when calcium is released into the muscle through neurochemical stimulation, the contracting process begins. The sarcomere contracts as the myosin filament walks along the actin filament, forming cross-bridges between the head of the myosin and a prepared site on the actin filament. In the contracted state, the actin and myosin filaments overlap along most of their lengths (Fig. 3-21).

The simultaneous sliding of many thousands of sarcomeres in series changes the length and force of the muscle (8). The amount of force that can be developed in the muscle is proportional to the number of cross-bridges formed. The shortening of many sarcomeres, myofibrils, and fibers develops tension running through the muscle and to the bone at both ends to create a movement.

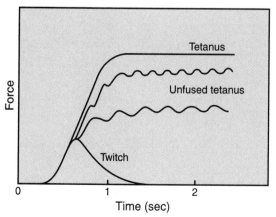

FIGURE 3-20 When a single stimulus is given, a twitch occurs. When a series of stimuli is given, muscle force rises to an uneven plateau or unfused tetanus. As the frequency of stimuli increases, the muscle force ultimately reaches a limit, or tetanus. (Adapted from McMahon, T. A. [1984]. *Muscles, Reflexes, and Locomotion*. Princeton, New Jersey: Princeton University Press.)

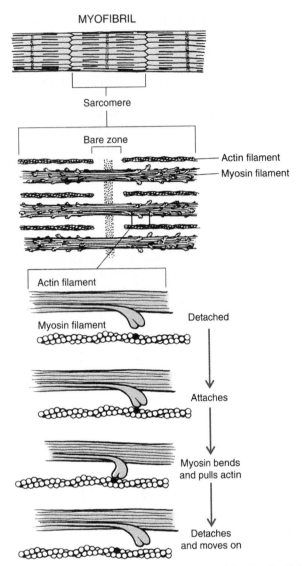

FIGURE 3-21 Shortening of the muscle has been explained by the sliding filament theory. Shortening takes place in the sarcomere as the myosin heads bind to sites on the actin filament to form a cross-bridge. The myosin head attaches and turns, moving the actin filament toward the center. It then detaches and moves on to the next actin site.

MECHANICAL MODEL OF MUSCLE

A series of experiments by A. V. Hill gave rise to a behavioral model that predicted the mechanical nature of muscle. This Hill model has three components that together act in a manner that describes the behavior of a whole muscle (23, 24). A schematic of configurations of the Hill model is presented in Figure 3-22. Hill used the techniques of a systems engineer to perform experiments that helped him identify key phenomena of muscle function. The model contained components referred to as the **contractile component** (CC), the **parallel elastic component** (PEC), and the **series elastic component** (SEC). Since this is a behavioral model, it is inappropriate to ascribe these mechanical components to specific structures in the muscle itself. However, the model has given great insight into how muscle func-

tions to develop tension and is often used as a basis for many computer models of muscle.

The contractile component is the element of the muscle model that converts the stimulation of the nervous system into a force. The contractile component has mechanical characteristics that determine the efficiency of a contraction, that is, how well the signal from the nervous system translates into a force. We have already discussed the first of these mechanical characteristics, the relationship between stimulation and activation. Two others, the force–velocity and force–length relationships, are discussed later in this chapter.

The elasticity inherent in muscle is personified by the series elastic and the parallel elastic components. Since the SEC is in series with the CC, any force produced by the CC is also applied to the SEC. It would first appear that the SEC is the tendon of the muscle, but the SEC represents the elasticity of all elastic elements in series with the force-generating structures of the muscle. The SEC is a highly nonlinearly elastic structure.

Muscle displays elastic behavior even when the CC is not producing force. An external force applied to a muscle causes the muscle to resist, but the muscle also stretches. This inactive elastic response is produced by structures that must be in parallel to the CC rather than in series to the CC. Thus, we have the PEC. The PEC is often associated with the fascia that surrounds the muscle and its compartments, but once again, this is a behavioral model and not a structural model, so this association cannot be made. The PEC, like the SEC, is highly nonlinear, increasing in stiffness as the muscle lengthens.

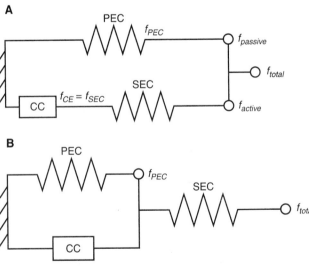

FIGURE 3-22 A. The most common form of the Hill muscle model. **B.** An alternative form. Because SEC is usually stiffer than PEC for most muscles, it generally does not matter which form of the model is used. (Adapted with permission from Winters, J. M. [2000]. Terminology and Foundations of Movement Science. In J. M. Winters, P. E. Crago [Eds.]. *Biomechanics and Neural Control of Posture and Movement.* New York: Springer-Verlag, 3–35.)

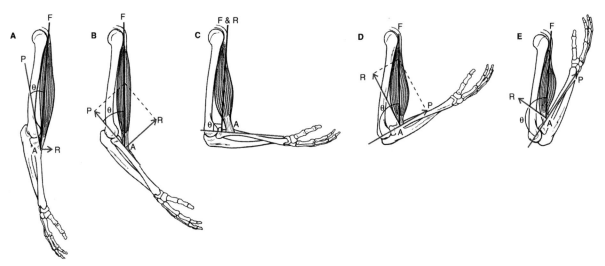

FIGURE 3-23 When muscle attachment angles are acute, the parallel component of the force (P) is highest and is stabilizing the joint. The rotatory component (R) is low **(A)**. The rotatory component increases to its maximum level at a 90° angle of attachment **(C)**. Beyond a 90° angle of attachment, the rotatory component diminishes and the parallel component increases to produce a dislocating force **(D** and **E)**.

FACTORS INFLUENCING MUSCLE FORCE

Angle of Attachment of Muscle

The muscle supplies a certain amount of tension that is transferred via the tendon or aponeurosis to the bone. Not all of the tension or force produced by the muscle will be put to use in generating rotation of the segment. Depending on the angle of insertion of the muscle, some force will be directed to stabilizing or destabilizing the segment by pulling the bone into or away from the joint.

Muscular force will be primarily directed along the length of the bone and into the joint when the tendon angle is acute or lying flat on the bone. When the forearm is extended, the tendon of the biceps brachii inserts into the radius at a low angle. Initiating an arm curl from this position requires greater muscle force than from other positions because most of the force generated by the biceps brachii is directed into the elbow rather than into moving the segments around the joint. Fortunately, the resistance offered by the forearm weight is at a minimum in the extended position. Thus the small muscular force available to move the segment is usually sufficient. Both the force directed along the length of the bone and that which is applied perpendicular to the bone to create joint movement can be determined by resolving the angle of the muscular force application into its respective parallel and rotary components. Figure 3-23 shows the parallel and rotatory components of the biceps brachii force for various attachment angles.

Even though muscular tension may be maintained during a joint movement, the rotary component and the torque will vary with the angle of insertion. Many neutral starting positions are weak, since most of the muscular force is directed along the length of the bone. As segments move through the midrange of the joint motion, the angle of insertion will usually increase and direct more of the muscular force into moving the segment. Consequently, when starting a weight-lifting movement from the fully extended position, less weight can be lifted than if the person started the lift with some flexion in the joint. Figure 3-24 shows the isometric force output of the shoulder flexors and extensors for a range of joint positions.

In addition, at the end of some joint movements, the angle of insertion may move past 90°, the point at which the moving force will again begin to decrease and the force along the length of the bone will act to pull the bone away from the joint. This dislocating force is present in the elbow and shoulder joints when there is a high degree of flexion in the joints.

Force–Time Characteristics

Somewhat related to the angle of muscular pull on the muscle is the force–time relationship in isometric muscle action.

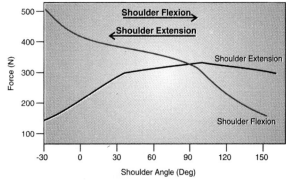

FIGURE 3-24 The isometric force output varies with the joint angle. As the shoulder angle increases, the shoulder extension force increases. The reverse happens with shoulder flexion force values, which decrease with an increase of the shoulder angle. (Adapted with permission from Kulig, K., et al. [1984]. Human strength curves. In R.L. Terjund [Ed.]. *Exercise and Sport Sciences Reviews*, 12: 417–466.)

When a muscle begins to develop tension through the contractile component of the muscle, the force increases nonlinearly over time because the passive elastic components in the tendon and the connective tissue stretch and absorb some of the force. After the elastic components are stretched, the tension that the muscle exerts on the bone increases linearly over time until maximum force is achieved.

The time to achieve maximum force and the magnitude of the force vary with a change in joint position. In one joint position, maximum force may be produced very quickly, while in other joint positions, it may occur later in the contraction. This reflects the changes in tendon laxity, not changes in the tension-generating capabilities of the contractile components. If the tendon is slack, the maximum force will occur later and vice versa.

Length–Tension Relationship

The magnitude of force produced by a muscle is also related to the length at which the muscle is held (14). The maximum tension that can be generated in the muscle fiber will occur when a muscle is activated at a length slightly greater than resting length, somewhere between 80 and 120% of the resting length. Fortunately, the length of most muscles in the body is within this maximum force production range. Figure 3-25 shows the length–tension relationship and demonstrates the contribution of active and passive components in the muscle.

Tension at Shortened Lengths

The tension-developing capacity drops off when the muscle is activated at both short and elongated lengths. When a muscle has shortened to half its length, it is not capable of generating much more contractile tension. At short lengths, there is less tension because the filaments have exceeded their overlapping capability, creating an incomplete activation of the cross-bridges, since fewer of these

can be formed (14) (Fig. 3-25). Thus, at the end of a joint movement or range of motion of a segment, the muscle is weak and incapable of generating large amounts of force.

Tension at Elongated Lengths

When a muscle is lengthened and then activated, muscle fiber tension is initially greater because the cross-bridges are pulled apart after initially joining (57). This continues until the muscle length is increased slightly past the resting length. When the muscle is lengthened further and contracted, the tension generated in the muscle will drop off because of slippage of the cross-bridges, resulting in fewer cross-bridges being formed (Fig. 3-25).

Contribution of the Elastic Components

The contractile component is not the only contributor to tension at different muscle lengths. The tension generated in a shortened muscle is shared by the series elastic component; that is, most tension develops in the tendon. The tension in the muscle is equal to the tension in the series elastic component when the muscle contracts in a shortened length.

As the tension-developing characteristics of the active components of the muscle fibers diminish with elongation, tension in the total muscle increases because of the contribution of the passive elements in the muscle. The series elastic component is stretched and tension is developed in the tendon and the cross-bridges as they are rotated back (27). Significant tension is also developed in the parallel elastic component as the connective tissue in the muscle offers resistance to the stretch. As the muscle is lengthened, passive tension is generated in these structures, so that the total tension is a combination of contractile and passive components (Fig. 3-25). At extreme muscle lengths, the tension in the muscle is almost exclusively elastic, or passive, tension.

Optimal Length for Tension

The optimal muscle length for generating muscle tension is slightly greater than the resting length because the contractile components are optimally producing tension and the passive components are storing elastic energy and adding to the total tension in the unit (19). This relationship lends support for placing the muscle on a stretch prior to using the muscle for a joint action. One of the major purposes of a windup or preparatory phase is to put the muscle on stretch to facilitate output from the muscle in the movement.

Force–Velocity Relationship

Muscle fibers will shorten at a specific speed or velocity while concurrently developing a force used to move a segment or external load. Muscles create an active force to match the load in shortening, and the active force continuously adjusts to the speed at which the contractile system moves (14). When load is low, the active force is adjusted by increasing the speed of contraction. With greater loads, the muscle adjusts the active force by reducing the speed of shortening.

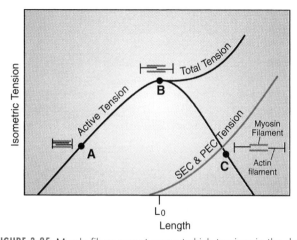

FIGURE 3-25 Muscle fibers cannot generate high tensions in the shortened state **(A)** because the actin and myosin filaments are maximally overlapped. The greatest tension in the muscle fiber can be generated at a length slightly greater than resting length **(B)**. In the elongated muscle **(C)**, the fibers are incapable of generating tension because the crossbridges are pulled apart. However, the total muscle tension increases because the elastic components increase their tension development.

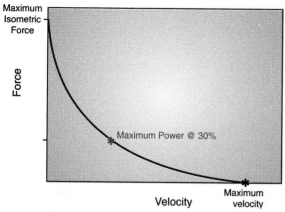

FIGURE 3-26 The force–velocity relationship in a concentric muscle action is inverse. The amount of tension or force-developing capability in the muscle decreases with an increase in velocity because fewer cross-bridges can be maintained. Maximum tension can be generated in the isometric or zero velocity condition, in which many cross-bridges can be formed. Maximum power can be generated in concentric muscle action with the velocity and force levels at 30% of maximum.

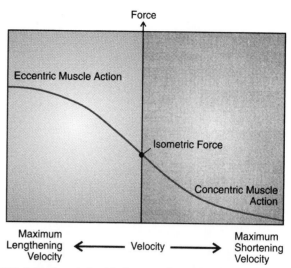

FIGURE 3-27 The relationship between force and velocity in eccentric muscle action is opposite to that of concentric muscle action. In eccentric muscle action, the force increases as the velocity of the lengthening increases. The force continues to increase until the eccentric action can no longer control lengthening of the muscle.

Force–Velocity Relationship in Concentric Muscle Actions

In concentric muscle action, velocity increases at the expense of a decrease in force and vice versa. The maximum force can be generated at zero velocity and the maximum velocity can be achieved with the lightest load. An optimal force can be created at zero velocity because a large number of cross-bridges are attached. As the velocity of the muscle shortening increases, the cycling rate of the cross-bridges increases, leaving fewer cross-bridges attached at one time (27). This equates to less force, and at high velocities, when all of the cross-bridges are cycling, the force production is negligible (Fig. 3-26).

Force–Velocity in the Muscle Fiber vs External Load

The force–velocity relationship relates to the behavior of muscle fiber, and it is sometimes confusing to relate this concept to an activity such as weightlifting. As an athlete increases the load in a lift, the speed of movement is likely to decrease. Although the force–velocity relationship is still present in the muscle fiber itself, the total system is responding to the increase in the external load or weight. The muscle may be generating the same amount of force in the fiber, but the addition of the weight slows the movement of the total system. In this case, the action velocity of the muscle is high, but the movement velocity of the high load is low (53).

Power

The product of force and velocity, **power**, is one of the major distinguishing features between successful and average athletes. Many sports require large power outputs, with the athlete expected to move his or her body or some external object very quickly. Since velocity diminishes with the increase of load, the most power can be achieved if the athlete produces one-third of maximum force at one-third

of maximum velocity (48,50). In this way, the power output is maximized even though the velocities or the forces may not be at their maximum level.

To train athletes for power, coaches must schedule high-velocity activities at 30% of maximum force (48). The development of power is also enhanced by fast-twitch muscle fibers, which are capable of generating four times more peak power than slow-twitch fibers.

Force–Velocity Relationships in Eccentric Muscle Actions

The force–velocity relationship in an eccentric muscle action is opposite to that in the shortening or concentric action. An eccentric muscle action is generated by antagonistic muscles, gravity, or some other external force. When a load greater than the maximum isometric strength value is applied to a muscle fiber, the fiber will begin to lengthen eccentrically. At the initial stages of lengthening, when the load is slightly greater than the isometric maximum, the speed of lengthening and the length changes in the sarcomeres will be small (14).

If a load is as high as 50% greater than the isometric maximum, the muscle will elongate at a high velocity. In eccentric muscle action the tension increases with the speed of lengthening because the muscle is stretching as it contracts (Fig. 3-27). The eccentric force–velocity curve will end abruptly at some lengthening velocity when the muscle can no longer control the movement of the load.

Electromyography

Electromyography (EMG) is the study of the electrical activity of muscle. The study of muscle from this perspective can be very valuable in providing information concerning the control of voluntary and/or reflexive

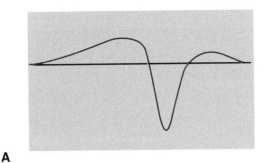

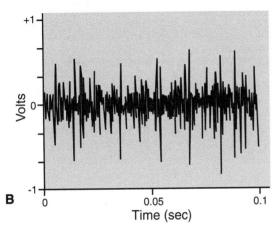

FIGURE 3-28 EMG records. **A.** A single action potential. **B.** A single EMG record containing many action potentials. The duration of the single action potential is much shorter than that of the EMG signal in **B**.

movements. The study of muscle activity during a particular task can yield insight into which muscles are active and when the muscles initiate and cease their activity. In addition, we can quantify the magnitude of the electrical response of the muscles during the task. However, there are limitations to the use of EMG, and these must be clearly understood if it is to be used correctly.

THE ELECTROMYOGRAM

The **electromyogram** is the profile of the electrical signal detected by an electrode on a muscle. That is, it is the measure of the action potential of the sarcolemma. The EMG signal is very complex, the composite of multiple action potentials of all active motor units superimposed on each other. Figure 3-28 illustrates the complexity of the signal. Note that the raw signal has both positive and negative components.

The amplitude of the EMG signal varies with a number of factors discussed in a later section. However, the amplitude increases as the intensity of the muscular contraction increases. This does not mean that there is a linear relationship between EMG amplitude and muscle force. In fact, increases in EMG activity do not necessarily indicate an increase in muscle force (56). Only in isometric contractions is there a close association between muscle electrical activity and muscle force (15).

RECORDING AN ELECTROMYOGRAPHIC SIGNAL

Electrodes

The EMG signal is recorded using an electrode. An electrode, which acts like an antenna, may be either indwelling or on the surface. The **indwelling electrode**, which may be either a needle or fine wire, is placed directly in the muscle. These electrodes are used for deep or small muscles. **Surface electrodes** are placed on the skin over a muscle and thus are mainly used for superficial muscles; they should not be used for deep muscles. The surface electrode is most often used in biomechanics and so most of the following discussion addresses surface electrodes.

Surface electrodes can be placed in either a monopolar or bipolar arrangement (Fig. 3-29). In a monopolar mode, one electrode is placed directly over the muscle in question and a second electrode goes over an electrically neutral site, such as a bony prominence. Monopolar recordings are nonselective relative to bipolar recordings, and while they are used in certain situations, such as static contractions, are poor in nonisometric movements. Bipolar electrodes are much more commonly used in biomechanics. In this case, two electrodes with a diameter of about 8 mm are placed over the muscle about 1.5 to 2 cm apart, and a third electrode is placed at an electrically neutral site. This arrangement uses a differential amplifier, which records the difference between the two recording electrodes. This differential technique removes any signal that is common to the inputs from the two recording electrodes.

The correct placement of electrodes is critical to a good recording. It is obvious that the electrodes must be placed so that the action potentials from the underlying muscle can be recorded. Therefore, electrodes should not be placed over tendinous areas of the muscle or over the motor point, that is, the point at which the nerve enters the muscle. Since action potentials propagate in both directions along the muscle from the motor point, signals recorded above the motor point have the potential to be attenuated because of cancellation of signals from both electrodes. There are various sources on standard locations for electrode placement (39).

Electrodes must also be oriented correctly, that is, parallel to the muscle fiber. The EMG signal is greatly affected when the electrodes are perpendicular rather than parallel to the fiber.

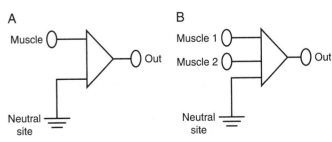

FIGURE 3-29 EMG electrodes can have either monopolar **(A)** or bipolar **(B)** configuration.

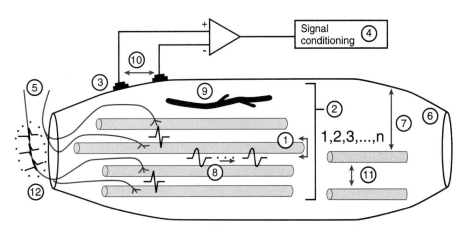

FIGURE 3-30 Some of the influences on the electromyographic signal. *1.* muscle fiber diameter. *2.* Number of muscle fibers. *3.* Electrode–skin interface. *4.* Signal conditioning. *5.* Number of active motor units. *6.* Tissue. *7.* Distance from skin surface to muscle fiber. *8.* Muscle fiber conduction velocity. *9.* Muscle blood flow. *10.* Interelectrode spacing. *11.* Fiber type and location. *12.* Motor unit firing rate. (Adapted with permission from Kamen, G., Caldwell, G. E. [1996]. Physiology and interpretation of the electromyogram. *Journal of Clinical Neurophysiology,* 13:366–384.)

When using surface electrodes, the resistance of the skin must be taken into consideration. For an electrical signal to be detected, this resistance should be very low. To obtain a low skin resistance, the skin must be thoroughly prepared by shaving the site, abrading the skin, and cleaning the skin with alcohol. When this is done, the electrodes can be placed properly. Surface electrodes are then placed using an electrolyte gel that also keeps the resistance low.

Amplification of the Signal

The EMG signal is relatively small, varying from 10 μ to 5 mV. It is therefore imperative that the signal be amplified, generally up to a level of ± 1 V. The usual type is the differential amplifier, which can amplify the EMG signal linearly without amplifying the noise or error in the signal. The noise in the signal can be obtained from sources other than the muscle, such as power line hum, machinery, or the amplifier itself. In addition, the amplifier must have high input impedance (resistance) and good frequency response and must be able to eliminate common noise from the signal. The International Society of Electrophysiological Kinesiology (ISEK) has determined a set of amplifier characteristics that are recommended for use in biomechanics. These characteristics are presented in a document published by ISEK (12).

Acquisition of the Signal

EMG signals are generally collected using an analog-to-digital (A/D) converter in conjunction with a computer. The A/D converter takes the analog or continuous EMG signal and digitizes it into estimates of the signal at discrete intervals. Knowledge of the frequency characteristics of the EMG signal itself is critical to selecting the rate at which the A/D converter samples the data. For the surface EMG signal, a sample rate of at least 1000 Hz (samples per second) or higher is required. If the sampling rate is less than 1000 Hz, the signal cannot be faithfully reproduced.

FACTORS AFFECTING THE ELECTROMYOGRAM

Any of a number of factors, both physiological and technical, can influence the interpretation of the EMG signal (32). It is essential to fully understand these factors before a knowledgeable interpretation of the EMG signal can be made. Figure 3-30 illustrates a number of these factors. Some, such as muscle fiber diameter, number of fibers, number of active motor units, muscle fiber conduction velocity, muscle fiber type and location, motor unit firing rate, muscle blood flow, distance from the skin surface to the muscle fiber, and tissue surrounding the muscle, may appear obvious because they all relate to the muscle itself. However, the other factors, including electrode–skin interface, signal conditioning, and electrode spacing, essentially relate to how the data are collected.

ANALYZING THE SIGNAL

It is difficult except under special circumstances to record a single action potential. Thus we are left with a signal comprising numerous action potentials from many motor units. Researchers are often interested in quantifying the EMG signal, and there are several procedures to do so (41). Most often, biomechanists first rectify the signal. **Rectification** involves taking the absolute value of the raw signal. That is, all values in the signal are positive. At this point, a **linear envelope** may be determined. This involves filtering out the high-frequency content of the signal to produce a smooth pattern that represents the volume of the activity. An alternative technique to the linear envelope is to integrate the rectified signal. When the signal is integrated, the EMG activity is summed over time so that the total accumulated activity can be determined over the chosen time period. Rectification, linear enveloping, and integration can be accomplished using electronic hardware, although they can also be done by computer. Figure 3-31 illustrates the results of these procedures.

In the procedures just described, the EMG signal was presented as a function of time or in the **time domain**. The EMG signal has also been analyzed in the **frequency domain** so that the frequency content of the signal can be determined. In this case, the power of the signal is plotted as a function of the frequency of the signal (Fig. 3-32). This profile is referred to as a frequency spectrum.

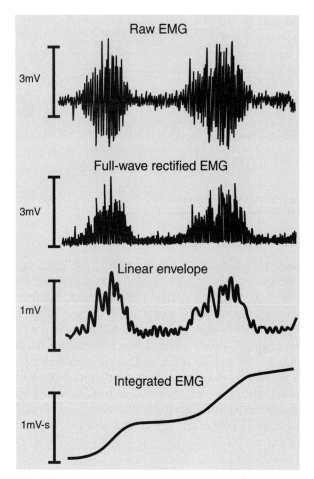

FIGURE 3-31 A raw EMG signal, full-wave rectified EMG signal, linear envelope, and integrated EMG signal.

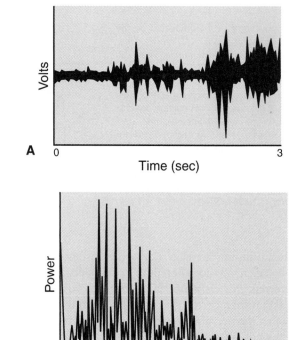

FIGURE 3-32 A raw EMG signal in the time domain **(A)** and frequency domain **(B)**.

Electromechanical Delay

When a muscle is activated by a signal from the nervous system, the action potential must travel the length of the muscle before tension can be developed in the muscle. Thus, there is a temporal disassociation or delay between the onset of the EMG signal and the onset of the development of force in the muscle. This is referred to as the **electromechanical delay** (EMD). This EMD portion of the EMG signal represents the activation of the motor units and the shortening of the series elastic component of the muscle and can be affected by mechanical factors that change the rate of series elastic shortening. These factors include the initial muscle length and muscle loading. It has been reported that athletes who have a high percentage of fast-twitch muscle fibers exhibit a short EMD (31). The actual duration of this delay is not known, and values in the literature range from 50 to 200 ms. Figure 3-33 illustrates this concept.

APPLICATIONS OF ELECTROMYOGRAPHY

Muscle Force–Electromyography Relationship

In isometric conditions, the relationship between muscle force and EMG activity is relatively linear (30,40). That is, for a given increment in muscle force, there is a concomi-

tant increase in EMG amplitude. These increases in EMG amplitude are probably produced by a combination of motor unit recruitment and increase in motor unit firing rate. However, many relationships, including both linear and curvilinear, between EMG and force have been suggested for different muscles (7) (Fig. 3-34).

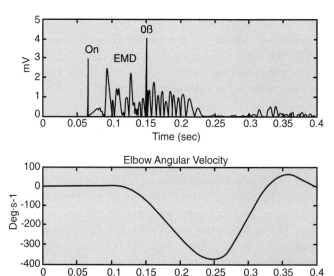

FIGURE 3-33 The electromechanical delay (EMD) of the biceps brachii during elbow flexion. **Top.** The EMG activity of the biceps brachii. **Bottom.** The elbow angular velocity profile (Reprinted with permission from Gabriel, D. A., Boucher, J. P. [1998]. Effects of repetitive dynamic contractions upon electromechanical delay. *European Journal of Physiology,* 79:37-40.)

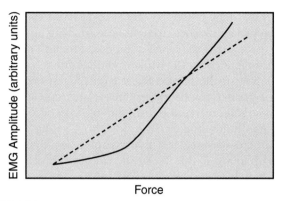

FIGURE 3-34 A linear relationship between EMG amplitude and external muscle force is frequently observed (***dotted line***). However, there are numerous exceptions that often result in a curvilinear relationship. (Adapted from a drawing by G. Kamen, University of Massachusetts at Amherst.)

In terms of concentric or eccentric contractions, descriptions of EMG–force relationships are controversial. The methodology of the studies that report such relationships is often questioned because of the predominant use of isokinetic dynamometers that constrain the joint velocity. In the literature, only a few studies have attempted to relate EMG and force during unconstrained movements (25,49).

Muscle Fatigue

EMG has greatly enhanced the study of muscle fatigue. Fatigue can result from either peripheral (muscular) or central (neural) mechanisms, although EMG cannot directly determine the exact site of the fatigue. This section briefly discusses local muscle fatigue. When a motor unit fatigues, there is a change in the frequency content and the amplitude of the EMG signal (6). The signal in the frequency domain shifts toward the low end of the frequency scale, and the amplitude increases (Fig. 3-35).

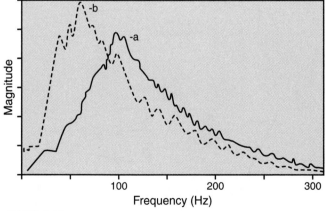

FIGURE 3-35 The frequency and amplitude changes during a sustained isometric contraction of the first dorsal interosseous muscle. (Adapted from Basmajian, J. V., DeLuca, C. J. [1985]. ***Muscles Alive: Their Functions Revealed by Electromyography*** [5th Ed.]. Baltimore: Williams & Wilkins, 205).

A number of physiological explanations have been proposed for these changes, including motor unit recruitment, motor unit synchronization, firing rate, and motor unit action potential rate. The shifts in the frequency domain are recoverable after sufficient rest, with the amount of rest dependent on the type and duration of loading. However, the recovery in the frequency spectrum of the signal does not appear to correspond to mechanical or physiological recovery of the muscle (47).

Clinical Gait Analysis

In the clinical setting, a gait analysis often involves EMG to determine which muscle group is used at a particular phase of the gait cycle (49). Generally, the raw or rectified EMG signal is used to determine when the muscles are active and when they are inactive, that is, to determine the activation order. Onsets and offsets of muscles should not be evaluated from any type of signal other than the raw or rectified signal, because further processing, such as filtering the data, distorts the onset or offset. More often, however, linear envelopes of EMG signals are used, after appropriate scaling, to determine amplitudes. Figure 3-36 illustrates typical EMG activity of lower extremity muscle groups during walking.

Ergonomics

Electromyography has been used in ergonomics for many applications. For example, studies have used EMG to investigate the effects of sitting posture, hand and arm movement, and armrests on the activity of neck and shoulder muscles of electronics assembly-line workers (54); to investigate the shoulder, back, and leg muscles during load carrying by varying load magnitude and the duration of load carrying (10); to study the erector spinae muscles of persons sitting in chairs with inclined seat pans (55); and to study postal letter sorting (13).

A particularly interesting use of EMG in ergonomics has been in the study of the low back in industry (44,45). This research has focused on proper lifting techniques and rehabilitation of workers who have low back problems. In addition, EMG has been used to study low back mechanics in exercise and during weight lifting.

LIMITATIONS OF ELECTROMYOGRAPHY

At best, EMG is a semiquantitative technique, because it gives only indirect information regarding the strength of the contraction of muscles. While there have been many attempts to quantify EMG, they have been largely unsuccessful. A second limitation is that it is difficult to obtain satisfactory recordings of dynamic EMG during movements such as walking and running. The EMG recording, therefore, is an indication of muscle activity only. One positive aspect of EMG recordings, however, is that they do reveal when the muscle is active and when it is not.

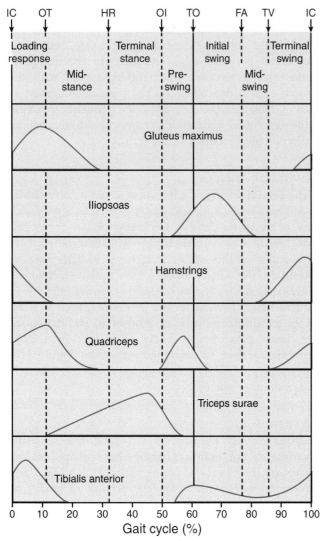

FIGURE 3-36 Typical EMG activity of the major lower extremity muscle groups during a stride cycle of walking. IC, initial contact; OT, opposite toe-off; HR, heel raise; OI, opposite initial contact; TO, toe-off; FA, feet adjacent; TV, tibial vertical. (Reprinted with permission from Whittle, M. W. [1996]. *Gait Analysis* [2nd ed.]. Oxford, UK: Butterworth-Heinemann, 68.)

Strengthening the Muscle

Strength is defined as the maximum amount of force produced by a muscle or muscle group at a site of attachment on the skeleton (38). Mechanically, strength is equal to maximum isometric torque at a specific angle. However, strength is usually measured by moving the heaviest possible external load through one repetition of a specific range of motion. The movement of the load is not performed at a constant speed, since joint movements are usually done at speeds varying considerably through the range of motion. Many variables influence strength measurement. Some of these include the muscle action (eccentric, concentric, isometric) and the speed of the limb movement

(33). Also, length–tension, force–angle, and force–time characteristics influence strength measurements as strength varies throughout the range of motion. Strength measurements are limited by the weakest joint position.

Training of the muscle for strength focuses on developing a greater cross-sectional area in the muscle and on developing more tension per unit of cross-section area (63). This holds true for all people, both young and old. Greater cross-section, or **hypertrophy**, associated with weight training is due to an increase in the size of the actual muscle fibers and more capillaries to the muscle that creates greater mean fiber area in the muscle (35,42). The size increase is attributed to increase in size of the actual myofibrils or separation of the myofibrils, as shown in Figure 3-37. Some researchers speculate that the actual muscle fibers may split (Fig. 3-37), but this has not been experimentally substantiated in humans (42). The increase in tension per unit of cross-section reflects the neural influence on the development of strength (52).

PRINCIPLES OF TRAINING

Genetic Predisposition

During strength training, the magnitude of the strength gains is related to numerous factors. First, there are genetic limits to the amount of strength obtainable; this is determined by distribution of fiber type and body type or musculoskeletal anthropometrics (63). These cannot be altered with training. Working within these genetic limits, one can directly control the strength gains through specific attention to training principles.

A

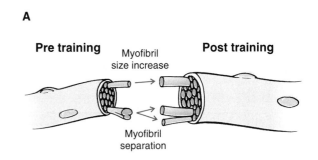

B

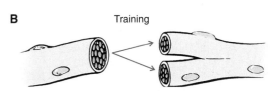

FIGURE 3-37 A. During strength training, the muscle fibers increase in cross-section as the myofibrils become larger and separate. **B.** It has been hypothesized that the fibers may also actually split; however, this has yet to be demonstrated in humans. (Adapted with permission from MacDougall, J. D. (1992). Hypertrophy or hyperplasia. In P. Komi (Ed.). *Strength and Power in Sport*. Boston: Blackwell Scientific, 230–238.)

Training Specificity

Training specificity, relating to the specific muscles, is also important in strength training. Only the muscles used in a specific movement pattern gain strength. This principle, specific adaptation to imposed demands, should direct the choice of lifts toward movement patterns related to the sport or activity in which the pattern might be used (63). This training specificity has a neurological basis, somewhat like learning a new motor skill—one is usually clumsy until the neurological patterning is established.

Figure 3-38 shows two sport skills, football lineman drives and basketball rebounding, along with lifts specific to the movement.

A learning process takes place in the early stages of strength training. This process continues into the later stages of training, but it has its greatest influence at the beginning of the program. It is in the beginning stages of a program that the novice lifter will demonstrate strength gains as a consequence of learning the lift rather than any noticeable increase in the physical determinants of

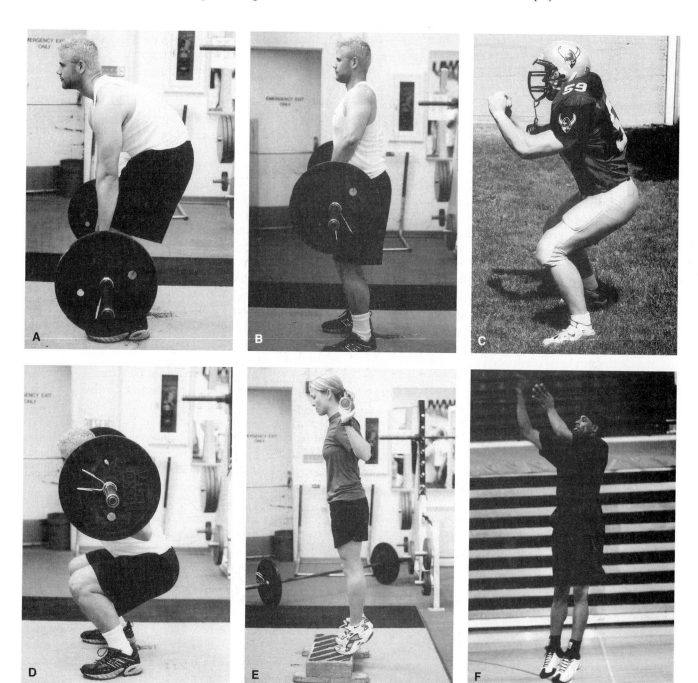

FIGURE 3-38 Weight-lifting exercises should be selected so that they reproduce some of the movements used in the sport. For the football lineman **(A–C),** the dead lift and the power clean include similar joint actions. Likewise, for the basketball player who uses jumping action, the squat and heel-raising exercises are good **(D–F).**

strength, such as increase in fiber size (16,63). This is the basis for using submaximal resistance and high-repetition lifting at the beginning of a strength-training program, so that the lift can first be learned safely.

In addition to the specificity of the pattern of joint movement, specificity of training of the muscle also relates to the speed of training. If a muscle is trained at slow speeds, it will improve strength at slow speeds but may not be strengthened at higher speeds. Thus, if power is the ultimate goal for an athlete, the strength-training routine should contain movements focusing on force and velocity components to maximize and emulate power. Once a strength base is established, power is obtained with high-intensity loads and a low number of repetitions (53).

Intensity

The intensity of the training routine is another important factor to monitor in the development of strength. Strength gains are directly related to the tension produced in the muscle. A muscle must be overloaded to a particular threshold before it will respond and adapt to the training (66). It is the amount of tension in the muscle rather than the number of repetitions that is the stimulus for strength. The amount of overload is usually determined as a percentage of the maximum amount of tension a muscle or muscle group can develop.

Athletes attempt to work at the highest percentage of their maximal lifting capability to increase the magnitude of their strength gains. If the athlete trains regularly using a high number of repetitions with low amounts of tension per repetition, the strength gains will be minimal because the muscle has not been overloaded beyond its threshold. The greatest strength gains are achieved when the muscle is worked near its maximum tension before it reaches a fatigue state (2 to 6 repetitions).

Rest

The quality and success of a strength-development routine are also directly related to the rest provided to the muscles between sets, between days of training, and prior to competition. Rest of skeletal muscle that has been stressed through resistive training is important for the recovery and rebuilding of the muscle fiber. As the skeletal muscle fatigues, the tension-development capability deteriorates, and the muscle is not operating at optimal overload.

Volume

The volume of work that a muscle performs may be the important factor in terms of rest of the muscle. Volume of work on a muscle is the sum of the number of repetitions multiplied by the load or weight lifted (63). Volume can be computed per week, month, or year and should include all of the major lifts and the number of lifts. In a week, the volume of lifting for two lifters may be the same even though their regimens are not the same. For example, one lifter lifts 3 sets of 10 repetitions at 100 lb for a volume of 3000 lb and another lifts 3 sets of 2 repetitions at 500 lb, also for a volume of 3000 lb.

At the beginning of a weight-training program, the volume is usually high. There are more sessions per week, more lifts per session, more sets per exercise, and more repetitions per set than later in the program (16). The volume decreases as one progresses through the training program. This is done by lifting fewer times per week, performing fewer sets per exercise, increasing the intensity of the lifts, and performing fewer repetitions.

The yearly repetition recommendation is 20,000 lifts, which can be divided into monthly and weekly volumes as the weights are increased or decreased (16). In a month or in a week, the volume of lifting varies to offer higher- and lower-volume days and weeks.

A lifter performing heavy resistance exercises with a low number of repetitions must allow 5 to 10 minutes between sets in order for the energy systems to be replenished (63). If the rest is less than 3 minutes, a different energy system is used, resulting in lactic acid accumulation in the muscle.

Bodybuilders use the short-rest and high-intensity training to build up the size of the muscle at the expense of losing some strength gains achieved with a longer rest period. If a longer rest period is not possible, it is believed that a high-repetition, low-resistance form of circuit training between the high-resistance lifts may reduce the buildup of lactic acid in the muscle. Bodybuilders also exercise at loads less than those of power lifters and weight lifters (6 to 12 RM). This is the major reason for the strength differences between the weightlifter (greater strength) and the bodybuilder (less strength).

The development of strength for performance enhancement usually follows a detailed plan that has been outlined in the literature for numerous sports and activities. A sample weight training cycle is presented in Table 3-1. The long-term picture usually involves some form of periodization during which the loads are increased and the volume of lifting is decreased over a period of months. As the athlete heads into a performance season, the lifting volume may be reduced by as much as 60%, which will actually increase the strength of the muscles. If an athlete stops lifting in preparation for a performance, strength can be maintained for at least 5 days and may be even higher after a few days of rest (63).

Strength Training for the Nonathlete

The principles of strength or resistance training have been discussed using the athlete as an example. It is important to recognize that these principles are applicable to rehabilitation situations, the elderly, children, and unconditioned individuals. Strength training is now recommended as part of one's total fitness development. The American College of Sports Medicine recommends at least one set of resistance training 2 days a week and including 8 to 12 exercises (1).

TABLE 3-1 Sample Weight-Training Cycle

Phase	Preparation Hypertrophy	Transition Basic Strength	Competition Strength/Power	Transition (active rest) Peak/Maintain
Sets	3–10	3–5	3–5	1–3
Repetitions	8–12	4–6	2–3	1–3
Days/wk	1–3	1–3	1–2	1
Times/day	1–3	1–3	1–2	1
Intensity cycle[a]	2:1–3:1	2:1–4:1	2:1–3:1	—
Intensity	Low	High	High	Very high to low
Volume	High	Moderate to high	Low	Very low

[a]Ratio of heavy training weeks to light training weeks.
Source: NSCA 1986, 8(6), 17–24.

Strength training is recognized as an effective form of exercise for the elderly. A marked strength decrement occurs with aging and is believed to be related to reduced activity levels (29). Strength training that is maintained into the later years may counteract atrophy of bone tissue and moderate the progression of degenerative joint alterations. The muscle groups identified for special attention in a weight-training program for the elderly include the neck flexors, shoulder girdle muscles, abdominals, gluteals, and knee extensors.

It is only the magnitude of the resistance that will vary in weight training for the athlete, elderly, young, and others. The conditioned athlete may perform a dumbbell lateral raise with a 50-lb weight in the hand, whereas an elderly person may simply raise the arm to the side using the arm weight as the resistance. High-resistance weight lifting must be implemented with caution, especially with the young and the elderly. Excessive loading of the skeletal system through high-intensity lifting can fracture bone in the elderly, especially in the individual with osteoporosis. The epiphyseal plates in the young are also susceptible to injury under high loads; thus, high-intensity programs for children are not recommended.

TRAINING MODALITIES

Isometric Exercise

There are various ways of loading the muscle, all of which have advantages and disadvantages in terms of strength development. Isometric training loads the muscle in one joint position so the muscle torque equals the resistance torque and no movement results (2). Individuals have demonstrated moderate strength gains using isometric exercises, and power lifters may use heavy-resistance isometric training to enhance muscle size.

Isometric exercise is also used in rehabilitation and with the unconditioned individual, since it is easier to perform than the concentric exercise. The major problem associated with isometric exercise is that there is minimal transfer to the real world, since most activities involve eccentric and concentric muscle actions. Furthermore, the isometric exercise only enhances the strength of the muscle group at the joint angle in which the muscle is stressed, which limits development of strength throughout the range of motion.

Isotonic Exercise

The most popular strength-training modality is isotonic exercise. An exercise is considered **isotonic** when the segment moves a specified weight through a range of motion. Although the weight of the barbell or body segment is constant, the actual load imposed on the muscle varies throughout the range of motion. In an isotonic lift, the initial load or resistance is overcome and then moved through the motion (2). The resistance cannot be heavier than the amount of muscle torque developed by the weakest joint position, since the maximum load lifted is only as great as this position. Examples of isotonic modalities are the use of free weights and multijoint machines, such as universal gyms, in which the external resistance can be adjusted (Fig. 3-39).

An isotonic movement can be produced with an eccentric or concentric muscle action. For example, the squat exercise involves eccentrically lowering a weight and concentrically raising the same weight. Even though the weight in an isotonic lift is constant, the torque developed by the muscle is not due to the changes in length–tension, force–angle, or the speed of the lift. To initiate flexion of the elbow while holding a 2.5-kg weight, a person generates maximum tension in the flexors at the beginning of the lift to get the weight moving. Remember that this is also one of the weakest joint positions because of the angle of attachment of the muscle. Moving through the midrange of the motion requires reduced muscular tension because the weight is moving and the musculoskeletal lever is more efficient. The resistive torque also peaks in this stage of the movement.

The isotonic lift may not adequately overload the muscle in the midrange, where it is typically the strongest. This is especially magnified if the lift is performed very

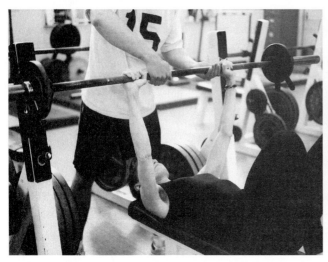
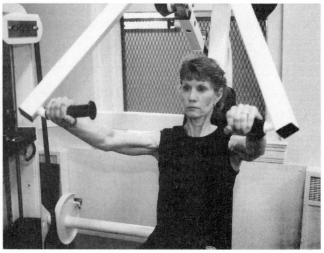

FIGURE 3-39 Two forms of isotonic exercises for the upper extremity. **Left.** The use of free weights (bench press). **Right.** The use of a machine.

quickly. If the person performs isotonic lifts with a constant speed (no acceleration) so that the midrange is exercised, the motive torque created by the muscle will match with the load offered by the resistance. Strength assessment using isotonic lifting is sometimes difficult, since specific joint actions are hard to isolate. Most isotonic exercises involve action or stabilization of adjacent segments.

Isokinetic Exercise

A third training modality is the **isokinetic** exercise, an exercise performed at a controlled velocity with varying resistance. This exercise must be performed on an isokinetic dynamometer allowing for isolation of a limb, stabilization of adjacent segments, and adjustment of the speed of movement, which typically ranges from 0 to 600°/second (Fig. 3-40).

When an individual applies a muscular force against the speed-controlled bar of the isokinetic device, an attempt is made to push the bar at the predetermined speed. As the individual attempts to generate maximum tension at the specific speed of contraction, the tension will vary because of changes in leverage and muscular attachment throughout the range of motion. Isokinetic testing has been used for quantifying strength in the laboratory and in the rehabilitation setting. An extensive body of literature presents a wide array of norms for isokinetic testing of different joints, joint positions, speeds, and populations.

The velocity of the devices will significantly influence the results. Therefore, testing must be conducted at a variety of speeds or at a speed close to that which will be used in activity. This is often the major limitation of isokinetic dynamometers. For example, the isokinetic strength of the shoulder internal rotators of a baseball pitcher may be assessed at 300°/second on the isokinetic dynamometer, but in fact, the actual speed of the

movement in the pitch has been shown to average 6000°/second (11). Isokinetic testing does allow for a quantitative measurement of power that has previously been difficult to measure in the field.

There are some drawbacks to using isokinetic testing and training. The movement at a constant velocity is not the type of movement typically found in the activities of daily living or in sport, and the cost of most isokinetic

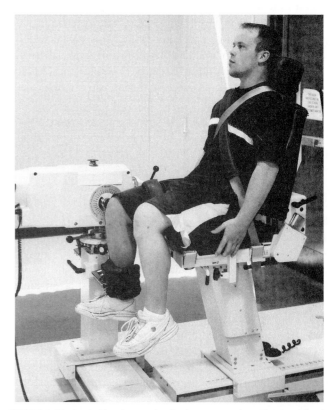

FIGURE 3-40 An isokinetic exercise for knee extension. The machine is the Biodex isokinetic dynamometer.

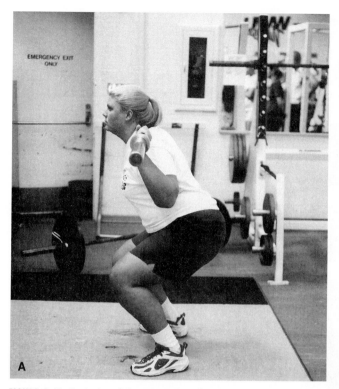 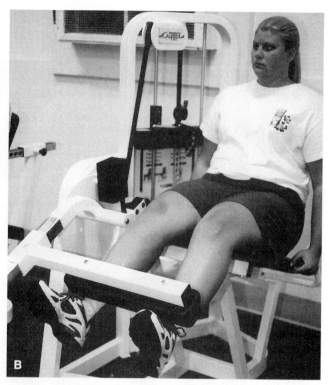

FIGURE 3-41 A. A close-link exercise for the quadriceps femoris muscles (squat). **B.** An open-link exercise for the same muscles (leg extension). Close-link exercises are more effective than open-link exercises.

systems and lack of mass usage make isokinetic training or testing prohibitive for many.

Close-Linked Exercise

While most therapists still use isokinetic testing for assessment, many have discontinued its use for training and have gone to close-linked training, in which individuals use body weight and eccentric and concentric muscle actions. A **close-linked exercise** is an isotonic exercise in which the end of the chain is fixed, as in the case of a foot or hand on the floor. An example of a close-linked exercise for the quadriceps is a simple squat movement with the feet on the floor (Fig. 3-41). It is believed that this form of exercise is more effective than an **open-linked exercise**, such as a knee extension on the isokinetic dynamometer or knee extension machine because it uses body weight, maintains muscle relationships, and is more transferable to normal human function.

Variable Resistive Exercise

The final training modality, **variable resistive exercise**, or dynamic accommodating exercise, is popular as a means of developing strength in the muscle. This training modality supposedly overloads the muscle group throughout the total range of motion (2). The goal is to load the muscle group near maximum potential at each point in the range of motion.

The Nautilus system is an example of a variable-resistance system in which the overload of the muscle is altered throughout the range of motion by means of a system of rotating cams that alter the mechanical advantage (Refer to Fig. 3-42 for an illustration of the Nautilus system). The shape of the cam is designed to match strength curves developed throughout a range of motion. Consequently, less resistance is offered to the muscle at the beginning of a lift than in the middle of the range of motion. At the end of the range of motion, the resistance is again decreased.

One of the drawbacks to the use of this type of training is that the cams used in the equipment do not produce resistances that match all individuals or the strength curves of all individuals (21). This type of training has been shown to be no more effective than the use of free-weight isotonic lifting, and similar strength gains have been reported for both types of training (5,43,60).

Another drawback of this type of training is the loss of contribution from adjacent segments, since this exercise is usually performed with the joint isolated. For example, to work the pectoralis major muscle in the specified arm machine, the muscle receives a good workout, as it is isolated in the horizontal flexion movement. But to use the horizontal flexion movement in an activity such as throwing, accompanying stabilization from the arm abductors, arm rotators, and forearm muscles is also needed. This synchrony between the stabilizers and primary muscles is lacking in many variable-resistance exercises. A trade-off may be in the reduction of injury with this type of lifting, since proper mechanical technique is less important than with free weights.

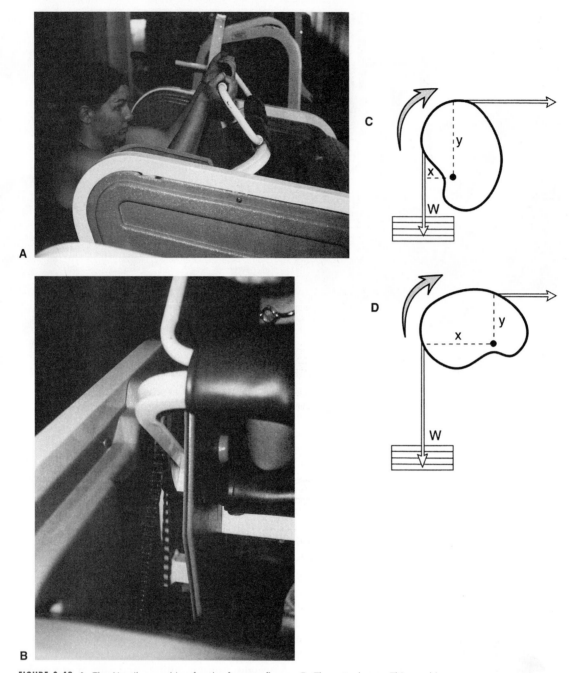

FIGURE 3-42 A. The Nautilus machine for the forearm flexors. **B.** The actual cam. This machine uses a cam system that changes the moment arm of the weight, making it easier (**C**) or harder (**D**) to lift.

Injury to Skeletal Muscle

CAUSE AND SITE OF MUSCLE INJURY

Injury to the skeletal muscle can occur through a bout of intense exercise, exercising a muscle over a long duration, or in eccentric exercise. The actual injury is usually a microinjury with small lesions in the muscle fiber. The result of a muscle strain or microtear in the muscle is manifested by pain or muscle soreness, swelling, possible anatomical deformity, and athletic dysfunction.

Muscles at greatest risk of strain are two-joint muscles, muscles limiting the range of motion, and muscles used

eccentrically (17). The two-joint muscles are at risk because they can be put on stretch at two joints (Fig. 3-43). Extension at the hip joint with flexion at the knee joint puts the rectus femoris on extreme stretch and renders it very vulnerable to injury.

Muscles used to terminate a range of motion are at risk because they are used to eccentrically slow a limb moving very quickly. Common sites where muscles are strained as they slow a movement are the hamstrings slowing hip flexion and the posterior rotator cuff muscles as they slow the arm in the follow-through phase of the throw (17).

While the muscle fiber itself may be the site of damage, it is believed that the source of muscle soreness immediately

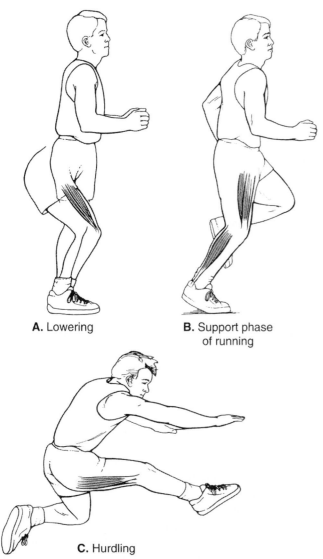

A. Lowering

B. Support phase of running

C. Hurdling

FIGURE 3-43 Muscles undergoing an eccentric muscle action are at increased risk for injury. **A.** The quadriceps femoris performing an eccentric muscle action in lowering as they control the knee flexion on the way down. **B.** The quadriceps and gastrocnemius eccentrically acting during the support phase of running. Two-joint muscles are also placed in injury-prone positions, making them more susceptible to strain. **C.** The hamstrings on extreme stretch when the hip is flexed and the knee is extended during hurdling.

following exercise and strain to the system is the connective tissue. This can be in the muscle sheaths, epimysium, perimysium, or endomysium, or it can be injury to the tendon or ligament (57). In fact, a common site of muscle strain is at the muscle–tendon junction because of the high tensions transmitted through this region. Injuries at this site are common in the gastrocnemius, pectoralis major, rectus femoris, adductor longus, triceps brachii, semimembranosus, semitendinosus, and biceps femoris (17).

It is important to identify those who are at risk for muscle strain. First, the chance of injury increases with muscular fatigue as the neuromuscular system loses its ability to control the forces imposed upon the system. This commonly results in an alteration in the mechanics

of movement and a shifting of shock-absorbing load responsibilities. Practice times should be controlled, and events late in the practice should not emphasize maximum load or stress conditions.

Second, an individual can incur a muscle strain at the onset of practice if it begins with muscles that are weak from recent usage (57). Muscles should be given ample time to recover from heavy usage. After extreme bouts of exercise, rest periods may have to be a week or more, but normally a muscle can recover from moderate usage in a day or two.

Third, if trained or untrained individuals perform a unique task for the first time, they will probably have pain, swelling, and loss of range of motion after performing the exercise. This swelling and injury are most likely to occur in the passive elements of the muscle and will generally lessen or be reduced as the number of practices increase (57).

Last, an individual with an injury is susceptible to a recurrence of the injury or development of an injury elsewhere in the system resulting from compensatory actions. For example, if the gastrocnemius is sore from a minor muscle strain, an individual may eccentrically load the lower extremity with a weak and inflexible gastrocnemius. This forces the person to pronate more during the support phase and run more on the balls of the feet, indirectly producing knee injuries or metatarsal fractures. With every injury there will be a functional substitution elsewhere in the system, and this is where the new injury will occur.

PREVENTING MUSCLE INJURY

Conditioning of the connective tissue in the muscle can greatly reduce the incidence of injury. Connective tissue responds to loading by becoming stronger. However, the rate of strengthening of connective tissue lags behind the rate of strengthening of the muscle. Therefore, base work with low load and high repetitions should be instituted for 3 to 4 weeks at the beginning of a strength and conditioning program to begin the strengthening process of the connective tissue before muscle strength is increased (58).

Different types of training influence the connective tissue in different ways. Endurance training has been shown to increase the size and tensile strength of both ligaments and tendons. Sprint training improves ligament weight and thickness, and heavy loading strengthens the muscle sheaths by stimulating the production of more collagen. When a muscle produces a maximum voluntary contraction, only 30% of the maximum tensile strength of the tendon is used (58). The remaining tensile strength serves as an excess to be used for very high dynamic loading. If this margin is exceeded, muscle injury occurs.

Other important considerations in preventing muscle injury are a warmup prior to beginning exercise routines, a progressive strength program, and attention to strength and flexibility balance in the musculoskeletal system. Finally, early recognition of signs of fatigue will also help prevent injury if corrective actions are taken.

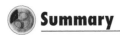
Summary

Skeletal muscle has four properties: irritability, contractility, extensibility, and elasticity. These properties allow muscle to respond to stimulation, shorten, lengthen beyond resting length, and return to resting length after a stretch, respectively.

Groups of muscles are contained in compartments that can be categorized by common function. The individual muscles in the group are covered by an epimysium and usually have a central portion called the belly. The muscle can be further divided internally into fascicles covered by the perimysium; the fascicles contain the actual muscle fibers covered by the endomysium. Muscle fibers can be organized in a fusiform arrangement, wherein the fibers run parallel and connect to a tendon at both ends, or in a penniform arrangement, wherein the fibers run diagonally to a tendon running through the muscle. In penniform muscle, the anatomical cross-section, situated at right angles to the direction of the fibers, is less than the physiological cross-section, the sum of all of the cross-sections in the fiber. In fusiform muscle, the anatomical and physiological cross-sections are equal.

Each muscle contains different fiber types that influence the muscle's ability to produce tension. Slow-twitch fiber types have slow contraction times and are well suited for prolonged, low-intensity workouts. Intermediate and fast-twitch fiber types are better suited for higher force outputs over shorter periods.

A muscle attaches to bone via an aponeurosis, or tendon. The tendon can withstand high tensile forces and respond stiffly to high rates of loading and less stiffly at lower loading rates. The tendon recoils during muscle contraction and delays the development of tension in the muscle. This recoiling action increases the load that a muscle can support. The tendon and the muscle are more prone to injury during an eccentric muscle action.

Muscles can perform a variety of functions, including producing movement, maintaining postures and positions, stabilizing joints, supporting internal organs, controlling pressures in the cavities, maintaining body temperature, and controlling entrances and exits to the body. Muscles also perform various roles, such as prime mover, agonist or antagonist, and stabilizer or neutralizer.

Muscle tension is generated to produce three types of muscle actions: isometric, concentric, and eccentric. The isometric muscle action is used to stabilize a segment; the concentric action creates a movement; and the eccentric muscle action controls a movement. The concentric muscle actions generate the lowest force output of the three, and the eccentric muscle action generates the highest.

Greater force can be developed in a concentric muscle action if it is preceded by an eccentric muscle action, or prestretch (stretch–shortening cycle). The muscle force is increased by facilitation via stored elastic energy and neurological facilitation. A quick short-range prestretch is optimal for developing maximum tension in fast-twitch fibers, and a slow, larger-range prestretch is beneficial for tension development in slow-twitch fibers.

Two-joint muscles are unique in that they act at two adjacent joints. Their effectiveness at one joint will depend on the positioning of the other joint, the moment arms at each joint, and the muscle synergies in the movement.

Each muscle fiber contains myofibrils that house the contractile unit of the muscle fiber, the sarcomere. It is at the sarcomere level that cross-bridging occurs between the actin and myosin filaments, resulting in shortening or lengthening of the muscle fiber.

A mechanical model of muscular contraction breaks the muscle down into active and passive components. The active component includes the contractile components found in the myofibrils and cross-bridging of the actin and myosin filaments. The passive or elastic components are in the tendon and the cross-bridges and in the sarcolemma and the connective tissue. Numerous factors influence the amount of force that can be generated by a muscle, including the angle of attachment of the tendon, the laxity or stiffness in the tendon that influences the force–time relationship, the length of the muscle, the contributions of the elastic component, and the velocity of the muscle action.

Electromyography is a technique whereby the electrical activity of muscle can be recorded. From EMG, we can gain insight into which muscles are active and when the muscles initiate and cease their activity. However, a number of concepts must be understood if one is to interpret the EMG signal clearly.

The development of strength in the muscle will be influenced by genetic predisposition, training specificity, training intensity, rest of the muscle during training, and the total training volume. Training principles apply to all groups, the conditioned and the unconditioned, and only the magnitude of the resistance need be altered. Muscles can be exercised isometrically, isotonically, isokinetically, or through variable-resistance exercise. Another important exercise consideration should be the decision on the use of open- or close-linked exercises.

Muscle injury is common and occurs most frequently in two-joint muscles and during eccentric muscle action. To prevent muscle injury, follow proper training and conditioning principles.

REVIEW QUESTIONS

True or False

1. ____ When one is creating a conditioning program for an elderly person, it is necessary to consider an entirely different set of principles.

2. ____ Muscles frequently act individually.

3. ____ The muscles of the thigh are contained within three compartments of fascia.

4. ____ The epimysium plays an important role in the transfer of muscle tension.

5. ____ A fascicle may contain as many as 2000 muscle fibers.

6. ____ The dark banding of the myofibril is made up of a thick protein called actin.

7. ____ A single contractile unit is a myofibril.

8. ____ It is established that actin filaments slide toward the middle of myosin filaments during contraction.

9. ____ The contraction process is initiated by the release of sodium ions.

10. ____ The magnitude of contractile force is directly proportional to the number of cross-bridges formed.

11. ____ In fusiform muscles the fibers are perpendicular to the tendon.

12. ____ The amplitude of the EMG recording indicates the amount of muscle tension developed.

13. ____ Monopolar EMG electrodes are most often used in biomechanics.

14. ____ The electromechanical delay refers to the time between the onset of the EMG signal and the initiation of movement.

15. ____ Muscle fatigue can be clearly demonstrated using EMG techniques.

16. ____ Full wave rectification of the EMG signal refers to applying a linear envelope to the signal.

17. ____ The likely site of injury in the muscle tendon unit is the aponeurosis.

18. ____ The ability of a muscle to respond to stimulation is its irritability.

19. ____ In most movements only a small percentage of a muscle's potential capability is used.

20. ____ In forearm flexion the triceps are the antagonists.

21. ____ In a slow stretch the actin–myosin cross-bridges contribute little to the elastic component.

22. ____ In abduction of the arm, the term that describes the contraction of the deltoid is eccentric.

23. ____ All of the force produced by a muscle is used in generating movement.

24. ____ When a muscle begins to develop tension, the increase in force is not linear.

25. ____ At extreme muscle lengths the actin–myosin cross-bridges provide an insignificant contribution to muscle tension.

Multiple Choice

1. The function of the perimysium is to ____.
   a. Protect muscle fibers
   b. Create pathways for nerves and blood cells
   c. Surround individual muscle fibers
   d. All of the above

2. The ____ is the focus of flexibility training because of the ability of the connective tissue to stretch.
   a. Endomysium
   b. Sarcomere
   c. Perimysium
   d. None of the above

3. Muscle fibers can be as much as ____ wide and ____ long.
   a. 10 mm, 20 cm
   b. 50 mm, 10 cm
   c. 100 mm, 50 cm
   d. None of the above

4. The dark banding of the myofibril is made up of a thick protein called ____.
   a. Actin
   b. Myosin
   c. Either A or B
   d. Neither A nor B

5. A single contractile unit is termed a ____.
   a. Myofibril
   b. Sarcolemma
   c. Sarcomere
   d. None of the above

6. Fusiform muscles can achieve high ____.
   a. Velocity
   b. Force
   c. Power
   d. None of the above

7. The biceps brachii is an example of ____ muscle.
   a. Pennate
   b. Fusiform
   c. Bipennate
   d. None of the above

8. Unipennate indicates ____.
   a. A single penniform muscle
   b. Muscle fibers running off one side of tendon
   c. A type of joint with only one degree of freedom
   d. None of the above

9. A rectified EMG signal that has been low pass filtered is called ____.
   a. Normalized
   b. Linear envelope
   c. Raw
   d. None of the above

10. Indwelling EMG electrodes are ____.
   a. Less specific than surface electrodes
   b. More specific than surface electrodes
   c. Able to capture a signal from wide range of muscle fibers
   d. None of the above

11. Postural muscles such as the upper back are primarily ____.
   a. Type 1
   b. Type 2
   c. Half type 1 and half type 2
   d. None of the above

12. The most likely site of injury in the muscle tendon unit is the ____.
   a. Muscle belly or myotendinous junction
   b. Aponeurosis
   c. Tendon–bone junction or myotendinous junction
   d. None of the above

13. The series elastic component in the Hill muscle model is comparable to ___.
   a. Fascia
   b. Myofibril
   c. Myosin filament
   d. None of the above

14. Typically the more ___ attachment site of a muscle is termed the ___.
   a. Distal, origin
   b. Proximal, insertion
   c. Proximal, origin
   d. Distal, insertion

15. EMG electrodes should be placed ___.
   a. Over the tendon
   b. Over the motor point
   c. Over the belly of the muscle
   d. None of the above

16. The ability of a muscle to respond to stimulation is its ___.
   a. Irritability
   b. Contractility
   c. Sensitivity
   d. None of the above

17. In the arm held in abduction, the term that describes the contraction of the deltoid is ___.
   a. Concentric
   b. Eccentric
   c. Isometric
   d. None of the above

18. In ___ movement the ___ is producing the movement force.
   a. Eccentric, agonist
   b. Concentric, agonist
   c. Concentric, antagonist
   d. None of the above

19. The order of maximum potential force output by contraction type is ___.
   a. Concentric, eccentric, isometric
   b. Eccentric, isometric, concentric
   c. Eccentric, concentric, isometric
   d. No difference in maximum potential force among contraction types

20. Muscle soreness and injury result most often from ___ muscle contractions.
   a. Concentric
   b. Isometric
   c. Eccentric
   d. None of the above

21. Maximum concentric force is generated at ___ velocity.
   a. Zero
   b. Moderate
   c. High
   d. Velocity is not related to maximum concentric force.

22. Maximum power is generated at ___ velocity.
   a. Zero
   b. Moderate
   c. High
   d. Velocity is not related to maximum power.

23. The term that describes growth in a muscle cross-section is ___.
   a. Hypertropia
   b. Hypertonia
   c. Hypertrophy
   d. Hypoglycemia

24. In the lowering phase of a squat, the ___ muscle is at highest risk of injury.
   a. Gastrocnemius
   b. Quadriceps
   c. Hamstring
   d. Soleus

25. EMG can give ___.
   a. Information about the force output of the muscle
   b. Information about muscle activation
   c. Neither A nor B
   d. Both A and B

26. EMG can be studied in ___.
   a. The time domain
   b. The frequency domain
   c. Neither A nor B
   d. Both A and B

REFERENCES

1. ACSM Position Stand (1990). The recommended quantity and quality of exercise for developing and maintaining cardiorespiratory and muscular fitness in healthy adults. *Medicine and Science in Sports and Exercise*, 22:265–274.
2. Ariel, G. (1984). Resistive exercise machines. In J. Terauds et al. (Eds.). *Biomechanics*. Eugene, OR: Microform Publications, 21–26.
3. Asmussen, E. (1952). Positive and negative muscular work. *Acta Physiologica Scandinavica*, 28:364–382.
4. Asmussen, E., Bonde-Petersen, F. (1974). Apparent efficiency and storage of elastic energy in human muscles during exercise. *Acta Physiologica Scandinavia*, 92:537–545.
5. Atha, J. (1981). Strengthening muscle. In D. I. Miller (Ed.). *Exercise and Sport Sciences Reviews*, 9:1–73.
6. Basmajian, J. V., DeLuca, C. J. (1985). *Muscles Alive: Their Functions Revealed by Electromyography* (5th ed.). Baltimore: Williams & Wilkins.
7. Bigland-Ritchie, B. (1980). EMG/force relations and fatigue of human voluntary contractions. In. D. I. Miller (Ed.). *Exercise and Sport Sciences Reviews*, 8:75–117.
8. Billeter, R., Hoppeler, H. (1992). Muscular basis of strength. In P. Komi (Ed.). *Strength and Power in Sport*. Boston: Blackwell Scientific, 39–63.
9. Bobbert, M. F., van Ingen Schenau, G. J. (1988). Coordination in vertical jumping. *Journal of Biomechanics*, 21:249–262.
10. Bobet, J., Norman, R. W. (1982). Use of the average electromyogram in design evaluation investigation of a whole-body task. *Ergonomics*, 25:1155–1163.
11. Cook, E. E., et al. (1987). Shoulder antagonistic strength ratios: A comparison between college-level baseball pitchers and nonpitchers. *Journal of Orthopaedic and Sports Physical Therapy*, 8:451–461.
12. Dainty, D. A., Norman, R. W. (Eds.). (1987). *Standardizing Biomechanics Testing in Sport*. Champaign, IL: Human Kinetics.

13. DeGroot, J. P. (1987). Electromyographic analysis of a postal sorting task. *Ergonomics*, 30:1079–1088.

14. Edman, K. A. P. (1992). Contractile performance of skeletal muscle fibers. In P. Komi (Ed.). *Strength and Power in Sport.* Boston: Blackwell Scientific, 96–114.

15. Fuglevand, A. J., et al. (1993). Impairment of neuromuscular propagation during human fatiguing contractions at submaximal forces. *Journal of Physiology*, 460:549–572.

16. Garhammer, J., Takano, B. (1992). Training for weight-lifting. In P. Komi (Ed.). *Strength and Power in Sport.* Boston: Blackwell Scientific, 357–369.

17. Garrett, W. E. (1991). Muscle strain injuries: Clinical and basic aspects. *Medicine and Science in Sports and Exercise*, 22:436–443.

18. Goldspink, G. (1992). Cellular and molecular aspects of adaptation in skeletal muscle. In P. Komi (Ed.). *Strength and Power in Sport.* Boston: Blackwell Scientific, 211–229.

19. Gowitzke, B. A. (1984). Muscles alive in sport. In M. Adrian, H. Deutsch (Eds.). *Biomechanics.* Eugene, OR: Microform Publications, 3–19.

20. Hay, J. G., Reid, J. G. (1988). *The Anatomical and Mechanical Bases of Human Motion.* Englewood Cliffs, NJ: Prentice-Hall.

21. Hay, J. G. (1992). Mechanical basis of strength expression. In P. Komi (Ed.). *Strength and Power in Sport.* Boston: Blackwell Scientific, 197–207.

22. Henneman, E., et al. (1965). Excitability and inhibitability of motor neurons of different sizes. *Journal of Neurobiology*, 28:599–620.

23. Hill, A. V. (1938). Heat and shortening and the dynamic constants of muscle. *Proceedings of the Royal Society of London (Biology)*, 126:136–195.

24. Hill, A. V. (1970). *First and Last Experiments in Muscle Mechanics.* Cambridge, UK: Cambridge University Press.

25. Hof, A. L., van den Berg, J. (1981). EMG to force processing: 1. An electrical analog of the Hill muscle model. *Journal of Biomechanics*, 14:747–758.

26. Huijing, P. A. (1992). Mechanical muscle models. In P. Komi (Ed.). *Strength and Power in Sport.* Boston: Blackwell Scientific, 130–150.

27. Huijing, P. A. (1992). Elastic potential of muscle. In P. Komi (Ed.). *Strength and Power in Sport.* Boston: Blackwell Scientific, 151–168.

28. Huxley, A. F. (1957). Muscle structure and theories of contraction. *Progress in Biophysics and Biophysical Chemistry*, 7:255–318.

29. Israel, S. (1992). Age-related changes in strength and special groups. In P. Komi (Ed.). *Strength and Power in Sport.* Boston: Blackwell Scientific, 319–328.

30. Jacobs, R., van Ingen Schenau, G. J. (1992). Control of an external force in leg extensions in humans. *Journal of Physiology*, 457:611–626.

31. Kamen, G., et al. (1981). Fractionated reaction time in power trained athletes under conditions of fatiguing isometric exercise. *Journal of Motor Behavior*, 13:117–129.

32. Kamen, G., Caldwell, G. E. (1996). Physiology and interpretation of the electromyogram. *Journal of Clinical Neurophysiology*, 13:366–384.

33. Knuttgen, H. G., Komi, P. (1992). Basic definitions for exercise. In P. Komi (Ed.). *Strength and Power in Sport.* Boston: Blackwell Scientific, 3–6.

34. Komi, P. V. (1984). Physiological and biomechanical correlates of muscle function: Effects of muscle structure and stretch–shortening cycle on force and speed. In R. L. Terjund (Ed.). *Exercise and Sport Sciences Reviews*, 12:81–121.

35. Komi, P. V. (1986). The stretch–shortening cycle and human power output. In N. L. Jones et al. (Eds.). *Human Muscle Power.* Champaign, IL: Human Kinetics, 27–40.

36. Komi, P. V. (1992). Stretch–shortening cycle. In P. Komi (Ed.). *Strength and Power in Sport.* Boston: Blackwell Scientific, 169–179.

37. Kornecki, S. (1992). Mechanism of muscular stabilization process in joints. *Journal of Biomechanics*, 25:235–245.

38. Kulig, K., et al. (1984). Human strength curves. In R. L. Terjund (Ed.). *Exercise and Sport Sciences Reviews*, 12: 417–466.

39. LeVeau, B., Andersson, G. (1992). Output forms: data analysis and applications. In G. L. Soderberg (Ed.). *Selected Topics in Surface Electromyography for the Use in the Occupational Setting.* Washington: National Institute for Occupational Safety and Health, U.S. Public Health Service, 70–102.

40. Lippold, O. C. J. (1952). The relation between integrated action potential in human muscle and its isometric tension. *Journal of Physiology*, 117:492–499.

41. Loeb, G. E., Gans, C. (1986). *Electromyography for Experimentalists.* Chicago: University of Chicago Press.

42. MacDougall, J. D. (1992). Hypertrophy or hyperplasia. In P. Komi (Ed.). *Strength and Power in Sport.* Boston: Blackwell Scientific, 230–238.

43. Manning, R. J., et al. (1990). Constant vs variable resistance training. *Medicine and Science in Sports and Exercise*, 22:397–401.

44. McGill, S. M. (1991). Electromyographic activity of the abdominal and low back musculature during the generation of isometric and dynamic axial trunk torque: Implications for lumbar mechanics. *Journal of Orthopaedic Research*, 9:91–103.

45. McGill, S. M., Sharrat, M. T. (1990). The relationship between intra-abdominal pressure and trunk EMG. *Clinical Biomechanics*, 5:59–67.

46. McMahon, T. A. (1984). *Muscles, Reflexes, and Locomotion.* Princeton, NJ: Princeton University Press, 3–25.

47. Mills, K. R. (1982). Power spectral analysis of electromyogram and compound muscle action potential during muscle fatigue and recovery. *Journal of Physiology*, 326:401–409.

48. Moritani, T. (1992). Time course of adaptations during strength and power training. In P. Komi (Ed.). *Strength and Power in Sport.* Boston: Blackwell Scientific, 226–278.

49. Olney, S. J., Winter, D. A. (1985). Predictions of knee and ankle moments of force in walking from EMG and kinematic data. *Journal of Biomechanics*, 18:9–20.

50. Perrine, J. J. (1986). The biophysics of maximal muscle power outputs: Methods and problems of measurement. In N. L. Jones et al. (Eds.). *Human Muscle Power.* Champaign, IL: Human Kinetics, 15–26.

51. Proske, U., Morgan, D. L. (1987). Tendon stiffness: Methods of measurement and significance for the control of movement. *Journal of Biomechanics*, 20:75–82.

52. Sale, D. G. (1986). Neural adaptation in strength and power training. In N. L. Jones et al. (Eds.). *Human Muscle Power.* Champaign, Ill: Human Kinetics, 289–308.

53. Schmidtbleicher, D. (1992). Training for power events. In P. Komi (Ed.). *Strength and Power in Sport.* Boston: Blackwell Scientific, 381–395.

54. Schuldt, K., et al. (1986). Effects of sitting work posture on static neck and shoulder muscle activity. *Ergonomics*, 29:1525–1537.

55. Soderberg, G. L., et al. (1986). An EMG analysis of posterior trunk musculature during flat and anteriorly inclined sitting. *Human Factors*, 28:483–491.

56. Solomonow, M., et al. (1990). Electromyogram power spectra frequencies associated with motor unit recruitment strategies. *Journal of Applied Physiology*, 68:1177–1185.

57. Stauber, W. T. (1989). Eccentric action of muscles: Physiology, injury, and adaptation. In K. Pandolf (Ed.). *Exercise and Sports Sciences Review*, 17: 157–185.

58. Stone, M. H. (1990). Muscle conditioning and muscle injuries. *Medicine and Science in Sports and Exercise*, 22:457–462.

59. Stone, M. H. (1992). Connective tissue and bone response to strength training. In P. Komi (Ed.). *Strength and Power in Sport*. Boston: Blackwell Scientific, 279–290.

60. Sylvester, L. J., et al. (1981). The effect of variable resistance and free weight-training programs on strength and vertical jump. *National Strength and Conditioning Association Journal*, 3:30–33.

61. Vanderhelm, F. C. T., Veenbaas, R. (1991). Modelling the mechanical effect of muscles with large attachment sites: Application to the shoulder mechanism. *Journal of Biomechanics*, 24:1151–1163.

62. Van Soest, A. J., et al. (1993). The influence of the biarticularity of the gastrocnemius muscle on vertical jumping achievement. *Journal of Biomechanics*, 26:1–8.

63. Weiss, L. W. (1991). The obtuse nature of muscular strength: The contribution of rest to its development and expression. *Journal of Applied Sport Science Research*, 5:219–227.

64. Wells, R. P. (1988). Mechanical energy costs of human movement: An approach to evaluating the transfer possibilities of two-joint muscles. *Journal of Biomechanics*, 21:955–964.

65. Zajac, F. E., Gordon, M. E. (1989). Determining muscle's force and action in multi-articular movement. In K. B. Pandolf (Ed.). *Exercise and Sports Sciences Reviews*, 17:187–230.

66. Zernicke, R. F., Loitz, B. J. (1992). Exercise-related adaptations in connective tissue. In P. Komi (Ed.). *Strength and Power in Sport*. Boston: Blackwell Scientific, 77–95.

ADDITIONAL READING

Armstrong, R. B. (1990). Initial events in exercise-induced muscular injury. *Medicine and Science in Sports and Exercise*, 22:429–435.

Bosco, C., et al. (1982). Effect of elastic energy and myoelectrical potentiation of triceps surae during stretch–shortening cycle exercise. *International Journal of Sports Medicine*, 3:137–140.

Burke, R. E. (1986). The control of muscle force: Motor unit recruitment and firing patterns. In N. L. Jones et al. (Eds.). *Human Muscle Power*. Champaign, IL: Human Kinetics, 97–110.

Edgerton, V. R., et al. (1986). Morphological basis of skeletal muscle power output. In N. L. Jones et al. (Eds.). *Human Muscle Power*. Champaign, IL: Human Kinetics, 43–64.

Enoka, R. M. (1988). *Neuromuscular Basis of Kinesiology*. Champaign, IL: Human Kinetics.

Faulkner, J. A., et al. (1986). Power output of fast and slow fibers from human skeletal muscle. In N. L. Jones et al. (Eds.). *Human Muscle Power*. Champaign, IL: Human Kinetics, 81–94.

Fleckstein, S. J., et al. (1988) Effects of limited knee-flexion range on peak hip moments of force while transferring from sitting to standing. *Journal of Biomechanics*, 21:915–918.

Goldstein, S. A., et al. (1987). Analysis of cumulative strain in tendons and tendon sheaths. *Journal of Biomechanics*, 20:1–6.

Green, H. J. (1986). Muscle power: Fiber type recruitment, metabolism, and fatigue. In N. L. Jones et al. (Eds.). *Human Muscle Power*. Champaign, IL: Human Kinetics, 65–80.

Grimby, L. (1986). Single motor-unit discharge during voluntary contraction and locomotion. In N. L. Jones et al. (Eds.). *Human Muscle Power*. Champaign, IL: Human Kinetics, 111–130.

Grimby, G. (1992). Clinical aspects of strength and power training. In P. Komi (Ed.). *Strength and Power in Sport*. Boston: Blackwell Scientific, 338–355.

Herring, S. A. (1990). Rehabilitation of muscle injuries. *Medicine and Science in Sports and Exercise*, 22:453–456.

Kannus, P., Yusada, K. (1992). Value of isokinetic angle-specific torque measurements in normal and injured knees. *Medicine and Science in Sports and Exercise*, 24:292–297.

Kibler, W. B. (1990). Clinical aspects of muscle injury. *Medicine and Science in Sports and Exercise*, 22:450–452.

Kirkendall, D. T. (1990). Mechanisms of peripheral fatigue. *Medicine and Science in Sports Exercise*, 22:444–449.

Mansour, J. M., Pereira, J. M. (1987). Quantitative functional anatomy of the lower limb with application to human gait. *Journal of Biomechanics*, 20:51–58.

Moore, K. L., Dalley, A. E. (1999). *Clinically Oriented Anatomy* (4th ed.). Baltimore: Lippincott Williams & Wilkins.

NSCA Round Table Discussion on Periodization. Part 2. (1986). *National Strength and Conditioning Association Journal*, 8:17–24.

Otten, E. (1988). Concepts and models of functional architecture in skeletal muscle. In K. B. Pandolf (Ed.). *Exercise and Sport Science Reviews*, 16:89–137.

Pittman, M. I., Peterson, L. (1989). Biomechanics of Skeletal Muscle. In M. Nordin, V. H. Frankel (Eds.). *Basic Biomechanics of the Musculoskeletal System* (2nd ed.). Philadelphia: Lea & Febiger, 89–111.

Rohl, L., et al. (1991). Tensile and compressive properties of cancellous bone. *Journal of Biomechanics*, 24:1143–1149.

Sargeant, A. J., et al. (1977). Functional and structural changes after disuse of human muscle. *Sport Science and Molecular Medicine*, 52:337–342.

Stein, R. B., et al. (1986). What is optimized in muscular movements? In N. L. Jones et al (Eds.). *Human Muscle Power*. Champaign, IL: Human Kinetics, 131–150.

Stothart, J. P. (1973). Relationship between selected biomechanical parameters of static and dynamic muscle performance. In S. Cerquigliani (Ed.). *Biomechanics*. Basel: Karger, 210–217.

Tesch, P. A. (1992). Training for bodybuilding. In P. Komi (Ed.). *Strength and Power in Sport*. Boston: Blackwell Scientific, 370–380.

Wilson, G. J., et al. (1992). Stretch-shorten cycle performance enhancement through flexibility training. *Medicine and Science in Sports and Exercise*, 24:116–123.

GLOSSARY

Actin: A protein of the myofibril, noticeable by its light banding. Along with myosin, it is responsible for the contraction and relaxation of the muscle.

Action Potential: The signal propagated of a neuron and muscle fibers.

Agonist: A muscle responsible for producing a specific movement through concentric muscle action.

Anatomical Cross-Section: The cross-section at a right angle to the direction of the fibers.

Antagonist: A muscle responsible for opposing the concentric muscle action of the agonist.

Aponeurosis: A flattened or ribbonlike tendinous expansion from the muscle that connects into the bone.

Assistant Mover: A muscle that helps to bring about a desired movement.

Belly: The fleshy central portion of a muscle.

Bipennate: A feather-shaped fiber arrangement, in which the fibers run off of both sides of a tendon running through the muscle.

Close-Linked Exercise: Exercises using eccentric and concentric muscle actions with the feet fixed on the floor. Movements begin with segments distal to the feet (trunk and thigh) and move toward the feet, as in the squat.

Compartment Syndrome: A condition in which the circulation and function of the tissues within a muscle compartment are impaired by an increase in pressure within the compartment.

Concentric: Muscle action in which tension causes visible shortening in the length of the muscle; positive work is performed.

Conduction Velocity: The speed at which an action potential is propagated.

Contractile Component: The active component in a muscle where behavioral shortening takes place.

Contractility: The ability of muscle tissue to shorten when the muscle tissue receives sufficient stimulation.

Contraction: The state of muscle when tension is generated across a number of actin and myosin filaments.

Cross-Bridge: The connection and intertwining of the actin and myosin filaments of the myofibrils.

Depolarization: A reduction in the potential of a membrane.

Eccentric: Muscle action in which tension is developed in the muscle and the muscle lengthens; negative work is performed.

Excitation–Contraction Coupling: Electrochemical stimulation of the muscle fiber that initiates the release of calcium and the subsequent cross-bridging between actin and myosin filaments, which leads to contraction.

Elastic: Capable of being stretched, compressed, or distorted and then returning to the original shape.

Elasticity: The ability of muscle tissue to return to its resting length once a stretch is removed.

Electromyography: The measurement of electrical activity of muscle.

Electromyogram: The recorded signal of the electrical activity of muscle.

Electromechanical Delay: The temporal disassociation or delay between the onset of the EMG signal and the onset of the development of force in the muscle.

Endomysium: The sheath surrounding each muscle fiber.

Epimysium: A dense, fibrous sheath covering an entire muscle.

Extensibility: The ability of muscle tissue to lengthen beyond resting length.

Fascia: Sheet or band of fibrous tissue.

Fascicle: A bundle or cluster of muscle fibers.

Fast-Twitch Fiber: Large skeletal muscle fiber innervated by the alpha-I motor neuron; has fast contraction times. There are two subtypes of fast-twitch fibers: the low oxidative and high glycolytic (Type IIb) and the medium oxidative and high glycolytic (Type IIa).

Fibers: Elongated cylindrical structures containing cells that constitute the contractile elements of muscle tissue.

Force–Velocity Relationship: The relationship between the tension development in the muscle and velocity of shortening or lengthening.

Frequency Domain: An analysis technique whereby the power of the signal is plotted as a function of the frequency of the signal.

Fusiform: Spindle-shaped fiber arrangement in a muscle.

Hyperpolarization: An increase in the potential of a membrane.

Indwelling Electrode: An EMG electrode that is placed directly in the muscle.

Inelastic: Lacking the ability to withstand compression, stretch, or distortion and return to the original shape or length.

Insertion: The more distal attachment site of the muscle.

Intensity: In weight training, the load or percentage of maximum lifting capacity lifted with each repetition.

Irritability: The capacity of muscle tissue to respond to a stimulus.

Isokinetic Exercise: An exercise in which concentric muscle action is generated to move a limb against a device that is speed controlled. Individuals attempt to develop maximum tension through the full range of motion at the specified speed of movement.

Isometric: Muscle action in which tension develops but there is no visible or external change in joint position; no external work is produced.

Isometric Exercise: An exercise that loads the muscle in one joint position.

Isotonic Exercise: An exercise in which an eccentric and/or concentric muscle action is generated to move a specified weight through a range of motion.

Length–Tension Relationship: The relationship between the length of the muscle and the tension produced by the muscle; highest tensions are developed slightly past resting length.

Linear Envelope: The process whereby a rectified EMG signal has most of the high-frequency components removed via a low pass filter.

Motor Unit: The nerve and all of the muscle fibers that it innervates.

Multipennate: A feather-shaped fiber arrangement in which the muscle fibers run diagonally off one or both sides of a tendon running through the muscle.

Myofibril: Rodlike strand contained within and running the length of the muscle fibers; contains the contractile elements of the muscle.

Myosin: A thick protein of the myofibril, noticeable by its dark banding. Along with actin, it is responsible for contraction and relaxation of the muscle.

Myotendinous Junction: The site where the muscle and tendon join, consisting of a layered interface as the myofibrils and the collagen fibers of the tendon meet.

Neuromuscular Junction (motor end plate): The synapse between the motor neuron and the muscle fiber.

Neutralizer: A muscle responsible for eliminating or canceling out an undesired movement.

Origin: The more proximal attachment site of a muscle.

Parallel Elastic Component: The passive component in a muscle model that behaviorally develops tension with elongation.

Penniform: A feather-shaped fiber arrangement in a muscle in which the fibers run diagonally to a tendon running through the muscle.

Perimysium: A dense connective tissue sheath covering the fascicles.

Physiological Cross-Section: Area that is the sum total of all of the cross-sections of fibers in the muscle; the area perpendicular to the direction of the fibers.

Plyometrics: A training technique that uses the stretch–shortening cycle to increase athletic power.

Power: The product of force and velocity.

Prime mover: The muscle that acts directly to bring about a desired movement.

Recoil: To spring back to the original position, as seen in the elastic components in the muscle.

Rectification: The process whereby the negative portion of a raw EMG signal is made positive so that the complete signal is positive.

Repolarization: A return to the resting potential of a membrane.

Resting Potential: The voltage across the membrane at steady-state conditions.

Sarcolemma: A thin plasma membrane covering the muscle that branches into the muscle, carrying nerve impulses.

Sarcomere: One contractile unit of banding on the myofibril, running Z-band to Z-band.

Sarcoplasm: The fluid enclosed within a muscle fiber by the sarcolemma.

Sarcoplasmic Reticulum: A membranous system within a muscle fiber that forms lateral sacs near the t-tubules.

Series Elastic Component: The passive component in a muscle model that behaviorally develops tension in contraction and during elongation.

Sliding Filament Theory: A theory describing muscle contraction whereby tension is developed in the myofibrils as the head of the myosin filament attaches to a site on the actin filament.

Slow-Twitch Fiber: Small skeletal muscle fiber innervated by the alpha-2 motor neuron, having a slow contraction time. This fiber is highly oxidative and poorly glycolytic.

Specificity: Training principle suggesting that specific training movements should be done in the same manner and position in which the movements are performed in the sport or activity.

Stabilizer: A muscle responsible for stabilizing an adjacent segment.

Strength: The maximum amount of force produced by a muscle or muscle group at a site of attachment on the skeleton; one maximal effort.

Stretch–Shortening Cycle: A common sequence of joint actions in which an eccentric muscle action, or pre-stretch, precedes a concentric muscle action.

Surface Electrode: An EMG electrode that is placed directly on the skin above the muscle that is being recorded.

Tendon: A fibrous cord, consisting primarily of collagen, by which muscles attach to bone.

Tetanus: The force response of muscle to a series of excitatory inputs resulting in a summation of twitch responses.

Time Domain: A parameter that is presented as a function of time.

T-tubule (transverse tubule): Structure in the sarcolemma that facilitates rapid communication between action potentials and myofilaments in the interior of the muscle.

Twitch: The force response of a muscle to a single stimulation.

Unipennate: A feather-shaped fiber arrangement in which the muscle fibers run diagonally off one side of the tendon.

Variable Resistive Exercise: Exercise performed on a machine that alters the amount of resistance through the range of motion.

Volume: In weight training, the sum of the number of repetitions multiplied by the load or weight lifted. Usually calculated over a week, month, or year.

4

Neurological Considerations for Movement

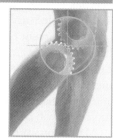

OBJECTIVES

After reading this chapter, the student will be able to:

1. Describe the anatomy of a motor unit including central nervous system pathways, the neuron structure, the neuromuscular junction, and the ratio of fibers to neurons that are innervated.

2. Explain the differences between the three motor unit Types: Type I, Type IIa, and Type IIB.

3. Discuss the characteristics of the action potential, emphasizing how a twitch or tetanus develops, as well as the influence of local graded potentials.

4. Describe the pattern of motor unit contribution to a muscle contraction through discussion of the size principle, synchronization, and rate coding of the motor unit activity.

5. Compare the myotatic, propriospinal, and supraspinal reflexes, and provide examples of each.

6. Describe the anatomy of the muscle spindle and the functional characteristics of the spindle during a stretch of the muscle or during gamma motor neuron influence.

7. Describe the anatomy of the Golgi tendon organ (GTO) and explain how the GTO responds to tension in the muscle.

8. Explain how weight training, bilateral training, or warmup influences the neurological activity in the muscle.

9. Identify the factors influencing flexibility, and provide examples of specific stretching techniques that are successful in enhancing flexibility.

10. Describe a plyometric exercise, detailing the neurological and structural contributions to the exercise.

I. **General Organization of the Nervous System**

II. **Motor Neurons**
   A. Structure of the Motor Neuron
   B. The Motor Unit
   C. Functional Characteristics of the Motor Unit

III. **Sensory Neurons**
   A. Foundations of Neural Control
   B. Sensory Receptors
      1. Muscle Spindle
      2. Golgi Tendon Organ
      3. Joint Sensory Receptors

IV. **Effect of Training on Neurological Input and Output**

V. **Stretching the Muscle**
   A. Flexibility Techniques
      1. Neurological Restrictions
      2. Structural Restrictions
      3. Proprioceptive Neuromuscular Facilitation

VI. **Plyometric Training**
   A. Neurological Influences
   B. Structural Influences
   C. Plyometric Examples

VII. **Summary**

Human movement is controlled and monitored by the nervous system. The nature of this control is such that many muscles may have to be activated to perform a vigorous movement like sprinting, or only a few muscles may have to be activated to push a doorbell or make a phone call. The nervous system is responsible for identifying the muscles that will be activated for a particular movement and then generating the stimulus to develop the level of force that will be required from that muscle.

Many human movements require stabilization of adjacent segments while a fine motor skill is performed. This requires a great deal of coordination on the part of the nervous system to stabilize such segments as the arm and forearm while very small, coordinated movements are created with the fingers, as in the act of writing.

Accuracy of movement is another task with which the nervous system is faced. The nervous system coordinates the muscles to throw a baseball with just the right amount of muscular force so that the throw is successful. Recognizing the difficulty of being accurate with a physical movement contributes to an appreciation of the complexity of neural control.

The neural network is extensive, since each muscle fiber is individually innervated by a branch of the nervous system. Information exits the muscle and provides input to the nervous system, and information enters the muscle to initiate a muscle activity of a specific nature and magnitude. Through this loop system, interconnected with many other loops from other muscles and with central nervous control, the nervous system is able to coordinate the activity of many muscles at once. Specific levels of force may be generated in several muscles simultaneously so that a skill such as kicking may be performed accurately and forcefully. Knowledge of the nervous system will be very helpful in improvement of muscular output, refinement of a skill or task, rehabilitation of an injury, and stretching a muscle group.

 # General Organization of the Nervous System

The nervous system consists of two parts, the central nervous system and the peripheral nervous system, both illustrated in Figure 4-1. The **central nervous system** consists of the brain and the spinal cord and should be viewed as the means by which human movement is initiated, controlled, and monitored.

The **peripheral nervous system** consists of all of the branches of nerves that lie outside the spinal cord. The peripheral nerves primarily responsible for muscular action are the **spinal nerves**, which enter on the posterior, or dorsal, side of the vertebral column and exit on the anterior, or ventral, side at each vertebral level of the spinal cord. Eight pairs of nerves enter and exit the cervical region, twelve pairs at the thoracic region, five at the

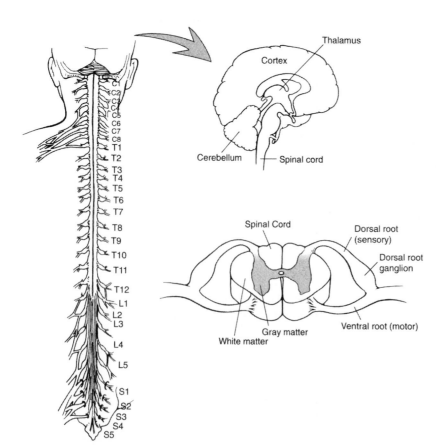

FIGURE 4-1 The central nervous system consists of the brain and the spinal cord. The peripheral nervous system consists of all of the nerves that lie outside the spinal cord. The 31 pairs of spinal nerves exit and enter the spinal cord at the various vertebral levels. Motor information leaves the spinal cord through the ventral root (anterior), and sensory information enters the spinal cord through the dorsal root (posterior).

Anterior View

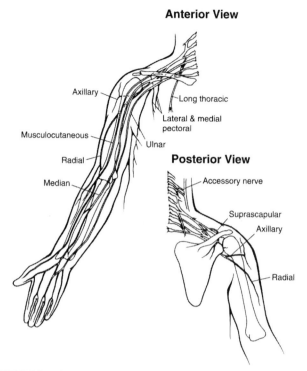

Posterior View

FIGURE 4-2 The upper extremity nerves. Nine nerves innervate the muscles of the upper extremity.

lumbar region, five in the sacral region, and one in the coccygeal region. The pathways of the nerves are presented for the upper and lower extremities in Figures 4-2 and 4-3, respectively.

The nerves entering the spinal cord on the dorsal, or back, side of the cord are called sensory neurons because they transmit information into the system from the muscle. The nerves exiting on the ventral, or front, side of the body are called **motor neurons** because they carry impulses away from the system to the muscle.

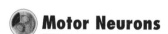 Motor Neurons

STRUCTURE OF THE MOTOR NEURON

The **neuron** is the functional unit of the nervous system carrying information to and from the nervous system. The structure of a neuron, specifically the motor neuron, warrants examination to clarify the process of muscular contraction. Figure 4-4 shows a close-up view of the neuron and the neuromuscular junction.

The motor neuron consists of a cell body containing the nucleus of the nerve cell. The **cell body**, or **soma**, of a motor neuron is usually contained within the gray matter of the spinal cord or in bundles of cell bodies just outside the cord, referred to as **ganglia**. The cell bodies are arranged in pools spanning one to three levels of the spinal cord and innervate portions of a single muscle or selected synergists.

Projections on the cell body, called **dendrites**, serve as receivers and bring information into the neuron from other neurons. The dendrites are bunched to form small bundles. A bundle will contain dendrites from other neurons and can consist of dendrites from different spinal cord levels or different neuron pools. The composition of the bundle will change as dendrites are added and subtracted. This arrangement facilitates cross-talk between neurons.

A large nerve fiber, the **axon**, branches out from the cell body and exits the spinal cord via the ventral root, where it is bundled together with other peripheral nerves. The axon of the motor neuron is fairly large, making it capable of transmitting nerve impulses at high velocities, up to 100 m/second. This large and rapidly transmitting motor neuron is also called an **alpha motor neuron**. The axon of the motor neuron is **myelinated**, or covered with an insulated shell. Actually, the myelination is sectioned, with **Schwann cells** insulating and enveloping a specific length along the axon, followed by a gap, termed the **node of Ranvier**, and then a repeat of the insulated Schwann cell covering.

When the myelinated motor neuron approaches a muscle fiber, it breaks off into unmyelinated terminals, or branches, called **motor endplates**, which embed into fissures, or clefts, near the center of the muscle fiber. This site is called the **neuromuscular junction**. The neuron does not make contact with the actual muscle fiber; instead, there is a small gap, termed the synaptic gap or **synapse**, between the terminal branch of the neuron and the muscle. This is the reason muscular contraction involves a chemical transmission, since the only way for a nerve impulse to reach the actual muscle fiber is some type of chemical transmission across the gap.

THE MOTOR UNIT

The structure of the **motor unit** was introduced in Chapter 3, in which we concentrated on the action of the muscles in the motor unit. In this section, we concentrate on the nervous system portion of the motor unit. The neuron, cell body, dendrites, axon, branches, and muscle fibers constitute the motor unit (Fig. 4-5). A neuron may terminate on as many as 2000 fibers in muscles, as in the gluteus maximus, or as few as 5 or 6 fibers, as in the orbicularis oculi of the eye. The typical ratio of neurons to muscle fibers is 1:10 for the eye muscles, 1:1600 for the gastrocnemius, 1:500 for the tibialis anterior, 1:1000 for the biceps brachii, 1:300 for the dorsal interossei in the hand, and 1:96 for the lumbricales in the hand (2). The average number of fibers per neuron is somewhere between 100 and 200 (2,27). The fibers innervated by each motor unit are not bunched together and are not all in the same fascicle but are spread throughout the muscle.

When a motor unit is activated sufficiently, all of the muscle fibers belonging to it will contract within a few

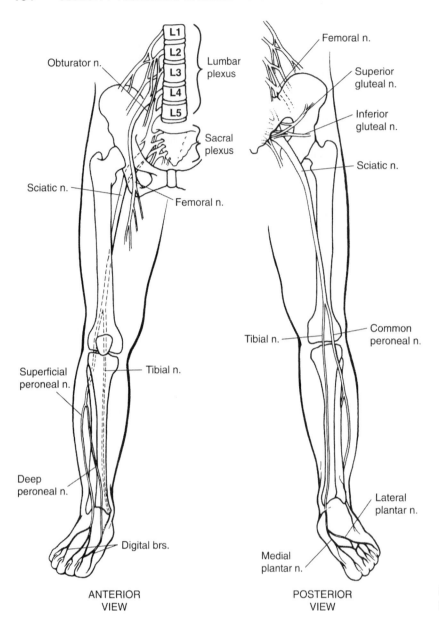

ANTERIOR
VIEW

POSTERIOR
VIEW

FIGURE 4-3 The lower extremity nerves. Twelve nerves innervate the muscles of the lower extremity.

milliseconds. This is referred to as the **all-or-none principle**. A muscle that has motor units with very low ratios of nerve to fiber allows finer control of the movement characteristics, such as is seen in eye and hand movements. Many lower extremity muscles have large neuron-to-fiber ratios suitable to functions in which large amounts of muscular output are required, such as in weight bearing and walking.

Three different types of motor units exist, corresponding to the three fiber types discussed in the previous chapter: slow-twitch oxidative (Type I), fast-twitch oxidative (Type IIa), and fast-twitch glycolytic (Type IIb). Micrographs of the three different fiber types are presented in Figure 4-6. Even at this level, there is considerable variation between the three fiber types. Certain muscles, like the soleus, consist primarily of Type I muscle fibers and motor units; whereas, muscles like the vastus lateralis are approximately 50% Type I and the remainder Type II.

These fiber and motor unit types are primarily genetically determined, but they can be enhanced through training. It has been shown that Type IIa muscle fibers can be converted to Type IIb fibers through specific training emphasizing power and quickness (17). It is not clear whether a transformation can be made from Type I to Type II through specific training.

All of the muscle fibers in a motor unit are of the same type. The fast-twitch glycolytic motor units (Type IIb) are innervated by very large alpha motor neurons that conduct the impulses at very fast velocities (>100 m/second) creating rapid contraction times in the muscle (approximately 30–40 ms) (8). As a result, these large motor units generate muscular activity that contracts fast, develops high tensions, and fatigues quickly. These motor units usually have large neuron-to-fiber ratios and are found in some of the largest muscles in the body, such as

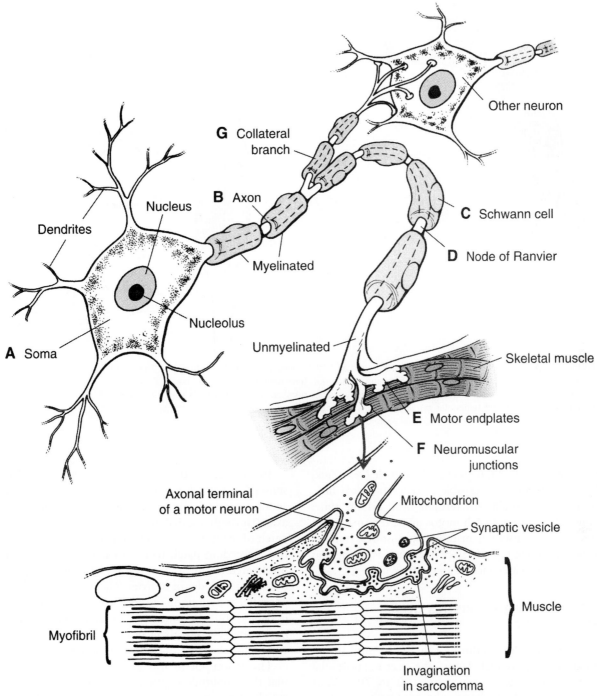

FIGURE 4-4 The cell body, or soma **(A)**, of the neuron is in or just outside the spinal cord. Traveling from the soma is the axon **(B)**, which is myelinated by Schwann cells **(C)** separated by gaps, the nodes of Ranvier **(D)**. On the ends of each axon, the branches become unmyelinated to form the motor end plates **(E)** that terminate at the neuromuscular junction **(F)** on the muscle. Neurons receive information from other neurons through collateral branches **(G)**.

the quadriceps femoris group. These motor units are useful in activities such as sprinting, jumping, and weight lifting.

The fast-twitch oxidative motor units (Type IIa) also have fast contraction times (approximately 30–50 ms), but they have the advantage over fast-twitch glycolytic motor units because they are more fatigue resistant (8). These

moderately-sized motor units are capable of generating moderate tensions over longer periods. The activity from these motor units is useful in activities such as swimming and bicycling and in job tasks in factories and among long-shoremen.

The slow-twitch oxidative motor units (Type I) transmit the impulses slowly (approximately 80 m/second),

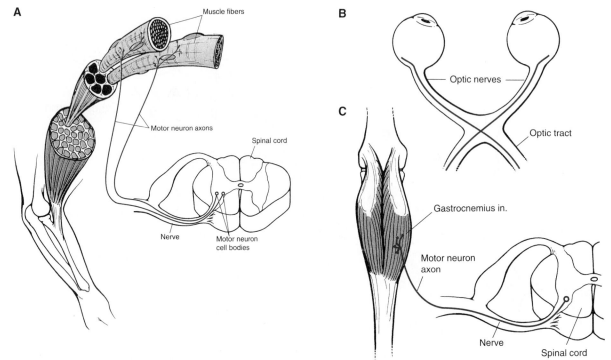

FIGURE 4-5 A. The motor unit consists of a neuron and all of the fibers innervated by that neuron. The motor neurons exit the anterior side of the spinal cord and branch out, terminating on a muscle fiber. **B.** Fine motor movements can occur when the motor unit services only a small number of muscle fibers, such as in the eye. **C.** When the motor unit terminates on large numbers of muscle fibers, such as in the gastrocnemius, finer movement capabilities are lost at the gain of more overall muscle activity.

generating slow contraction times in the muscle (>70/ms) (8). These motor units are capable of generating very little tension but can sustain this tension over a long time. Consequently, the slow-twitch motor units, the smallest of the three types, are useful in maintaining postures, stabilizing joints, and doing repetitive activities such as typing and gross muscular activities such as jogging.

FUNCTIONAL CHARACTERISTICS OF THE MOTOR UNIT

The nerve impulse travels through the motor unit in the form of an action potential. At rest, the electrical potential across the membrane, approximately 60 to 70 mV, is negative in the inside of the membrane. Upon activation by the central or peripheral nervous system, the action potential travels down through the motor unit via rapid depolarization, repolarization, and hyperpolarization.

In depolarization, the membrane potential decreases and moves closer to zero and a positive voltage of approximately 30 mV, as there is an exchange of ions across the membrane. This is followed by repolarization as the voltage moves back in the negative direction and hyperpolarization as the voltage becomes more negative than in the resting condition. The exchange of ions, the generation of the action potential, and the voltage change associated with depolarization are presented in Figure 4-7.

In unmyelinated axons, the sodium (Na$^+$) and potassium (K$^+$) channels are distributed along the axon, and the action potential is propagated along the length of the axon through local depolarization of each neighboring patch of membrane. Each patch of membrane thus causes the succeeding patch to produce an action potential. In myelinated axons, however, the Na$^+$ channels are concentrated at the nodes of Ranvier. The generation of an action potential at each node results in depolarization of the next node and thus the generation of an action potential at the next node. The net effect of myelination is to increase the conduction velocity of the action potential.

The action potential is a propagated impulse, meaning that the amplitude of the impulse remains the same as it travels down the axon to the motor endplate. At the motor endplate, the action potential traveling down through the nerve becomes a muscle action potential traveling through the muscle. Externally these two action potentials are indistinguishable. Eventually the muscle action potential initiates the development of the cross-bridging and shortening within the muscle sarcomere. The total process is referred to as excitation–contraction coupling (see Chapter 3).

Each action potential generates a twitch response in the muscle. If action potentials are in close enough sequence, the tensions generated by one muscle twitch will be summed with other twitches to form a tetanus, or constant tension in the muscle fiber (see Fig. 3-20). This level

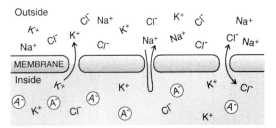

Exchange of Ions Across Membrane

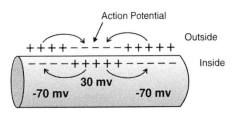

Action Potential Generated Through Change in Electrical Potential

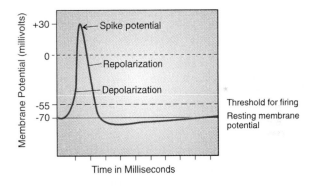

Recording of Action Potential

FIGURE 4-7 The action potential travels down the nerve as the permeability of the nerve membrane changes, allowing an exchange of sodium (Na⁺) and potassium (K⁺) ions across the membrane. This creates a voltage differential that is negative on the outside of the membrane. This negative voltage, or action potential, travels down the nerve until it reaches the muscle and stimulates a muscle action potential that can be recorded.

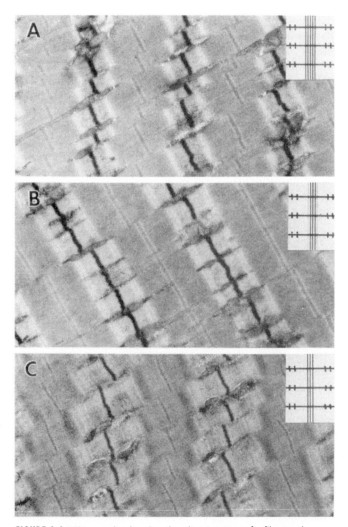

FIGURE 4-6 Micrographs showing the ultrastructure of a fiber to demonstrate actual structural differences between the three fiber Types. Type I fibers **(A)** have bands of equal density; Type IIa fibers have bands of nonuniform density, and Type II fibers **(B)** have only three bands (Courtesy of J. Friden, Goeteberg University, Sweden).

of tension will decline as the motor unit becomes incapable of regenerating the individual twitch responses fast enough.

The action potential in a motor unit can be facilitated or inhibited by the input it receives from the many neurons that are connecting to it within the spinal cord. As shown in Figure 4-8, a motor unit receives synaptic input from other neurons and from **interneurons**, which are small, connecting branches that can be both excitatory and inhibitory. The input is in the form of a **local graded potential** that unlike the action potential, does not maintain its amplitude as it travels along. Thus, the stimulus has to be sufficient to reach its destination on another neuron and be large enough to generate a response in the neuron with which it has interfaced.

The alpha motor neuron has many collateral branches interacting with other neurons, and the number of collateral branches is highest in the distal muscles. An inhibitory interneuron receiving input from these collaterals is the

Renshaw cell, also in the spinal cord. The Renshaw cell is considered one of the key elements in organizing muscular response in the agonists, antagonists and synergists when it is stimulated sufficiently by a collateral branch (18,19).

The tension or force generated by a muscle is determined by the number of motor units actively stimulated at the same time and by the frequency at which the motor units are firing. **Recruitment**, the term used to describe the order of activation of the motor units, is the prime mechanism for force production in the muscle. It usually follows an orderly pattern in which pools of motor units

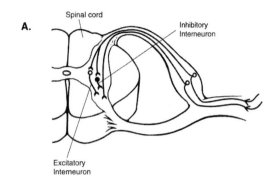

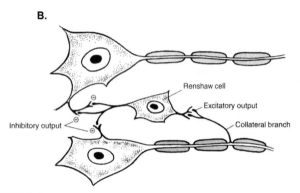

FIGURE 4-8 A. The action potential traveling through a motor unit can be altered by input from interneurons, which are small connecting nerve branches that generate a local graded potential; the potential may or may not institute a change in the connecting neuron. The interneurons may produce an excitatory local graded potential, which facilitates the action potential, or an inhibitory local graded potential sufficient to inhibit the action potential. **B.** A special interneuron, the Renshaw cell, receives excitatory information from a collateral branch of another neuron, stimulating an inhibitory local graded potential.

are sequentially recruited (9). There is a functional pool of motor units for each task, whereby separate recruitment sequences can be initiated to stimulate the three different types of motor units (Type I, IIa, IIb) for the performance of different actions within the same muscle.

The sequence of motor unit recruitment usually follows the **size principle**, whereby the small, slow-twitch motor neurons are recruited first, followed by recruitment of the fast-twitch oxidative and finally the large, fast-twitch glycolytic motor units (9). This is because the small motor neurons have lower thresholds than the large motor neurons. Thus, the small motor neurons are used over a broad tension range before the moderate or large fibers are recruited.

In walking, for example, the low-threshold motor units are used for most of the gait cycle, except for some brief recruitment of the intermediate motor units during peak activation times. The high threshold, fast-twitch motor units are not usually recruited unless there is a rapid change of direction or a stumble.

In running, more motor units are recruited, with some high-threshold units recruited for the peak output times in the cycle. Furthermore, the low-threshold units are recruited for activities such as walking and jogging, and the fast-twitch fibers are recruited in activities such as weight lifting (9,14). Recruitment sequences for walking and for different exercise intensities are presented in Figure 4-9.

The motor units are recruited **asynchronously**, whereby the activation of a motor unit is temporally spaced but is summed with the preceding motor unit activity. If the tension is held isometrically over a long time, some of the larger motor neurons will be activated. Likewise, in vigorous, rapid movements, both small and large motor neurons will be activated.

The motor unit recruitment pattern proceeds from small to large motor neurons, slow to fast, small force to large force, and fatigue-resistant to fatigable muscles. Once a motor unit is recruited, it will remain active until the force declines, and when the force declines, the motor units are deactivated in reverse order of activation, with the large motor neurons going first. Also, the motor unit recruitment pattern is established in the muscle for a specific movement pattern (31). If the joint position changes and a new pattern of movement is required, the recruitment pattern will change because different motor units are recruited. However, the order of recruitment from small to large will remain the same.

There is some evidence that alternative recruitment patterns may be initiated by input from the excitatory and inhibitory pathways. This is done through interneurons that alter the threshold response of the slow- and fast-twitch units. The threshold level of the fast-twitch motor unit can be lowered via excitatory interneurons.

In ballistic movements involving rapid alternating movements, there appears to be **synchronous** or concurrent activation of the motor unit pool whereby large motor units are recruited along with the small motor neurons. This synchronous firing has also been shown to occur as a result of weight training. It is believed that in athletic performance requiring a wide range of muscular output, the neuromuscular sequence may in fact be reversed, with the fast-twitch fibers recruited first in vigorous muscle actions (5,9).

The frequency of motor unit firing can also influence the amount of force or tension developed by the muscle. This is known as **frequency coding** or **rate coding** and involves intermittent high-frequency bursts of action potentials or impulses ranging from 3 to 50 impulses/second (27). With increased rate coding, the rate of impulses increases in a linear fashion and only after all of the motor units are recruited (4).

In the small muscles, all of the motor units are usually recruited and activated when the external force of the muscle is at levels of only 30 to 50% of the maximum voluntary contraction level. Beyond this level, the force output in the muscle is increased through increases in rate coding, allowing for the production of a smooth, accurate contraction.

In the large muscles, recruitment of motor units takes place all through the total force range, so that some muscles

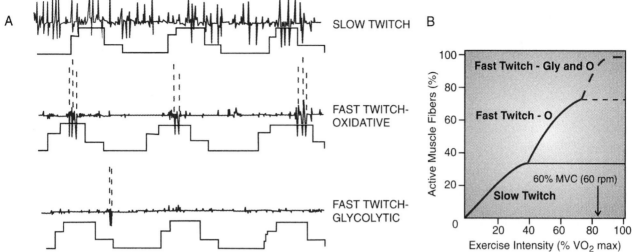

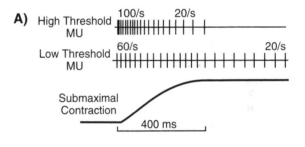

FIGURE 4-9 The order of activation of the motor units, termed recruitment, usually follows the size principle: the small slow-twitch fibers are recruited first, followed by the fast-twitch oxidative and last by the fast-twitch gly-colytic fibers. **A.** the muscle activity for the three muscle Types for three support phases in walking. Slow-twitch fibers are used for most of the gait cycle, with some recruitment of fast-twitch fibers at peak activation times. (Reprinted with permission from Grimby, L. [1986]. Single motor unit discharge during voluntary contraction and locomotion. In N. L. Jones et al. [Eds.]. *Human Muscle Power*. Champaign, IL: Human Kinetics, 111–129). **B.** Similar recruitment pattern, with slow-twitch fibers recruited for up to 40% of the exercise intensity, at which point the fast-twitch oxidative fibers are recruited. It is not until 80% of exercise intensity is reached that the fast-twitch glycolytic fibers are recruited (Reprinted with permission from Sale, D. G. [1987]. Influence of exercise and training on motor unit activation. *Exercise and Sport Science Reviews*, 16:95–151, 1987.)

are still recruiting more motor units at 100% of maximum voluntary contraction. The deltoid and the biceps brachii are examples of muscles still recruiting motor units at 80 to 100% of maximum output of the muscle.

The rate coding also varies with fiber type and changes with the type of movement. Examples of the rate coding of both high- and low-threshold fibers in two muscle contractions is illustrated in Figure 4-10. In ballistic movements, the higher-threshold fast-twitch motor units fire at higher rates than the slow-twitch units. To produce rapid accelerations of the segments, the fast-twitch motor units increase the firing rates more than the slow-twitch motor units (14). The high-threshold fast-twitch fibers cannot be driven for any considerable length of time, but it is believed that trained athletes can drive the high-threshold units longer by maintaining the firing rates. This results in the ability to produce a vigorous contraction for a limited time. Eventually, the frequency of motor unit firing will decrease during any continuous muscular contraction, whether vigorous or mild.

🌀 Sensory Neurons

The body requires an input system to provide feedback on the condition and changing characteristics of the musculoskeletal system and other body tissues, such as the skin. Sensors collect information on such events as stretch in the muscle, heat or pressure on the muscle, tension in the muscle, and pain in the extremity. These sensors send

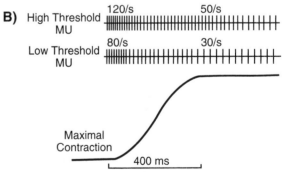

FIGURE 4-10 A. Tension development in the muscle is influenced by the frequency at which a motor unit is activated, termed rate coding. In a submaximal muscle contract and hold, the high-threshold fast-twitch fibers increase firing rates in the ramp phase more than the low-threshold units. The frequency of motor unit firing drops off during the hold phase, and the high-threshold units cease firing. **B.** In a more vigorous contract and hold, the rate coding increases and is maintained further into the contraction by both the high and low threshold motor units (Reprinted with permission from Sale, D. G. [1987]. Influence of exercise and training on motor unit activation. *Exercise and Sport Science Reviews*, 16:95–151, 1987.).

information to the spinal cord, where the information is processed and used by the central nervous system in the adjustment or initiation of motor output to the muscles. These sensors are connected to the spinal cord via **sensory neurons**.

FOUNDATIONS OF NEURAL CONTROL

When the sensory information from one of these receptors brings information into the cord, triggering a predictable motor response, it is termed a **reflex**. A simple reflex arc is shown in Figure 4-11. Some reflexes have sensory information entering and motor information leaving the spinal cord at the same level, creating a **monosynaptic reflex arc**. An example of this reflex is the stretch or **myotatic reflex**, stimulated by sensory neurons responding to stretch in the muscle, which in turn initiates an increase in the motor input to the same muscle (35).

Other reflexes using a simple reflex arc are the **flexor reflex**, which initiates a quick withdrawal response after receiving sensory information indicating pain, and the **cutaneous reflex**, which causes relaxation of a muscle after receiving stimuli on the skin in the form of massage and heat. Knowledge of the cutaneous reflex is beneficial for athletic trainers and physical therapists using heat and massage to create relaxation in a segment or joint.

Reflexes that bring information into the spinal cord and are processed through both sides and different levels of the spinal cord are termed **propriospinal**. An example of this type of reflex is the **crossed extensor reflex**, which is initiated by receiving or expecting to receive a painful stimulus, such as stepping on a nail. This sensory information is processed in the spinal cord by creating a flexor and withdrawal response in the pained limb and an increase or excitation in the extension muscles of the other limb.

Another propriospinal reflex is the **tonic neck reflex**, stimulated by movements of the head that create a motor response in the arms. When the head is rotated to the left, this reflex stimulates an asymmetric response of extension of the same-side arm (left) and a flexion of the opposite arm (right). Also, when the head flexes or extends, this reflex initiates flexion or extension of the arms, respectively.

Another type of reflex is the **supraspinal reflex**, which brings information into the spinal cord and processes it in the brain. The result is a motor response. The **labyrinthine righting reflex** is an example of this type of reflex. This reflex is stimulated by leaning, being upside down, or falling out of an upright posture. The response from the upper centers is to stimulate a motor response from the neck and limbs to maintain or move to an upright position. This complex reflex involves many levels of the spinal cord as well as the upper centers of the nervous system. Examples of these various reflex actions are presented in Figure 4-12.

SENSORY RECEPTORS

The main sensory receptors for the musculoskeletal system are the **proprioceptors**, which transform mechanical distortion in the muscle or joint, such as any change in joint position, muscle length, or muscle tension, into nerve impulses that enter the spinal cord and stimulate a motor response (35).

Muscle Spindle

The **muscle spindle** is a proprioceptor, found in higher abundance in the belly of the muscle, lying parallel to the muscle fibers, and actually connecting into the fascicles via connective tissue (Fig. 4-13). The fibers of the muscle spindle are termed intrafusal as compared to muscle fibers that are termed extrafusal. The **intrafusal fibers** of the spindle are contained within a capsule, forming a spindle shape, hence the name muscle spindle. Some muscles, such as those of the eye, hand, and upper back, have hundreds of spindles, while other muscles, such as the latissimus dorsi and other shoulder muscles, may have only a handful of spindles (35). Every muscle has some spindles. However, the muscle spindle is absent from some of the Type IIb fast-twitch glycolytic muscle fibers within some muscles.

Each spindle capsule may contain as many as 12 intrafusal fibers, which can be either of two types: nuclear bag or nuclear chain (35). Both types of fibers have noncontractile centers that contain the nuclei of the fiber and contractile ends that can be innervated, creating shortening upon receipt of motor input. Also, both fiber types have sensory nerve fibers exiting from the equatorial region or center of the fibers, taking information into the system through the dorsal root of the spinal cord.

The **nuclear bag fiber** has a large cluster of nuclei in its center. It is also thicker, and its fibers connect to the capsule and to the actual connective tissue of the muscle fiber itself. The contractile poles of the nuclear bag fiber are innervated by a gamma or fusimotor motor neuron, smaller than the alpha motor neuron that innervates the muscle fibers. These neurons in the ventral horn of the spinal column are

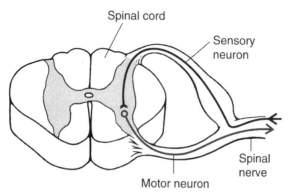

FIGURE 4-11 A simple reflex arc. Sensory information from receptors is brought into the cord, where it initiates a motor response sent back out to the extremities. The stretch reflex is a reflex arc that sends sensory information into the cord in response to stretch of the muscle; the cord sends back motor stimulation to the same muscle, causing a contraction.

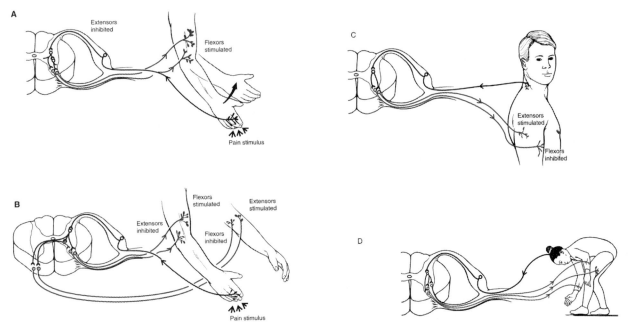

FIGURE 4-12 Examples of reflex actions (a reflex is a motor response developed in the central nervous system after sensory input is received). **A.** The flexor reflex is triggered by sensory information registering pain, which facilitates a quick flexor withdrawal from the pain source. **B.** The crossed extensor reflex is also initiated by pain; it works with the flexor reflex to create flexion on the stimulated limb and extension on the contralateral limb. **C.** The tonic neck reflex is stimulated by head movements; it creates flexion or extension of the arms, depending on the direction of the neck movement. **D.** The labyrinthine righting reflex is stimulated by body positioning; it causes movements of the limbs and neck to maintain a balanced, upright posture.

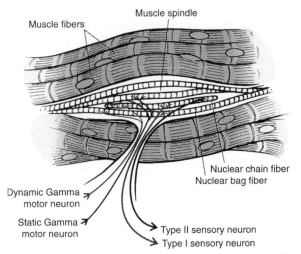

FIGURE 4-13 The muscle spindle lies parallel with the muscle fibers. Within each spindle capsule are the spindle fibers, which can be either of two Types: nuclear chain or nuclear bag fibers. Both Types have contractile ends that are innervated by gamma motor neurons. Sensory information responding to stretch leaves the middle portion of both the chain and bag fibers through the Type Ia sensory neuron and from the ends of the nuclear chain fibers via the Type II sensory neuron.

intermingled with the alpha motor neurons. Each **gamma motor neuron** innervates multiple muscle spindles. The gamma motor neuron to the nuclear bag fiber is often termed the dynamic gamma motor neuron.

Exiting from the equatorial region of the nuclear bag fiber is the Type Ia or **primary afferent** motor neuron.

There is one Type Ia afferent motor neuron per muscle spindle that sends information into the spinal cord via the dorsal horn of the spinal cord. The cell body, or soma, of these sensory neurons lies just outside the spinal cord, is large in diameter, and discharges in response to stretch in the muscle.

The **nuclear chain fiber** is smaller, with the nuclei arranged in rows in the equatorial region. The nuclear chain fiber does not connect to the actual muscle fiber but only makes connection with the spindle capsule. The ends of the nuclear chain fiber are also contractile and are innervated by a gamma motor neuron sometimes referred to as the static gamma or static fusimotor motor neuron.

The nuclear chain fiber has two types of sensory neurons exiting from the noncontractile portion of the fiber. In the middle of the nuclear chain fiber, the Type Ia primary afferent sensory neuron exits, taking information into the spinal cord. This sensory neuron is identical to the one leaving from the nuclear bag fiber.

From the polar ends of the nuclear chain fiber, a Type II or **secondary afferent** sensory neuron exits, traveling into the dorsal horn of the spinal cord. This sensory neuron is medium sized and is stimulated by stretch in the muscle, responding at a higher threshold of stretch than the Type I sensory neuron. There are generally one or two Type II sensory neurons per muscle spindle. However, some muscle spindles and even some muscles (10–20%) have no Type II sensory neurons (35).

The muscle spindle responds to stretch of the muscle fiber because the nucleated middle portion of the muscle spindle fibers, containing the Type I spiral and the Type II flower spray sensory neuron endings also stretches and elongates. The Type I sensory neurons are more sensitive to stretch, or change in length, in the muscle because of a lower threshold, so they are the first to respond to the muscle stretch. As the muscle is stretched, the Type I generates a sensory impulse. If the muscle is stretched more rapidly, the impulses increase proportionally to the rate of stretch and fire at a higher rate. At the end of the stretch, when there is a pause in the motion, the Type I sensory impulse firing level will drop to a lower level and then fire at a constant rate. This represents a static response of muscle stretch in a fixed position.

When a stretch is imposed on the muscle, the Type I sensory neuron sends impulses into the spinal cord and connects with interneurons, generating an excitatory local graded potential that is sent back to the muscle being stretched. If the stretch is vigorous enough, a local graded impulse will be sent back to the same muscle with sufficient magnitude to initiate a contraction via the alpha motor neurons. This reflex arc known as the **stretch reflex** is characterized by a quick muscular contraction following a rapid stretch of that same muscle group. The Type Ia loop is illustrated in Figure 4-14. It is also termed **autogenic facilitation** because of the facilitation of the alpha motor neurons of the same muscle. The stretch reflex primarily recruits slow-twitch muscle fibers.

The information coming into the spinal cord via the Type I sensory neuron is also sent to the cerebellum and cerebral sensory areas to be used as feedback on muscle length and velocity. Additional connections are made in the spinal cord with inhibitory interneurons, creating a **reciprocal inhibition**, or relaxation of the antagonistic muscles (18). Other excitatory interneuron connections are made with the alpha motor neurons of synergistic muscles to facilitate their muscle activity along with the agonist.

When the Type II, or secondary, afferent neuron is stimulated, it has a different response from that of the Type I sensory neuron. It produces a sensory input in response to stretch or change in length in the muscle, and it is a good feedback indicator of the actual length in the muscle because its sensory impulses do not diminish when the muscle is held in a stationary position.

The Type II sensory information enters the dorsal root of the spinal cord and produces an inhibitory local graded potential in the same muscle that was stretched. This lowers the excitability in the muscle and can cause relaxation of the muscle if the stretch is substantial enough.

The innervation of the ends of the spindle fibers by the gamma motor neuron alters the response of the muscle spindle considerably. The first important effect of gamma innervation of the spindle is that it does not allow the spindle discharge to cease when a muscle is shortened. If the muscle shortened with no gamma innervation of the ends of the spindle, the spindle activity would be silenced by the removal of the external stretch on the muscle. The gamma motor neurons create a contraction at the ends of the spindle fibers, elongating the middle portion of the spindle in the same way an external stretch of the muscle

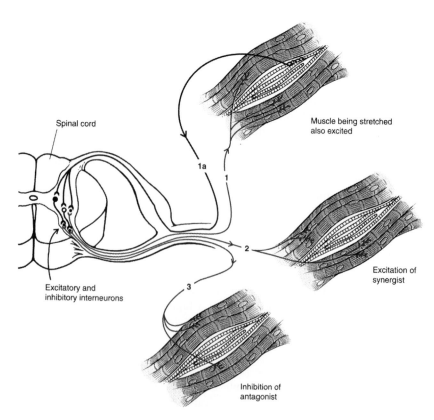

FIGURE 4-14 The Type Ia loop initiated by a stretch of the muscle. Responding proportionally to the rate of stretch, the muscle spindle sends impulses to the spinal cord via the Type Ia sensory neuron. Within the cord, connections with interneurons produce a local graded potential that inhibits the antagonistic muscles and excites the synergists and the muscle in which the stretch occurred. This is the typical stretch reflex response, also termed autogenic facilitation.

would (35). This is called **gamma bias**, or resetting of the muscle spindle.

The second major input from the gamma motor neuron innervation of the muscle spindle is an indirect enhancement of the motor impulses being sent to the muscle via the alpha neuron pathways. This adds to the impulses coming down through the system, alters the gain, and increases the potential for full activation via the alpha pathways. It is a main contributor to coordinating the output and patterning of the alpha motor neurons.

In anticipation of lifting something heavy, the alpha and gamma motor neurons will establish a certain level of excitability in the system for accommodating the heavy resistance. If the object lifted is much lighter than anticipated, the gamma system will act to reduce the output of the Type I afferent. It will make a quick adjustment in the alpha motor neuron output to the muscle and reduce the number of motor units activated.

Finally, the gamma motor neuron is activated at a lower threshold than the alpha motor neuron and can therefore initiate responses to postural changes by resetting the spindle and activating the alpha output (16). The afferent pathways, the gamma pathways, and the alpha pathways are all part of the **gamma loop**, shown in Figure 4-15.

Golgi Tendon Organ

Another important proprioceptor significantly influencing muscular action is the **Golgi tendon organ** (GTO). This structure monitors force or tension in the muscle. As illustrated in Figure 4-16, the GTO lies at the musculoskeletal junction. It is a spindle-shaped collection of collagen fascicles surrounded by a capsule that continues inside the fascicles to create compartments. The collagen fibers of the GTO are connected directly to **extrafusal fibers** from the muscles (35).

Two sensory neurons exit from a site between the collagen fascicles. When the collagen is compressed through a stretch or contraction of the muscle fibers, the Type Ib nerve endings of the GTO generate a sensory impulse proportional to the amount of deformation created in them. The response to the load and the rate of change in the load are linear. Several muscle fibers insert in one GTO, and any tension generated in any of the muscles will generate a response in the GTO.

In a stretch of the muscle, the tension in the individual GTO is generated along with all other GTOs in the tendon. Consequently, the GTO response is more sensitive in tension than in stretch. This is because the GTO measures load bearing in series with the muscle fibers but is parallel to the tension developed in the passive elements during stretch (20). Thus, contraction has a lower threshold than stretch.

The GTO generates an inhibitory local graded potential in the spinal cord known as the **inverse stretch reflex**. If the graded potential is sufficient, relaxation or autogenic inhibition will be produced in the muscle fibers connected in series with the GTO stimulated. The alpha motor neuron output to muscles undergoing a high velocity stretch or producing a high resistance output is reduced.

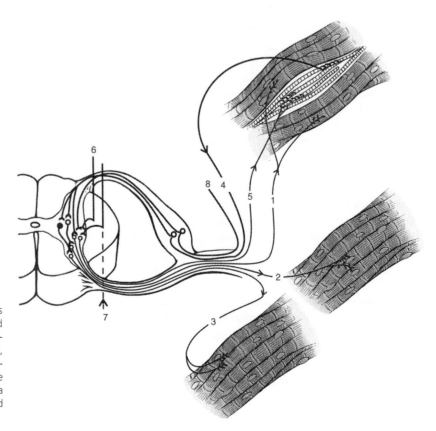

FIGURE 4-15 The Type Ia loop in which information is sent from the spindle (4), causing inhibition (3) and excitation of synergists and agonists (2, 1). It is facilitated by input from the gamma motor neuron (5), which initiates a contraction of the ends of the spindle fibers, creating an internal stretch of the spindle fibers. The gamma motor neuron receives input via the upper centers or other interneurons in the cord (6, 7, 8).

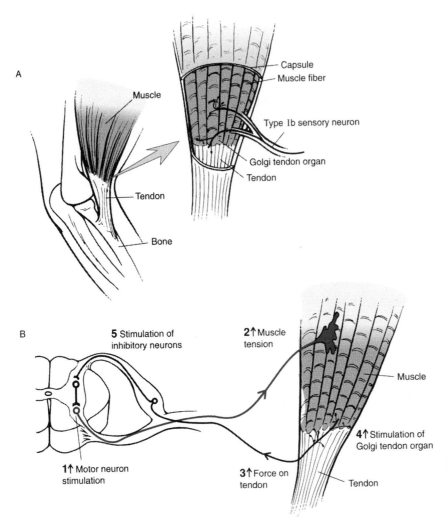

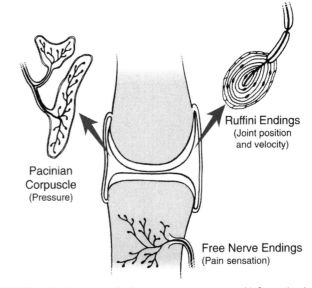

FIGURE 4-16 A. The Golgi tendon organ (GTO) is at the muscle–tendon junction. **B.** When there is tension at this site, the GTO sends information into the spinal cord via Type Ib sensory neurons. The sensory input from the GTO facilitates relaxation of the muscle via stimulation of inhibitory interneurons. This response is as the inverse stretch reflex, or autogenic inhibition.

The GTO response is seen as a critical determinant to maximum lifting levels in weight training. It also may be responsible for uncoordinated action in the inexperienced performer by shutting down a muscle at the inappropriate time in the sequence. This is a simplistic description of the impact of GTO input. The GTO response can be inhibited in extreme circumstances, such as when a mother lifts a car off a child.

Joint Sensory Receptors

There is limited information on the sensory neuron input from the joint receptors placed in and around the synovial joints (Fig. 4-17). One such receptor, the **Ruffini ending**, lies in the joint capsule and responds to change in joint position and velocity of movement of the joint (29). The **pacinian corpuscle** is another joint receptor in the capsule and connective tissue that responds to pressure created by the muscles and to pain within the joint (29). These joint receptors, as well as other receptors in the ligaments and tendons, provide continuous input to the nervous system about the conditions in and around the joint.

FIGURE 4-17 A number of other sensory receptors send information into the central nervous system. In the joint capsules and connective tissue is found the pacinian corpuscle, which responds to pressure, and the Ruffini endings, which respond to changes in joint position. Also, free nerve endings around the joints create pain sensations.

Effect of Training on Neurological Input and Output

During training of the muscular system, a neural adaptation modifies the activation levels and patterns of the neural input to the muscle. In strength training, for example, significant strength gains can be demonstrated after approximately 4 weeks of training. This strength gain is not due to an increase in muscle fiber size but is rather a learning effect in which neural adaptation has occurred (32).

The effect of the neural adaptation is an improved muscular contraction of higher quality through coordination of motor unit activation. The neural input to the muscle, as a consequence of maximal voluntary contractions, is increased to the agonists and synergists, and there is greater inhibition of the antagonists. This neural adaptation, or learning effect, levels off after about 4 to 5 weeks of training. Increases in strength beyond this point are usually due to structural changes and physical increases in the cross-section of the muscle. The influence of training on both the electromechanical delay and the amount of electromyographic activity is presented from the work of Hakkinen and Komi (15) in Figure 4-18.

Specificity of training is important for enhancement of neural input to the muscles. If one limb is trained at a time, greater force production can be attained with more neural input to the muscles of that limb than if two limbs are trained at once. The loss of both force and neural input to the muscles through bilateral training is termed **bilateral deficit** (3,9). In fact, training of one limb will even neurologically enhance the activity and increase the voluntary strength in the other limb.

When working with athletes who use the limbs asymmetrically, as in running or throwing, the trainer should incorporate some unilateral limb movements into the conditioning program. Participants in sports or activities that use both limbs together, such as weight lifters, should train bilaterally.

Specificity of training also determines the fiber type that is enhanced and developed. Through resistive training, Type II fibers can be enhanced through reduction in central inhibition and increased neural facilitation. This may serve to resist fatigue in short-term, high-intensity exercise in which the fatigue is brought on by the inability to maintain optimal nerve activation.

Even a short warmup (5–10 minutes) preceding an event or performance will influence neural input by increasing the motor unit activity (22). Another factor enhancing the neural input to the muscle is the use of an antagonistic muscle contraction that precedes the contraction of the agonist, such as seen in preparatory movements in a skill (e.g., backswing, lowering). This diminishes the inhibitory input to the agonist and allows for more neural input and activation in the agonist contraction.

A stretch of a muscle before it contracts produces some neural stimulation of the muscle via the stretch reflex arc. Athletes who must produce power, such as jumpers and sprinters, have been shown to have excitable systems where the reflex potentiation is high (22).

In summary, the neural input to the muscle can be enhanced through training to increase the number of active motor units contributing, alter the pattern of firing, and increase the reflex potentiation of the system (28). Likewise, immobilization of the muscle can create the opposite response by lowering neural input to the muscle and decreasing reflex potentiation.

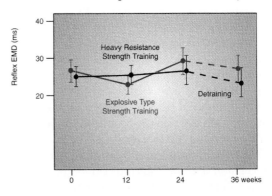

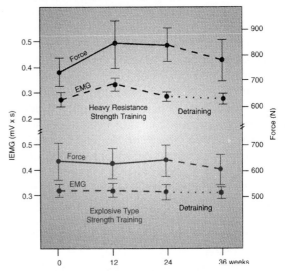

FIGURE 4-18 A. Explosive strength training has been shown to decrease the electromechanical delay (EMD) in the muscle contraction after 12 weeks of training. However, the EMD increases again if training continues to 24 weeks and drops off slightly with detraining. The influence of heavy resistance training on EMD is negligible. **B.** The IEMG increases in the early weeks during heavy resistance training but not with explosive training. It is believed that some neural adaptation occurs in the early stages of specific types of resistance training, which facilitates an early increase in force production. (Reprinted with permission from Hakkinen, K., and Komi, P. V. [1986]. Training-induced changes in neuromuscular performance under voluntary and reflex conditions. *European Journal of Applied Physiology*, 55:147–155.)

Stretching the Muscle

FLEXIBILITY TECHNIQUES

Flexibility is an essential component of physical fitness. Increased flexibility has been shown to improve efficiency of movement, reduce the incidence of muscle strain, improve posture, and generally improve skill in certain sports. Flexibility, as it is used in this section, is defined as the terminal range of motion of a segment. This can be obtained actively through some voluntary contraction of an agonist creating the joint movement (**active range of motion**) or passively, as when the agonist muscles are relaxed as the segment is moved through a range of motion by an external force, such as another person or object (**passive range of motion**) (33,38).

Many components contribute to one's flexibility or lack thereof. First, joint structure is a determinant of flexibility; it will limit the range of motion in some joints and produce the termination or end point of the movement. This is true in a joint such as the elbow, in which the movement of extension is terminated by bony contact between the olecranon process and fossa on the back of the joint. A person who can hyperextend the forearm at the elbow is not one who is exceptionally flexible but is someone who has either a deep olecranon fossa or a small olecranon process. Bony restrictions to range of motion are present in a variety of joints in the body but this type of restriction is not the main mechanism limiting or enhancing joint flexibility.

Soft tissue around the joint is another factor contributing to flexibility. As a joint nears the ends of the range of motion, the soft tissue of one segment will be compressed by the soft tissue of the adjacent segment. This compression between adjacent tissue components will eventually contribute to the termination of the range of motion.

This means that obese individuals and individuals with large amounts of muscle mass or hypertrophy will usually demonstrate lower levels of flexibility. However, the hypertrophied individual can obtain good flexibility in a joint by applying a greater force at the end of the range of motion that can compress the restrictive soft tissue to a greater degree. The obese individual who lacks strength will definitely be limited in flexibility because of an inability to produce the force necessary to achieve the greater range of motion.

Ligaments restrict range of motion and flexibility by offering maximal support at the end of the range of motion. For example, the ligaments of the knee terminate the extension of the leg. An individual who can hyperextend the knees is commonly called double jointed but actually has slightly long ligaments that allow more than the usual joint motion.

The main factors influencing flexibility are the actual physical length of the antagonistic muscle or muscles and the level of neurological innervation in a muscle being stretched. Both of these factors can be influenced by specific types of flexibility training.

Neurological Restrictions

When a muscle is stretched, three neurological mechanisms restrict the range of motion. First, the Type Ia primary afferent sensory neuron initiates the stretch reflex, creating increased muscular activity through alpha motor neuron innervation. This response is proportional to the rate of stretch. Thus, the faster the stretch, the more the same muscle contracts. After the stretch is completed, the Type Ia sensory neurons will drop to a lower firing level, reducing the level of motor neuron activation or resistance in the muscle. A flexibility technique that enhances this response is **ballistic stretching**, in which the segments are bounced to achieve the terminal range of motion. This type of stretching is not recommended for the improvement of flexibility because of the stimulation of the Type Ia neurons and the increase in the resistance in the muscle. However, ballistic stretching is a component of many common movements, such as a preparatory windup in baseball or the end of the follow-through in a kick.

A better stretching technique for the improvement of range of motion is **static stretching**, in which the limb is moved slightly beyond the terminal position slowly and then maintained in that position for at least 30 seconds (6). Moving the limb slowly decreases the response of the Type Ia sensory neuron, and holding the position at the end significantly reduces the Type Ia input, allowing minimal interference to the joint movement.

The second neurological factor in flexibility is the input of the Type II secondary afferent sensory neuron. This sensory input will be facilitated by change in length in the muscle, producing relaxation of the stretched muscle through the generation of a local graded potential that is also inhibitory.

The third neurological input is the inverse stretch reflex produced by the GTO. The GTO response occurs mainly in the active stretch, when the limb is voluntarily moving into the terminal joint position. If the stretch is extreme, the GTO will initiate the inverse stretch reflex, which may relax the muscle being stretched or the muscle being contracted to produce the stretch, depending on the level of the tensions generated in each GTO.

Structural Restrictions

The primary restriction to the stretch of a muscle is found in the connective tissue and tendons in and around the muscle (13,26). This includes the fascia, epimysium, perimysium, endomysium, and tendons. The actual muscle fibers do not play a significant role in the elongation of a muscle through flexibility training. To understand how the connective tissue responds to a stretch, it is necessary to examine the stress–strain characteristics of the muscle unit.

When a stretch is first imposed, the muscle creates a linear response to the load through elongation in all parts of the muscle. This is the elastic phase of external stretch. If the external load is removed from the muscle during this phase of stretching, it will return to its original length within a few hours and no residual or long-term increase in muscle length will remain. The stretching techniques working the elastic response of the muscle are common; they include short-duration, repetitive joint movements. These stretches, usually preceding an activity, will produce some increase in muscle length for use in the practice or game but will not produce any long-term improvement in flexibility.

If a muscle is put in a terminal position and maintained in the position for an extended period, the tissue enters the plastic region of response to the load, elongating and undergoing plastic deformation (37). This plastic deformation is a long-term increase in the length of the muscle and will carry over from day to day (24). A model describing the behavior of the elastic and plastic elements acting in a stretch is presented in Figure 4-19.

To create increases in length due to plastic or long-term elongation, the muscle should be stretched while it is warm, and the stretch should be maintained for a long time under a low load (29,30). Thus, to gain long-term benefits from stretching, the stretch should occur after a practice or workout, and individual stretches should be held in the terminal joint positions for an extended period.

Cooling of a warm muscle enhances the permanent elongation of the tissues in that muscle. It is recommended that the joint positions be held for at least 30 seconds and ideally up to a minute. However, in muscles that are inflexible and require extra attention, stretching should occur for longer times, 6 to 10 minutes (34). To avoid any significant tissue damage, stretching with pain should not take place.

Proprioceptive Neuromuscular Facilitation

The enhancement of permanent elongation of the muscle tissue can be attained through the use of a static stretch. Another technique, **proprioceptive neuromuscular facilitation** (PNF), can be used to stimulate relaxation of the stretched muscle so that the joint can be moved through a greater range of motion (21). This technique, used in rehabilitation settings, can also be put to good use with athletes and individuals who have limited flexibility in certain muscle groups, such as the hamstrings (30).

PNF incorporates various combination sequences using relaxation and contraction of the muscles being stretched. A simple PNF exercise is passive movement of an individual's limb into the terminal range of motion, have him or her contract back isometrically against the manual resistance applied by a partner, and then relax and move further into the stretch. Repeating this cycle can achieve a significant increase in the terminal range of motion (12). This procedure increases the range of motion because the input from the Type Ia afferent from the muscle spindle is reduced by the resetting of the spindle (16).

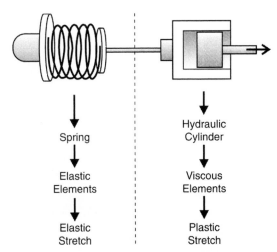

FIGURE 4-19 When a repetitive stretch of short duration is applied to the muscle, the connective tissue and muscle respond like a spring, with a short-term elongation of the tissue but a return to the original length after a short time. In a long-term sustained stretch, especially while the muscle is warm, the tissues behave more hydraulically, as a long-term deformation of the tissues takes place. (Reprinted with permission from Sapega, A. A., Quedenfeld, T. C., Moyer, R. A., and Butler, R. A. [1981]. Biophysical factors in range of motion exercises. *Physician and Sports Medicine*, 9:57–64.)

The process can be enhanced even more if a contraction of the agonist occurs at the end of the range of motion. This sets up an increase in the relaxation of the antagonist or the muscle being stretched. For example, passively move the foot into plantarflexion to stretch the dorsiflexors. Contract the dorsiflexors isometrically against resistance applied by a partner on the top of the foot. Move the foot farther into plantarflexion and then contract the plantar flexors. Both of these techniques will produce the greatest increase in the range of motion. Examples of PNF exercises for the muscles of the hip and shoulder joint are presented in Figure 4-20.

Plyometric Training

The purpose of **plyometric training** is to improve the velocity of a performance. Plyometric training has been effective in increasing power output from athletes in sports such as volleyball, basketball, high jumping, long jumping, throwing, and sprinting. Plyometrics builds on the idea of specificity of training, whereby a muscle trained at higher velocities will function better at those velocities.

The plyometric exercise consists of rapidly stretching a muscle and immediately following with a contraction of the same muscle (3). Plyometric exercises improve power output in the muscle through facilitation of the neurological input to the muscle and through increased muscle tension generated in the elastic components of the muscle. An examination of both these factors in greater detail follows.

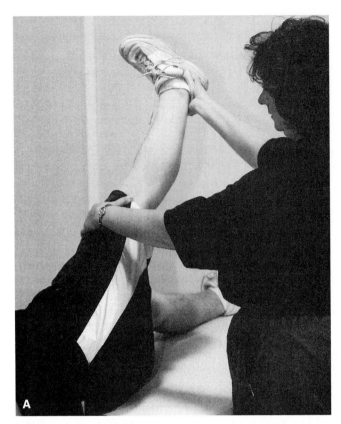
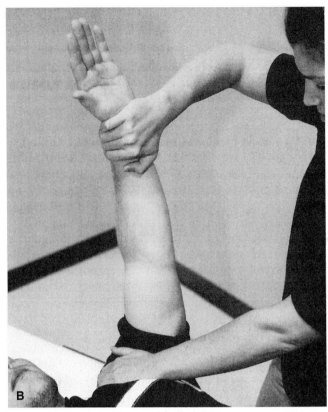

FIGURE 4-20 Proprioceptive neuromuscular facilitation (PNF) stretching is effective for increasing flexibility in areas such as the hip and shoulder. Examples of PNF exercises for the muscles of the hip and shoulder are provided. **A.** At the hip, the thigh moves through a diagonal pattern, with manual resistance applied at the foot and the thigh. **B.** In the shoulder, the arm moves into flexion, with manual resistance offered at the hand.

NEUROLOGICAL INFLUENCES

The neurological basis for plyometrics is the input from the stretch reflex via the Type Ia sensory neuron. Rapid stretching of the muscle produces excitation of the alpha motor neurons contracting that muscle. This excitation is increased with the velocity of the stretch and is maximum at the conclusion of a rapid stretch, after which the excitation levels drop. Thus, if a muscle can be rapidly stretched and immediately contracted with no pause at the end of the stretch, this reflex loop will produce maximum facilitation. If an individual pauses at the end of the stretch, this myoneural input will be greatly diminished. The myoelectric enhancement of the muscle being stretched accounts for approximately 25 to 30% of the increase of the force output in the plyometric stretch–contract sequence (23).

STRUCTURAL INFLUENCES

The factor accounting for most of the increases in output (70–75%) as a consequence of plyometric exercise is the restitution of elastic energy in the muscle (23). When a muscle is stretched, elastic potential energy is stored in the connective tissue and tendon and in the cross-bridges as they are rotated back with the stretch (1). With a vigorous short-term stretch, maximal recovery of the elastic potential energy is returned to the succeeding contraction of that same muscle. The net result of this short-range pre-stretch with a small time period between the stretch and the contraction is that larger forces can be produced for any given velocity, enhancing the power output of the system (7). Implementation of this technique suggests that a quick stretch through a limited range of motion should be followed immediately with a vigorous contraction of the same muscle.

Plyometric Examples

A plyometric exercise program includes a series of exercises imposing a rapid stretch followed by a vigorous contraction. Since the muscle is undergoing a vigorous eccentric contraction, attention should be given to the number of exercises and the load imposed through the eccentric contraction (11,25). It is suggested that plyometric exercises be done on yielding surfaces and not more than 2 days a week. Injury rates will be higher in the use of plyometric training if these factors are not taken into account. Further, plyometric training should be used very conservatively when the participants lack strength in

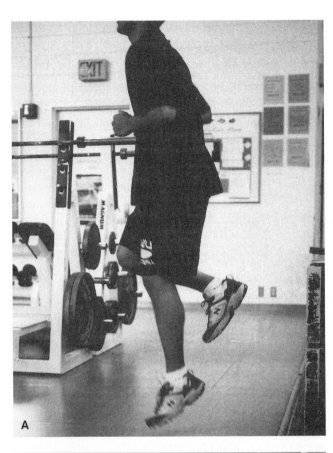
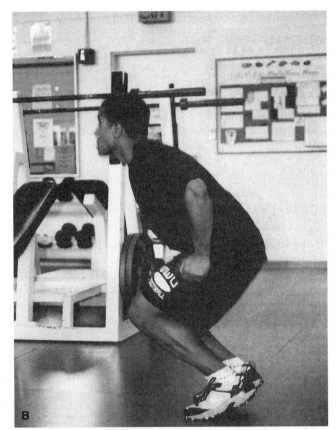
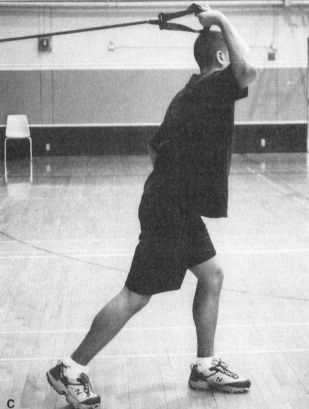
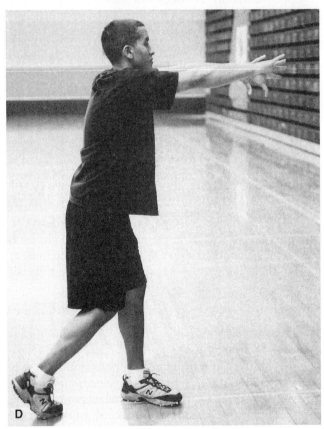

FIGURE 4-21 Plyometric exercises can be developed for any sport or region of the body by use of a stretch–contract cycle in exercise. Examples of plyometric exercises for the lower extremity include bounding **(A)** and depth **(B)** jumps. For the upper extremity, the use of surgical tubing **(C)** and medicine ball throws **(D)** are good exercises.

the muscles being trained. A strength base should be developed first. It is suggested that an individual be able to squat 60% of body weight 5 times in 5 seconds before beginning plyometrics (10). This is done to see if eccentric and concentric muscle actions can be reversed quickly.

Lower extremity plyometric exercises include activities such as single-leg bounds, depth jumps from various heights, stair hopping, double-leg speed hops, split jumps, bench jumps, and quick countermovement jumping. The height from which the plyometric jump is performed is an important consideration. Heights can range from 0.25 to 1.5 m and should be based on the fitness level of the participant. A height is too high if a quick, vigorous rebound cannot be achieved shortly after landing.

Plyometric exercises can be done 1 to 2 times per week by a conditioned athlete. A sample plyometric workout may include 3 to 5 low intensity exercises (10–20 repetitions), such as jumping in place or double-leg hops; 3 to 4 moderate intensity exercises (5–10 repetitions) including single-leg hops, double-leg hops over a hurdle or bounding; and 2 to 3 high-intensity exercises, including depth jumping (5–10 repetitions). In the beginning, the height of the box for depth jumping should be limited to avoid injury, since the amount of force to be absorbed and controlled will increase with each height increase.

Upper extremity activities can best be implemented with surgical tubing or material that can be stretched. The muscle can be pulled into a stretch by the surgical tubing, after which the muscle can contract against the resistance offered by the tubing. For example, hold surgical tubing in a diagonal position across the back and simulate a throwing motion with the right hand while holding the left hand in place. The arm will generate a movement against the surgical tube resistance and then be drawn back into a quick stretch by the tension generated in the tubing. These resistive tubes or straps can be purchased in varying resistances, offering compatibility with a variety of different strength levels.

Other forms of upper extremity plyometrics include catching a medicine ball and immediately throwing it. This puts a rapid stretch on the muscle in the catch that is followed by a concentric contraction of the same muscles in the throw. Figure 4-21 shows specific plyometric exercises.

Summary

The nervous system controls and monitors human movement by transmitting and receiving signals through an extensive neural network. The central nervous system, consisting of the brain and the spinal cord, works with the peripheral nervous system via 31 pairs of spinal nerves that lie outside the spinal cord. The main signal transmitter of the nervous system is the motor neuron, which carries the impulse to the muscle.

The nerve impulse travels to the muscle as an action potential, and when it reaches the muscle, a similar action potential develops in the muscle, eventually initiating a muscle contraction. The actual tension in the muscle is determined by the number of motor units actively stimulated at one time.

Sensory neurons play an important role in the nervous system by providing feedback on the characteristics of the muscle or other tissues. When a sensory neuron brings information into the spinal cord and initiates a motor response, it is termed a reflex. The main sensory neurons for the musculoskeletal system are the proprioceptors. One proprioceptor, the muscle spindle, brings information into the spinal cord about any change in the muscle length or velocity of a muscle stretch. Another important proprioceptor is the GTO, which responds to tension in the muscle.

Flexibility, an important component of fitness, is influenced by a neurological restriction to stretching that is produced by the proprioceptive input from the muscle spindle. Another area of training that uses the neurological input from the sensory neurons is plyometrics. A plyometric exercise is one that involves a rapid stretch of a muscle that is immediately followed by a contraction of the same muscle.

REVIEW QUESTIONS

True or False

1. ____ The nervous system consists of two major parts.

2. ____ The central nervous system consists of all of the branches of nerves that lie outside the spinal chord.

3. ____ The sensory nerves enter the spinal cord on the dorsal side.

4. ____ Motor neurons send signals from the motor units to the spinal cord.

5. ____ There are 33 pairs of spinal nerves that enter and exit the spinal cord.

6. ____ The body of the nerve cell is also called the soma.

7. ____ Projections on the cell body called dendrites serve as receivers and bring information into the neuron from other neurons.

8. ____ A bundle of dendrites will contain dendrites from one neuron pool only.

9. ____ The neuron contacts the muscle fiber at the neuromuscular junction.

10. ____ The muscle fibers innervated by each motor unit are concentrated in one section of the muscle.

11. ____ When a motor unit is initially activated, most of the fibers will contract immediately.

12. ____ Muscle fiber type is basically genetic, but it has been shown that specific training can transform Type I fibers to Type II fibers.

13. ____ The amplitude of a nerve action potential impulse varies with the demand for muscle tension.

14. ___ The small motor neurons are used over a broad tension range before the moderate or large motor neurons are recruited.

15. ___ Rate coding increases only after all of the motor units are recruited.

16. ___ Stepping on a sharp object will initiate a retrospinal reflex.

17. ___ Resetting of the muscle spindle is also known as gamma bias.

18. ___ Anticipation of lifting something heavy stimulates both the alpha and gamma motor neurons.

19. ___ The sensory impulse generated by the Golgi tendon organ is directly proportional to the amount of deformation erected in them.

20. ___ Strength gain during the first 4 weeks of a strength training program is typically the result of neural adaptation.

21. ___ Training of one limb can increase the strength of the contralateral limb.

22. ___ PNF uses rapid contractions.

23. ___ It is suggested that plyometric training be done no more than 1 day per week.

24. ___ The primary factor influencing flexibility is joint structure.

25. ___ To reduce the Type Ia response to stretching, a person should use a bouncing technique.

Multiple Choice

1. Motor neurons ___.
   a. Send signals from the motor units
   b. Send signals to the motor units
   c. Receive signals from the periphery
   d. None of the above

2. ___ nerves innervate the muscles of the upper extremity.
   a. 6
   b. 9
   c. 10
   d. 12

3. Bundles of cell bodies just outside of the spinal cord are called ___.
   a. Dendrites
   b. Ganglia
   c. Myelin
   d. None of the above

4. The axon of motor neurons is fairly large, making it capable of transmitting impulses up to ___ m/second.
   a. 50
   b. 100
   c. 150
   d. 200

5. When the motor neuron approaches a muscle fiber, it breaks off into unmyelinated terminals called ___.
   a. Nerve endings
   b. Synaptic gaps
   c. Motor endplates
   d. None of the above

6. The signal in the motor neuron ___.
   a. Moves directly into the muscle
   b. Is transmitted chemically
   c. Causes the muscle to contract
   d. None of the above

7. A neuron may terminate on as many as ___ or as few as ___ fibers.
   a. 100, 20
   b. 500, 6
   c. 2000, 5
   d. 4000, 100

8. A muscle with a low nerve to fiber ratio will have ___.
   a. More power
   b. More control
   c. Both a and b
   d. None of the above

9. A single motor unit may innervate ___ fibers.
   a. Type I and Type II
   b. Type IIa and Type IIb or Type I
   c. Both a and b
   d. None of the above.

10. Large alpha neurons typically innervate Type ___ muscle fibers.
    a. I
    b. IIa
    c. IIb
    d. Any of the above

11. At rest the electrical potential on the inside of the nerve membrane has a value of ___.
    a. 70m/v
    b. −70m/v
    c. 90m/v
    d. −90m/v

12. The sequence of motor unit recruitment is usually ___.
    a. I, IIa, IIb
    b. IIb, IIa, I
    c. IIa, IIb, I
    d. IIb, IIa, I

13. The labyrinthine righting reflex is an example of a ___ reflex.
    a. Simple
    b. Propriospinal
    c. Balancing
    d. Supraspinal

14. Proprioceptors transform mechanical distortion of (the) ___ into nerve impulses.
    a. Muscle tension
    b. Joints
    c. Muscle length
    d. All of the above

15. The cutaneous reflex causes a(n) ___.
    a. Increase in motor input to the same muscle
    b. Quick withdrawal response
    c. Relaxation
    d. Both a and b.

16. The muscle spindle is ___.
    a. A proprioceptor
    b. Perpendicular to the muscle fibers
    c. Intrafusal
    d. Both a and c

17. Sensory impulses from type ___ sensory neurons do not diminish when the muscle is stationary.
    a. Ia
    b. II
    c. A and b
    d. Both types maintain a steady impulse level

18. The contractile ends of the sensory neurons are innervated by ___ motor neurons.
    a. Alpha
    b. Beta
    c. Gamma
    d. Depends on type of neuron

19. In autogenic facilitation a local graded potential ___ the agonist and ___ the antagonist.
    a. Inhibits, excites
    b. Excites, inhibits
    c. Inhibits, inhibits
    d. Depends on what is causing movement

20. The GTO monitors ___.
    a. Muscle length
    b. Movement
    c. Joint position
    d. Muscle tension

21. The GTO is responsible for ___.
    a. Determining range of motion
    b. Autogenic facilitation
    c. Autogenic inhibition
    d. None of the above

22. Ruffini endings are located in the ___.
    a. Ligaments
    b. Muscles
    c. Tendons
    d. Joint capsules

23. The pacinian corpuscle responds to ___ and ___.
    a. Joint position, velocity
    b. Velocity, pressure
    c. Pressure, pain
    d. Pain, velocity

24. It is recommended that muscles needing large improvements in flexibility be held in the terminal position for up to ___.
    a. 60 seconds
    b. 90 seconds
    c. 6 minutes
    d. 26 minutes

25. Plyometric training uses ___ to improve performance.
    a. The elastic components
    b. Hypertrophy
    c. Enhanced neurological input
    d. A and c

REFERENCES

1. Asmussen, E., Bonde-Peterson, F. (1974). Storage of elastic energy in skeletal muscles in man. *Acta Physiologica Scandinavia*, 91:385–392.

2. Basmajian, J. V. (1978). *Muscles Alive: Their Functions Revealed by Electromyography* (4th Ed.). Baltimore: Williams & Wilkins.

3. Bedi, J. F., et al. (1987). Increase in jumping height associated with maximal vertical depth jumps. *Research Quarterly for Exercise and Sport*, 58(1):11–15.

4. Bigland-Ritchie, B., et al. (1983). Changes in motor neuron firing rates during sustained maximal voluntary contractions. *Journal of Physiology*, 340:335–346.

5. Billeter, R., Hoppeler, H. (1992). Muscular basis of strength. In P. Komi (Ed.). *Strength and Power in Sport*. Boston: Blackwell Scientific, 39–63.

6. Blanke, D. (1982). Flexibility training: Ballistic, static, or proprioceptive neuromuscular facilitation. *Archives of Physical Medicine Rehabilitation*, 63:261–263.

7. Bosco, C., et al. (1982). Neuromuscular function and mechanical efficiency of human leg extensor muscles during jumping exercises. *Acta Physiologica Scandinavia*, 114:543–550.

8. Burke, R. E. (1981). Motor units: Anatomy, physiology, and functional organization. In J. M. Brookhart, V. B. Mountcastle (Eds.). *Handbook of Physiology: The Nervous System*. Bethesda, MD: American Physiological Society, 345–422.

9. Burke, R. E. (1986). The control of muscle force: Motor unit recruitment and firing patterns. In N. L. Jones et al. (Eds.). *Human Muscle Power*. Champaign, IL: Human Kinetics, 97–109.

10. Chu, D. (1983). Plyometrics: The link between strength and speed. *National Strength and Conditioning Association Journal*, 5:20–21.

11. Chu, D., Plummer, L. (1985). The language of plyometrics. *National Strength and Conditioning Association Journal*, 6:30–31.

12. Entyre, B. R., Abraham, L. D. (1986). Reflex changes during static stretching and two variations of proprioceptive neuromuscular facilitation techniques. *Electroencephalography and Clinical Neurophysiology*, 63:174–179.

13. Garrett, W. E., et al. (1987). Biomechanical comparison of stimulated and nonstimulated skeletal muscle pulled to failure. *American Journal of Sports Medicine*, 15:448–454.

14. Grimby, L. (1986). Single motor unit discharge during voluntary contraction and locomotion. In N. L. Jones et al. (Eds.). *Human Muscle Power*. Champaign, IL: Human Kinetics, 111–129.

15. Hakkinen, K., Komi, P. V. (1986). Training-induced changes in neuromuscular performance under voluntary and reflex conditions. *European Journal of Applied Physiology*, 55:147–155.

16. Hardy, L., Jones, D. (1986). Dynamic flexibility and proprioceptive neuromuscular facilitation. *Research Quarterly for Exercise and Sport*, 51:625–635.

17. Howald, H. (1982). Training-induced morphological and functional changes in skeletal muscle. *International Journal of Sports Medicine*, 3:1–12.

18. Hultborn, H., et al. (1971). Recurrent inhibition of interneurons monosynaptically activated from group Ia afferents. *Journal of Physiology*, 215:613–636.

19. Hultborn, H. (1972). Convergence on interneurons in the reciprocal Ia inhibitory pathway to motor neurons. *Acta Physiologica Scandinavica*, 84 (Suppl.): 375.

20. Jansen, J. K., Rudford, T. (1964). On the silent period and Golgi tendon organs of the soleus muscle of the cat. *Acta Physiologica Scandinavica*, 62:364–379.

21. Knot, M., Voss, D. E. (1968). *Proprioceptive Neuromuscular Facilitation: Patterns and Techniques* (2nd Ed.). New York: Harper and Row.

22. Koceja, D. M., Kamen, G. (1992). Segmental reflex organization in endurance-trained athletes and untrained subjects. *Medicine and Science in Sports and Exercise*, 24(2):235–241.

23. Komi, P. V. (1986b). The stretch-shortening cycle and human power output. In N. L. Jones et al. (Eds.). *Human Muscle Power*. Champaign, IL: Human Kinetics, 27–42.

24. Kottke, F. J., et al. (1966). The rationale for prolonged stretching for correction of shortening of connective tissue. *Archives of Physical Medicine and Rehabilitation*, 47:345–352.

25. Lundin, P. (1985). A review of plyometric training. *National Strength and Conditioning Association Journal*, 7(3):69–74.

26. McHugh, M. P., et al. (1992). Viscoelastic stress relaxation in human skeletal muscle. *Medicine Science and Sports Exercise*, 24(12):1375–1382.

27. Moritani, T., DeVries, H. A. (1979). Neural factors versus hypertrophy in the time course of muscle strength gain. *American Journal of Physical Medicine*, 58(3):115–130.

28. Moritani, T. (1993). Neuromuscular adaptations during the acquisition of muscle strength, power, and motor tasks. *Journal of Biomechanics*, 26:95–107.

29. Newton, R. A. (1982). Joint receptor contributions to reflexive and kinesthetic responses. *Physical Therapy*, 62(1):23–29.

30. Osternig, L. R., et al. (1990). Differential responses to proprioceptive neuromuscular facilitation (PNF) stretch techniques. *Medicine and Science in Sports and Exercise*, 22:106–111.

31. Sale, D. G. (1987). Influence of exercise and training on motor unit activation. In K. B. Pandolf (Ed.). *Exercise and Sport Science Reviews*, 16:95–151.

32. Sale, D. G. (1988). Neural adaptation to resistance training. *Medicine and Science in Sport and Exercise*, 20:S135–145.

33. Sandy, S. P., et al. (1982). Flexibility training: Ballistic, static, or proprioceptive neuromuscular facilitation? *Archives of Physical Medicine and Rehabilitation*, 6:132–138.

34. Sapega, A. A., et al. (1981). Biophysical factors in range of motion exercises. *Physician and Sports Medicine*, 9:57–64.

35. Smith, J. L. (1976). Fusimotor loop properties and involvement during voluntary movement. In J. Keogh, R. S. Hutton (Eds.). *Exercise and Sport Sciences Reviews*, 4:297–333.

36. Stern, R. M., et al. (1980). *Psychophysiological Recording*. New York: Oxford Press.

37. Taylor, D. C., et al. (1990). Viscoelastic properties of muscle-tendon units: The biomechanical effects of stretching. *American Journal of Sports Medicine*, 18:300–309.

38. Wallin, D. V., et al. (1985). Improvement of muscle flexibility: A comparison between two techniques. *American Journal of Sports Medicine*, 13:263–268.

ADDITIONAL READING

Asmussen, E. (1979). Muscle fatigue. *Medicine Science and Sports*, 11:313–321.

Aura, O., Komi, P. V. (1987). Coupling time in stretch-shortening cycle: Influence on mechanical efficiency and elastic characteristics of leg extensor muscles. In B. Jonsson (Ed.). *Biomechanics XA*. Champaign, IL: Human Kinetics, 507–511.

Beaulieu, J. E. (1981). Developing a stretching program. *Physician and Sports Medicine*, 9(11):5–65.

Bobbert, M. F., et al. (1987). Drop jumping. I. The influence of jumping techniques on the biomechanics of jumping. *Medicine and Science in Sports and Exercise*, 19(4):332–338.

Close, J. D. (1973). *Functional Anatomy of the Extremities*. Springfield, IL: Charles C. Thomas.

Cracraft, J. D., Petajan, J. H. (1977). Effect of muscle training on the pattern of firing of single motor units. *American Journal of Physical Medicine*, 56:183–194.

Edgerton, V. R. (1976). Neuromuscular adaptation to power and endurance work. *Canadian Journal of Applied Physiology*, 56:296–301.

Hakkinen, K., et al. (1985). Changes in isometric force and relaxation time, electromyographic and muscle fibre characteristics of human skeletal muscle during strength training and detraining. *Acta Physiologica Scandinavia*, 125:573–585.

Hickson, R. C., et al. (1988). Potential for strength and endurance training to amplify endurance performance. *Journal of Applied Physiology*, 65:2285–2290.

LaBan, M. M. (1962). Collagen tissue: Implications of its response to stress in vitro. *Archives of Physical Medicine and Rehabilitation*, 43:461–466.

Ozguven, N. H., Berme, N. (1988). An experimental and analytical study of impact forces during human jumping. *Journal of Biomechanics*, 21:1061–1066.

Person, R. S., Kudina, L. P. (1972). Discharge frequency and discharge pattern of human motor units during voluntary contraction of muscle. *Electroencephalography and Clinical Neurophysiology*, 32:471–483.

Sullivan, M. K., et al. (1992). Effect of pelvic position and stretching method on hamstring muscle flexibility. *Medicine Science and Sports Exercise*, 24:1383–1389.

Stein, R. B., et al. (1986). What is optimized in muscular movements? In N. L. Jones et al. (Eds.). *Human Muscle Power*. Champaign, IL: Human Kinetics, 131–150.

Tesch, P. A., et al. (1983). Influence of lactate accumulation of EMG frequency spectrum during repeated concentric contractions. *Acta Physiologica Scandinavia*, 119:61–67.

GLOSSARY

Action Potential: An electrical current that travels through the nerve or muscle as the membrane potential changes due to the exchange of ions.

Active Range of Motion: The range of motion achieved through some voluntary contraction of an agonist creating the joint movement.

All-or-None Principle: The stimulation of a muscle fiber that will cause the action potential to travel over either the whole muscle fiber (activation threshold) or none of the muscle fiber.

Alpha Motor Neuron: An afferent neuron with a large cell body in or near the spinal cord from which a long axon projects from the spinal cord to the muscle fibers which it innervates.

Asynchronous: Describing events that do not occur at the same time. In skeletal muscle contraction, the spacing of the activation of the motor unit.

Autogenic Facilitation: Internally generated excitation of the alpha motor neurons through stretch or some other input.

Axon: Neuron process carrying nerve impulses away from the cell body of the neuron. The pathway through which the nerve impulse travels.

Ballistic Stretching: Moving a limb to the terminal range of motion through rapid movements initiated by strong muscular contractions and continued by momentum.

Bilateral Deficit: The loss of both force and neural input to the muscles through bilateral training of both limbs.

Cell Body: The portion of the neuron that contains the nucleus and a well-marked nucleolus. The cell body receives information through the dendrites and sends information through the axon. Also called the soma.

Central Nervous System: The brain and the spinal cord.

Crossed Extensor Reflex: Reflex causing extension of a flexed limb when stimulated by rapid flexion or withdrawal by the contralateral limb.

Cutaneous Reflex: Reflex that causes relaxation of the muscle upon receiving stimuli in the form of heat or massage.

Dendrites: Processes on the neuron that receive information and transmit information to the cell body of the neuron.

Extrafusal Fiber: Fibers outside the muscle spindle; muscle fibers.

Flexor Reflex: Reflex initiated by a painful stimulus that causes a withdrawal or flexion of the limb away from the stimulus.

Frequency Coding: See Rate Coding.

Gamma Bias: Readjustment of the muscle spindle length by contracting the ends of the intrafusal fiber. Initiated by voluntary control, such as when anticipating the receipt of a heavy weight.

Gamma Loop: A reflex arc that works with the stretch reflex, in which descending motor pathways synapse with both alpha and gamma motor neurons of the muscle fiber and the muscle spindle.

Gamma Motor Neuron: A neuron that innervates the contractile ends of the muscle spindle.

Ganglia: Nerve cell bodies outside the central nervous system.

Golgi Tendon Organ: A sensory receptor located at the muscle–tendon junction that responds to tension generated during both stretch and contraction of the muscle. Initiates the inverse stretch reflex if the activation threshold is reached.

Interneuron: Small, connecting neuron in the spinal cord; can be excitatory or inhibitory.

Intrafusal Fiber: Fibers that are inside the muscle spindle.

Inverse Stretch Reflex: Reflex initiated by high tension in the muscle, which inhibits contraction of the muscle through the Golgi tendon organ, causing relaxation of a vigorously contracting muscle.

Labyrinthine Righting Reflex: Reflex stimulated by tilting or spinning of the body, which alters the fluid in the inner ear. The body responds to restore balance by bringing the head to the neutral position or thrusting arms and legs out for balance.

Local Graded Potential: An excitatory or inhibitory signal in the nerve or muscle that is not propagated.

Monosynaptic Reflex Arc: The reflex arc whereby a sensory neuron is stimulated and facilitates the stimulation of a spinal motor neuron.

Motor End Plates: A flattened expansion in the sarcolemma of the muscle that contains receptors to receive the expansions from the axonal terminals; also called the neuromuscular junction.

Motor Neurons: Neurons that carry impulses from the brain and spinal cord to the muscle receptors.

Motor Unit: A motor neuron and all of the muscle cells it stimulates.

Muscle Spindle: An encapsulated sensory receptor that lies parallel to muscle fibers; responds to stretch of the muscle.

Myelinated: Nerve fibers having a myelin sheath composed of a fatty insulated lipid substance.

Myotatic Reflex: Reflex initiated by stretching the muscle, which facilitates a contraction of the same muscle via muscle spindle stimulation; also called the stretch reflex.

Neuromuscular Junction: Region where the motor neuron comes into close contact with the skeletal muscle; also called the motor endplate.

Neuron: A conducting cell in the nervous system that specializes in generating and transmitting nerve impulses.

Node of Ranvier: Gaps in the myelinated axon where the axon is enclosed only by processes of the Schwann cells.

Nuclear Bag Fiber: An intrafusal fiber within the muscle spindle having a large clustering of nuclei in the center. The Type Ia afferent neurons exit from the middle portion of this fiber.

Nuclear Chain Fiber: An intrafusal fiber within the muscle spindle with nuclei arranged in rows. Both Type Ia and the Type II sensory neurons exit from this fiber.

Pacinian Corpuscle: Sensory receptor in the skin that is stimulated by pressure.

Passive Range of Motion: The degree of motion that occurs between two adjacent segments through external manipulation, such as gravity or manual manipulation.

Peripheral Nerve System: All nerve branches lying outside the brain and spinal cord.

Plyometric Training: Exercise that uses the stretch–contract sequence of muscle activity.

Primary Afferent: Sensory nerve fibers from the muscle spindle that are sensitive to stretch and respond to stretch by initiating the stretch reflex.

Proprioceptive Neuromuscular Facilitation: Rehabilitation technique that enhances the response from a muscle through a series of contract–relax exercises.

Proprioceptor: A sensory receptor in the joint, muscle, or tendon that can detect stimuli.

Propriospinal Reflex: Reflex processed on both sides and at different levels of the spinal cord; an example is the crossed extensor reflex.

Rate Coding: The frequency of the discharge of the action potentials. Also referred to as frequency coding.

Reciprocal Inhibition: Relaxation of the antagonistic muscle(s) while the agonist muscles produce a joint action.

Recruitment: A system of motor unit activation.

Reflex: Involuntary response to a stimuli.

Renshaw Cell: Interneuron that receives excitatory input from collateral branches of other neurons and then produces an inhibitory effect on other neurons.

Ruffini Ending: Sensory receptors in the joint capsule that respond to change in joint position.

Schwann Cells: Cells that cover the axon and produce myelination, which is numerous concentric layers of the Schwann cell plasma membrane.

Secondary Afferent: Sensory nerve fibers from the muscle spindle that are sensitive to stretch, and that facilitate flexors and inhibit extensor activity.

Sensory Neuron: Neuron that carries impulses from the receptors in the body into the central nervous system.

Size Principle: The principle that describes the order of motor unit recruitment as a function of size.

Soma: The portion of the nerve cell that contains the nucleus and well-marked nucleolus. The soma receives information from the dendrites and sends information through the axon; also called the cell body.

Spinal Nerves: The 31 pairs of nerves that arise from the various levels of the spinal cord.

Static Stretching: Moving a limb to the terminal range of motion slowly and then holding the final position.

Stretch Reflex: Reflex initiated by stretching the muscle, which facilitates a contraction of the same muscle via muscle spindle stimulation; also called the myotatic reflex.

Supraspinal Reflex: Reflex brought into the spinal cord but processed in the brain; example is the labyrinthine righting reflex.

Synapse: The junction or point of close contact between two neurons or between a neuron and a target cell.

Synchronous: Describes events occurring at the same time. In muscular contraction, the concurrent activation of motor units.

Tonic Neck Reflex: Reflex stimulated by head movements, which stimulates flexion and extension of the limbs. The arms flex with head flexion and extend with neck extension.

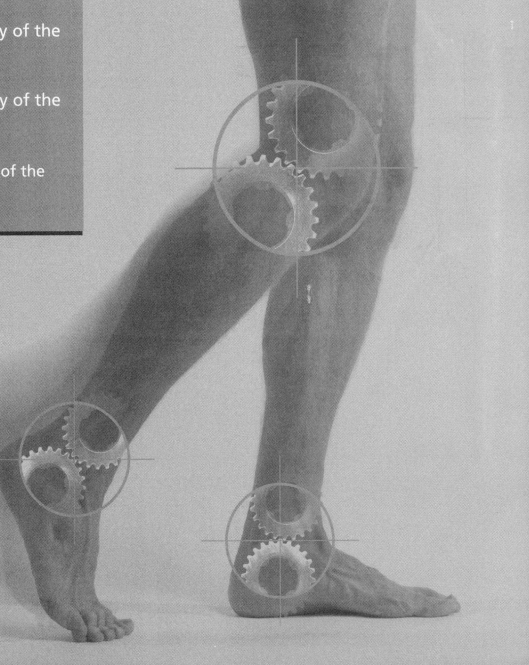

Functional Anatomy

5

Functional Anatomy of the Upper Extremity

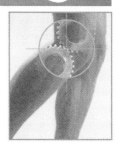

OBJECTIVES

After reading this chapter, the student will be able to:

1. Describe the structure, support, and movements of the joints of the shoulder girdle, shoulder joint, elbow, wrist, and hand.

2. Describe the scapulohumeral rhythm in an arm movement.

3. Identify the muscular actions contributing to shoulder girdle, elbow, wrist, and hand movements.

4. Explain the differences in muscle strength across the different arm movements.

5. Identify common injuries to the shoulder, elbow, wrist, and hand.

6. Develop a set of strength and flexibility exercises for the upper extremity.

7. Identify the upper extremity muscular contributions to activities of daily living (i.e., rising from a chair), throwing, swimming, and swinging a golf club.

8. Describe some common wrist and hand positions used in precision or power.

Introduction

The upper extremity is interesting from a functional anatomy perspective because of the interplay among the various joints and segments necessary for smooth, efficient movement. Movements of the hand are made more effective through proper hand positioning by the elbow, shoulder joint, and **shoulder girdle**. Also, forearm movements occur in concert with both hand and shoulder movements. These movements would not be half as effective if the movements occurred in isolation.

The Shoulder Complex

The shoulder complex has many articulations, each contributing to the movement of the arm through coordinated joint actions. Observing the motion of the **scapula** is the best way of understanding the actions of two of the shoulder articulations: the **sternoclavicular joint** and the **acromioclavicular joint**. Arm movements, on the other hand, take place at the **glenohumeral joint**. While it is possible to create a small amount of movement at any one of these articulations in isolation, usually movement is generated at all three of these joints concomitantly as the arm is raised or lowered or if any other significant arm action is produced (50).

ANATOMICAL AND FUNCTIONAL CHARACTERISTICS OF THE JOINTS OF THE SHOULDER

Sternoclavicular Joint

The only point of skeletal attachment of the upper extremity to the trunk occurs at the sternoclavicular joint. At this joint the **clavicle** is joined to the manubrium of the sternum. A close view of the sternoclavicular joint is shown in Figure 5-1. This gliding synovial joint has a fibrocartilaginous disc (51). The joint is reinforced by three ligaments: the interclavicular, the costoclavicular, and the sternoclavicular ligaments, of which the costoclavicular ligament is the main support for the joint (42). The joint is also reinforced and supported by muscles, such as the short, powerful subclavius. Additionally, a

strong joint capsule contributes to making the joint resilient to **dislocation** or disruption.

Movements of the clavicle at the sternoclavicular joint occur in three directions, giving it three degrees of freedom. The clavicle can move superiorly and inferiorly in movements referred to as **elevation** and **depression**, respectively. These movements take place between the clavicle and the meniscus in the sternoclavicular joint and have a range of motion of approximately 30 to 40° (51).

The clavicle can also move anteriorly and posteriorly via movements termed protraction and retraction, respectively. These movements occur between the sternum and the meniscus in the joint through a range of motion of approximately 30°. Finally, the clavicle can rotate anteriorly and posteriorly along its long axis through approximately 40 to 50° (51).

Acromioclavicular Joint

The clavicle is connected to the scapula at its distal end via the acromioclavicular (AC) joint. This is a small gliding synovial joint that is not present in all individuals. It frequently has a fibrocartilaginous disc like the sternoclavicular joint (42). It is at this joint that most of the movements of the scapula on the clavicle occur. The acromioclavicular joint is illustrated in Figure 5-2.

The AC joint lies over the top of the humeral head and can serve as a bony restriction to arm movements above the head. The joint is reinforced with a dense capsule and

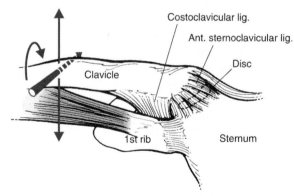

FIGURE 5-1 The sternoclavicular joint is a sturdy, well-reinforced joint that allows movement in three planes. Movements include elevation and depression, protraction and retraction, and rotation.

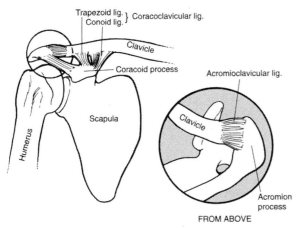

FIGURE 5-2 The acromioclavicular joint is a small joint that allows movement of the scapula on the clavicle. It is vulnerable to injury when forces come up through the arm and the shoulder.

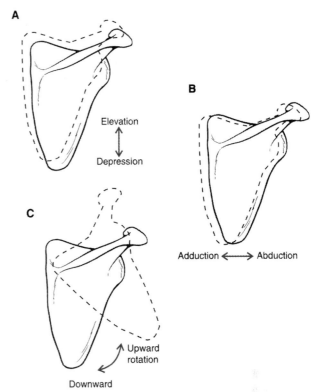

FIGURE 5-3 Scapular movements take place in three directions. **A.** Elevation and depression of the scapula occur with a shoulder shrug or when the arm raises. **B.** Abduction (protraction) and adduction (retraction) occur when the scapulae are drawn away from or toward the vertebrae, respectively, or when the arm is brought in front or behind the body, respectively. **C.** The scapula also rotates upward and downward as the arm raises and lowers, respectively.

a set of acromioclavicular ligaments lying above and below the joint. Close to the AC joint is the important coracoclavicular ligament, which assists scapular movements by serving as an axis of **rotation**.

The movement of the scapula at the acromioclavicular joint can occur in three directions, as shown in Figure 5-3. The scapula can move anteriorly and posteriorly about a vertical axis; these motions are known as **protraction** or **abduction** and **retraction** or **adduction**, respectively. Protraction and retraction occur as the acromion process moves on the meniscus in the joint and as the scapula rotates about the medial coracoclavicular ligament. There can be anywhere from 30 to 50° of protraction and retraction of the scapula (42).

The second scapular movement occurs when the base of the scapula swings laterally and medially in the frontal plane. These actions are termed upward and downward rotation. This movement occurs as the clavicle moves on the meniscus in the joint and as the scapula rotates about the trapezoid portion of the lateral coracoclavicular ligament. This movement can occur through a range of motion of approximately 60° (51).

The third and final movement potential, or degree of freedom, is the scapular movement up and down, termed elevation and depression. This movement occurs at the acromioclavicular joint and is not assisted by rotations about the coracoclavicular ligament. The range of motion at the acromioclavicular joint for elevation and depression is approximately 30° (51,42).

The scapula movements also depend on the movement and position of the clavicle. The movements at the sternoclavicular joint are opposite to the movements at the acromioclavicular joint for elevation, depression, protraction, and retraction. For example, as elevation occurs at the acromioclavicular joint, depression occurs at the sternoclavicular joint and vice versa. This is not true for rotation, since the clavicle will rotate in the same direction along its length. The clavicle does rotate in different directions to accommodate the movements of the scapula: anteriorly with protraction and elevation and posteriorly with retraction and depression.

Scapulothoracic Joint

The scapula interfaces with the thorax via the **scapulothoracic joint**. This is not a typical articulation, connecting bone to bone. It is a physiological joint (51). The scapula actually rests on two muscles, the serratus anterior and the subscapularis, both connected to the scapula and moving across each other as the scapula moves. Underneath these two muscles lies the thorax.

The scapula moves across the thorax as a consequence of actions at the acromioclavicular and the sternoclavicular joints, giving a total range of motion for the scapulothoracic articulation of approximately 60° of motion for 180° of arm abduction or flexion. Approximately 65% of this range of motion occurs at the sternoclavicular joint, and 35% occurs as a result of acromioclavicular joint motion (51).

Glenohumeral Joint

The final articulation in the shoulder complex is the shoulder joint, or the glenohumeral joint, illustrated in

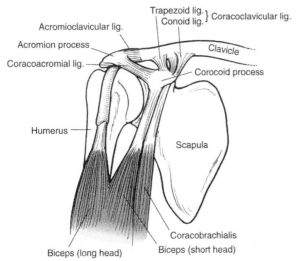

FIGURE 5-4 The glenohumeral joint is a ball-and-socket joint that relies on the muscles, ligaments, and other soft tissue for support. It is one of the most mobile joints in the body.

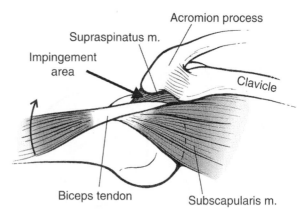

FIGURE 5-5 The impingement area of the shoulder contains structures that can be damaged with repeated overuse. The actual impingement occurs in the abducted position with the arm rotated.

Figure 5-4. Motions at the shoulder joint are represented by the movements of the arm. This is a synovial ball-and-socket joint, offering the greatest range of motion and movement potential of any joint in the body. The reason for the laxity and the excessive range of motion allowed in the joint is the structural makeup, that is, a lax joint capsule and limited ligamentous support.

The joint contains a small, shallow socket called the **glenoid fossa**. This socket is only one-fourth the size of the humeral head that must fit into it. The joint cavity is deepened by a rim of fibrocartilage referred to as the **glenoid labrum**. This structure receives supplementary reinforcement from the surrounding ligaments and tendons. The labrum varies from individual to individual and is even absent in some cases (39). The glenoid labrum increases the contact area to 75%. The joint capsule has approximately twice the volume of the humeral head, allowing the arm to be raised through a considerable range of motion (16).

Ligaments
Because there is minimal contact between the glenoid fossa and the head of the humerus, the shoulder joint largely depends on the ligamentous and muscular structures for stability. On the anterior side of the joint, support is provided by the capsule, the glenoid labrum, the glenohumeral ligaments, three reinforcements in the capsule, the coracohumeral ligament, fibers of the subscapularis, and the pectoralis major. These muscles blend into the joint capsule (16). Both the coracohumeral and the middle glenohumeral ligament support and hold up the relaxed arm. They also offer functional support through abduction, external rotation, and extension (42). Posteriorly, the joint is reinforced by the capsule, the glenoid labrum, and fibers from the teres minor and infraspinatus, which also blend into the capsule. Location and support action of ligaments of the shoulder girdle and shoulder joint are included in Appendix A.

The superior aspect of the shoulder joint is often termed the impingement area. The glenoid labrum, the coracohumeral ligament, and the muscles support the superior portion of the shoulder joint, and the supraspinatus and the long head of the biceps brachii reinforce the capsule. Above the supraspinatus muscle lie the **subacromial bursae** and the coracoacromial ligament. These form an arch underneath the acromioclavicular joint. This area and a typical impingement position are presented in Figure 5-5.

A **bursa** is a fluid-filled sac found at strategic sites around the synovial joints that reduces the friction in the joint. The supraspinatus muscle and the bursae in this area are compressed as the arm rises above the head and can be irritated if the compression is of sufficient magnitude or duration. The inferior portion of the shoulder joint is minimally reinforced by the capsule and the long head of the triceps brachii.

Movement Characteristics
The range of motion of the arm at the shoulder joint is considerable for the aforementioned structural reasons (Fig. 5-6). The arm can move through approximately 180° of flexion to approximately 60° of hyperextension in the sagittal plane (7,51). The amount of flexion can be limited if the shoulder joint is also externally rotated. With the joint in maximal external rotation, the arm can be flexed through only 30° (7). Also, during passive flexion and extension, there is accompanying anterior and posterior translation, respectively, of the head of the humerus on the glenoid (17).

The arm can also abduct through 180°. The abduction movement can be limited by the amount of internal rotation occurring simultaneously with abduction. If the joint is maximally rotated internally, the arm can produce only about 60° of abduction (7). As the arm adducts down to the anatomical or neutral position, it can continue past the neutral position for approximately 75° of hyperadduction across the body.

The arm can rotate both internally and externally 90°, for a total of 180° of rotation (16). Rotation is limited by

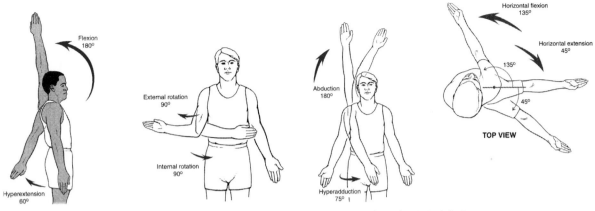

FIGURE 5-6 The shoulder has considerable range of motion. The arm can move through 180° of flexion or abduction, 60° of hyperextension, 75° of hyperadduction, 90° of internal and external rotation, 135° of horizontal flexion, and 45° of horizontal extension.

abduction of the arm. In anatomical position, the arm can rotate through the full 180°, but in 90° of abduction, the arm can rotate only through 90° (7). Finally, the arm can move across the body in an elevated position for 135° of **horizontal flexion** or adduction and 45° of **horizontal extension** or abduction (51).

Extreme range of motion is required in many activities, such as throwing, tennis, swimming, and gymnastics (52). Some athletes who commonly produce movements using extreme joint positions can have a loose shoulder joint such that the humeral head can actually lose contact with the glenoid cavity in the terminal or extreme positions. At these extreme joint positions, the joint capsule and the ligaments surrounding the shoulder joint are strained. With continued motion at the terminal joint positions, the humeral head can be forced over the glenoid labrum rim into a dislocated or subluxated position, from which it will usually slip back into the socket (50).

With the arm in the anatomical position, the ligaments and many of the supporting muscles are loose. If the arm is externally rotated in this position, the capsule is tightened (18). Internal rotation in this position does not tighten the capsule.

The inferior portion of the glenohumeral joint capsule is loose, allowing the arm to abduct and externally rotate through a significant range of motion. As the arm moves into abduction through 45°, the subscapularis and the lower glenohumeral ligament begin to tighten and support the joint (44). The joint can be stabilized even more with the addition of greater external rotation. This stabilization continues up to 90° of abduction with the activity level of the subscapularis diminishing.

Other muscles, such as the supraspinatus, infraspinatus, and teres minor, also provide stability of the glenohumeral joint through 90° of abduction by compressing the humeral head in the socket. Their contribution to the stability in the joint diminishes with greater than 90° of abduction. However, in extreme abduction with external rotation, the shoulder joint is in a close-packed position

with the ligaments tight around the joint, offering some stability (42).

COMBINED MOVEMENT CHARACTERISTICS OF THE SHOULDER COMPLEX

The movement potential of each joint was examined in the previous section. This section examines the movement of the shoulder complex as a whole, sometimes referred to as scapulohumeral rhythm.

Anytime the arm is raised in flexion or abduction, there are accompanying scapular and clavicular movements. A posterior view of the relationship between the arm and scapular movements is shown in Figure 5-7.

In the first 30° of abduction or the first 45 to 60° of flexion, the scapula moves either toward the vertebral column or away from the vertebral column to seek a position of stability on the thorax (42). After stabilization has been achieved, the scapula moves laterally, anteriorly, and superiorly in the movements described as upward rotation, protraction, or abduction and elevation. The clavicle also rotates posteriorly, elevates, and protracts as the arm moves through flexion or abduction (12).

In the early stages of abduction or flexion, the movements are primarily at the glenohumeral joint except for the stabilizing motions of the scapula. Past 30° of abduction or 45 to 60° of flexion, the ratio of glenohumeral to scapular movements becomes 5:4. That is, there is 5° of humeral movement for every 4° of scapular movement on the thorax (38,42). For the total range of motion through 180° of abduction or flexion, the glenohumeral to scapula ratio is 2:1; thus, the 180° range of motion is produced by 120° of glenohumeral motion and 60° of scapular motion (16). The contributing joint actions to the scapular motion are 20° produced at the acromioclavicular joint, 40° produced at the sternoclavicular joint, and 40° of posterior clavicular rotation (12).

As the arm abducts to 90°, the greater tuberosity on the humeral head approaches the coracoacromial arch,

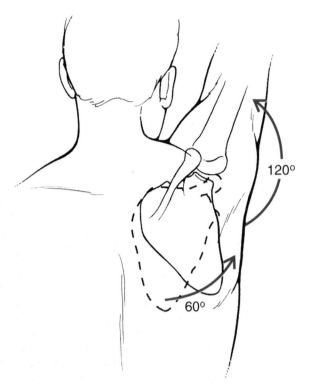

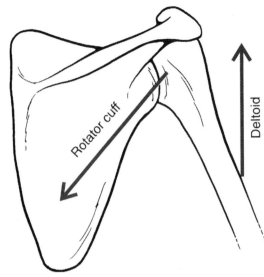

FIGURE 5-8 For efficient flexion or abduction of the arm, the deltoid and the rotator cuff work together. In the early stages of abduction and flexion through 90°, the rotator cuff applies a force to the humeral head that keeps the head depressed and stabilized in the joint while the deltoid applies a force to elevate the arm. This relationship changes in the upper range of motion as the rotator cuff activity drops off.

FIGURE 5-7 The movement of the arm is accompanied by movements of the shoulder girdle. The working relationship between the two is known as the scapulohumeral rhythm. The arm can move through only 30° of abduction and 45 to 60° of flexion with minimal scapular movements. Past these points, the scapula movements occur concomitantly with the arm movements. For 180° of flexion or abduction, approximately 120° of motion occurs in the glenohumeral joint and 60° of motion occurs as a result of scapular movement on the thorax.

compression of the soft tissue begins to limit further abduction, and the tuberosity makes contact with the acromion process (12). If the arm is externally rotated, 30° more abduction can occur as the greater tuberosity is moved out from under the arch. Abduction is limited even more and can occur through only 60° with arm internal rotation, since the greater tuberosity is held under the arch (12). Also, full abduction cannot be achieved without some extension of the upper trunk to assist the movement.

MUSCULAR ACTIONS

The insertion, action, and nerve supply for each individual muscle of the shoulder joint and shoulder girdle are outlined in Appendix B. Special interactions between the muscles are presented in this section.

The muscles contributing to shoulder abduction and flexion are similar. The deltoid generates about 50% of the muscular force for elevation of the arm in abduction or flexion. The contribution of the deltoid increases with increased abduction. The muscle is most active through 90 to 180° (37). However, the deltoid has been shown to be most resistant to fatigue in the range of motion through 45 to 90° of abduction, making this range of motion most popular for arm-raising exercises.

When the arm elevates, the **rotator cuff** (teres minor, subscapularis, infraspinatus, supraspinatus) also plays an important role, since the deltoid cannot abduct or flex the arm without stabilization of the humeral head (51). The rotator cuff as a whole is also capable of generating flexion or abduction with about 50% of the force normally generated in these movements (16).

In the early stages of arm flexion or abduction, the teres minor works with the deltoid to depress the humeral head and stabilize it so that the deltoid can raise the arm (42). The muscle force of the teres minor is equal and opposite to that of the deltoid, so a force couple is formed. The subscapularis and the infraspinatus join a little later in flexion or abduction to assist with the humeral head stabilization (6,25). The latissimus dorsi also contracts eccentrically to assist with the stabilization of the humeral head and increases in activity as the angle increases (25). The interaction between the deltoid and the rotator cuff in abduction and flexion is shown in Figure 5-8. The inferior and medial force of the rotator cuff allows the deltoid to elevate the arm.

Above 90° of flexion or abduction, the rotator cuff force decreases, leaving the shoulder joint more vulnerable to injury (16). However, one of the rotator cuff muscles, the supraspinatus, remains a major contributor above 90° of flexion or abduction. In the upper range of motion, the deltoid begins to pull the humeral head down and out of the joint cavity, thus creating a subluxating force (42). Motion through 90 to 180° of flexion or abduction requires external rotation in the joint. If the humerus externally rotates 20° or more, the biceps brachii can also abduct the arm (16).

When the arm is abducted or flexed, the shoulder girdle must protract or abduct, elevate, and upwardly rotate with posterior clavicular rotation to maintain the glenoid fossa in the optimal position. As shown in Figure 5-9, the serratus anterior and the trapezius work as a force couple

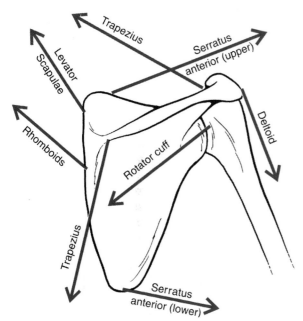

FIGURE 5-9 The direction of pull of various shoulder girdle muscles, the deltoid, and the rotator cuff for the resting arm. Notice the line of pull of the trapezius and the serratus anterior, which work together to produce abduction, elevation, and upward rotation of the scapula necessary in arm flexion or abduction. Likewise, notice the pull of the levator scapulae and the rhomboid, which also assist in elevation of the scapula.

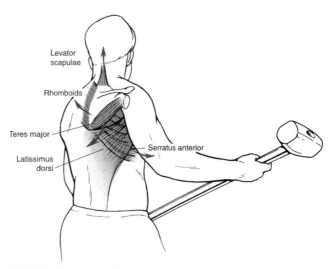

FIGURE 5-10 Lowering the arm against a resistance uses the latissimus dorsi and teres major working as a force coupled with the rhomboid. Other muscles that contribute to the lowering action are the pectoralis major, pectoralis minor, levator scapulae, and serratus anterior.

to create the lateral, superior, and rotational motions of the scapula (16). These muscle actions take place after the deltoid and the teres minor have initiated the elevation of the arm and continue up through 180°, with the greatest muscular activity through 90 to 180° (37). The serratus anterior is also responsible for holding the scapula to the thorax wall and preventing any movement of the medial border of the scapula off the thorax.

If the arm is slowly lowered, producing adduction or extension of the arm with accompanying retraction, depression, and downward rotation of the shoulder girdle with forward clavicular rotation, the muscle actions are eccentric. Therefore, the movement is controlled by the muscles previously described in the arm abduction and flexion section. However, if the arm is forcefully lowered or if it is lowered against external resistance, such as a weight machine, the muscle action will be concentric.

In a concentric adduction or extension against external resistance, such as in a swimming stroke, the muscles responsible for creating these joint actions are the latissimus dorsi, teres major, and sternal portion of the pectoralis major. The teres major is active only against a resistance, whereas the latissimus dorsi has been shown to be active in these movements even when no resistance is offered (9).

As the arm is adducted or extended, the shoulder girdle retracts, depresses, and downwardly rotates with forward clavicular rotation. The rhomboid muscle downwardly rotates the scapula and works with the teres major and the latissimus dorsi in a force couple to control the arm and scapular motions during lowering. Other muscles actively contributing to the movement of the scapula back to the resting position while working against resistance are the

pectoralis minor, which depresses and downwardly rotates the scapula, and the middle and lower portions of the trapezius, which contribute to the retraction of the scapula with the rhomboid. These muscular interactions are illustrated in Figure 5-10.

Two other movements of the arm, very important in many sport skills and in the efficient movement of the arm above 90° (measured from arm at the side), are internal and external rotation. An example of both external and internal rotation in a throwing action is shown in Figure 5-11. External rotation is an important component of the preparatory, or cocking, phase of an overhand throw, and internal rotation is important in the force application and follow-through phase of the throw.

External rotation, necessary when the arm is above 90°, is produced by the infraspinatus and the teres minor (42). The activity of both of these muscles increases with external

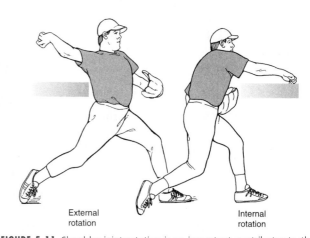

FIGURE 5-11 Shoulder joint rotation is an important contributor to the overhand throw. In the preparatory, or cocking, phase, the arm externally rotates to increase the range of motion and the distance over which the ball will travel. Internal rotation is an active contributor to the force application phase. The movement continues in the follow-through phase as the arm slows down.

rotation in the joint (22). Since the infraspinatus is also an important muscle in humeral head stabilization, it fatigues early in elevated arm activities.

Internal rotation is produced primarily by the subscapularis, latissimus dorsi, teres major, and portions of the pectoralis major. The teres major is an active contributor to internal rotation only when the movement is produced against resistance. The muscles contributing to the internal rotation joint movement are capable of generating a large force, yet the internal rotation in most upper extremity actions never require or use much internal rotation force (42).

The shoulder girdle movements accompanying internal and external rotation depend on the position of the arm. In an elevated arm position, the shoulder girdle movements described in conjunction with abduction and flexion are necessary. Rotation produced with the arm in the neutral or anatomical position requires minimal shoulder girdle assistance. It is also in this position that the full range of rotation through 180° can be obtained. This is so because as the arm is raised, muscles used to rotate the humerus are also used to stabilize the humeral head, which will be restrained in rotation in the upper range of motion. Specifically, internal rotation is difficult in elevated arm positions, since the tissue under the acromion process is very compressed by the greater tuberosity (37).

Two final joint actions that are actually combinations of elevated arm positions are horizontal flexion or adduction and horizontal extension or abduction. Since the arm is elevated, the same muscles described earlier for abduction and flexion also contribute to these movements of the arm across the body.

Muscles contributing more significantly to horizontal flexion are the pectoralis major and the anterior head of the deltoid. This movement brings the arms across the body in the elevated position and is important in power movements of upper extremity skills. Horizontal extension in which the arm is brought back in the elevated position is produced primarily by the infraspinatus, teres minor, and posterior head of the deltoid. This joint action is common in the backswing and preparatory actions in upper extremity skills (51).

STRENGTH OF THE SHOULDER MUSCLES

The shoulder muscles can generate the greatest strength output in adduction when muscle fibers of the latissimus dorsi, teres major, and the pectoralis major contribute to the movement. The adduction strength of the shoulder muscles is twice that for abduction, even though the abduction movement and muscle group are used more frequently in activities of daily living and sport (51).

The movement capable of generating the next greatest level of strength after the adductors is an extension movement that uses the same muscles that contribute to arm adduction. The extension action is slightly stronger than its opposite movement, flexion. Following flexion, the next strongest joint action is abduction, illustrating the fact that shoulder joint actions are capable of generating greater force output in the lowering phase using the adductors and extensors than in the raising phase, when the flexors and abductors are used.

The weakest joint actions in the shoulder are rotational, with external rotation being weaker than internal rotation. The strength output of the rotators is influenced by arm position, and the greatest internal rotation strength can be obtained with the arm in the neutral position. The greatest external rotation strength can be obtained with the shoulder in 90° of flexion. However, with the arm elevated to 45°, both internal and external rotation strength outputs are greater in 45° of abduction than 45° of flexion (15). External rotation is important in the upper 90° of arm elevation, providing stability to the joint. Internal rotation creates instability in the joint, especially in the upper elevation levels, as it compresses the soft tissue in the joint.

Muscle activity in the shoulder complex generates high forces in the shoulder joint itself. The rotator cuff muscle group as a whole, capable of generating a force 9.6 times the weight of the limb, generates maximum forces at 60° of abduction (51). Since each arm constitutes approximately 7% of body weight, the rotator cuff generates a force in the shoulder joint equal to approximately 70% of body weight. At 90° of abduction, the deltoid generates a force averaging 8 to 9 times the weight of the limb, creating a force in the shoulder joint ranging from 40 to 50% of body weight (51). In fact, the forces in the shoulder joint at 90° of abduction have been shown to be close to 90% of body weight. These forces can be significantly reduced if the forearm is flexed to 90° at the elbow.

CONDITIONING

The shoulder muscles are easy to stretch and strengthen because of the mobility of the joint. The examples include both active and passive stretches. In the active stretches, the individual can move the limb to the terminal position without any external force, while in passive stretches, an external force is imposed. The external force is usually a weight or force created manually by the other limb.

In the strengthening categories, both manual resistance and weight lifting illustrations offer suggestions for the poorly conditioned individual and in the rehabilitation setting as well as for any individual with access to a weight-training facility. A manual resistance exercise requires another individual to apply an external force while the subject moves through the desired range of motion. The benefit of manual resistance exercising is that the external force applied by a partner can be readily adjusted to the level the subject can handle. It is a good technique for individuals who lack strength in specific regions. Another technique for a weak muscle group is to begin exercises using body parts such as an arm or leg as the resistance.

The muscles acting on the shoulder joint and shoulder girdle usually work in combination, making it difficult to isolate a specific muscle in an exercise. Examples of stretching, manual resistance, and weight training for the shoulder abductors and flexors are presented in Figure 5-12.

Examples for shoulder adductors and extensors are shown in Figure 5-13. A rowing action is good for the trapezius, levator scapula, and rhomboid muscles, while a push-up motion is effective for the serratus anterior and pectoralis minor (30).

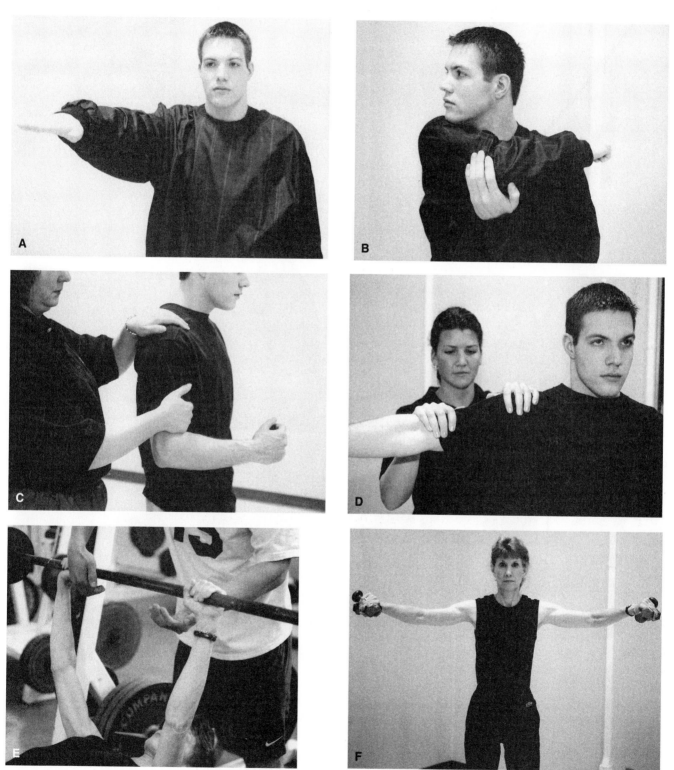

FIGURE 5-12 Flexibility (A and B), Manual Resistance (C and D), and Weight Training (E and F). Illustrations of stretching, manual resistance and weight training examples for shoulder flexion. **(A, C, E)** and abduction **(B, D, F)**. The flexors and abductors can be stretched as the arm is brought horizontally across the chest. Manual resistance in flexion and abduction can be applied to the humerus as the arm is brought forward and up, respectively. A good weight training exercise for the flexors is the bench press and for the abductors, a lateral fly.

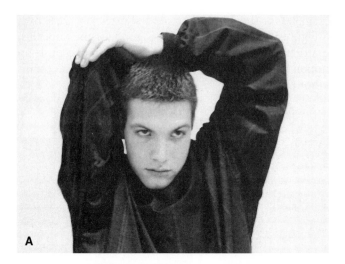

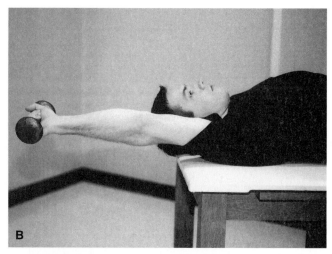

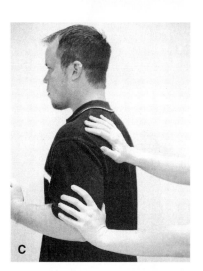

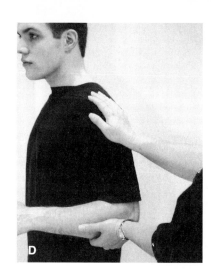

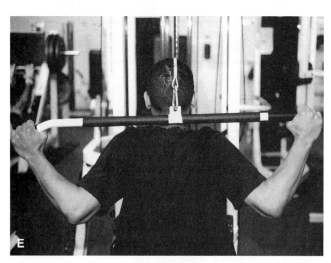

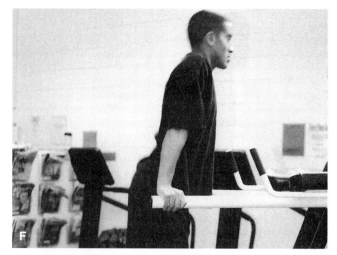

FIGURE 5-13 Flexibility (A and B), Manual Resistance (C and D), and Weight Training (E and F). Flexibility exercises for the extensors and adductors include **(A)** a passive stretch imposed by the other arm and **(B)** a stretch imposed by a lightweight dumbbell. Manual resistance can be applied to the posterior humerus as the arm is pulled back into hyperextension **(C)** or at the elbow as the arm is pulled down into adduction **(D)**. Two good weight-training exercises for the extensors and adductors are the **(E)** lateral pull down and **(F)** dips.

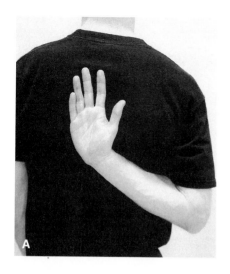
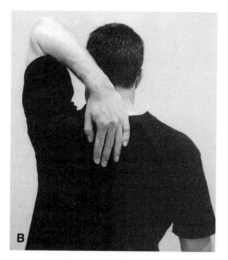
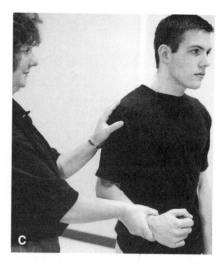
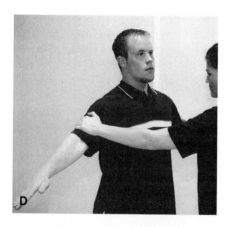
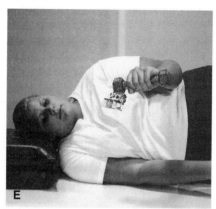
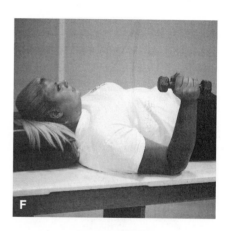
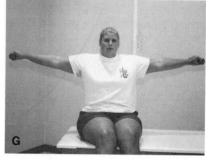

FIGURE 5-14 Flexibility (A and B), Manual Resistance (C and D), and Weight Training (E to G). Exercises for the rotator cuff usually include some shoulder rotation exercises. The scratch test is a good flexibility exercise that stretches the rotator cuff when the scratch is made behind the back **(A)** or over the head **(B)**. The rotator cuff can be strengthened with manual resistance **(C)** applied to the lower forearm as the arm rotates externally. Another good manual resistance exercise is resistance applied to the humerus **(D)** as the arm is being raised in abduction. The arm should be rotated internally 20 to 30° in this exercise. High-resistance exercises for the rotator cuff include dumbbell rotation exercises in external rotation **(E)**, internal rotation **(F),** and arm rotation exercises with dumbbells from the abducted position **(G)**.

An important muscle group in a stretching or strengthening routine of the shoulder complex is the rotator cuff, because these muscles stabilize the shoulder joint and perform a wide variety of shoulder movements. It is essential that exercises for this muscle group be included in any shoulder exercise protocol. Examples of rotator cuff exercises are presented in Figure 5-14. The final example, for the shoulder girdle, includes exercises for the abductors, adductors, and elevators (Fig. 5-15).

Some resistance exercises may irritate the shoulder joint and should be avoided by individuals with specific injuries to that area. Any lateral dumbbell raise using the deltoid may cause impingement in the coracoacromial area. This impingement is magnified if the shoulder is internally rotated. A solution for those wishing to avoid impingement or who have injuries in this area is to rotate the arm externally and then perform the lateral raise (12). It is important to recognize that when an adjustment like this is made, the muscle activity and the forces generated internally will also change. External rotation during a lateral raise will alter the activity of the deltoid and facilitate activity in the internal rotators.

Exercises like the bench press and push-ups should be avoided by individuals with instability in the anterior or posterior portion of the shoulder joint caused by adduction and internal rotation. Likewise, stress on the anterior

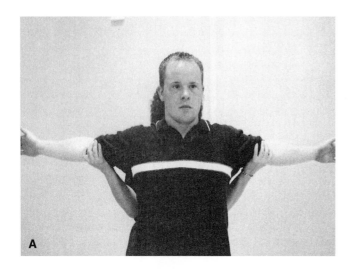

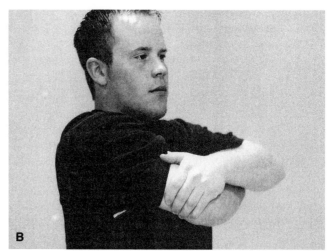

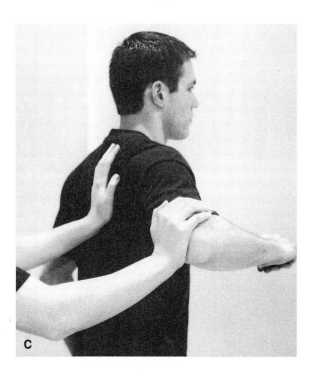

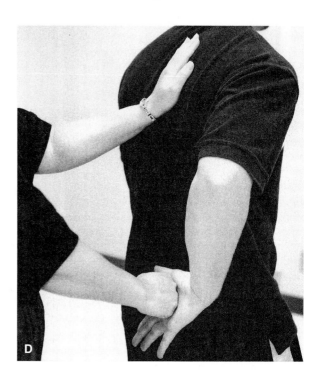

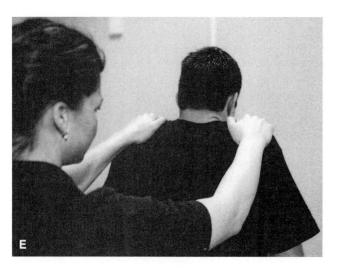

FIGURE 5-15 Flexibility (A and B), Manual Resistance (C and D), and Weight Training (E to H). The abductors of the shoulder girdle can be stretched in a horizontal extension partner stretch **(A)**. The adductors can be passively stretched as the arm is pulled across the body **(B)**. Manual resistance exercises for the shoulder girdle require special attention to isolating a specific movement. The adductors can be strengthened by stabilizing the upper back and applying resistance to the posterior distal humerus as it is horizontally extended **(C)**. With pressure on the scapula, the adductors can also be exercised with pressure placed on the hand as the arm is pulled back **(D)**. The elevators can be isolated in a manual resistance exercise with pressure placed on top of the shoulder in a shrug action **(E)**. Weight-training exercises for the shoulder girdle include a push-up for the abductors **(F)**, bent-over row for the adductors **(G)**, and dumbbell shrugs for the elevators **(H)**.

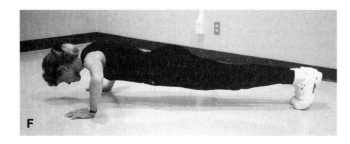

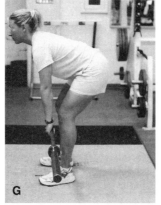

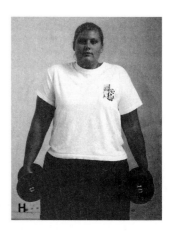

FIGURE 5-15 (CONTINUED)

portion of the capsule is produced by the pullover exercise that moves from an extreme flexed, abducted, and externally rotated position. Other exercises to be avoided by individuals with anterior capsule problems are behind-the-neck pull-downs, horizontal flexion–extension movements, and rowing exercises. The risks in these three exercises can be minimized if no external rotation is maintained or even if some internal rotation is maintained in the joint. The external rotation position produces strain on the anterior portion of the shoulder (12). In an exercise such as the squat, which uses the lower extremity musculature, the position of the shoulder in external rotation may even prove to be harmful because of the strain on the anterior capsule created by weights held in external rotation. Attempts should be made to minimize this joint action by balancing a portion of the weight on the trapezius or to use alternative exercises, such as the dead lift.

Finally, if an individual is having problems with rotator cuff musculature, heavy lifting in an abduction movement should be minimized or avoided. This is because the rotator cuff muscles must generate a large force during the abduction action to support the shoulder joint and complement the activity of the deltoid. Heavy weight lifting above the head should be avoided to reduce strain on the rotator cuff muscles (28).

CONTRIBUTION OF SHOULDER MUSCULATURE TO SPORT SKILLS OR MOVEMENTS

To fully appreciate the contribution of a muscle or muscle group to an activity, the activity or movement of interest must be evaluated and studied. This will provide an understanding of the functional aspect of the movement, ideas for training and conditioning of the appropriate musculature, and a better comprehension of injury sites and mechanisms. Selected activities are presented in this section. These are examples of a functional anatomy description of a movement and are gathered primarily from electromyographic research. It is important to note that these examples do not include all of the muscles that may be active in these activities but only the major contributing muscles.

Activities of Daily Living

The first example is a daily living activity of pushing up to get out of a chair or a wheelchair (Fig. 5-16). This activity places a tremendous load on the upper extremity muscles, as the full body weight is supported in the transfer from a sitting to a standing position (14). Three pushup techniques are presented. First, if you simply push up out of a chair or wheelchair, the muscle primarily used is the triceps brachii, followed by the pectoralis major, with some minimal contribution from the latissimus dorsi (Fig. 5-16A). If you alter the technique and push up, using the arms exclusively, with the elbows flexed to 90°, the triceps brachii will still be extensively used (3). In this case (Fig. 5-16B), the activity of the pectoralis major will decrease and the activity of the latissimus dorsi will increase, reversing their order of contribution as compared to the first method (Fig. 5-16A). Finally, if a push from a position using the arms exclusively is done with the elbow maximally flexed and the arm abducted, the muscular output from all three of these muscles must be maximum, making this the most difficult of the three pushup techniques (Fig. 5-16C) (3).

Freestyle Swimming

A second activity, freestyle or front crawl swimming, incorporates many shoulder movements and uses shoulder muscles as the primary source of force generation in the activity. The activity and the muscles contributing to freestyle swimming are presented in Figure 5-17.

The freestyle swimming technique can be broken down into two basic phases: (*a*) pull-through or propulsion and (*b*) recovery. In the pull-through phase, the propelling forces are generated by the motion of the arm through the water. Both internal rotation and adduction are the primary movements in this phase, generated predominantly by the latissimus dorsi, teres major, and pectoralis major muscles (31,34). These muscles are active throughout the pull-through phase, with activity maximal at the mid-pull position. The pull-through phase is terminated at full adduction and internal rotation of the arm.

The recovery phase is initiated when the arm begins to abduct and externally rotate to bring it out of the

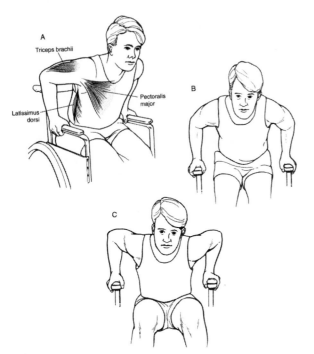

	Push-up Actions Types of Raising/Push-up Activities		
Muscles	Chair Raise	Long Sit Elbow Flex	Long Sit Elbow Flex + ABD
Latissimus dorsi	*	**	***
Pectoralis major	**	*	***
Triceps brachii	***	***	***

*= Low activity; **= moderate activity; ***= high activity.

FIGURE 5-16 A. If you push up out of a chair, the muscle primarily used is the triceps brachii with some contribution from the pectoralis major and minimal assistance from the latissimus dorsi. **B.** From the long sitting position with the elbows flexed, the triceps is still active, but there is more contribution from the latissimus dorsi. **C.** If the arms are abducted, all three muscles are very active in the raising movement.

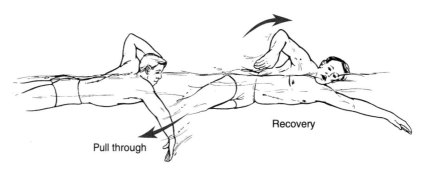

	Swimming Muscle Actions Phases	
Muscle	Pull Through	Recovery
Deltoid	*	***
Infraspinatus		***
Latissimus dorsi	***	
Pectoralis major	***	
Serratus anterior		***
Supraspinatus		***
Teres major	***	

*= Low activity; **= moderate activity; ***= high activity

FIGURE 5-17 The shoulder muscles are significant contributors to swimming action, generating most of the muscular power. In the pull-through phase of swimming the latissimus dorsi and the pectoralis major are very active. In the recovery phase as the arm is lifted out of the water, the deltoid, infraspinatus, serratus anterior, and the supraspinatus are active.

water to prepare for another stroke. The main muscles active in the recovery phase are the supraspinatus and infraspinatus (abduction and external rotation of the humerus), middle deltoid (abduction), and serratus anterior (very active in the hand lift as it rotates the scapula). The role of the serratus anterior is crucial, since it is operating at near-maximal levels during the stroke. It is believed that impingement in the swimmer's shoulder may be a result of serratus anterior fatigue producing scapular rotation that is out of synchrony with humeral abduction, thereby creating the impingement in the subacromial area (31,34).

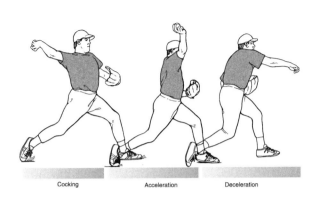

Cocking   Acceleration   Deceleration

| | Throwing Muscle Actions | | |
| | Phases | | |
Muscles	Cocking	Acceleration	Deceleration
Biceps brachii	**	*	***
Brachialis	**	*	***
Deltoid	****	**	***
Infraspinatus	***	**	**
Latissimus dorsi	**	***	*
Pectoralis major	**	***	
Rhomboid	*	*	***
Serratus anterior	**	***	
Subscapularis	***	***	
Supraspinatus	***	**	***
Teres minor	***	**	**
Trapezius	*	*	***
Triceps brachii	*	***	

*= Low activity; **= moderate activity; ***= high activity

FIGURE 5-18 Although throwing uses the lower extremity to develop a significant portion of the power, upper extremity musculature also contributes to the activity. In the cocking phase, the arm is drawn back behind the body. In this phase, numerous muscles are active, with the infraspinatus, subscapularis, teres minor, and supraspinatus the most active. In the acceleration phase, the latissimus dorsi, pectoralis major, serratus anterior, subscapularis, and triceps brachii are active. In the follow-through or deceleration phase, there is substantial activity in the biceps brachii, brachialis, supraspinatus, and trapezius.

Overhand Throwing

The third activity for evaluation in terms of shoulder musculature is throwing. This is an overhead pattern common to many sports, including football, baseball, and track and field, among others. This pattern is illustrated in Figure 5-18. Throwing places a great deal of strain on the shoulder joint and requires significant upper extremity muscular action to control and contribute to the throwing movement even though the lower extremity is a major contributor to the power generation in a throw.

The throwing action described in this section is a pitch in baseball from the perspective of a right-hand thrower. Throwing, or pitching, can be divided into three basic phases. First, during the cocking or preparatory phase, the front leg strides forward and the hand and ball are moved as far back behind the body as possible. This is accomplished through abduction of the arm to 90°, external rotation of the arm, scapula retraction or adduction, and forearm flexion. Also, the body is propelled forward through extension of the lower extremity and rotation of the trunk to move the hand even farther behind the body. This phase ends when the arm reaches 90° of abduction with maximal external rotation (13,31).

The muscular activity in the cocking phase is minimal in the early stages but becomes substantial at the end of the phase, when the arm is maximally externally rotated and the trunk is beginning to rotate to the left as it moves forward. In the early part of the cocking phase, the deltoid and the supraspinatus muscles are active in producing the abduction of the arm. The infraspinatus and the teres minor are also active, assisting with abduction and initiating the external rotation action. The subscapularis is also minimally active to assist during the shoulder abduction. The trapezius and the rhomboid muscles retract or adduct

the scapula during the cocking phase, although their level of activity is minimal (31).

During the late cocking phase, when the front, or left, stride foot contacts the ground and the shoulder is nearing maximal external rotation, other muscles are beginning to contribute to the movement. The latissimus dorsi and the pectoralis major muscles demonstrate a rapid increase in activity as they eccentrically act to slow the backward arm movement and concentrically act to initiate forward movement. The activity in these two muscles increases as tension is developed through stretching of the muscle fibers. This is an example of the stretch-shortening cycle discussed in a previous chapter. Likewise, the triceps brachii activity also increases to slow forearm flexion, and the serratus anterior activity increases to control the scapular movements. The biceps brachii also reaches its peak activity as elbow flexion reaches its maximum level, producing reciprocal muscle activity within the triceps brachii (23).

Muscles previously active in the early portion of the cocking phase also change their level of activity as the arm nears the completion of this phase. Teres minor and infraspinatus activity increase at the end of the cocking phase to generate maximal external rotation. The activity of the supraspinatus increases as it maintains the abduction late into the cocking phase. Subscapularis activity also increases to maximum levels in preparation for the acceleration of the arm forward. The deltoid is the only muscle whose activity diminishes late in the cocking phase (31).

At the end of the cocking phase, the external rotation motion is terminated by the anterior capsule and ligaments and the actions of the subscapularis, pectoralis major, triceps brachii, teres major, and latissimus dorsi muscles. Consequently, in this phase of throwing, the anterior capsule and ligaments and the tissue of the specified muscles are at greatest risk for injury (13,31). Examples of injuries developing in this phase are tendinitis of the insertion of the subscapularis and strain of the pectoralis major, teres major, or latissimus dorsi muscle.

The second phase of the throw is termed the acceleration phase. It is an explosive action characterized by the initiation of elbow extension, arm internal rotation with maintenance of 90° of abduction, scapula protraction or abduction, and some horizontal flexion as the arm moves forward. The muscles most active in the acceleration phase are those that act late in the cocking phase, including the subscapularis, latissimus dorsi, teres major, and pectoralis major (generating the horizontal flexion and the internal rotation movements); the serratus anterior (pulling the scapula forward into protraction or abduction); and the triceps brachii (initiating and controlling the extension of the forearm). Muscles minimally active during the acceleration phase are the biceps brachii, the trapezius, the infraspinatus, and the teres minor (23,31). Sites of irritation and strain in this phase of the throw are found at the sites of the muscular attachment and in the subacromial area. This area is subjected to compression during adduction and internal rotation in this phase.

The last phase of throwing is the follow-through or deceleration phase. In this phase, the arm travels across the body in a diagonal movement and eventually stops over the opposite knee. This phase begins after the ball is released. In the early portion of this phase, after maximum internal rotation in the joint is achieved, there is a very quick muscular action resulting in external rotation and horizontal flexion of the arm. Following this into the later stages of the follow-through are trunk rotation and replication of the shoulder and scapular movements of the cocking phase. This includes an increase in the activity of the deltoid as it attempts to slow the horizontally flexed arm; the latissimus dorsi as it creates further internal rotation; the trapezius, which creates slowing of the scapula; and the supraspinatus, to maintain the arm abduction and continue to produce internal rotation (23,31). In this phase of throwing, the posterior capsule and corresponding muscles are at risk for injury, since they are being rapidly stretched.

Golf Swing

The golf swing presents a more complicated picture of shoulder muscle function because the left and right arms must work in concert. That is, the arms produce opposite movements and use opposing muscles. The golf swing can be divided into four phases: (*a*) takeaway; (*b*) forward swing; (*c*) acceleration; and (*d*) follow-through. These phases and their muscular actions are shown in Figure 5-19.

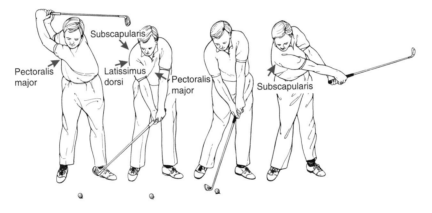

Golf Muscle Actions

| | Phases | | | |
Muscles	Takeaway	Forward Swing	Acceleration	Follow Through
L. deltoid	*	*	*	*
R. deltoid	*	*	*	*
L. infraspinatus			**	
R. infraspinatus			*	
L. latissimus dorsi		**	***	**
R. latissimus dorsi		**	***	
L. pectoralis major			***	**
R. pectoralis major		***	***	**
L. subscapularis	**	**	***	***
R. subscapularis		**	***	***
L. supraspinatus				
R. supraspinatus	**	*		*

*= Low activity; **= moderate activity; ***= high activity

FIGURE 5-19 The upper extremity muscle activity in the takeaway and forward swing phases of the golf swing is moderate, with only the pectoralis major registering high activity in the forward swing phase. However, in the acceleration phase, the muscular activity is high in the latissimus dorsi, pectoralis major, and subscapularis on both sides of the body. Finally, high activity is seen in the subscapularis in the follow-through.

In the takeaway phase for a right-handed golfer, the club is brought up and back behind the body as the left arm comes across the body and the right arm abducts minimally. The shoulder muscular activity in this phase is minimal except for moderate subscapularis activity on the left arm to produce internal rotation and marked activity from the supraspinatus on the right side to abduct the arm (31).

In the next phase, the forward swing, movement of the club is initiated by moderate activity from the latissimus dorsi and subscapularis muscles on the left side. On the right side, there is accompanying high activity from the pectoralis major, moderate activity from the latissimus dorsi and subscapularis, and minimal activity from the supraspinatus and deltoid. This phase brings the club around to shoulder level through continued internal rotation of the left arm and the initiation of internal rotation with some adduction of the right arm.

The acceleration phase begins when the arms are at approximately shoulder level and continues until the club makes contact with the ball. On the left side, there is substantial muscular activity in the pectoralis major, latissimus dorsi, and subscapularis as the arm is extended and maintained in internal rotation. On the right side, there is even greater activity from these same three muscles as the arm is brought vigorously downward (31).

Once contact with the ball is made, the follow-through phase begins with continued movement of the arm and club across the body to the left side. This action must be decelerated. In the follow-through phase, there is some minimal activity from the supraspinatus and the deltoid on the right side as the arm moves up and across the body. The left side has high activity in the subscapularis and moderate activity in the pectoralis major, latissimus dorsi, and infraspinatus as the upward movement of the arm is curtailed and slowed (31). It is here, in the follow-through phase, that considerable strain can be placed on the posterior portion of the right shoulder and the anterior portion of the left shoulder during the rapid deceleration.

INJURY POTENTIAL IN THE SHOULDER COMPLEX

The shoulder complex is subject to a wide variety of injuries that can be incurred in two ways. The first type of injury is through trauma. This type of injury usually occurs when contact is made with an external object, such as the ground or another individual. The second type of injury is through repetitive joint actions that create inflammatory sites in and around the joints or muscular attachments. When examining the various types of injuries to an anatomical region, pay close attention to the cause of the injury. By paying close attention, you may work on injury reduction through recognition and elimination of factors predisposing an individual to injury.

Many injuries to the shoulder girdle are traumatic, a result of impacts during falls or contact with an external object. The sternoclavicular joint can **sprain** or dislocate anteriorly if an individual falls on the top of the shoulder in the area of the middle deltoid. An individual with a sprain to this joint has pain in horizontal extension movements of the shoulder, such as in the golf swing or the backstroke in swimming (48).

Anterior **subluxations** of this joint in adolescents have also occurred spontaneously during throwing because they have greater mobility in this joint than adults. A posterior dislocation or subluxation of the sternoclavicular joint can be quite serious, since the trachea, esophagus, and numerous veins and arteries lie below this structure. This injury occurs as a consequence of force to the sternal end of the clavicle. The individual may have symptoms such as choking, shortness of breath, or difficulty in swallowing (48). Overall, the sternoclavicular joint is well reinforced with ligaments, and fortunately, injury in the form of sprains, subluxations, and dislocations is not common.

The clavicle is frequently a site of injury by direct trauma received through contact in football or some other sport. The most common injury is a **fracture** to the middle third of the clavicle. This injury is incurred by falling on the shoulder or outstretched arm or receiving a blow on the shoulder so that a force is applied along the shaft of the clavicle. Other less common fractures occur to the medial clavicle as a result of direct trauma to the lateral end of the clavicle or as a result of direct trauma to the tip of the shoulder (48). Clavicular fractures in adolescents heal quickly and effectively; whereas, in adults the healing and repair process is not as efficient or effective. This is related to the differences in the level of skeletal maturation. In adolescents, new bone is being formed at a much faster rate than in the mature individual.

Injuries to the acromioclavicular joint can cause a considerable amount of disruption to shoulder movements. Again, if you fall on the point of the shoulder, the acromioclavicular joint can subluxate or dislocate. This can also occur if you fall on your elbow or on an outstretched arm. This joint is also frequently subjected to overuse injuries in sports using the overhand pattern, such as throwing, tennis, and swimming. Other sports that repeatedly load the joint in the overhead position, such as weight lifting and wrestling, may also cause the overuse syndrome. The consequences of overuse of the joint are capsule injury, an **ectopic calcification** in the joint, and possible **degeneration** of the cartilage (48).

The scapula rarely receives sufficient force to cause an injury. However, if an athlete or an individual falls on the upper back, it is possible to fracture the scapula and bruise the musculature so that arm abduction is quite painful. Another site of fracture on the scapula is the **coracoid process**, which can be fractured with separation of the acromioclavicular joint. Throwers can also acquire **bursitis** at the inferomedial border of the scapula, causing pain as the scapula moves through the cocking and acceleration phases in the throw. The pain is diminished in the follow-through phase.

Activities such as weight lifting (bench press, push-ups), lifting above the head, playing tennis, and carrying a backpack can produce trauma to the brachial nerve plexus by means of a traction force (i.e., a pulling force). If the long thoracic nerve is impinged, isolated paralysis of the serratus anterior can cause movement of the medial border of the scapula away from the thorax and a decreased ability to abduct and flex at the shoulder joint (48).

The shoulder joint is commonly injured either through direct trauma or repeated overuse. Dislocation or subluxation in the glenohumeral joint is frequent because of the lack of bony restraint and the dependence on soft tissue for restraint and support of the joint. The glenoid fossa faces anterolaterally, creating more stability in the posterior joint than the anterior. Thus the most common direction of dislocation is anterior. Anterior and inferior dislocations account for 95% of dislocations (33).

The usual cause of the dislocation is contact or some force applied to the arm when it is abducted and externally rotated overhead. This drives the humeral head anteriorly, possibly tearing the capsule or the glenoid labrum. The rate of recurrence of dislocation depends on the age of the individual and the magnitude of the force producing the dislocation (19). The recurrence rate for the general population is 33 to 50%, increasing to 66 to 90% in individuals less than 20 years of age (37). In fact, the younger the age at the first dislocation, the more likely is a recurrent dislocation. Also, if a relatively small amount of force created the dislocation, a recurrent dislocation is more likely.

Recurrent dislocations also depend on the amount of initial damage and whether the glenoid labrum was also damaged (36). A tear to the glenoid labrum, similar to tearing the meniscus in the knee, results in clicking and pain with the arm overhead (50). An anterior dislocation also makes it difficult to rotate the arm internally, so that the contralateral shoulder cannot be touched with the hand on the injured side.

Posterior dislocations of the shoulder are rare (2%) and usually associated with a force applied with an adducted and internally rotated arm with the hand below shoulder level (50). The clinical signs of a posterior dislocation are inability to abduct and externally rotate the arm.

Soft tissue injuries at the shoulder joint are numerous and are associated most often with overhead motions of the arm, such as in throwing, swimming, and racket sports. The rotator cuff muscles, active in controlling the humeral head and motion during the overhand pattern, are very susceptible to injury.

In an upper extremity throwing pattern, when the arm is in the preparatory phase with the shoulder abducted and externally rotated, the anterior capsule and specifically the subscapularis muscle are susceptible to strain or tendinitis at the insertion on the lesser tuberosity (41). In late cocking and early acceleration phase, the posterior portion of the capsule and posterior labrum are susceptible to injury as the anterior shoulder is tightened, driving the head of the humerus backward (6). In the follow-through phase, when the arm is brought horizontally across the body at a very high speed, the posterior rotator cuff, infraspinatus and teres minor, are very susceptible to muscle strain or tendinitis on the greater tuberosity insertion site as they work to decelerate the arm (11).

The most common mechanism of injury to the rotator cuff occurs when the greater tuberosity pushes against the underside of the acromion process. This **impingement syndrome** occurs during the acceleration phase of the overhand throwing pattern, when the arm is internally rotating while still maintained in the abducted position. This condition occurs in the range of 70 to 120° of flexion or abduction and is most common in such activities as the tennis serve, throwing, and butterfly and crawl strokes in swimming (16). If an athlete maintains the shoulder joint in an internally rotated position, impingement is more likely to occur. It is also commonly injured in wheelchair athletes or in individuals transferring from the wheelchair to a bed or chair (5,10). The supraspinatus muscle, lying in the subacromial space, is compressed and can be torn with impingement, and with time, calcific deposits can be laid down in the muscle or tendon. This irritation can occur with any overhead activity, creating a painful arc of arm motion through 60 to 120° of abduction or flexion (42).

Another injury that is a consequence of impingement is **subacromial bursitis**. This injury results from an irritation of the bursae above the supraspinatus muscle and underneath the acromion process (16). It also develops in wheelchair propulsion because of greater than normal pressures in the joint and abnormal distribution of stress in the subacromial area (5).

Finally, the tendon of the long head of the biceps brachii can become irritated when the arm is forcefully abducted and rotated. **Bicipital tendinitis** develops as the biceps tendon is subluxated or irritated within the bicipital groove. In throwing, the arm externally rotates to 160° in the cocking phase, and the elbow moves through 50° of motion. Since the biceps brachii acts on the shoulder and is responsible for decelerating the elbow in the final 30° of extension, it is often maximally stressed (4). In a rapid throw, the long head of the biceps brachii may also be responsible for tearing the anterosuperior portion of the glenoid labrum. Irritation to the biceps tendon is manifested in a painful arc syndrome similar to that of the rotator cuff injury.

In summary, the shoulder complex provides us with the greatest mobility of any region in the body, but as a consequence of this great mobility, it is an unstable area in which numerous injuries may occur. In spite of the high probability of injury, successful rehabilitation following surgery is quite common. It is important to maintain the strength and flexibility of the musculature surrounding the shoulder complex, since there is considerable dependence on the musculature and soft tissue for support and stabilization.

The Elbow and Radioulnar Joints

The role of forearm movement, generated at the elbow or **radioulnar joint**, is to assist the shoulder in applying force and in controlling the placement of the hand in space. The combination of shoulder and elbow–radioulnar joint movements affords the capacity to place the hand in many positions, allowing tremendous versatility. Whether you are working above your head, shaking someone's hand, writing a note, or tying your shoes, hand position is important and is generated by the working relationship between the shoulder complex and the forearm.

ANATOMICAL AND FUNCTIONAL CHARACTERISTICS OF THE JOINTS OF THE ELBOW

The elbow is considered a stable joint, with structural integrity, good ligamentous support, and good muscular support. The elbow has three joints allowing motion between the three bones of the arm and forearm (humerus, radius, ulna). Movement between the forearm and the arm takes place at the ulnar-humeral and radiohumeral articulations, while movements between the radius and the ulna take place at the radioulnar articulations (42). The ulnar-humeral, radiohumeral, and proximal radioulnar articulations are shown in Figure 5-20.

Ulnar-Humeral Joint

The **ulnar-humeral joint** is the articulation between the ulna and the humerus and is the major contributing joint to flexion and extension of the forearm. The joint is the union between the spoollike **trochlea** on the distal end of the humerus and the **trochlear notch** on the ulna. On the front of the ulna is the **coronoid process**, which makes contact in the **coronoid fossa** of the humerus, limiting flexion in the terminal range of motion. Likewise, on the posterior side of

the ulna is the **olecranon process**, which makes contact with the **olecranon fossa** on the humerus, terminating extension. An individual who can hyperextend at the elbow joint may have a small olecranon process or a large olecranon fossa, which allows more extension before contact occurs.

The trochlear notch of the ulna fits snugly around the trochlea, offering good structural stability. The trochlea is covered with articular cartilage over the anterior, inferior, and posterior surfaces and is asymmetrical, with an oblique posterior projection (49). In the extended position, the asymmetrical trochlea creates an angulation of the ulna laterally referred to as a valgus position. This is termed the **carrying angle** and ranges from 10 to 15° in males and 20 to 25° in females (49). Measurement of the carrying angle is shown in Figure 5-21. As the forearm flexes, this valgus position is reduced and may even result in a varus position with full flexion.

Radiohumeral Joint

The second joint participating in flexion and extension of the forearm is the **radiohumeral joint**. At the distal end of the humerus is the articulating surface for this joint, the **capitulum**, which is spheroidal and covered with cartilage

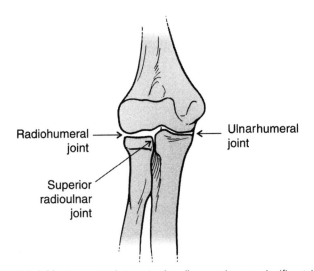

FIGURE 5-20 Three articulations in the elbow region are significant in terms of movement. Flexion and extension at the elbow joint occur at the ulnar-humeral and radiohumeral articulations. Pronation and supination occur at the superior and inferior radioulnar articulations (superior shown).

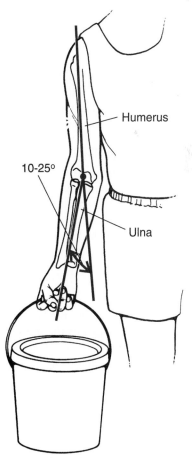

FIGURE 5-21 In the extended position, the ulna and humerus form the carrying angle because of asymmetry in the trochlea. The carrying angle is measured as the angle between a line describing the long axis of the ulna and a line describing the long axis of the humerus. The angle ranges from 10 to 25°.

on the anterior and inferior surfaces. The top of the round radial head butts up against the capitulum, allowing radial movement around the humerus during flexion and extension. The capitulum acts as a buttress for lateral compression and other rotational forces absorbed during throwing and other rapid forearm movements.

Radioulnar Joint

The third articulation, the radioulnar joint, establishes movement between the radius and the ulna in **pronation** and **supination**. There are actually two radioulnar articulations, the superior in the elbow joint region and the inferior near the wrist. Also, midway between the elbow and the wrist is another fibrous connection between the radius and the ulna, recognized by some as a third radioulnar articulation.

The superior or proximal radioulnar joint consists of the articulation between the radial head and the radial fossa on the side of the ulna. The radial head rotates in a fibrous osseous ring and can turn both clockwise and counterclockwise, creating movement of the radius relative to the ulna (8). In the neutral position, the radius and ulna lie next to each other, but in full pronation the radius has crossed over the ulna diagonally. As the radius crosses over in pronation, the distal end of the ulna moves laterally. The opposite occurs during supination.

An **interosseous membrane** connecting the radius and ulna runs the length of the two bones. This fascia increases the area for muscular attachment and ensures that the radius and ulna maintain a specific relationship to each other. It also transmits forces received distally from the radius to the ulna. The membrane is taut in a semiprone position (8).

Medial and Lateral Epicondyles

Two final structural components in the elbow region are the **medial** and **lateral epicondyles**. These are prominent landmarks on the medial and lateral sides of the humerus. These extensions of the humerus serve as a site of muscular attachment for many of the hand muscles and are also sites of overuse injury.

Ligaments

The elbow joint is supported on the medial and lateral sides by collateral ligaments. The medial, or ulnar, collateral ligament connects the ulna to the humerus and offers support and resistance to valgus stresses imposed upon the elbow joint. Support in the valgus direction is very important in the elbow joint, since most forces are directed medially, creating a valgus force. Consequently, the ulnar collateral ligament is taut in all joint positions. There is also a set of collateral ligaments on the lateral side of the joint, termed the lateral or radial collateral ligaments. Since varus stresses are rare, these ligaments are not as significant in supporting the joint (51).

A ligament that is important for the function and support of the radius is the **annular ligament**. This ligament wraps around the head of the radius and attaches to the side of the ulna. The annular ligament holds the radius in the elbow joint while still allowing it to turn in pronation and supination. The insertion and stabilizing actions of ligaments supporting the elbow joint region are reviewed in Appendix A.

Movement Characteristics

The three joints of the elbow complex do not all reach a close-packed position (i.e., position of maximum joint surface contact and ligamentous support) at the same point in the range of motion. Close-packed position for the radiohumeral is achieved when the forearm is flexed to 80° and in the semiprone position (8). The fully extended position is the close-packed position for the ulnar-humeral joint. Thus, when the ulnar-humeral articulation is most stable in the extended position, the radiohumeral articulation is loose-packed and least stable. The proximal radioulnar joint is in its close-packed position in the semiprone position, complementing the close-packed position of the radiohumeral (8).

The range of motion at the elbow in flexion and extension is approximately 145° of active flexion, 160° of passive flexion, and 5 to 10° of hyperextension (8). An extension movement is limited by the joint capsule and the flexor muscles. It is also terminally restrained by bone-on-bone impact with the olecranon process.

Flexion at the joint is limited by soft tissue, the posterior capsule, the extensor muscles, and the bone-on-bone contact of the coronoid process with its respective fossa. A significant amount of hypertrophy or fatty tissue will limit the range of motion in flexion considerably. Approximately 100 to 140° of flexion and extension is required for most daily activities, though the total range of motion is 30 to 130° of flexion (29).

The range of motion for pronation is approximately 70°, limited by the ligaments, the joint capsule, and soft tissue compressing as the radius and ulna cross. Range of motion for supination is 85° and is limited by ligaments, the capsule, and the pronator muscles. Approximately 50° of pronation and 50° of supination are required to perform most daily activities (51).

MUSCULAR ACTIONS

There are 24 muscles that cross the elbow joint, some of which act on the elbow joint exclusively and others that act at the wrist and finger joints (2). Most of these muscles are capable of producing as many as three movements at the elbow, wrist, or phalangeal joints. However, one movement is usually dominant, and it is the movement with which the muscle or muscle group is associated. The location, action, and nerve supply of the muscles acting at the elbow joint can be found in Appendix B.

The elbow flexors (biceps brachii, brachialis, brachioradialis, pronator teres, extensor carpi radialis) become more effective as elbow flexion increases, because their mechanical advantage increases with an increase in the magnitude of the moment arm (2). The strongest flexor of the group is the brachialis, the workhorse of elbow flexion, because it is the only pure elbow flexor and does more work than the other muscles (42). The brachialis's output is not influenced by pronation or supination of the forearm, reaching its maximum output at approximately 120° of flexion (43). It is active in all positions, at all speeds, with or without resistance.

The biceps brachii has a long head that originates at the supraglenoidal tuberosity of the scapula and a short head that attaches to the coracoid process of the scapula, making it a two-joint muscle. At the distal end of the biceps brachii, the muscle inserts into the radial tuberosity of the radius, which can be moved with supination and pronation of the forearm. Consequently, the contribution of the biceps brachii to forearm flexion depends on both the position of the arm and the position of the forearm in pronation and supination.

The biceps brachii is most effective as a flexor in the supine forearm position. The influence of pronation on the tendon of the biceps brachii is illustrated in Figure 5-22. The activity of this muscle drops off in the semiprone position, where it becomes active only against resistance. In the prone position, the biceps brachii minimally contributes even against resistance. It has also been shown to make the most contribution to the flexion action during the middle 90° of flexion, that is, from 30 to 120° of flexion (45).

The contribution of the biceps brachii can be increased if the arm is extended or hyperextended at the shoulder

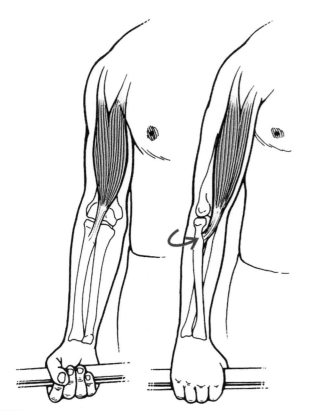

FIGURE 5-22 When the forearm is pronated, the attachment of the biceps brachii to the radius is twisted under. This position interferes with the flexion-producing action of the biceps brachii, which is more efficient in producing flexion when the forearm is supinated and the tendon is not twisted under the radius.

joint, at which the insertion of the long head of the biceps brachii is put on stretch. The output from the biceps brachii is maximal at approximately 120° of forearm flexion and can be increased further with the forearm supinated and the arm extending (43).

The brachioradialis is a muscle with a small volume and very long fibers. It is a very efficient muscle used mainly with rapid elbow flexion movements and against resistance. The brachioradialis has been shown to produce the greatest activity at 120° of flexion with the forearm in the supine position (43). The brachioradialis does not increase its activity when the arm is semiprone or prone.

In the extensor muscle group is the powerful triceps brachii, the strongest arm muscle of all. The triceps brachii has great strength potential and work capacity because of its muscle volume (2). The triceps brachii has three portions: the long head, medial head, and lateral head. Of these three, only the long head crosses the shoulder joint, making it dependent partially on shoulder position for its effectiveness. The long head is the least active of the triceps. However, it can be increasingly more involved with shoulder flexion as its insertion on the shoulder is stretched.

The medial head of the triceps brachii is considered the workhorse of the extension movement because it is active in all positions, at all speeds, and against maximal or minimal resistance. The lateral head of the triceps brachii, although the strongest of the three heads, is relatively inactive unless movement occurs against resistance (42). The output of the triceps brachii is not influenced by forearm positions of pronation and supination.

A third movement of the forearm occurring at the radioulnar articulations is pronation produced by the pronator quadratus and pronator teres. The activity and the overall contribution of the pronator quadratus are considerably greater than those of the pronator teres. The pronator quadratus is more active regardless of forearm position, whether the activity is slow or fast or working against a resistance or not. The pronator teres is called upon to become more active when the pronation action becomes rapid or against a high load. The pronator teres is most active at 60° of forearm flexion (43).

The final movement of the forearm, supination, is produced by the supinator muscle and under special circumstances by the biceps brachii. The supinator is the only muscle contributing to a slow unresisted supination action in all forearm positions. The biceps brachii can supinate during rapid or rested movements when the elbow is flexed. The flexion action of the biceps brachii is neutralized by actions from the triceps brachii, allowing contribution to the supination action. At 90° of flexion, the biceps brachii becomes a very effective supinator.

The muscles surrounding the elbow joint are also positioned to create forces in the mediolateral direction. The muscles on the lateral side of the joint, the anconeus, brachioradialis, extensor carpi radialis, extensor digitorum communis, and extensor carpi ulnaris, create a valgus force. The muscles on the medial side of the joint, the pronator teres, flexor carpi radialis, flexor digitorum superficialis, and flexor carpi ulnaris, create varus forces (2). These muscles should be considered and included in a conditioning program when stability at the elbow joint is required.

STRENGTH OF THE FOREARM MUSCLES

The flexor muscle group is almost twice as strong as the extensors at all joint positions, making us better pullers than pushers. The joint forces created by a maximum isometric flexion in an extended position is equal to approximately two times body weight.

The semiprone elbow position is the position at which maximum strength in flexion can be developed, followed by the supine position and finally, the pronated position (35). The semiprone position is most commonly used in daily activities. Semiprone flexion exercises should be included in a conditioning routine to take advantage of the strong position of the forearm.

Extension strength is greatest from a position of 90° of flexion (51). This is a common forearm position for daily living activities and for power positions in upper extremity sport skills. Finally, pronation and supination strength is greatest in the semiprone position, with the torque dropping off considerably at the fully pronated or fully supinated position.

The load-carrying capacity of the elbow joint is considerable. In a pushup, the peak axial forces on the elbow joint average 45% of body weight (1). These forces depend on hand position, with the force reduced to 42.7% of body weight with the hands farther apart than normal (1).

CONDITIONING

The effectiveness of exercises used to strengthen or stretch will depend on the various positions of the arm and the forearm. In stretching the muscles, the only positions putting any form of stretch on the flexors and extensors must incorporate some hyperextension and flexion at the shoulder joints. Stretching these muscles while the arm is in the neutral position is almost impossible because of the bony restrictions to the range of motion.

The flexor and extensor muscles can be strengthened through manipulation of the length–tension relationship in the muscle, that is, by placing the arm in hyperextension when working the flexors and in flexion when working the extensors. The use of a stretch–contract sequence in a strength exercise will facilitate the activity and output from the muscles.

The position of the forearm is also important in forearm strengthening activities. The forearm position in which the flexors and extensors are the strongest is semiprone. For the flexors specifically, the biceps brachii can be brought more or less into the exercise by supinating or pronating, respectively. Numerous exercises are available for both the flexors and extensors, examples of which are provided in Figures 5-23 and 5-24.

The pronators and supinators offer a greater challenge in the prescription of strength or resistive exercises (Fig. 5-25). Stretching these muscle groups presents no problem, since a maximal supination position will adequately stretch the pronation musculature and vice versa. Also, low-resistance exercises can be implemented by applying a force in a turning action (for example, to a doorknob or some other immovable object). However, high-resistance exercises necessitate the use of creativity, since there are no standardized sets of exercises for these muscles.

CONTRIBUTION TO SPORTS SKILLS OR MOVEMENTS

Activities of Daily Living

The forearm musculature, specifically the forearm extensor muscles, is very important for rising from a chair. As shown in Figure 5-16, pushing up from a chair and many wheelchair activities require a great amount of extension at the elbow joint. Thus, it is important to strengthen the triceps brachii muscle in the elderly and in wheelchair-bound individuals (3).

Throwing

In throwing, the forearm flexors and extensors are active throughout the action (Fig. 5-18). In the cocking phase of the throw, the biceps brachii and the brachialis are active as the forearm flexes and the arm is abducted. The activity of the triceps brachii begins at the end of the cocking phase, when the arm is in maximum external rotation and the elbow is maximally flexed. There is a cocontraction of the biceps brachii and the triceps brachii at this time. Additionally, the forearm is pronated to 90° at the end of the cocking phase via the pronator teres and pronator quadratus (23).

In the acceleration phase of throwing, the activity of the triceps brachii increases significantly as the forearm is rapidly extended, and the activity continues until a high forearm extension velocity is achieved. The activity of both the biceps brachii and the brachialis drops off rapidly in the acceleration phase (23).

Just after release, the negative acceleration, or slowing down, phase begins and is marked by a rapid drop-off in the activity of the triceps brachii. There is a very rapid increase in the activity of the biceps brachii and the brachialis in the follow-through phase as these muscles attempt to reduce the tensile loads on the rapidly extending forearm. It is in this portion of the throwing action that the biceps brachii is most susceptible to strain (4). The overall activity of the biceps brachii and the brachialis increases with corresponding increases in speed of the throw.

INJURY POTENTIAL IN THE FOREARM

There are two categories of injuries at the elbow joint: traumatic or high-force injuries and repetitive or overuse injuries. The elbow joint is subjected to traumatic injuries

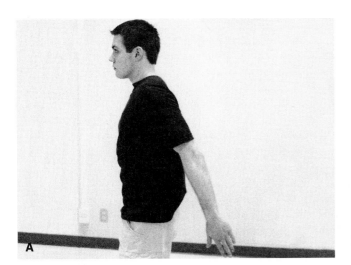

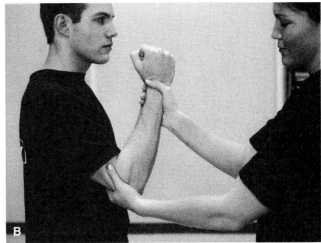

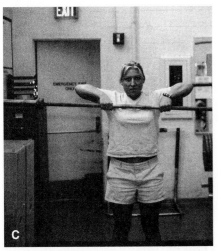

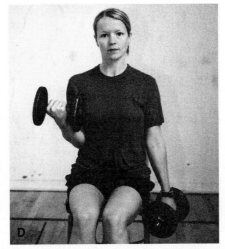

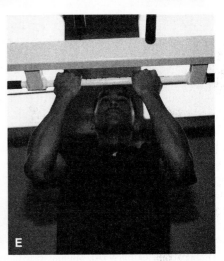

FIGURE 5-23 Flexibility (A), Manual Resistance (B), and Weight Training (C to E). Only the biceps brachii, which crosses the shoulder joint, can be stretched to any significant degree. A stretch can be imposed by hyperextending the arm with the elbow extended **(A)**. A good manual resistance exercise is one in which the elbow is stabilized and resistance is applied at the wrist region as the forearm is pulled into flexion **(B)**. The flexors are an easy group to weight train using exercises like the upright row **(C)**, dumbbell curls **(D)**, and the pull-up **(E)**.

caused by the absorption of a high force, such as in falling, but most of the injuries at the elbow joint result from repetitive activities, such as throwing or throwing-type actions. The high-impact or traumatic injuries will be presented first, followed by the more common overuse injuries.

One of the injuries occurring as a consequence of absorbing a high force is a dislocation. These injuries usually occur in sports such as gymnastics, football, and wrestling. The athlete falls on an outstretched arm, causing a posterior dislocation (21). With the dislocation, a fracture in the medial epicondyle is common. Other areas that may fracture with a fall include the olecranon process, the head of the radius, and the shaft of the radius, the ulna, or both. Additionally, spiral fractures of the humerus can be incurred through a fall.

Direct blows to any muscle can culminate in a condition known as myositis ossificans. In this injury, the body deposits **ectopic bone** in the muscle in response to the severe bruising and repeated stress to the muscle tissue. Although it is most common in the quadriceps femoris in

the thigh, the brachioradialis muscle in the forearm is the second most common area of the body to develop this condition (21).

A high muscular force can create a **rupture** of the long head of the biceps brachii, commonly seen in adults. The joint movements facilitating this injury are arm hyperextension, forearm extension, and forearm pronation. If these three movements occur concomitantly, the strain on the biceps brachii may be significant. Finally, falling on the elbow can irritate the olecranon bursa, causing **olecranon bursitis**. This injury looks very disabling because of the swelling but is actually minimally painful (8).

The repetitive or overuse injuries occurring at the elbow are usually associated with throwing or some overhead movement, such as the tennis serve. Throwing places stringent demands upon the medial side of the elbow joint. Through the high-velocity actions of the throw, large tensile forces develop on the medial side of the elbow joint, compressive forces develop on the lateral

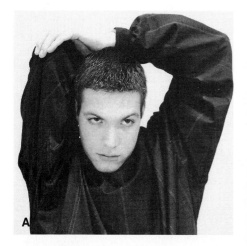
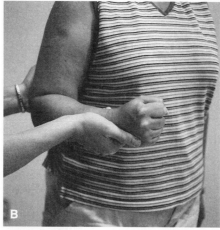
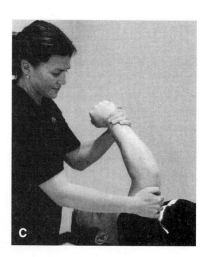
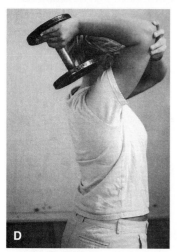
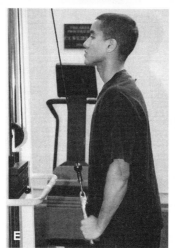
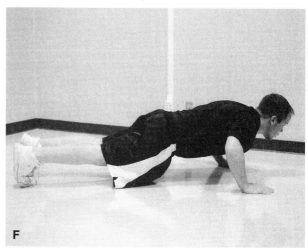

FIGURE 5-24 Flexibility (A), Manual Resistance (B and C), and Weight Training (D to F). The triceps brachii can be stretched by pulling the arm up behind the head with the elbow flexed **(A)**. Manual resistance can be used to strengthen the triceps brachii by stabilizing the elbow and applying resistance at the wrist as the individual extends **(B)**, or the same exercise can be performed from the supine position **(C)**. Common weight-training exercises for the forearm extensors include the french curl **(D)**, the triceps press **(E)**, and the push-up **(F)**.

side of the joint, and shear forces occur on the posterior side of the joint. A maximal valgus force is applied to the medial side of the elbow during the latter part of the cocking phase and through the initial portion of the acceleration phase. This force is responsible for creating the **medial tension syndrome**, or pitcher's elbow (21). This excessive valgus force is responsible for sprain or rupture of the ulnar collateral ligaments, medial **epicondylitis**, **tendinitis** of the forearm or wrist flexors, avulsion fractures to the medial epicondyle, and **osteochondritis dissecans** to the capitulum or olecranon (21,51).

Medial epicondylitis is an irritation of the insertion site of the wrist flexor muscles attached to the medial epicondyle. They are stressed with the valgus force accompanied by wrist actions. Osteochondritis dissecans, a lesion in the bone and articular cartilage, commonly occurs on the capitulum as a result of compression during the valgus position that forces the radial head up against the capitulum. During the valgus overload, coupled with forearm

extension, the olecranon process can be wedged against the fossa, creating an additional site for osteochondritis dissecans and breakdown in the bone. Additionally, the olecranon is subject to high tensile forces and can develop a **traction apophysitis**, or bony outgrowth, similar to that seen with the patellar ligament of the quadriceps femoris group (21).

The lateral overuse injuries to the elbow usually occur as a consequence of overuse of the wrist extensors at their attachment site on the lateral epicondyle. The overuse of the wrist extensors occurs as they eccentrically slow down or resist any flexion movement at the wrist. Lateral epicondylitis, or tennis elbow, is associated with force overload resulting from improper technique or use of a heavy racket. If the backhand stroke in tennis is executed with the elbow leading or if the performer hits the ball consistently off-center, the wrist extensors and the lateral epicondyle will become irritated (26). Also, a large racket grip or tight strings may increase the load on the epicondyle by the extensors.

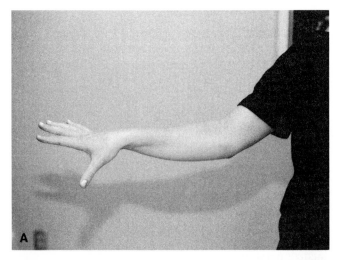

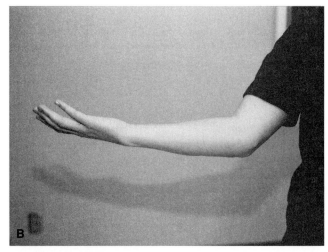

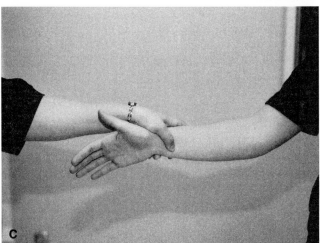

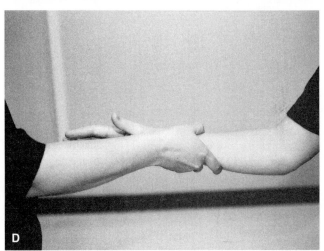

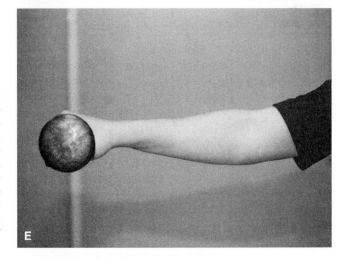

FIGURE 5-25 Flexibility (A and B), Manual Resistance (C and D), and Weight Training (E). The pronators and supinators are not usually included in a stretching or strengthening routine, but there is much to be gained by including them. To stretch the supinators, turn the hand from the supine position until the palm is facing posteriorly **(A)**. To stretch the pronators, move the forearm into the maximum supination position close to anatomical position **(B)**. The supinators and pronators can be strengthened with manual resistance by applying resistance on the outside of the forearm during supination **(C)** or on the inside of the forearm during pronation **(D)**. The elbow should be flexed to reduce contribution from the shoulder rotators. Higher-resistance exercises can be performed for both supination and pronation using a dumbbell **(E)**.

 ## The Wrist and Fingers

The hand is primarily used for manipulation activities requiring very fine movements incorporating a wide variety of hand and finger postures. Consequently, there is much interplay between the wrist joint positions and efficiency of finger actions. The hand region has many stable yet very mobile segments, with complex muscle and joint actions.

ANATOMICAL AND FUNCTIONAL CHARACTERISTICS OF THE JOINTS OF THE WRIST AND HAND

Beginning with the most proximal joints of the hand and working distally to the tips of the fingers offers the best perspective on the interaction between segments and joints in the hand. All of the joints of the hand are illustrated in Figure 5-26. To review the anatomical structures

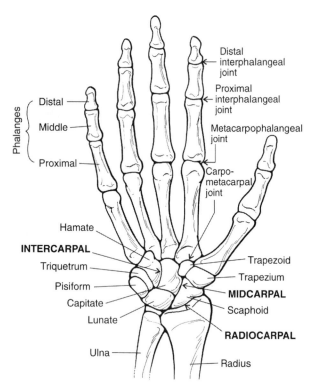

Phalanges: Distal, Middle, Proximal

Distal interphalangeal joint
Proximal interphalangeal joint
Metacarpophalangeal joint
Carpo-metacarpal joint

Hamate
INTERCARPAL
Triquetrum
Pisiform
Capitate
Lunate
Ulna

Trapezoid
Trapezium
MIDCARPAL
Scaphoid
RADIOCARPAL
Radius

FIGURE 5-26 The wrist and hand can perform both precision and power movements because of numerous joints controlled by a large number of muscles. Most of the muscles originate in the forearm and enter the hand as tendons.

in the wrist and hand, refer to Appendix A for ligamentous structure and Appendix B for muscular location, action, and innervation.

Radiocarpal Joint

The wrist joint, or **radiocarpal joint**, is the articulation where movement of the whole hand occurs. The radiocarpal joint involves the broad distal end of the radius and two carpals, the scaphoid and the lunate. There is also minimal contact and involvement with the triquetrum. This ellipsoid joint allows movement in two planes: flexion–extension and radial–ulnar flexion.

Distal Radioulnar Joint

Adjacent to the radiocarpal joint but not participating in any wrist movements is the distal radioulnar articulation. The ulna makes no actual contact with the carpals and is separated by a fibrocartilage disc. This arrangement is important so that the ulna can glide on the disc in pronation and supination while not influencing wrist or carpal movements.

Midcarpal and Intercarpal Joints

To understand wrist joint function, it is necessary to examine the structure and function at the joints between the carpals. There are two rows of carpals, the proximal row, containing the three carpals that participate in wrist

joint function (lunate, scaphoid, triquetrum) and the pisiform bone, which sits on the medial side of the hand, serving as a site of muscular attachment. In the distal row there are also four carpals, the trapezium interfacing with the thumb at the saddle joint, the trapezoid, the capitate, and the hamate.

The articulation between the two rows of carpals is called the **midcarpal joint**, and the articulation between a pair of carpal bones is referred to as an **intercarpal joint**. All of these are gliding joints in which translation movements are produced concomitantly with wrist movements. However, the proximal row of carpals is more mobile than the distal row (46). A concave transverse arch runs across the carpals, forming the floor and walls of the carpal tunnel, through which the tendons of the flexors and the median nerve travel.

The scaphoid may be one of the most important carpals, since it supports the weight of the arm, transmits forces received from the hand to the bones of the forearm, and is a key participant in wrist joint actions. The scaphoid supports the weight of the arm and transmits forces when the hand is fixed and the forearm weight is applied to the hand. Because the scaphoid interjects into the distal row of carpals, it sometimes will move with the proximal row and other times with the distal row.

When the hand flexes at the wrist joint, the movement begins at the midcarpal joint. This joint accounts for 60% of the total range of flexion motion (42), and 40% of wrist flexion is attributable to movement of the scaphoid and lunate on the radius. The total range of motion for wrist flexion is 70 to 90°, although it is reported that only 10 to 15° of wrist flexion is needed for most daily activities involving the hand (51). Wrist flexion range of motion will be reduced if flexion is performed with the fingers flexed because of the resistance offered by the finger extensor muscles.

Wrist extension is also initiated at the midcarpal joint, where the capitate moves quickly and becomes close-packed with the scaphoid. This action draws the scaphoid into movements of the second row of carpals. This reverses the role of the midcarpal and radiocarpal joints to the extension movement, with more than 60% of the movement now produced at the radiocarpal joint and more than 30% at the midcarpal joint (42). This switch is attributed to the fact that the scaphoid moves with the proximal row of carpals in the flexion movement and with the distal row of carpals in extension. The range of motion for extension is approximately 70 to 80°, with approximately 35° of extension needed for daily activities (46). The range of motion of wrist extension will be reduced if the extension is performed with the fingers extended.

The hand can also move laterally in radial and ulnar flexion or deviation. These movements are created as the proximal row of carpals glides over the distal row. In the radial flexion movement, the proximal carpal row moves toward the ulna and the distal row moves toward the radius. The opposite occurs for ulnar flexion. The range of motion for radial flexion is approximately 15 to 20° and for ulnar flexion is about 30 to 40° (51).

The close-packed position for the wrist, in which maximal support is offered, is in a hyperextended position. The close-packed position for the midcarpal joint is radial flexion. Both of these positions should be considered when selecting positions that maximize stability in the hand. For example, in racket sports, the wrist will be most stable in a slightly hyperextended position. Also, when one falls on the hand with the arm outstretched and the wrist hyperextended, the wrist and specifically the scaphoid carpal bone are especially susceptible to injury because they are in the close-packed position.

Carpometacarpal Joints

Moving distally, the next articulation is the carpometacarpal (CMC) joint, which connects the carpals with each of the five fingers via the metacarpals. Each metacarpal and phalanx is also called a ray. They are numbered from the thumb to the little finger, with the thumb being the first ray and the little finger the fifth. The CMC articulation is the joint providing the most movement for the thumb and the least movement for the fingers.

For the four fingers, the CMC joint offers very little movement, being a gliding joint that moves directionally with the carpals. The movement is very restricted at the second and third CMC but increases to allow as much as 10 to 30° of flexion and extension at the CMC joint of the ring and little fingers (51). There is also a concave transverse arch across the metacarpals of the fingers similar to that of the carpals. This arch facilitates the gripping potential of the hand.

The CMC joint of the first ray, or thumb, is a saddle joint consisting of the articulation between the trapezium and the first metacarpal. It provides the thumb with most of its range of motion, allowing for 50 to 80° of flexion and extension, 40 to 80° of abduction and adduction, and 10 to 15° of rotation (43). The thumb sits at an angle of 60 to 80° to the arch of the hand and has a wide range of functional movements (20).

The thumb can touch each of the fingers in the movement of opposition and is very important in all gripping and prehension tasks. Opposition can take place through a range of motion of approximately 90°. Without the thumb, specifically the movements allowed at the CMC joint, the function of the hand would be very limited.

Metacarpophalangeal Joints

The metacarpals connect with the phalanges to form the **metacarpophalangeal joints** (MCP). Again, the function of the MCP joints of the four fingers differs from that of the thumb. The MCP joints of the four fingers are condyloid joints allowing movements in two planes: flexion–extension and abduction–adduction. The joint is well reinforced on the dorsal side by the dorsal hood of the fingers, on the palmar side by the palmar plates that span the joint, and on the sides by the collateral ligaments or deep transverse ligaments.

The fingers can flex through 70 to 90°, with most flexion in the little finger and least in the index finger (42). Flexion, which determines grip strength, can be more effective and produces more force when the wrist joint is held in 20 to 30° of hyperextension, a position that increases the length of the finger flexors.

Extension of the fingers at the MCP joints can take place through about 25° of motion. The extension can be limited by the position of the wrist. That is, finger extension is limited with the wrist hyperextended and enhanced with the wrist flexed.

The fingers spread in abduction and are brought back together in adduction at the MCP joint. Approximately 20° of abduction and adduction is allowed (46). Abduction is extremely limited if the fingers are flexed, since the collateral ligaments become very tight and restrict this movement. Thus, fingers can be abducted when extended and then cannot be abducted or adducted when flexed around the object.

The MCP for the thumb is a hinge joint allowing motion in only one plane. The joint is reinforced with collateral ligaments and the palmar plates but is not connected with the other fingers via the deep transverse ligaments. Approximately 30 to 90° of flexion and 15° of extension can take place at this joint (46).

Interphalangeal Joints

The most distal joints in the upper extremity link are the interphalangeal articulations (IP). Each finger has two IP joints, the proximal interphalangeal (PIP) and the distal **interphalangeal joints** (DIP). The thumb has one IP joint and consequently has only two sections or phalanges, the proximal and distal phalanges. The fingers, however, have three phalanges, the proximal, middle, and distal. The IP joints are hinge joints allowing for movement in one plane only (flexion and extension), and they are reinforced on the lateral sides of the joints by collateral ligaments that restrict movements other than flexion and extension. The range of motion in flexion of the fingers is 110° at the PIP joint and 90° at the DIP joint and the IP joint of the thumb (51,46).

As with the MCP joint, the flexion strength at these joints determines grip strength. It can be enhanced with the wrist hyperextended by 20° and is impaired if the wrist is flexed. Various finger positions can be obtained through antagonistic and synergistic actions from other muscles so that all fingers can flex or extend at the same time. There can also be extension of the MCP with flexion of the IP and vice versa. There is usually no hyperextension allowed at the IP joints unless an individual has long ligaments that allow extension because of joint laxity.

MUSCULAR ACTIONS

Most of the muscles acting at the wrist and finger joints originate outside the hand in the region of the elbow joint and are termed extrinsic muscles (see Appendix B). These muscles enter the hand as tendons that can be quite long, as in the case of some finger tendons that eventually terminate on the distal tip of a finger. The tendons are held in place on the dorsal and palmar wrist area by extensor and flexor retinacula. These are bands of fibrous tissue running transversely across the distal forearm and wrist. During wrist and finger movements, the tendons move through considerable distances but are still maintained by the retinacula.

In addition to the muscles originating in the forearm, intrinsic muscles originating within the hand create movement at the MCP and IP joints. The four intrinsic muscles of the thumb form the fleshy region in the palm known as the **thenar eminence**. Three intrinsic muscles of the little finger form the smaller **hypothenar eminence**, the fleshy ridge on the little finger side of the palm.

The wrist flexors (flexor carpi ulnaris, flexor carpi radialis, palmaris longus) are all fusiform muscles originating in the vicinity of the medial epicondyle on the humerus. These muscles run about halfway along the forearm before becoming a tendon. The flexor carpi radialis and flexor carpi ulnaris contribute the most to wrist flexion. The palmaris longus is variable and may be as small as a tendon or even absent in about 13% of the population (42). The strongest flexor of the group, the flexor carpi ulnaris, gains some of its power by encasing the pisiform bone and using it as a sesamoid bone to increase mechanical advantage and reduce the overall tension on the tendon. Since most activities require the use of a small amount of wrist flexion, attention should always be given to the conditioning of this muscle group.

The wrist extensors (extensor carpi ulnaris, extensor carpi radialis longus, extensor carpi radialis brevis) originate in the vicinity of the lateral epicondyle. These muscles become tendons about a third of the way along the forearm. The wrist extensors also act and create movements at the elbow joint. Thus, elbow joint position is important for wrist extensor function. The extensor carpi radialis longus and extensor carpi radialis brevis create flexion at the elbow joint and thus can be enhanced as a wrist extensor with extension at the elbow. The extensor carpi ulnaris creates extension at the elbow and is enhanced as a wrist extensor in elbow flexion. Also, wrist extension is an important action accompanying and supporting a gripping action using finger flexion. Thus, the wrist extensor muscles are active with this activity.

The wrist flexors and extensors pair up to produce ulnar and radial flexion. Ulnar flexion is produced by the ulnaris wrist muscles, consisting of the flexor carpi ulnaris and the extensor carpi ulnaris. Likewise, radial flexion is produced by the flexor carpi radialis, extensor carpi radialis longus, and extensor carpi radialis brevis. Radial flexion joint movement, although having half the range of motion of ulnar flexion, is important in many racket sports, since it creates the close-packed position of the wrist and so stabilizes the hand (46).

Finger flexion is performed primarily by the flexor digitorum profundus and flexor digitorum superficialis. These extrinsic muscles originate in the vicinity of the medial epicondyle. The flexor digitorum profundus cannot independently flex each finger. Thus, flexion at the middle, ring, and little fingers will usually occur together, since the flexor tendons all arise from a common tendon and muscle. However, the index finger can independently flex because of the separation of the flexor digitorum profundus muscle and tendon for this digit.

The flexor digitorum superficialis is capable of flexing each finger independently. The fingers can be independently flexed at the PIP but not at the DIP. Flexion of the little finger is also assisted by one of the intrinsic muscles, the flexor digiti minimi brevis. Flexion of the fingers at the metacarpophalangeal articulation is produced by the lumbricales and the interossei, two sets of intrinsic muscles lying in the palm and between the metacarpals. These muscles also produce extension at the interphalangeal joints, since they attach to the fibrous extensor hood running the length of the dorsal surface of the fingers. Consequently, to achieve full flexion of the MCP, PIP, and DIP joints, the long finger flexors must override the extension component of the lumbricales and interossei. This is easier if tension is taken off the extensors by some wrist extension.

Extension of the fingers is created primarily by the extensor digitorum muscle. This muscle originates at the lateral epicondyle and enters the hand as four tendon slips that branch off at the metacarpophalangeal articulation. The tendons create a main slip that inserts into the extensor hood and two collateral slips that connect into adjacent fingers. The extensor hood, formed by the tendon of the extensor digitorum and fibrous connective tissue, wraps around the dorsal surface of the phalanges and runs the total length of the finger to the distal phalanx. The structures in the finger are shown in Figure 5-27.

Since the lumbricales and interossei connect into this hood, they also assist with extension of the PIP and DIP joints. Their actions are facilitated as the extensor digitorum contracts, applying tension to the extensor hood and stretching these muscles (46).

Abduction of fingers two, three, and four is performed by the dorsal interossei. The dorsal interossei consist of four intrinsic muscles lying between the metacarpals. They connect to the lateral sides of digits two and four and to both sides of digit three. The little finger, digit five, is abducted by one of its intrinsic muscles, the abductor digiti minimi brevis.

The three palmar interossei, lying on the medial side of digits two, four, and five, pull the fingers back into adduction. The middle finger is adducted by the dorsal interossei, which is connected to both sides of the middle finger. Abduction and adduction movements are necessary for grasping, catching, and gripping objects. When the fingers are flexed, abduction is severely limited by the tightening

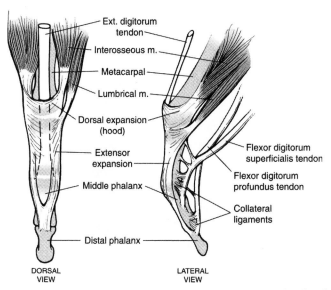

FIGURE 5-27 There are no muscle bellies in the fingers. On the dorsal surface of the fingers is the extensor expansion and the extensor hood, to which the finger extensors attach. Tendons of the finger flexors travel the ventral surface of the fingers. The fingers flex and extend as tension is generated in the tendons via muscular activity in the upper forearm.

of the collateral ligament and the limited length–tension relationship in the interossei, which are also flexors of the metacarpophalangeal joint.

The thumb has eight muscles controlling and generating an expansive array of movements. The muscles of the thumb are presented in Appendix B. Opposition is the most important movement of the thumb because it provides the opportunity to pinch, grasp, or grip an object by bringing the thumb across to meet any of the fingers. Although all of the hypothenar muscles contribute to opposition, the main muscle responsible for initiating the movement is the opponens pollicis. The little finger is also assisted in opposition by the opponens digiti minimi.

STRENGTH OF THE HAND AND FINGERS

Strength in the hand is usually associated with grip strength, and there are many ways to grasp or grip an object. A firm grip requiring maximum output will use the extrinsic muscles, whereas fine movements, such as a pinch, will use more of the intrinsic muscles to fine-tune the movements.

The strength of a grip can be enhanced by the position of the wrist. Placing the wrist in ulnar flexion increases the strength output of the PIP and DIP flexor muscles to the greatest extent, followed by wrist hyperextension and lastly wrist flexion. Thus, a grip can be strengthened if the wrist is placed in a position of slight ulnar flexion and hyperextension. Likewise, the grip can be loosened if the wrist is put in a flexion position. Grip strength at approximately 40° of wrist hyperextension is more than three times that of grip strength measured in

40° of wrist flexion (51). The strength of the grip may increase with specific wrist positioning, but the incidence of strain or impingement on structures around the wrist also increases. The neutral position of the wrist is the safest position, since it reduces strain on the wrist structures.

The strongest muscles in the hand region, capable of the greatest work capacity, in order from high to low are the flexor digitorum profundus, the flexor carpi ulnaris, the extensor digitorum, the flexor pollicis longus, the extensor carpi ulnaris, and the extensor carpi radialis longus. Two muscles that are weak and capable of little work capacity are the palmaris longus and the extensor pollicis longus.

CONDITIONING

There are three main reasons people condition the hand region. First, the fingers can be strengthened to enhance the grip strength in athletes who participate in racket sports, individuals who work with implements, and individuals who lack the ability to grasp or grip objects. Second, the muscles acting at the wrist joint are usually strengthened and stretched to facilitate a wrist position for racket sports or to enhance wrist action in a throwing or striking event, such as volleyball. The final reason for conditioning the hand region is to reduce or prevent injury. The tension developed in the hand and finger flexor and extensor muscles places considerable strain on the medial and lateral aspect of the elbow joint. Some of this strain can be reduced through stretching and strengthening exercises.

Overall, the conditioning of the hand region is relatively simple and can be done in a very limited environment with minimal equipment. Examples of some flexibility and resistance exercises for the wrist flexors and extensors and the fingers are presented in Figures 5-28 and 5-29, respectively. Wrist curls and tennis ball–gripping exercises are the most popular for this region.

CONTRIBUTION TO SPORT SKILLS OR MOVEMENTS

The wrist joint can provide a dynamic contribution to a skill or movement or stabilization of the joint in a fixed position. In golf, for example, the wrist actively flexes radially via the flexor carpi radialis and extensor carpi radialis muscles in the preparatory phase and ulnar flexes via the opposite muscle groups in the power phase. These same joint actions are seen in the baseball batting swing and are significant contributors to the success of both events.

Wrist extension draws the hand back, and wrist flexion snaps the hand forward in activities such as serving and spiking in volleyball, dribbling in basketball, and throwing a baseball. Even though the speed of the flexion and extension movement may be determined by contributions

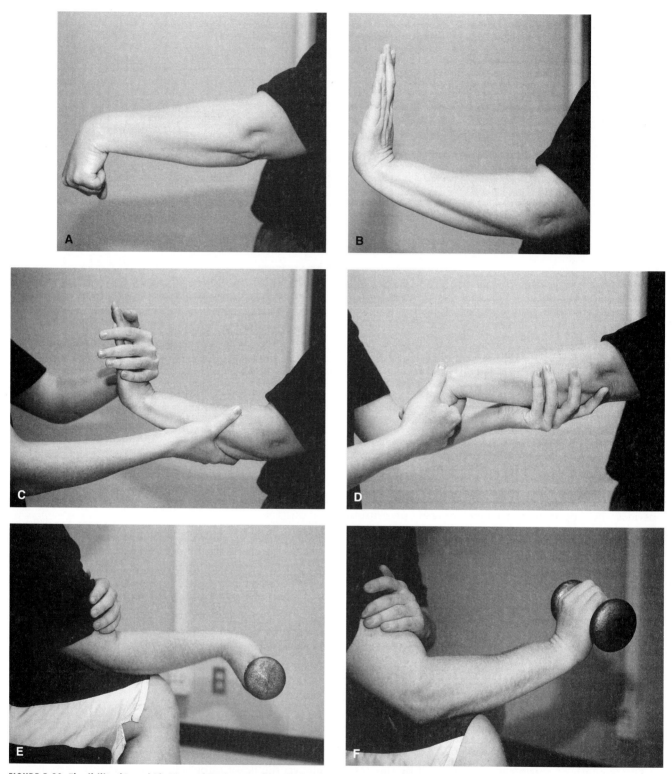

FIGURE 5-28 Flexibility (A and B), Manual Resistance (C and D), and Weight Training (E and F). Stretch the wrist extensors and flexors by placing the hand in extreme flexion **(A)** or hyperextension **(B)**, respectively. The extensors and flexors can be strengthened with manual exercises by applying pressure on the top of the hand during extension **(C)** or holding the hand as it moves into flexion **(D)**. The flexors can be further strengthened with wrist curls **(E)** and the extensors with the use of the reverse wrist curl **(F)**.

from adjacent joints, strengthening of the wrist flexor and extensor muscles enhances the force production.

Commonly, the wrist is maintained in a position so that an efficient force application can occur. In tennis and racket sports, for example, the wrist is held either in the neutral position or in a slightly radially flexed position. If the wrist is held stationary, the force applied to the ball by the racket will not be lost through movements occurring at the wrist. This position is maintained by both wrist flexor and wrist extensor muscles.

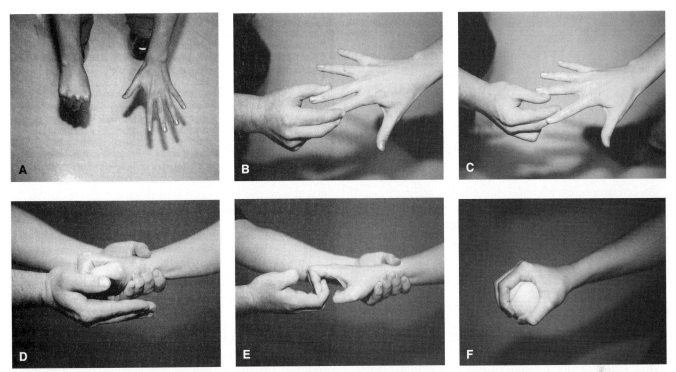

FIGURE 5-29 Flexibility (A), Manual Resistance (B to E), and Weight Training (F). The finger muscles can be stretched by opening and closing the fingers **(A)**. They can be strengthened by applying resistance to the fingers as they abduct **(B)** or adduct **(C)**. Resistance over the top as they extend **(D)** and underneath as the fingers attempt to form a fist **(E)** also strengthens them. Squeezing a tennis ball **(F)** is also good.

Another example of maintaining wrist position is in the volleyball underhand pass, in which the wrist is maintained in an ulnar flexed position. This opens up a broader area for contact and locks the elbows so they maintain an extended position upon contact. Finally, the wrist must be maintained in a stable, static position to achieve maximal performance from the fingers. Thus, while playing a piano or typing, the wrist must be maintained in the optimal position for finger usage. This is usually a slight hyperextended position via the wrist extensors. However, all of these wrist positions, while allowing for stability or creating more efficient muscle action, also create additional stress on the joint and may result in an overuse injury to the region.

In the hand, grip strength and the type of grip are the most important contributions to sport skills or daily activities, and both involve maintaining a static position of the fingers and the thumb. In a grip, the fingers flex to wrap around an object. If a **power grip** is needed, the fingers will flex more, with the most powerful grip being the fist position with flexion at all three finger joints, the MP, PIP, and DIP. If a fine **precision grip** is required, there may be only limited flexion at the PIP and DIP joints and only one or two fingers may be involved, such as in pinching and writing (51). Examples of both power and precision grips are shown in Figure 5-30.

It is really the thumb that determines whether a fine precision position or power position is generated. If the thumb remains in the plane of the hand in an adducted position and the fingers flex around an object, a power position is created. An example of this is the grip used in the javelin throw and in the golf swing. This power position still allows

for some precision, important in directing the golf club or the javelin.

Power in the grip can be enhanced by producing a fist with the thumb wrapped over the fully flexed fingers. With this grip, there is minimal if any precision. In addition, most power positions of the fingers are accompanied by ulnar flexion and extension at the wrist joint.

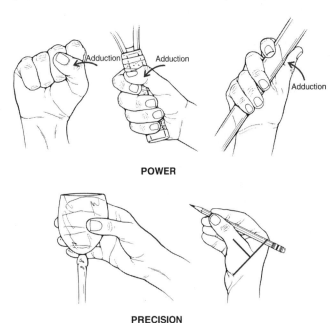

FIGURE 5-30 If power is needed in grip, the fingers flex at all three joints to form a fist. Also, if the thumb adducts, the grip is more powerful. A precision grip usually involves slight flexion at a small number of finger joints with the thumb perpendicular to the hand.

In activities requiring precise actions, the thumb is held more perpendicular to the hand and moved into opposition, with limited flexion at the fingers. An example of this type of position is in pitching, writing, and pinching. In a pinch or prehensile grip, greater force can be generated if the pulp of the thumb is placed against the pulps of the index and long fingers. This pinch is 40% stronger than the pinch grip with the tips of the thumb and fingers (24).

Finally, the dynamic actions of the fingers in a wide variety of activities, such as writing, tying shoes, and playing a musical instrument, require coordinated action between flexors, extensors, abductors, and adductors of all of the fingers. An analysis of the muscular actions contributing to an activity such as playing a piano is beyond the scope of this text.

INJURY POTENTIAL IN THE HAND AND FINGERS

Many injuries can occur to the hand as a result of absorbing a blunt force, as in impact with a ball, the ground, or another object. Injuries of this type in the wrist region usually are associated with a fall forcing the wrist into extreme flexion or extension. In this case, extreme hyperextension is the most common injury. This can result in a sprain of the wrist ligaments, a strain of the wrist muscles, a fracture of the scaphoid (70%) or other carpals (30%), a fracture of the distal radius, or a dislocation between the carpals and the wrist or other carpals (27).

The distal end of the radius is one of the most frequently fractured areas of the body, since the bone is not dense and the force of the fall is absorbed by the radius. A common fracture of the radius, Colles' fracture, is a diagonal fracture that forces the radius into more radial flexion and shortens it. These injuries are associated mainly with activities such as hockey, fencing, football, rugby, skiing, soccer, bicycling, parachuting, mountain climbing, and hang gliding, in which the chance of a blunt macrotrauma is greater than in other activities.

Examples of injuries to the fingers and the thumb as a result of blunt impact are fractures, dislocations, and tendon avulsions. The thumb can be injured by jamming it or forcing it into extension, causing severe strain of the thenar muscles and the ligaments surrounding the MCP joint. **Bennett's fracture** is a common fracture to the thumb at the base of the first metacarpal. Thumb injuries due to jamming by the pole are common in skiing (47). Thumb injuries are also common in biking (40).

Fingers are also frequently fractured or dislocated by an impact on the tip of the finger forcing it into extreme flexion or extension. Fractures are relatively common in the proximal phalanx and rare in the middle phalanx. High-impact collisions with the hand, such as are seen in boxing and the martial arts, result in more fractures or dislocations of the ring and little fingers, since they are least supported in a fist position.

Finger flexor or extensor mechanisms can be disrupted with a blow forcing the finger into extreme positions.

Mallet finger is an avulsion injury to the extensor tendon at the distal phalanx due to forced flexion resulting in the loss of the ability to extend the finger. **Boutonniere deformity**, caused by avulsion or stretching of the middle branch of the extensor mechanism, creates a stiff and immobile PIP articulation (42). Avulsion of the finger flexors is called **jersey finger** and is caused by forced hyperextension of the distal phalanx. The finger flexors can also develop nodules, a **trigger finger**. This results in snapping during flexion and extension of the fingers. These finger and thumb injuries are also commonly associated with the sports and activities listed above due to the incidence of impact occurring to the hand region.

There are also overuse injuries associated with repetitive use of the hand in sports, work, or other activities. **Tenosynovitis** of the radial flexors and thumb muscles is common in activities such as canoeing, rowing, rodeo, tennis, and fencing. Tennis and other racket sports, golf, throwing, javelin, and hockey, in which the wrist flexors and extensors are used to stabilize the wrist or create a repetitive wrist action, are susceptible to tendinitis of the wrist muscles inserting into the medial and lateral epicondyles. Medial or lateral epicondylitis may also result from this overuse. Medial epicondylitis is associated with overuse of the wrist flexors, while lateral epicondylitis is associated with overuse of the wrist extensors.

A disabling overuse injury to the hand is **carpal tunnel syndrome**. Next to low back injuries, carpal tunnel syndrome is one of the most frequent work injuries reported by the medical profession. The floor and sides of the carpal tunnel are formed by the carpals, and the top is formed by the transverse ligament. Traveling through this tunnel are all of the wrist flexor tendons and the median nerve (Fig. 5-31). Through repetitive actions at the wrist, usually repeated wrist flexion, the wrist flexor tendons may be inflamed to the point where there is pressure and constriction of the median

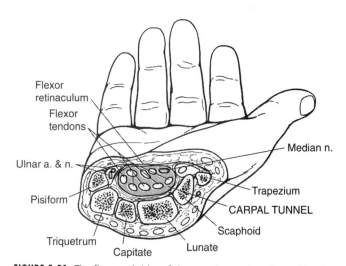

FIGURE 5-31 The floor and sides of the carpal tunnel are formed by the carpals, and the top of the tunnel is covered by ligament and the flexor retinaculum. Within the tunnel are wrist flexor tendons and the median nerve. Overuse of the wrist flexors can impinge the median nerve, causing carpal tunnel syndrome.

nerve. The median nerve innervates the radial side of the hand, specifically the thenar muscles of the thumb. Impingement of this nerve can cause pain, atrophy of the thenar muscles, and tingling sensations in the radial side of the hand.

To eliminate this condition, the source of the irritation must be removed by examining the workplace environment; a wrist stabilizing device can be applied to reduce the magnitude of the flexor forces; or a surgical release can be administered. It is recommended that the wrist be maintained in a neutral position while performing tasks in the workplace to avoid carpal tunnel syndrome.

Ulnar nerve injuries can also result in loss of function to the ulnar side of the hand, specifically the ring and little finger. Damage to this nerve can occur as a result of trauma to the elbow or shoulder region. Ulnar neuropathy is associated with activities such as cycling (32).

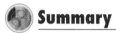 Summary

The upper extremity is much more mobile than the lower extremity, even though they have structural similarities. There are similarities in the connection into girdles, the number of segments, and the decreasing size of the bones toward the distal end of the extremities.

The shoulder complex consists of the sternoclavicular joint, the acromioclavicular joint, and the glenohumeral joint. The sternoclavicular joint is very stable, allowing the clavicle to move in elevation and depression, protraction and retraction, and rotation. The acromioclavicular joint is a small joint that allows the scapula to protract and retract, elevate and depress, and rotate up and down. The glenohumeral joint provides movement of the humerus through flexion and extension, abduction and adduction, medial and lateral rotation, and combination movements of horizontal abduction and adduction and circumduction. A final articulation, the scapulothoracic joint, is termed a physiological joint because of the lack of connection between two bones. It is here that the scapula moves on the thorax.

There is considerable movement of the arm at the shoulder joint. The arm can move through 180° of abduction, flexion, and rotation because of the interplay between movements occurring at all of the articulations. The timing of the movements between the arm, scapula, and clavicle is termed the scapulohumeral rhythm. Through 180° of elevation (flexion or abduction), there is approximately 2:1 degrees of humeral movement to scapular movement.

The muscles creating movement of the shoulder and shoulder girdle are also important for maintaining stability in the region. In abduction and flexion, for example, the deltoid produces about 50% of the muscular force for the movement, but it requires assistance from the rotator cuff (teres minor, subscapularis, infraspinatus, supraspinatus) to stabilize the head of the humerus

so that elevation can occur. Also, the shoulder girdle muscles contribute as the serratus anterior and the trapezius assist to stabilize the scapula and produce accompanying movements of elevation, upward rotation, and protraction.

To extend the arm against resistance, the latissimus dorsi, teres major, and pectoralis major act on the humerus and are joined by the rhomboid and the pectoralis minor, which retract, depress, and downwardly rotate the scapula. Similar muscular contributions are made by the infraspinatus and teres minor in external rotation of the humerus and the subscapularis, latissimus dorsi, teres major, and pectoralis major in internal rotation.

The shoulder muscles can generate considerable force in adduction and extension. The next strongest movement is flexion, and the weakest movements are abduction and rotation. The muscles surrounding the shoulder joint are capable of generating high forces, in the range of eight to nine times the weight of the limb.

Conditioning of the shoulder muscles is relatively easy because of the mobility of the joint. Numerous strength and flexibility exercises are used to isolate specific muscle groups or to replicate an upper extremity pattern used in a skill. Special exercise considerations for individuals with shoulder injury should exclude any exercise creating impingement in the joint.

Shoulder muscles are very important contributors to specific sport skills and movements. In the push-up, for example, the pectoralis major, latissimus dorsi, and triceps brachii are important contributors. In swimming, the latissimus dorsi, teres major, pectoralis major, supraspinatus, infraspinatus, middle deltoid, and serratus anterior make important contributions. In throwing, the deltoid, supraspinatus, infraspinatus, teres minor, subscapularis, trapezius, rhomboid, latissimus dorsi, pectoralis major, teres major, and deltoid all contribute.

Injury to the shoulder complex can be acute in the case of dislocations of the sternoclavicular or glenohumeral joints and fractures of the clavicle or humerus. Injuries can also be chronic, as with bursitis and tendinitis. Common injuries associated with impingement of the shoulder joint are subacromial bursitis, bicipital tendinitis, and tears in the supraspinatus muscle.

The elbow and the radioulnar joints assist the shoulder in applying force and placing the hand in a proper position for the desired action. The joints making up the elbow joint are the ulnar-humeral and radiohumeral joints, where flexion and extension occur, and the superior radioulnar joint, where pronation and supination of the forearm occur. The region is well supported by ligaments and the interosseous membrane running between the radius and the ulna. The joint structures allow approximately 145 to 160° of flexion and 70 to 85° of pronation and supination.

There are 24 muscles spanning the elbow joint, and these can be further classified into flexors (biceps brachii, brachioradialis, brachialis, pronator teres, extensor carpi radialis), extensors (triceps brachii, anconeus), pronators (pronator quadratus, pronator teres), and supinators (biceps brachii, supinator). The flexor muscle group is considerably stronger than the extensor group. Maximum flexion strength can be developed from the semiprone forearm position. Extension strength is maximum in a flexion position of 90°. Pronation and supination strength is also maximum from the semiprone position.

The arm muscles are used in a variety of different skills and movements. For example, the triceps brachii is an important contributor to rising from a chair, wheelchair activities, and throwing. Likewise, the biceps brachii and the pronator muscles are important in various phases of throwing.

The elbow and forearm are vulnerable to injury as a result of falling or repetitive overuse. In absorbing high forces, the elbow can dislocate or fracture or muscles can rupture. Through overuse, injuries such as medial or lateral tension syndrome can produce epicondylitis, tendinitis, or avulsion fractures.

The wrist and hand consist of complex structures that work together to provide fine movements used in a variety of daily activities. The main joints of the hand are the radiocarpal joint, the inferior radioulnar joint, the midcarpal and intercarpal joints, the carpometacarpal joints, the metacarpophalangeal joints, and the interphalangeal joints. The hand is capable of moving through 70 to 90° of wrist flexion, 70 to 80° of extension, 15 to 20° of radial flexion, and 30 to 40° of ulnar flexion. The fingers can flex through 70 to 110°, depending on the actual joint of interest (MCP or IP), 20 to 30° of hyperextension, and 20° of abduction. The thumb has special structural and functional characteristics that are related to the role of the carpometacarpal joint.

The extrinsic muscles acting on the hand enter the region as tendons. The muscles work in groups to produce wrist flexion (flexor carpi ulnaris, flexor carpi radialis, palmaris longus), extension (extensor carpi ulnaris, extensor carpi radialis longus, extensor carpi radialis brevis), ulnar flexion (flexor carpi ulnaris, extensor carpi ulnaris), and radial flexion (flexor carpi radialis, extensor carpi radialis longus, extensor carpi radialis brevis). Finger flexion is produced by the flexor digitorum profundus and flexor digitorum superficialis, while extension is produced primarily by the extensor digitorum. The fingers are abducted by the dorsal interossei and adducted by the palmar interossei.

Strength in the fingers is important in activities and sports in which a firm grip is essential. Grip strength can be enhanced by placing the thumb in a position parallel with the fingers (fist position). When precision is required, the thumb should be placed perpendicular to the fingers. The muscles of the hand can be exercised via a series of exercises that incorporates various wrist and finger positions.

The fingers and hand are frequently injured because of their vulnerability, especially when performing activities such as catching balls. Sprains, strains, fractures, and dislocations are common results of injuries sustained by the fingers or hands in the absorption of an external force. Other common injuries in the hand are associated with overuse, including medial or lateral tendinitis or epicondylitis and carpal tunnel syndrome.

REVIEW QUESTIONS

True or False

1. ____ The upper extremity attaches to the trunk at the acromioclavicular joint.

2. ____ Some individuals have no acromioclavicular joint.

3. ____ A typical bone-to-bone joint is also called a physiological joint.

4. ____ Muscular support in the superior aspect of the shoulder is provided by the long head of the biceps muscle.

5. ____ Arm extension is severely limited by internal rotation.

6. ____ If the arm is elevated, the shoulder will be more stable if it is externally rotated.

7. ____ The forces in the shoulder joint at 90° of abduction have been shown to be up to 50% of body weight.

8. ____ An active stretch uses an external force.

9. ____ There are many exercises for specific muscles of the shoulder.

10. ____ Exercises like the behind-the-neck pull-down should be avoided by people with anterior shoulder problems.

11. ____ For pushing up out of a chair, the primary upper extremity muscle used is the triceps brachii.

12. ____ Tendinitis at the insertion of the subscapularis is typically caused during the cocking phase of throwing.

13. ____ Shoulder girdle injuries are primarily due to overuse or impingement.

14. ____ Approximately 95% of shoulder dislocations are in the posterior direction.

15. ____ The elbow region consists of three joints.

16. ____ The asymmetry of the trochlea creates a valgus position in the extended position.

17. ____ The interosseous membrane runs from the proximal radioulnar joint to about halfway to the distal radioulnar joint.

18. ____ The interosseous membrane serves as a site for muscular attachment.

19. ____ The joints of the elbow complex do not all reach a close-packed position at the same point in the range of motion.

20. ____ Twelve muscles cross the elbow.

21. ____ Forces in the elbow increase with grip width on a bench press exercise.

22. ____ The distal radioulnar joint does not participate in any wrist movements.

23. ____ In racket sports the wrist will be more stable in the neutral position.

24. ___ Each hand has 12 phalanges.

25. ___ The interphalangeal articulation is an example of a hinge joint.

Multiple Choice

1. The clavicle can move in ___ directions at the sternoclavicular joint.
   a. 1
   b. 2
   c. 3
   d. Does not move

2. The acromioclavicular joint attaches the clavicle to the ___.
   a. Shoulder
   b. Humerus
   c. First rib
   d. Scapula

3. The ___ ligament assists scapular movements by acting as an axis of rotation.
   a. Acromioclavicular
   b. Coracoclavicular
   c. Sternoclavicular
   d. None of above

4. The glenoid fossa is approximately ___ of the size of the humeral head.
   a. 10%
   b. 25%
   c. 50%
   d. 60%

5. Stability in the glenohumeral joint is derived primarily from the ___.
   a. Joint contact area
   b. Vacuum in the joint
   c. Ligaments and muscles
   d. All of the above

6. The impingement area of the shoulder joint is in the ___ aspect.
   a. Superior
   b. Inferior
   c. Posterior
   d. Anterior

7. The function of a bursa is to ___.
   a. Distribute load
   b. Maintain joint stability
   c. Reduce friction
   d. All of the above

8. With the arm in the neutral position, ___ rotation will ___ the shoulder capsule.
   a. Internal, tighten
   b. Internal, loosen
   c. External, tighten
   d. External, loosen

9. The muscles of the rotator cuff are the ___.
   a. Infraspinatus, supraspinatus, serratus anterior, teres minor
   b. Infraspinatus, teres minor, teres major, subscapularis
   c. Subscapularis, teres minor, teres major, infraspinatus
   d. None of the above

10. If the arm is adducted against gravity, the action is ___, while if it is lowered against an external force, such as a weight machine, the action is ___.
   a. eccentric, concentric
   b. eccentric, eccentric
   c. concentric, eccentric
   d. concentric, concentric

11. A solution to impingement problems during the lateral raise would be to ___ the arm.
   a. Internally rotate
   b. Externally rotate
   c. Horizontally flex
   d. None of the above

12. Persons with rotator cuff problems should avoid heavy lifting in the ___ movement.
   a. Flexion
   b. Extension
   c. Abduction
   d. Adduction

13. It is believed that impingement in a swimmer's shoulder may be due to ___ fatigue.
   a. Latissimus dorsi
   b. Deltoid
   c. Teres major
   d. Serratus anterior

14. The ___ articulation is the major contributing joint to flexion and extension of the forearm.
   a. Ulnar-humeral
   b. Radiohumeral
   c. Radioulnar
   d. All of the above

15. The medial collateral ligament connects the ___ to the ___.
   a. Humerus, radius
   b. Humerus, ulna
   c. Radius, ulna
   d. None of the above

16. The annular ligament wraps around the head of the ___.
   a. Humerus
   b. Ulna
   c. Lateral epicondyle
   d. None of the above

17. The ulnar-humeral articulation is in the close-packed position when it is ___.
   a. Flexed 80° and semiprone
   b. Extended
   c. Flexed 90°
   d. Extended and semiprone

18. Approximately ___ of pronation and ___ of supination is required for daily living activities.
   a. 90°, 75°
   b. 75°, 90°
   c. 25°, 25°
   d. 50°, 50°

19. The strongest elbow flexor is the ___.
   a. Biceps brachii
   b. Brachialis
   c. Brachioradialis
   d. Pronator teres

20. In the hand there are ___ rows of carpals with ___ bones in each row.
   a. 2, 4
   b. 2, 3
   c. 3, 4
   d. 3, 2

21. The midcarpal joint accounts for ___ percent of the total range of extension movement.
   a. 10
   b. 40
   c. 60
   d. 75

22. Most of the muscles acting at the wrist and fingers are considered ___.
   a. Concentric
   b. Eccentric
   c. Intrinsic
   d. Extrinsic

23. An avulsion injury to the extensor tendon at the distal phalanx is called a ___.
   a. Boutonnière deformity
   b. Jersey finger
   c. Mallet finger
   d. Bennett's finger

24. Carpal tunnel syndrome is an irritation of the ___.
   a. Lateral nerve
   b. Median nerve
   c. Flexor retinaculum
   d. Ulnar nerve

25. To avoid carpal tunnel syndrome it is recommended that the wrist be maintained in a ___ position.
   a. Neutral
   b. Flexed
   c. Extended
   d. Radially flexed

REFERENCES

1. An, K. N., et al. (1992). Intersegmental elbow joint load during pushup. *Biomedical Scientific Instrumentation*, 28:69–74.

2. An, K. N., et al. (1981). Muscles across the elbow joint: A biomechanical analysis. *Journal of Biomechanics*, 14:659–669.

3. Anderson, D. S., et al. (1984). Electromyographic analysis of selected muscles during sitting pushups. *Physical Therapy*, 64:24–28.

4. Andrews, J. R., et al. (1985). Glenoid labrum tears related to the long head of the biceps. *American Journal of Sports Medicine*, 13:337–341.

5. Bayley, J. C., et al. (1987). The weight-bearing shoulder. *Journal of Bone and Joint Surgery*, 69-A:676–678.

6. Blackburn, T. A., et al. (1990). EMG analysis of posterior rotator cuff exercises. *Athletic Training*, 25(1):40–45.

7. Blakely, R. L., Palmer, M. L. (1984). Analysis of rotation accompanying shoulder flexion. *Physical Therapy*, 64:1214–1216.

8. Bowling, R. W., Rockar, P. (1985). The elbow complex. In J. Gould, G. J. Davies (Eds.). *Orthopaedics and Sports Physical Therapy*. St. Louis: Mosby, 476–496.

9. Broome, H. L., Basmajian, J. V. (1970). The function of the teres major muscle: An electromyographic study. *Anatomical Record*, 170:309–310.

10. Burnham, R. S., et al. (1993). Shoulder pain in wheelchair athletes. *American Journal of Sports Medicine*, 21:238–242.

11. Duda, M. (1985). Prevention and treatment of throwing arm injuries. *Physician and Sports Medicine*, 13:181–186.

12. Einhorn, A. R. (1985). Shoulder rehabilitation: Equipment modifications. *Journal of Orthopaedic and Sports Physical Therapy*, 6:247–253.

13. Fleisig, G. S., et al. (1991). A biomechanical description of the shoulder joint during pitching. *Sports Medicine Update*, 6:10–24.

14. Gellman, H., et al. (1988). Late complications of the weight-bearing upper extremity in the paraplegic patient. *Clinical Orthopaedics and Related Research*, 233:132–135.

15. Hageman, P. A., et al. (1989). Effects of position and speed on eccentric and concentric isokinetic testing of the shoulder rotators. *Journal of Orthopaedic and Sports Physical Therapy*, 11:64–69.

16. Halbach, J. W., Tank, R. T. (1985). The shoulder. In J. A. Gould, G. J. Davies (Eds.). *Orthopaedic and Sports Physical Therapy*. St. Louis: C.V. Mosby, 497–517.

17. Harryman, D. T., et al. (1990). Translation of the humeral head on the glenoid with passive glenohumeral motion. *Journal of Bone and Joint Surgery*, 72-A:1334–1343.

18. Heinrichs, K. I. (1991). Shoulder anatomy, biomechanics and rehabilitation considerations for the whitewater slalom athlete. *National Strength and Conditioning Association Journal*, 13:26–35.

19. Henry, J. H., Genung, J. A. (1982). Natural history of glenohumeral dislocation—revisited. *American Journal of Sports Medicine*, 10:135–137.

20. Imaeda, T., et al. (1992). Functional anatomy and biomechanics of the thumb. *Hand Clinics*, 8:9–15.

21. Ireland, M. L., Andrews, J. R. (1988). Shoulder and elbow injuries in the young athlete. *Clinics in Sports Medicine*, 7:473–494.

22. Jiang, C. C., et al. (1987). Muscle excursion measurements and moment arm determinations of rotator cuff muscles. *Biomechanics in Sport*, 13:41–44.

23. Jobe, F. W., et al. (1984). An EMG analysis of the shoulder in pitching. *American Journal of Sports Medicine*, 12:218–220.

24. Jones, L. A. (1989). The assessment of hand function: A critical review of techniques. *Journal of Hand Surgery*, 14A:221–228.

25. Kronberg, M., et al. (1990). Muscle activity and coordination in the normal shoulder. *Clinical Orthopaedics and Related Research*, 257:76–85.

26. Kulund, D. N., et al. (1979). The long-term effects of playing tennis. *Physician and Sports Medicine*, 7:87–91.

27. Mayfield, J. K. (1980). Mechanism of carpal injuries. *Clinical Orthopaedics and Related Research*, 149:45–54.

28. McCann, P. D., et al. (1993). A kinematic and electromyographic study of shoulder rehabilitation exercises. *Clinical Orthopaedics and Related Research*, 288:179–188.

29. Morrey, B. F., et al. (1981). A biomechanical study of normal and functional elbow motion. *Journal of Bone and Joint Surgery*, 63-A:872–877.

30. Moseley, J. B., et al. (1992). EMG analysis of the scapular muscles during a shoulder rehabilitation program. *American Journal of Sports Medicine*, 20:128–134.

31. Moynes, D. R., et al. (1986). Electromyography and motion analysis of the upper extremity in sports. *Physical Therapy*, 66:1905–1910.

32. Munnings, F. (1991). Cyclist's palsy. *Physician and Sports Medicine*, 19:113–119.

33. Nitz, A. J. (1986). Physical therapy management of the shoulder. *Physical Therapy*, 66:1912–1919.

34. Nuber, G. W., et al. (1986). Fine wire electromyography analysis of muscles of the shoulder during swimming. *American Journal of Sports Medicine*, 14:7–11.

35. Ober, A. G. (1988). An electromyographic analysis of elbow flexors during sub-maximal concentric contractions. *Research Quarterly for Exercise and Sport*, 59:139–143.

36. Pappas, A. M., et al. (1983). Symptomatic shoulder instability due to lesions of the glenoid labrum. *American Journal of Sports Medicine*, 11:279–288.

37. Peat, M., Graham, R. E. (1977). Electromyographic analysis of soft tissue lesions affecting shoulder function. *American Journal of Physical Medicine*, 56:223–240.

38. Poppen, N. K., Walker, P. S. (1976). Normal and abnormal motion of the shoulder. *Journal of Bone and Joint Surgery*, 58-A:195–200.

39. Prodromos, C. C., et al. (1990). Histological studies of the glenoid labrum from fetal life to old age. *Journal of Bone and Joint Surgery*, 72-A:1344–1348.

40. Shea, K. G., et al. (1991). Shifting into wrist pain. *Physician and Sports Medicine*, 19:59–63.

41. Simon, E. R., Hill, J. A. (1989). Rotator cuff injuries: An update. *Journal of Orthopaedic and Sports Physical Therapy*, 10:394–398.

42. Soderberg, G. L. (1986). *Kinesiology: Application to Pathological Motion*. Baltimore: Williams & Wilkins, pp. 109–128.

43. Stewart, O. J., et al. (1981). Influence of resistance, speed of movement, and forearm position on recruitment of the elbow flexors. *American Journal of Physical Medicine*, 60(4):165–179.

44. Turkel, S. J., et al. (1981). Stabilizing mechanisms preventing anterior dislocation of the glenohumeral joint. *Journal of Bone and Joint Surgery*, 63(8):1208–1217.

45. Van Zuylen, E. J., Van Velzen, A. (1988). A biomechanical model for flexion torques of human arm muscles as a function of elbow angle. *Journal of Biomechanics*, 21:183–189.

46. Wadsworth, C. T. (1985). The wrist and hand. In J. A. Gould, G. J. Davies (Eds.). *Orthopaedic and Sports Physical Therapy*. St. Louis: Mosby, 437–475.

47. Wadsworth, L. T. (1992). How to manage skier's thumb. *Physician and Sports Medicine*, 20:69–78.

48. Whiteside, J. A., Andrews, J. R. (1992). On-the-field evaluation of common athletic injuries: 6. Evaluation of the shoulder girdle. *Sports Medicine Update*, 7:24–28.

49. Yocum, L. A. (1989). The diagnosis and nonoperative treatment of elbow problems in the athlete. *Office Practice of Sports Medicine*, 8:437–439.

50. Zarins, B., Rowe, R. (1984). Current concepts in the diagnosis and treatment of shoulder instability in athletes. *Medicine and Science in Sports and Exercise*, 16:444–448.

51. Zuckerman, J. D., Matsea III, F. A. (1989). Biomechanics of the shoulder. In M. Nordin and V. H. Frankel (Eds). *Biomechanics of the Musculoskeletal System*. Philadelphia: Lea & Febiger, 225–248.

ADDITIONAL READING

An, K. N., et al. (1983). Tendon excursion and moment arm of index finger muscles. *Journal of Biomechanics*, 16:419–426.

Andrews, J. R., Whiteside, J. A. (1993). Common elbow problems in the athlete. *Journal of Sports Physical Therapy*, 17:289–295.

Baker, C. L., et al. (1990). Arthroscopic evaluation of acute initial anterior shoulder dislocations. *American Journal of Sports Medicine*, 18:25–280.

Barmakian, J. T. (1992). Anatomy of the joints of the thumb. *Hand Clinics*, 8:683–691.

Basmajian, J. V. (1969). Recent advances in the functional anatomy of the upper limb. *American Journal of Physical Medicine*, 18:165–177.

Basset, R. W., et al. (1990). Glenohumeral muscle force and moment mechanics in a position of shoulder instability. *Journal of Biomechanics*, 23:405–412.

Blakely, R. L., Palmer, M. L. (1986). Analysis of shoulder rotation accompanying a proprioceptive neuromuscular facilitation approach. *Physical Therapy*, 66:1224–1227.

Bowers, K. D. (1979). Treatment of acromioclavicular sprains in athletes. *Physician and Sports Medicine*, 11:79–89.

Boyd, H. B., Sisk, D. (1972). Recurrent posterior dislocation of the shoulder. *Journal of Bone and Joint Surgery*, 54-A:779–786.

Brewer, B. J. (1972). Aging of the rotator cuff. *American Journal of Sports Medicine*, 7:102–110.

Brown, L. P., et al. (1988). Upper extremity range of motion and isokinetic strength of the internal and external shoulder rotators in major league baseball players. *American Journal of Sports Medicine*, 16:577–585.

Brunet, M. E., et al. (1982). Rotator cuff impingement syndrome in sports. *Physician and Sports Medicine*, 10:86–94.

Bryan, R. S., Dobyns, J. H. (1979). Fractures of the carpal bones other than the lunate and navicular. *Clinical Orthopaedics and Related Research*, 149:107–111.

Carmichael, S. W., Hart, D. L. (1985). Anatomy of the shoulder joint. *Journal of Orthopaedic and Sports Physical Therapy*, 6:225–228.

Carson, W. G. (1989). Rehabilitation of the throwing shoulder. *Clinics in Sports Medicine*, 8:657–689.

Coleman, A. E. (1982). In-season strength training in major league baseball players. *Physician and Sports Medicine*, 10:125–132.

Constant, C. R. (1990). Injuries to the elbow. *Journal of Royal College of Edinburgh*, 35(Suppl):S31–S32.

Conwell, E. (1970). Injuries to the wrist. *Clinical Symposia*, 22:3–30.

Cook, E. E., et al. (1987). Shoulder antagonistic strength ratios: A comparison between college-level baseball pitchers and non-pitchers. *Journal of Orthopaedic and Sports Physical Therapy*, 8:451–461.

Craig, S. M. (1992). Anatomy of the joints of the fingers. *Hand Clinics*, 8:693–700.

Danzig, L., et al. (1982). Evaluation of unstable shoulders by computed tomography. *American Journal of Sports Medicine*, 10:138–141.

Dobyns, J. H., et al. (1978). Sports stress syndromes of the hand and wrist. *American Journal of Sports Medicine*, 6:236–253.

Donatelli, R., Greenfield, B. (1987). Case study: Rehabilitation of a stiff and painful shoulder: A biomechanical approach. *Journal of Orthopaedic and Sports Physical Therapy*, 9:118–126.

Ellenbecker, T. S., Derscheid, G. L. (1989). Rehabilitation of overuse injuries of the shoulder. *Clinics in Sports Medicine*, 8:583–604.

Ellenbecker, T. S., et al. (1988). Concentric versus eccentric isokinetic strengthening of the rotator cuff. *American Journal of Sports Medicine*, 16:64–69.

Engle, R. P., Canner, G. C. (1989). Posterior shoulder instability: Approach to rehabilitation. *Journal of Orthopaedic and Sports Physical Therapy*, 10(12):488–494.

Ferrari, D. A. (1990). Capsular ligaments of the shoulder. *American Journal of Sports Medicine*, 18:20–24.

Fisk, G. R. (1980). An overview of the injuries of the wrist. *Clinical Orthopaedics and Related Research*, 149:137–143.

Gerdle, B., et al. (1988). Changes in the surface electromyogram during increasing isometric shoulder forward flexions. *European Journal of Applied Physiology*, 57:404–408.

Gerdle, B., et al. (1989). Muscular fatigue during repeated isokinetic shoulder forward flexions in young females. *European Journal of Applied Sciences*, 58:666–673.

Gerdle, B., et al. (1988). Surface EMG recordings during maximum static shoulder forward flexion in different positions. *European Journal of Applied Physiology*, 57:415–419.

Gowan, D., et al. (1987). A comparative electromyographic analysis of the shoulder during pitching. *American Journal of Sports Medicine*, 15:486–490.

Gregg, J. R., et al. (1979). Serratus anterior paralysis in the young athlete. *Journal of Bone and Joint Surgery*, 61-A:825–832.

Hagberg, M. (1981). Electromyographic signs of shoulder muscular fatigue in two elevated arm positions. *American Journal of Physical Medicine*, 60:111–121.

Hagberg, C., Hagberg, M. (1989). Surface EMG amplitude and frequency dependence on exerted force for the upper trapezius muscle: A comparison between right and left sides. *European Journal of Applied Physiology*, 58:641–645.

Hart, D. L., Carmichael, S. W. (1985). Biomechanics of the shoulder. *Journal of Orthopaedic and Sports Physical Therapy*, 16:229–278.

Howell, S. M., et al. (1985). Clarification of the role of the supraspinatus muscle in shoulder function. *Journal of Bone and Joint Surgery*, 68:398–404.

Imaeda, T., et al. (1993). Anatomy of trapeziometacarpal ligament. *Journal of Hand Surgery*, 18A:226–231.

Jobe, F. W., Bradley, J. P. (1989). The diagnosis and nonoperative treatment of shoulder injuries in athletes. *Office Practice of Sports Medicine*, 8:419–433.

Jobe, F. W., Moynes, D. R. (1982). Delineation of diagnostic criteria and a rehabilitation program for rotator cuff injuries. *American Journal of Sports Medicine*, 10:336–339.

Jobe, F. W., et al. (1983). An EMG analysis of the shoulder in throwing and pitching. *American Journal of Sports Medicine*, 11:3–5.

Jones, L., Hunter, I. W. (1992). Changes in pinch force with bidirectional load forces. *Journal of Motor Behavior*, 24:157–164.

Kauer, J. M. (1980). Functional anatomy of the wrist. *Clinical Orthopaedics and Related Research*, 149:9–19.

Knudsen, D. V. (1989). Hand forces and impact effectiveness in the tennis forehand. *Journal of Human Movement Studies*, 17:1–7.

Knudsen, D. V. (1991). Factors affecting force loading on the hand in the tennis forehand. *Journal of Sports Medicine and Physical Fitness*, 31:527–531.

Knudsen, D. V., White, S. C. (1989). Forces on the hand in the tennis forehand drive: Application of force sensing resistors. *International Journal of Sport Biomechanics*, 5:324–331.

Kuhlman, J. R., et al. (1992). Isokinetic and isometric measurement of strength of external rotation and abduction of the shoulder. *Journal of Bone and Joint Surgery*, 74-A:1320–1333.

Landerjerit, B., Maton, B. (1988). In vivo muscular force analysis during the isometric flexion of a monkey's elbow. *Journal of Biomechanics*, 21:577–584.

Martin, P. E., Heise, G. D. (1992). Archery bow grip force distribution: Relationships with performance and fatigue. *International Journal of Sport Biomechanics*, 8:305–319.

Minamikawa, Y., et al. (1993). Stability and constraint of the proximal interphalangeal joint. *Journal of Hand Surgery*, 18A:198–204.

Moynes, D. R. (1983). Prevention of injury to the shoulder through exercises and therapy. *Clinics in Sports Medicine*, 2:413–422.

Neer, C. S., Foster, C. R. (1980). Inferior capsular shift for involuntary inferior and multi-directional instability of the shoulder. *Journal of Bone and Joint Surgery*, 62-A:897–907.

Nemeth, G., et al. (1990). Electromyogram (EMG) recordings from the sub-scapularis muscle: Description of a technique. *Journal of Orthopaedic Research*, 8:151–153.

Nicholson, G. G. (1989). Rehabilitation of common shoulder injuries. *Clinics in Sports Medicine*, 8:657–689.

Nicholson, G. G. (1985). The effects of passive joint mobilization on pain and hypomobility associated with adhesive capsulitis of the shoulder. *Journal of Orthopaedic and Sports Physical Therapy*, 6:238–246.

Nielsen, A. J. (1981). Case study: Myofascial pain of the posterior shoulder relieved by spray and stretch. *Journal of Orthopaedic and Sports Physical Therapy*, 3:21–26.

Nikolaou, P. K., et al. (1987). Biomechanical and historical evaluation of muscle after controlled strain injury. *American Journal of Sports Medicine*, 15:9–14.

O'Driscoll, S. W., et al. (1992). Elbow subluxation and dislocation. *Clinical Orthopaedics and Related Research*, 280:186–197.

Otis, J. C., et al. (1990). Torque production in the shoulder of the normal young adult male. *American Journal of Sports Medicine*, 18:119–123.

Pappas, A. (1990). Elbow problems associated with baseball during childhood and adolescence. *American Journal of Sports Medicine*, 11:30–41.

Paulos, L. E., Franklin, J. L. (1990). Arthroscopic shoulder decompression development and application. *American Journal of Sports Medicine*, 18:235–244.

Pearl, M. L., et al. (1992). An electromyographic analysis of the shoulder during cones and planes of arm motion. *Clinical Orthopaedics and Related Research*, 284:116–127.

Peat, M. (1986). Functional anatomy of the shoulder complex. *Physical Therapy*, 66:1855–1865.

Perry, J. (1978). Normal upper extremity kinesiology. *Physical Therapy*, 58:265–269.

Regan, W. D., et al. (1991). Biomechanical study of ligaments around the elbow joint. *Clinical Orthopaedics and Related Research*, 271:170–179.

Richards, R. R., et al. (1993). Measurement of wrist, metacarpophalangeal joint, and thumb extension strength in a normal population. *Journal of Hand Surgery*, 18A:253–261.

Sarrafian, S. K., et al. (1977). Study of wrist motion in flexion and extension. *Clinical Orthopaedics and Related Research*, 126:153–159.

Schenkman, M., De Cartaya, V. R. (1987). Kinesiology of the shoulder complex. *Journal of Orthopaedic and Sports Physical Therapy*, 8:438–450.

Silfverskiold, J., Waters, R. L. (1991). Shoulder pain and functional disability in spinal cord injury patients. *Clinical Orthopaedics and Related Research*, 272:141–145.

Soderberg, G. J., Blaschak, M. J. (1987). Shoulder internal and external rotation peak torque production. *Journal of Orthopaedic and Sports Physical Therapy*, 8:518–524.

Stroyan, M., Wilk, K. E. (1993). The functional anatomy of the elbow complex. *Journal of Sport Physical Therapy*, 17:279–288.

Tank, R., Halbach, J. (1982). Physical therapy evaluation of the shoulder complex in athletes. *Journal of Orthopaedic and Sports Physical Therapy*, 3:108–119.

Taylor, D. C., et al. (1990). Viscoelastic properties of muscle tendon units. *American Journal of Sports Medicine*, 18:300–309.

Thein, L. A. (1989). Impingemen syndrome and its conservative management. *Journal of Sports Physical Therapy*, 11:183–191.

Tibone, J. E., et al. (1986). Surgical treatment of tears of the rotator cuff in athletes. *Journal of Bone and Joint Surgery*, 68-A:887–891.

Tolbert, J. R., et al. (1985). Kinetics of normal and prosthetic wrists. *Journal of Biomechanics*, 18:887–897.

Van Woensel, W., Arwert, H. (1993). Effects of external load and abduction angle on EMG level of shoulder muscles during isometric action. *Electromyographic Clinical Neurophysiology*, 33:185–191.

Veeger, H. E. J., et al. (1990). Inertia and muscle contraction parameters for musculoskeletal modeling of the shoulder mechanism. *Journal of Biomechanics*, 24:615–629.

Volz, R. G., et al. (1980). Biomechanics of the wrist. *Clinical Orthopaedics and Related Research*, 149:112–117.

Wadsworth, C. T. (1983). Clinical anatomy and mechanics of the wrist and hand. *Journal of Orthopaedics and Sports Physical Therapy*, 4:206–216.

Walmsley, R. P., Szybbo, C. (1987). A comparative study of the torque generated by the shoulder internal and external rotator muscles in different positions and at varying speeds. *Journal of Orthopaedic and Sports Physical Therapy*, 9:217–222.

Wilson, F. (1983). Valgus extension overload in the pitching elbow. *American Journal of Sports Medicine*, 11:123–132.

Youm, Y., et al. (1978). Kinematics of the wrist. *Journal of Bone and Joint Surgery*, 60-A:423–432.

Youm, Y., et al. (1978). Kinematic investigation of normal MCP joint. *Journal of Biomechanics*, 11:109–118.

Zemel, N. P. (1992). Metacarpophalangeal joint injuries in the fingers. *Hand Clinics*, 8:745–754.

GLOSSARY

Abduction: Sideways movement away from the midline or sagittal plane.

Acromioclavicular Joint: Articulation between the acromion process of the scapula and the lateral end of the clavicle.

Adduction: Sideways movement toward the midline or sagittal plane; return movement from abduction.

Annular Ligament: Ligament inserting on the anterior and posterior margins of the radial notch; supports the head of the radius.

Bennett's Fracture: Longitudinal fracture of the base of the first metacarpal.

Bicipital Tendinitis: Inflammation of the tendon of the biceps brachii.

Boutonnière Deformity: A stiff proximal interphalangeal articulation caused by injury to the finger extensor mechanism.

Bursa: A fibrous fluid-filled sac between bones and tendons or other structures that reduces friction during movement.

Bursitis: Inflammation of a bursa.

Capitulum: Eminence on the distal end of the lateral epicondyle of the humerus; articulates with the head of the radius at the elbow.

Carpal Tunnel Syndrome: Pressure and constriction of the median nerve caused by repetitive actions at the wrist.

Carpometacarpal Joint: Articulation between the carpals and the metacarpals in the hand.

Carrying Angle: Angle between the ulna and the humerus with the elbow extended; 10 to 25°.

Clavicle: An S, shaped long bone articulating with the scapula and the sternum.

Coracoid Process: A curved process arising from the upper neck of the scapula; overhangs the shoulder joint.

Coronoid Fossa: Cavity in the humerus that receives the coronoid process of the ulna during elbow flexion.

Coronoid Process: Wide eminence on proximal end of ulna; forms anterior portion of trochlear fossa.

Degeneration: Deterioration of tissue; a chemical change in the body tissue; change of tissue to a less functionally active form.

Depression: Movement of the segment downward (scapula, clavicle); return of the elevation movement.

Dislocation: Bone displacement; separation of the bony surfaces in a joint.

Ectopic Bone: Bone formation that is displaced away from the normal site.

Ectopic Calcification: Hardening of organic tissue through deposit of calcium salts in areas away from the normal sites.

Elevation: Movement of a segment upward, e.g., scapula, clavicle.

Epicondylitis: Inflammation of the epicondyle or tissues connecting to the epicondyle, e.g., medial or lateral epicondylitis.

Fracture: A break in a bone.

Force Couple: Two forces, equal in magnitude, acting in opposite directions, that produce rotation about an axis.

Glenohumeral Joint: The articulation between the head of the humerus and the glenoid fossa on the scapula.

Glenoid Labrum: Ring of fibrocartilage around the rim of the glenoid fossa that deepens the socket in the shoulder and hip joints.

Glenoid Fossa: Depression in the lateral superior scapula that forms the socket for the shoulder joint.

Horizontal Extension (Abduction): Movement of an elevated segment (arm, leg) away from the body in the posterior direction.

Horizontal Flexion (Adduction): Movement of an elevated segment (arm, leg) toward the body in the anterior direction.

Hypothenar Eminence: The ridge on the palm on the ulnar side created by the presence of intrinsic muscles acting on the little finger.

Impingement Syndrome: Irritation of structures above the shoulder joint due to repeated compression as the greater tuberosity is pushed up against the underside of the acromion process.

Intercarpal Joint: Articulation between the carpal bones.

Interosseous Membrane: A thin layer of tissue running between two bones (radius and ulna, tibia and fibula).

Interphalangeal Joint: Articulation between the phalanx of the fingers and toes.

Jersey Finger: Avulsion of a finger flexor tendon through forced hyperextension.

Lateral Epicondyle: Projection from the lateral side of the distal end of the humerus giving attachment to the hand and finger extensors.

Mallet Finger: Avulsion injury to the finger extensor tendons at the distal phalanx; produced by a forced flexion.

Medial Epicondyle: Projection from the medial side of the distal end of the humerus giving attachment to the hand and finger flexors.

Medial Tension Syndrome: Also termed pitcher's elbow, medial pain brought on by excessive valgus forces, which may cause ligament sprain, medial epicondylitis, tendinitis, or avulsion fractures to the medial epicondyle.

Metacarpophalangeal Joint: Articulation between the metacarpals and the phalanges in the hand.

Midcarpal Joint: Articulation between the proximal and distal row of carpals in the hand.

Olecranon Bursitis: Irritation of the olecranon bursae caused commonly by falling on the elbow.

Olecranon Fossa: A depression on the posterior distal humerus; creates a lodging space for the olecranon process of the ulna in forearm extension.

Olecranon Process: Projection on the proximal posterior ulna; fits into the olecranon fossa during forearm extension.

Osteochondritis Dissecans: Inflammation of bone and cartilage resulting in splitting of pieces of cartilage into the joint (shoulder, hip).

Pitcher's Elbow: Also termed medial tension syndrome, medial pain brought on by excessive valgus forces that may cause ligament sprain, medial epicondylitis, tendinitis, or avulsion fracture to the medial epicondyle.

Power Grip: A powerful hand position produced by flexing the fingers maximally around the object at all three finger joints and the thumb adducted in the same plane as the hand.

Precision Grip: A fine-movement hand position produced by positioning the fingers in a minimal amount of flexion with the thumb perpendicular to the hand.

Pronation: Inward rotation of a body segment (forearm).

Protraction: Also called abduction, movement of the scapula forward and away from the vertebral column.

Radiocarpal Joint: Articulation between the radius and the carpals (scaphoid and lunate).

Radiohumeral Joint: Articulation between the radius and the humerus.

Radioulnar Joint: Articulation between the radius and the ulna (superior and inferior).

Retinaculum: Fibrous band that contains tendons or other structures.

Retraction: Also called adduction, movement of the scapula backward and toward the vertebral column.

Rotation: Movement of a segment about an axis.

Rotator Cuff: Four muscles surrounding the shoulder joint, the infraspinatus, supraspinatus, teres minor, and subscapularis.

Rupture: An injury in which the tissue is torn or disrupted in a forcible manner.

Scapulohumeral Rhythm: The movement relationship between the humerus and the scapula during arm raising movements; the humerus moves 2° for every 1° of scapular movement through 180° of arm flexion or abduction.

Scapula: A flat, triangular bone on the upper posterior thorax.

Scapulothoracic joint: A physiological joint between the scapula and the thorax.

Shoulder Girdle: An incomplete bony ring in the upper extremity formed by the two scapulae and clavicles.

Sprain: An injury to a ligament surrounding a joint; rupture of fibers of a ligament.

Sternoclavicular Joint: Articulation between the sternum and the clavicle.

Strain: Injury to the muscle, tendon, or muscle–tendon junction due to overstretching or excessive tension applied to the muscle; tearing and rupture of the muscle or tendon fibers.

Subacromial Bursae: The bursae between the acromion process and the insertion of the supraspinatus muscle.

Subacromial Bursitis: Inflammation of the subacromial bursae, common to impingement syndrome.

Subluxation: An incomplete or partial dislocation between two joint surfaces.

Supination: Outward rotation of a body segment (forearm).

Tendinitis: Inflammation of a tendon.

Tenosynovitis: Inflammation of the sheath surrounding a tendon.

Thenar Eminence: Ridge or mound on the radial side of the palm formed by the intrinsic muscles acting on the thumb.

Traction Apophysitis: Inflammation of the apophysis (process, tuberosity) created by a pulling force of tendons.

Trigger Finger: Snapping during flexion and extension of the fingers created by nodules on the tendons.

Trochlea: Medial portion of the distal end of the humerus; articulates with the trochlear notch of the ulna.

Trochlear Notch: A deep groove in the proximal end of the ulna; articulates with the trochlea of the humerus.

Ulnohumeral Joint: Articulation between the ulna and the humerus; commonly called the elbow.

6

Functional Anatomy of the Lower Extremity

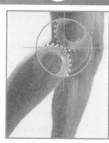

OBJECTIVES

After reading this chapter, the student will be able to:

1. Describe the structure, support, and movements of the hip, knee, ankle, and subtalar joints.

2. Identify the pelvic and sacral movements accompanying the movements of the thigh and the trunk.

3. Explain how changes in the femoral neck angles will influence hip position.

4. Identify the muscular actions contributing to movements at the hip and knee joints.

5. Compare the movements of the thigh in terms of flexibility and strength.

6. Identify the lower extremity muscular contributions to walking, running, stair climbing, cycling, and lifting.

7. Describe how alterations in the alignment in the lower extremity influences function at the knee, hip, ankle, and foot.

8. Discuss various loads that the hip, knee, ankle, and foot must absorb and transmit in daily activities.

9. Identify the muscular contributions to specific movements at the knee, ankle, and foot.

10. List and describe some of the common injuries to the hip, knee, ankle, and foot.

11. Develop a set of strength and flexibility exercises for the hip, knee, and ankle joints.

12. Differentiate between pronation and supination during both weight bearing and non–weight bearing.

13. Discuss the structure and function of the arches of the foot.

The lower extremity is subject to high forces that are generated via repetitive contacts between the foot and the ground. At the same time, the lower extremity is responsible for supporting the mass of the trunk and the upper extremities. The lower limbs are connected to each other and to the trunk by the **pelvic girdle**. This establishes a link between the extremities and the trunk that must always be considered when examining movements and the muscular contributions to movements in the lower extremity.

Movement in any part of the lower extremity, pelvis, or trunk will influence every aspect of the lower extremity. Thus, a foot position or movement can influence the position or movement at the knee or hip of either limb, or a pelvic position can influence actions throughout the lower extremity. It is important to evaluate movement and actions in both limbs, the pelvis, and the trunk rather than focus on a single joint to understand lower extremity function for the purpose of rehabilitation, sport performance, or exercise prescription.

For example, in a simple kicking action, it is not just the kicking limb that is critical to the success of the skill. The contralateral limb plays a very important role in stabilization and support of body weight. The pelvis establishes the correct positioning for the lower extremity and trunk positioning determines the efficiency of the lower extremity musculature. Likewise, in evaluating a limp in walking, attention should not be focused exclusively on the limb in which the limp occurs, since something happening in the other extremity may cause the limp.

The Pelvic and Hip Complex

COMPARISON OF SHOULDER AND PELVIC GIRDLES

The upper extremity is similar to the lower extremity in that both upper and lower limbs are connected to the trunk via a bony ring or girdle. Figure 6-1 demonstrates the two girdles, the shoulder girdle and the pelvic girdle. The upper and lower extremity girdles possess a large flat bone on the dorsal surface, and they both come in close contact anteriorly via a small strut. Also, the proximal segments in the upper and lower extremities both consist of the largest bone in the extremity, the humerus and the femur, respectively. Likewise, the next adjacent segments consist of two long bones: the radius and the ulna in the forearm and the tibia and fibula in the shank.

Finally, the hand and the foot contain a similar number of short bones, the carpals and the tarsals, respectively. These short bones are connected to a series of long bones in the hand and foot, the metacarpals and metatarsals, respectively, and the phalanges. The hand and the foot have a similar number of joints that are primarily of the same type.

Functionally, the arm and fingers have movement capacities similar to those of the thigh and toes. Conversely, the movement characteristics of the forearm and hand vary somewhat from those of the leg and foot.

A few major functional differences between the upper and lower extremities should be pointed out before we take a closer look at their individual structures and functions. The two girdles, shoulder and pelvic, connecting the upper and lower extremities to the trunk, connect in different ways, creating one of the main functional differences between upper and lower extremities. The upper extremity connects to the trunk via the sternum, and the shoulder girdle forms an incomplete ring, since the scapulae do not make contact with each other in the back. On the other hand, the lower extremity connects to the trunk via the sacrum, and a complete ring is formed by the pelvic girdle, since the sides of the pelvis are connected to each other anteriorly and posteriorly (Fig. 6-1). This has major functional consequences, allowing independent motion of the right and left upper extremity and dependent motion of the right and left lower extremity. Thus, a movement of the right arm will have minimal influence on the function of the left arm, while a movement of the left leg will have a direct effect on the function of the right limb.

The upper and lower extremities also have different functional roles to play, with the lower extremity involved

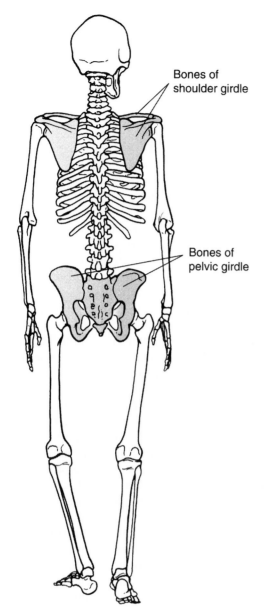

FIGURE 6-1 The upper and lower extremities are similar in many respects. Both have girdles that serve as the attachment site for the limbs. Both shoulder and pelvic girdles protect, serve as attachment sites for muscles, and participate in arm and thigh movements by moving to accommodate the shoulder and hip joints, respectively.

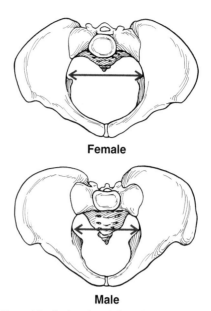

FIGURE 6-2 The pelvis of a female is lighter, thinner, and wider than that of a male. The female pelvis also flares out in the front and has a wider sacrum in the back.

primarily with weight bearing, walking, posture, and most gross motor activities. The upper extremity participates in activities that require skills in manipulation, dexterity, striking, catching, and fine motor abilities.

The pelvic girdle, including the hip joint, plays an integral role in supporting the weight of the body while offering mobility by increasing the range of motion in the lower extremity. The pelvic girdle is a site of muscular attachment for 28 trunk and thigh muscles, none of which are positioned to act solely on the pelvic girdle (77). Like the shoulder girdle, the pelvis must be oriented to place the hip joint in a favorable position for lower extremity movement. Therefore, concomitant movement of the

pelvic girdle and the thigh at the hip joint is necessary for efficient joint actions.

The pelvic girdle and hip joints are part of a closed kinetic chain system whereby forces travel up from the lower extremity through the hip and the pelvis into the trunk or down from the trunk through the pelvis and the hip to the lower extremity. Finally, pelvic girdle and hip joint positioning contribute significantly to the maintenance of balance and standing posture by employing continuous muscular action to fine-tune and ensure equilibrium.

The pelvic region is one area of the body where there are noticeable differences between the sexes in the general population. As illustrated in Figure 6-2, females generally have pelvic girdles that are lighter, thinner, and wider than their counterparts in the male (36). The female pelvis flares out more laterally in the front. The female **sacrum** is also wider in the back, creating a broader pelvic cavity than in males. This skeletal difference is discussed later in this chapter, since it has a direct influence on muscular function in and around the hip joint.

ANATOMICAL AND FUNCTIONAL CHARACTERISTICS OF THE JOINTS

The bony attachment of the lower extremity to the trunk occurs via the pelvic girdle (Fig. 6-3). The pelvic girdle consists of a fibrous union of three bones: the superior **ilium**, the posteroinferior **ischium**, and the anteroinferior **pubis**. These are separate bones at birth but are fully fused, or ossified, by the time the person is 15 to 17 years of age.

The right and left sides of the pelvis connect anteriorly at the **pubic symphysis**, a cartilaginous joint that has a fibrocartilage disc connecting the two pubic bones. The ends of each pubic bone are also covered with hyaline cartilage.

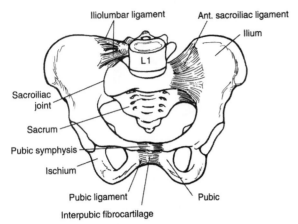

Iliolumbar ligament   Ant. sacroiliac ligament

Ilium

L1

Sacroiliac joint

Sacrum

Pubic symphysis

Ischium

Pubic ligament   Pubic

Interpubic fibrocartilage

FIGURE 6-3 The pelvic girdle supports the weight of the body, serves as an attachment site for numerous muscles, contributes to the efficient movements of the lower extremity, and helps maintain balance and equilibrium. The girdle consists of two coxal bones, each created through the fibrous union of the ilium, ischium, and pubic bones. The right and left coxal bones are joined anteriorly at the pubic symphysis, and connect posteriorly via the sacrum and the two sacroiliac joints.

This joint is firmly supported by a **pubic ligament** that runs along the anterior, posterior, and superior sides of the joint. Movement at this joint is limited, maintaining a firm connection between right and left sides of the pelvic girdle.

The pelvis is connected to the trunk at the **sacroiliac joint**, a strong synovial joint containing fibrocartilage and powerful ligamentous support (Fig. 6-3). The articulating surface on the sacrum faces posteriorly and laterally and articulates with the ilium, which faces anteriorly and medially (95).

The sacroiliac joint transmits the weight of the body to the hip and is subject to loads from the lumbar region or from the ground. It is also an energy absorber of shear forces during gait (77). There are three sets of ligaments supporting the left and right sacroiliac joints, and these ligaments are the strongest in the body (see Appendix A).

Even though the sacroiliac joint is well reinforced by very strong ligaments, movement occurs at the joint. The amount of movement allowed at the joint varies considerably between individuals and sexes. Males have thicker and stronger sacroiliac ligaments and consequently do not have mobile sacroiliac joints. In fact, 3 in 10 males have fused sacroiliac joints (95).

In females, the sacroiliac joint is more mobile because there is more laxity in the ligaments supporting the joint. This laxity may increase with monthly cycles of the hormones, and the joint is extremely lax and mobile during pregnancy (32).

Another reason the sacroiliac joint is more stable in males is related to positioning differences in the center of gravity. In the standing position, body weight forces the sacrum down, tightening the posterior ligaments and forcing the sacrum and ilium together. This provides stability to the joint and is the close-packed position for the sacroiliac joint (77).

In females, the center of gravity is in the same plane as the sacrum, while in males, the center of gravity is more anterior. Thus, in males, a greater load is placed on the sacroiliac joint, which in turn creates a tighter and more stable joint (95).

Motion at the sacroiliac joint can best be described by sacral movements. The movement of the sacrum accompanying each specific trunk movement is presented in Figure 6-4. The triangular sacrum is actually five fused vertebrae that will move with the pelvis and trunk. The top of the sacrum, the widest part, is the base of the sacrum, and when this base moves anteriorly, it is termed **sacral flexion** (77). Clinically, this is also referred to as **nutation**. This movement occurs with extension of the trunk or with flexion of the thigh.

Sacrum extension, or **counternutation**, occurs as the base moves posteriorly with trunk flexion or thigh extension. The sacrum also rotates along an axis running diagonally across the bone. Right rotation is designated if the anterior surface of the sacrum faces to the right and left rotation if the anterior surface faces to the left. This sacral torsion is produced by the piriformis muscle in a side-bending exercise of the trunk (77).

In addition to the movement between the sacrum and the ilium, there is movement of the pelvic girdle as a whole. These movements, shown in Figure 6-5, accompany trunk and thigh movements to facilitate positioning of the hip joint and the lumbar vertebrae. Although muscles will facilitate the movements of the pelvis, no one set of muscles acts on the pelvis specifically; thus, pelvic movements occur as a consequence of movements of the thigh or the lumbar vertebrae.

Movements of the pelvis are described by monitoring the ilium, specifically, the anterior, superior, and anterior inferior iliac spines on the front of the ilium. **Anterior tilt** of the pelvis occurs when the trunk flexes or the thighs extend and is defined as a forward tilting and downward movement of the pelvis. This anterior tilt can be created by protruding the abdomen and creating a swayback position in the low back. **Posterior tilt** is created through trunk extension, flattening of the low back, or thigh flexion, and it occurs as the pelvis moves posteriorly.

The pelvis can also tilt laterally, and will naturally try to move through a right lateral tilt when weight is supported by the left limb. Lateral pelvis tilt is sometimes referred to clinically as pelvic obliquity. This movement is controlled by muscles, in particular the gluteus medius, so that it is not pronounced unless the controlling muscles are weak. Thus, right and left lateral tilt will occur with weight bearing and any lateral movement of the thigh or trunk.

Finally, the pelvic girdle will rotate to the left and right as unilateral leg movements take place. As the right limb swings forward in a walk, run, or kick, the pelvis rotates to the left.

The final joint in the pelvic girdle complex is the hip joint, which can be generally characterized as stable yet mobile. The hip , which has 3 degrees of freedom (df), is a

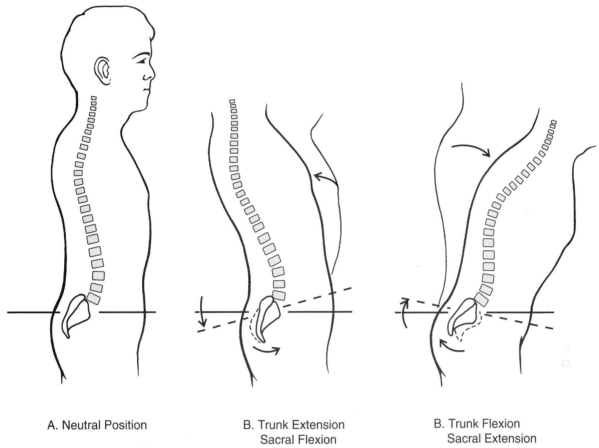

A. Neutral Position   B. Trunk Extension   B. Trunk Flexion
                              Sacral Flexion   Sacral Extension

FIGURE 6-4 A. In the neutral position, the sacrum is placed in the close-packed position by the force of gravity. The sacrum responds to movements of both the thigh and the trunk. **B.** When the trunk extends or the thigh flexes, the sacrum will flex. Flexion of the sacrum occurs when the wide base of the sacrum moves anteriorly. **C.** During trunk flexion or thigh extension, the sacrum extends as the base moves posteriorly. The sacrum will also rotate to the right or left with lateral flexion of the trunk (not shown).

ball-and-socket joint consisting of the articulation between the **acetabulum** on the pelvis and the head of the femur. The structure of the hip joint is illustrated in Figure 6-6.

The acetabulum is the concave surface of the ball and socket, facing anteriorly, laterally, and inferiorly (69,79). Interestingly, the three bones forming the pelvis, the ilium, ischium, and pubis, make their fibrous connections with each other in the acetabular cavity. The cavity is lined with articular cartilage that is thicker at the edge and thickest on the top part of the cavity (44,69). There is no cartilage on the underside of the acetabulum. As with the shoulder, a rim of fibrocartilage called the **acetabular labrum** encircles the acetabulum. This structure serves to deepen the socket and increase stability (91).

The spherical head of the femur fits snugly into the acetabular cavity. Both the femoral head and the acetabulum have large amounts of spongy trabecular bone that facilitates the distribution of the forces absorbed by the hip joint (69). The head is also lined with articular cartilage that is thicker in the middle central portions of the head, where most of the load is supported. The cartilage on the head thins out at the edges, where the acetabular cartilage is thick (69). Approximately 70% of the head of the femur

articulates with the acetabulum, in comparison to 20 to 25% for the head of the humerus with the glenoid cavity.

Surrounding the whole hip joint is a loose but strong capsule that is reinforced by ligaments and the tendon of the psoas muscle. The capsule is densest in the front and top of the joint, where the stresses are the greatest, and is quite thin on the back side and bottom of the joint (85).

Three ligaments blend with the capsule and receive nourishment from the joint. The insertions and actions of these ligaments can be found in Appendix A. The **iliofemoral ligament**, or Y-ligament, is strong and supports the anterior hip joint in the standing posture, resisting extension, **internal rotation**, and some **external rotation** (91). This ligament is capable of supporting most of the body weight. Also, **hyperextension** may be so limited by this ligament that it may not actually occur in the hip joint itself but rather as a consequence of anterior pelvic tilt.

The second ligament on the front of the hip joint, the **pubofemoral ligament**, primarily resists **abduction**, with some resistance to external rotation. The final ligament on the outside of the joint is the **ischiofemoral ligament**, on the posterior capsule, where it resists **adduction** and internal rotation (91). None of the ligaments surrounding the

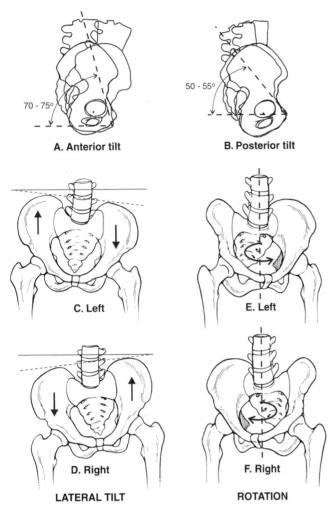

FIGURE 6-5 The pelvis moves in six directions in response to a trunk or thigh movement. Anterior tilt of the pelvis accompanies trunk flexion or thigh extension **(A)**. Posterior tilt accompanies trunk extension or thigh flexion **(B)**. Left **(C)** and right **(D)** lateral tilt accompany weight bearing on the right and left limbs, respectively, or lateral movements of the thigh or trunk. Left **(E)** and right **(F)** rotation accompany left and right rotation of the trunk, respectively, or unilateral leg movement.

hip joint resist during flexion movements, and all are loose during flexion. This makes flexion the movement with the greatest range of motion.

The femur is held away from the hip joint and the pelvis by the femoral neck. The neck is formed by cancellous trabecular bone with a thin cortical layer for strength. The cortical layer is reinforced on the lower surface of the neck, where greater strength is required in response to greater tension forces. Also, the medial femoral neck is the portion responsible for withstanding ground reaction forces. The lateral portion of the neck resists compression forces created by the muscles (69).

The femoral neck joins up with the shaft of the femur, which slants medially down to the knee. The shaft is very narrow in the middle, where it is reinforced with the thickest layer of cortical bone. Also, the shaft bows anteriorly to offer the optimal structure for sustaining and supporting high forces (85).

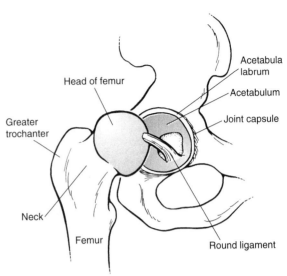

FIGURE 6-6 The hip is a stable joint with considerable mobility in three directions. It is formed by the concave surface of the acetabulum on the pelvis and the large head of the femur.

The femoral neck is positioned at a specific angle in both the frontal and transverse planes to facilitate congruent articulation within the hip joint and to hold the femur away from the body. The **angle of inclination** is the angle of the femoral neck with respect to the shaft of the femur in the frontal plane. This angle is approximately 125° (85) (Fig. 6-7). This angle is larger at birth by almost 20 to 25°, and it gets smaller as the person matures and assumes weight-bearing positions. It is also believed that the angle continues to reduce by approximately 5° in later adult years.

The range of the angle of inclination is usually within 90 to 135° (69). The angle of inclination is important because it determines the effectiveness of the hip abductors, the length of the limb, and the forces imposed on the hip joint. An angle of inclination greater than 125° is termed **coxa valga**. This increase in the angle of inclination lengthens the limb, reduces the effectiveness of the hip abductors, increases the load on the femoral head, and decreases the stress on the femoral neck (91). **Coxa vara**, in which the angle of inclination is less than 125°, shortens the limb, increases the effectiveness of the hip abductors, decreases load on the femoral head, and increases stress on the femoral neck. This **varus** position gives the hip abductors a mechanical advantage needed to counteract the forces produced by body weight. The result is reductions in the load imposed upon the hip joint and in the amount of muscular force needed to counteract the force of body weight (85).

The angle of the femoral neck in the transverse plane is termed the angle of **anteversion** (Fig. 6-8). Normally the femoral neck is rotated anteriorly 12 to 14° with respect to the femur (91). Anteversion in the hip increases the mechanical advantage of the gluteus maximus, making it more effective as an external rotator (79). If there is

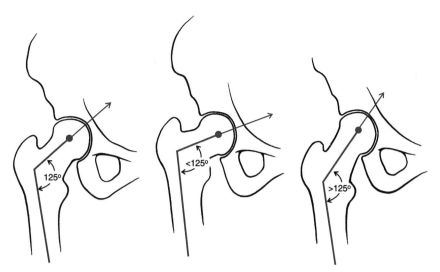

FIGURE 6-7 The angle of inclination of the neck of the femur is approximately 125°. If the angle is less than 125°, it is termed coxa vara. When the angle is reduced, the limb is shortened, the abductors are more effective, and there is less load on the femoral head but more load on the femoral neck. When the neck angle is greater than 125°, it is termed coxa valga. This position lengthens the limb, reduces the effectiveness of the abductors, increases the load on the femoral head, and decreases the load on the neck.

excessive anteversion in the hip joint, in which it rotates beyond 14° to the anterior side, the head of the femur is uncovered and a person must assume an internally rotated posture or gait to keep the femoral head in the joint socket. The toeing-in accompanying excessive anteversion is illustrated in Figure 6-8. Other accompanying lower extremity adjustments to excessive anteversion include an increase in the **Q-angle**, patellar problems, long legs, more **pronation** at the **subtalar joint**, and an increase in lumbar curvature (69,85).

If the angle of anteversion is reversed so that it moves posteriorly, it is termed **retroversion** (Fig. 6-8). Retroversion

creates an externally rotated gait, a supinated foot, and a decrease in the Q-angle (85).

The hip is a stable joint even though the acetabulum is not deep enough to cover all of the femoral head. The acetabular labrum deepens the socket to increase stability, and the joint is in a close-packed position in full extension when the lower body is stabilized on the pelvis. The joint is stabilized by gravity during stance, when body weight presses the femoral head against the acetabulum (85). There is also a difference in atmospheric pressure in the hip joint, creating a vacuum and suction of the femur up into the joint. Even if all of the ligaments and muscles

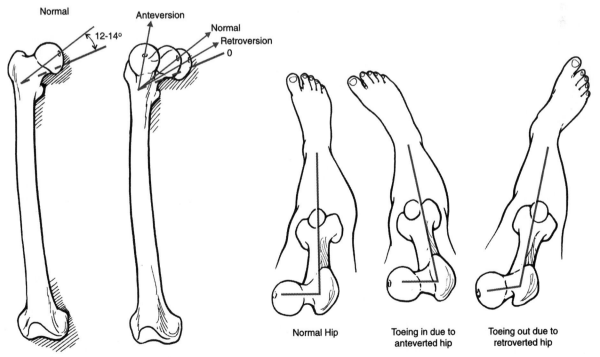

FIGURE 6-8 The angle of the femoral neck in the frontal plane is called the angle of anteversion. The normal angle is approximately 12 to 14° to the anterior side. If this angle increases, a toe-in position is created in the extremity. If the angle of anteversion is reversed so the femoral neck moves posteriorly, it is termed retroversion. Retroversion causes toeing out.

were removed from around the hip joint, the femur would still remain in the socket (42).

Strong ligaments and muscular support in all directions support and maintain stability in the hip joint. At 90° of flexion with a small amount of rotation and abduction, there is maximum congruence between the femoral head and the socket. This is a stable and comfortable position and is common in sitting. A position of instability for the hip joint is in flexion and adduction, as when the legs are crossed (42).

The hip joint allows the thigh to move through a wide range of motion in three directions (Fig. 6-9). The thigh can move through 70 to 140° of flexion and 4 to 15° of hyperextension in the sagittal plane (30,69). These measurements are made with respect to a fixed axis and vary considerably if measured with respect to the pelvis (2).

A wide range of hip flexion and extension is used in daily activities. Roughly 80 to 100° of flexion and exten-

sion is required to lower into or rise out of a chair, respectively (35). To climb a stair, 63° of flexion is used, while only 24 to 30° of hip flexion is required in descent of the same stair (35,85). These values change with a corresponding increase or decrease in the rise height of the stairs.

In walking, the maximum amount of hip flexion is 35 to 40°, achieved during late swing prior to heel strike (69). Full extension is required at the hip as the heel lifts off the ground. If thigh extension is limited or impaired, compensatory joint actions at the knee or in the lumbar vertebrae will accommodate the lack of hip extension.

Flexion of the thigh occurs freely with the knees flexed but is severely limited by the **hamstrings** if the flexion occurs with knee extension (42). Hyperextension is limited by the anterior capsule, the strong hip flexors, and the iliofemoral ligament.

The thigh can abduct through approximately 30° and can adduct 25° beyond the anatomical position (42). Most activities require 20° of abduction and adduction (42). Walking requires roughly 12° of abduction and adduction (85). Maximum abduction of the thigh occurs in swing just after toe-off, while maximum adduction is present through most of the support or stance phase (42). To bend down and pick something up from the squat position or tie a shoe requires 18 to 20° of abduction (85). Abduction is limited by the adductor muscles, and adduction is limited by the tensor fascia latae muscle.

Finally, the thigh can internally rotate through 70° and externally rotate through 90° from the anatomical position (42). The range of motion for rotation at the hip can be enhanced by the position of the thigh. Both internal and external rotation ranges of motion can be increased by flexing the thigh (42). In gait, the thigh externally rotates through 8 to 10° in the swing phase. The thigh internally rotates 4 to 6°, beginning just before heel strike and lasting into late stance (69). To bend down and pick something up requires 10 to 15° of external rotation (85). Both internal and external rotation are limited by their antagonistic muscle group and the ligaments of the hip joint.

COMBINED MOVEMENTS OF THE PELVIS AND THIGH

There is no movement in the pelvic girdle similar to the scapulohumeral rhythm seen in the upper extremity. This is because the right and left lower limbs do not move independently of each other as do the upper limbs. Also, the pelvis moves concomitantly with the lumbar vertebrae or with the thigh. Finally, thigh movements are not limited as much by the acetabulum as the humerus is by the scapula.

Although the thigh can move without pelvic movement, the pelvis and the thigh will commonly move together unless the trunk restrains pelvic activity. For example, if the pelvis is tilted anteriorly from a relaxed standing posture, flexion of both thighs and hyperextension, or swayback, in the lumbar spine will occur. Conversely, the thighs will

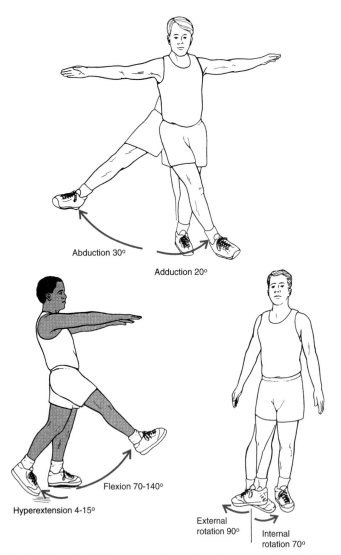

FIGURE 6-9 The thigh can move through a wide range of motion in three directions. The thigh moves through approximately 70 to 140°, 4 to 15° of hyperextension, 30° of abduction, 20° of adduction, 90° of external rotation, and 70° of internal rotation.

hyperextend and the lumbar vertebrae will flex or flatten out as a result of a posterior tilt.

If the trunk is stabilized by lying prone or supine or by hanging, the pelvis will be stabilized and a different combination of movements will occur. Flexion of the thigh in the supine position, such as in a double straight-leg raise, does not produce anterior tilt of the pelvis if the trunk muscles can stabilize the pelvis. If not, the hip flexors will produce hyperextension of the lumbar vertebrae that will in turn tilt the pelvis anteriorly. Thigh flexion with the knee flexed and the feet flat on the ground, such as in the case of a curl-up, will produce a posterior tilt of the pelvis. Likewise, flexing both limbs in a hanging position will produce a posterior tilt of the pelvis, since the pelvis is stabilized by the trunk.

Hyperextension of both thighs from the prone face-down position will produce anterior tilt of the pelvis, due again to the trunk stabilization. Finally, swinging both legs into extension from the supported hanging position will also result in an anterior tilt of the pelvis.

Since many lower extremity movements occur unilaterally, the combined movements of the pelvis and thigh are different from those just described for bilateral movement of the limbs. For example, if one thigh flexes forward and the other limb is supporting the body weight, such as in walking or kicking, the pelvis will rotate to the opposite side of the flexing thigh, posteriorly tilt, and laterally flex to the support limb side. With the thigh in hyperextension and the opposite limb supporting the body weight, such as in toe-off in the gait cycle or in the preparatory phase of a kick, the pelvis will rotate in the swing-leg direction, anteriorly tilt, but still laterally tilt to the support limb side (91). Many of these pelvic movements are counteracted and dampened by arm swinging and trunk rotation that absorb some of the pelvic activity.

MUSCULAR ACTIONS

Thigh flexion is used in walking and running to bring the leg forward. It is also an important movement in climbing stairs and walking uphill and is forcefully used in kicking. Little emphasis is placed on training the hip joint for the flexion movements, since most consider flexion at the hip to play a minor role in activities. However, hip flexion is very important for sprinters, hurdlers, high jumpers, and others who must develop quick leg action. Elite athletes in these activities usually have proportionally stronger hip flexors and abdominal muscles than do less skilled athletes. Recently, more attention has been given to training of the hip flexors in long distance runners as well, because it has been shown that fatigue in the hip flexors during running may alter gait mechanics and lead to injuries that may be avoidable with better conditioning of this muscle group.

The strongest hip flexor is the iliopsoas muscle, which consists of the psoas major, psoas minor, and iliacus (85). The iliopsoas is a two-joint muscle acting on both the lumbar spine of the trunk and the thigh. If the trunk is stabilized, the iliopsoas will produce flexion at the hip joint that is slightly facilitated with the thigh abducted and externally rotated. If the thigh is fixed, the iliopsoas will produce hyperextension of the lumbar vertebrae and flexion of the trunk.

The iliopsoas becomes more active in the midrange of the flexion movement. For example, in the double-leg raise, the initial part of the leg raise action will be facilitated by the abdominals and the iliopsoas, with the iliopsoas activity increasing after the movement is initiated in the middle range of motion. Likewise, in a curl-up or sit-up, the abdominals will contribute significantly through the first 45° of trunk flexion, and then the iliopsoas will be active through the midrange. This does not seem to change even if one moves from a straight-leg sit-up to a bent-knee curl-up, although the iliopsoas activity will be increased if the feet are held by a partner.

Iliopsoas activity during a sit-up or curl-up should be controlled by preceding the activity with a posterior pelvic tilt so that a swayback or lumbar hyperextension position is avoided. The loss of iliopsoas muscle function will only slightly impair thigh flexion, since some of the flexion can be initiated by the abdominals and other flexors. The impairment does increase with increasing angles of flexion, demonstrating the importance of the iliopsoas in the middle range of motion.

The rectus femoris is another hip flexor whose contribution depends on knee joint positioning. This is also a two-joint muscle, since it acts as an extensor of the knee joint as well. It is called the kicking muscle because it is in maximal position for output at the hip during the preparatory phase of the kick, when the thigh is drawn back into hyperextension and the leg is flexed at the knee. This position puts the rectus femoris on stretch and into an optimal length–tension relationship for the succeeding joint action, in which the rectus femoris makes a powerful contribution to both hip flexion and knee extension. During the kicking action, the rectus femoris is very susceptible to injury and avulsion at its insertion site, the anterior inferior spine on the ilium. Loss of function of the rectus femoris will diminish thigh flexion strength as much as 17% (55).

The three other secondary flexors of the thigh are the sartorius, the pectineus, and the tensor fascia latae (see Appendix B). The sartorius is a two-joint muscle originating at the anterior superior iliac spine and crossing the knee joint to the medial side of the proximal tibia. It is a weak fusiform muscle producing abduction and external rotation in addition to the flexion action of the hip. Knee extension will put this muscle on stretch.

The pectineus is one of the upper groin muscles. It is primarily an adductor of the thigh except in walking, actively contributing to thigh flexion. It is accompanied by the tensor fascia latae, which is generally an internal rotator. However, during walking, the tensor fascia latae aids thigh flexion. The tensor fascia latae is considered a two-joint muscle, since it attaches to the fibrous band of fascia, the **iliotibial band**, running down the lateral thigh and attaching across the knee joint on the lateral aspect of the proximal tibia. Thus, this muscle will be stretched in knee extension.

During thigh flexion, the pelvis is pulled anteriorly by these muscles unless stabilized and counteracted by the trunk. The iliopsoas muscle will pull the pelvis anteriorly, and so will the tensor fascia latae. If either of these muscles is tight, pelvic torsion, pelvic instability, or a functional short leg may occur.

Extension of the thigh is important in the support of the body weight in stance, as it maintains and controls the hip joint actions in response to gravitational pull. Thigh extension also assists in propelling the body up and forward in walking, running, or jumping by producing hip joint actions that counteract gravity. The extensors attach to the pelvis and consequently play a major role in stabilizing the pelvis in the anterior and posterior directions.

The muscles contributing in all conditions of extension at the hip joint are the hamstrings. The two medial hamstrings, the semimembranosus and the semitendinosus, are not as active as the lateral hamstring, the biceps femoris, considered the workhorse of extension at the hip.

Since all of the hamstrings cross the knee joint, producing both flexion and rotation of the lower, their effectiveness as hip extensors will depend on positioning at the knee joint. With the knee joint extended, the hamstrings are put on stretch for optimal action at the hip. The hamstring output also increases with increasing amounts of thigh flexion; however, the hamstrings can be lengthened to a position of muscle **strain** if the leg is extended with the thigh in maximal flexion.

The hamstrings also control the pelvis by pulling down on the ischial tuberosity, creating a posterior tilt of the pelvis. In this manner, the hamstrings are responsible for maintaining upright posture. Tightness in the hamstrings can create significant postural problems by flattening the low back and producing a continuous posterior tilt of the pelvis.

In level walking or in low-output hip extension activities, the hamstrings are the predominant muscles contributing to the extension movement. Loss of function in the hamstrings will produce significant impairment in hip extension.

If the resistance in extension is increased or if a more vigorous hip extension is needed, the gluteus maximus is recruited as a major contributor (91). This occurs in running up hills, climbing stairs, rising out of a deep squat, sprinting, and rising from a chair. It also occurs in an optimal length–tension position with thigh hyperextension and external rotation (91).

The gluteus maximus appears to dominate the pelvis during gait rather than contribute significantly to the generation of extension forces. Since the thigh is almost extended during the walking cycle, the function of the gluteus maximus is more trunk extension and posterior tilt of the pelvis. At foot strike when the trunk flexes, the gluteus maximus will prevent the trunk from pitching forward. Since the gluteus maximus also externally rotates the thigh, internal rotation will place the muscle on

stretch. Loss of function of the gluteus maximus muscle will not significantly impair the extension strength of the thigh, since the hamstrings dominate production of extension strength (55).

Finally, since the flexors and extensors control the pelvis anteroposteriorly, it is important that they be balanced in both strength and flexibility so that the pelvis is not drawn forward or backward as a result of one group being stronger or less flexible.

Abduction of the thigh is an important movement in many dance and gymnastics skills. During gait, abduction and the abduction muscles are more important in their role as stabilizers of the pelvis and thigh. The abductors can raise the thigh laterally in the frontal plane, or if the foot is on the ground, they can move the pelvis on the femur in the frontal plane. When abduction occurs, such as in doing the splits on the ground, both hip joints will displace the same number of degrees in abduction, even though only one limb may have moved. The relative angle between the thigh and the trunk will be the same in both hip joints in abduction because of the pelvic shift in response to abduction initiated in one hip joint.

The main abductor of the thigh at the hip joint is the gluteus medius. This multipennate muscle contracts during the stance in a walk, run, or jump to stabilize the pelvis so that it does not drop to the nonstance limb. The effectiveness of the gluteus medius muscle is determined by its mechanical advantage. It is more effective if the angle of inclination of the femoral neck is less than 125°, taking the insertion further away from the hip joint, and it is also more effective for the same reason in the wider pelvis (79). As the mechanical advantage of the gluteus medius increases, the stability of the pelvis in gait will also improve.

The gluteus minimus, tensor fascia latae, and piriformis also contribute to abduction of the thigh, with the gluteus minimus being the most active of the three. A 50% reduction in the function of the abductors will result in a slight to moderate impairment in abduction function (55). If the abductors are weak, there will be an excessive tilt in the frontal plane, with a higher pelvis on the weaker side (51). Additionally, the shear forces across the sacroiliac joint will greatly increase and the individual will walk with greater side-to-side sway.

The adductor muscle group works to bring the thigh across the body, as seen commonly in dance, soccer, gymnastics, and swimming. The adductors, like the abductors, also work to maintain the pelvic position during gait. The adductors as a group constitute a large muscle mass, with all of the muscles originating on the pubic bone and running down the inner thigh. Although the adductors are important in specific activities, it has been shown that a 70% reduction in the function of the thigh adductors will result in only a slight or moderate impairment in hip function (55).

The adductor muscles include the gracilis, on the medial side of the thigh; the adductor longus, on the anterior side of the thigh; the adductor brevis, in the middle of the thigh; and the adductor magnus, on the posterior side of the inner thigh. High in the groin is the pectineus, previously discussed briefly in its role as hip flexor. The adductors are active during the swing phase of gait as they work to swing the limb through (91).

The adductors work with the abductors to balance the pelvis. The abductors on one side of the pelvis will work with the adductors on the opposite side to maintain pelvic positioning and prevent tilting. The abductors and adductors must be balanced in strength and flexibility so that the pelvis can be balanced side to side. Figure 6-10 illustrates how imbalances in abduction and adduction can tilt the pelvis. If the abductors overpower the adductors through contracture or a strength imbalance, the pelvis will tilt to the side of the strong, contracted abductor. Adductor contracture or strength imbalances will produce a similar effect in the opposite direction.

External rotation of the thigh is important in preparation for power production in the lower extremity because it follows the trunk during rotation. The muscles primarily responsible for external rotation are the gluteus maximus,

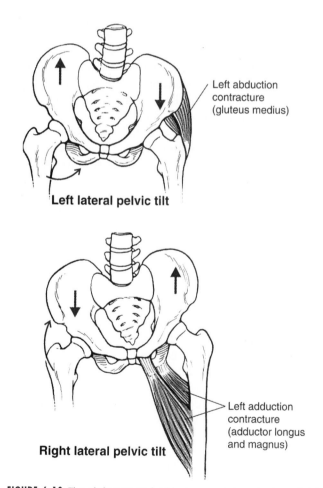

Left lateral pelvic tilt

Left abduction contracture (gluteus medius)

Right lateral pelvic tilt

Left adduction contracture (adductor longus and magnus)

FIGURE 6-10 The abductors and adductors work in pairs to maintain pelvic height and levelness. If an abductor or adductor muscle group is stronger than the contralateral group, the pelvis will tilt to the strong side. This will also happen with contracture of the muscle group.

the obturator externus, and the **quadriceps femoris**. The obturator internus, inferior and superior gemellus, and piriformis contribute to external rotation when the thigh is extended. Since most of these muscles attach to the anterior face of the pelvis, they also exert considerable control over the pelvis and the sacrum.

Internal rotation of the thigh is basically a weak movement. It is a secondary movement for all of the muscles contracting to produce this joint action. The two muscles most involved in internal rotation are the gluteus medius and the gluteus minimus. Internal rotation is also aided by contractions of the gracilis, adductor longus, adductor magnus, tensor fascia latae, semimembranosus, and semitendinosus.

STRENGTH AND FORCE OF THE HIP JOINT

The hip muscles can generate the greatest strength output in extension. The most massive muscle in the body, the gluteus maximus, combines with the hamstrings to produce hip extension. Extension strength is maximum with the hip flexed to 90° and diminishes by about half as the hip flexion angle approaches the 0° or neutral position (91). Extension strength also depends on knee position, since the hamstrings cross the knee joint. The hamstrings' contribution to hip extension strength is enhanced with the knees extended (42).

Many muscles contribute to hip flexion strength, but many of the muscles do so secondarily to other main roles. Hip flexion strength is primarily generated with the powerful iliopsoas muscle, though its strength diminishes with trunk flexion. Additionally, the flexion strength of the thigh can be enhanced if flexion at the knee joint increases the contribution of the rectus femoris to flexion strength.

Abduction strength is maximal from the neutral position and diminishes more than half at 25° of abduction (91). This reduction is associated with decreases in muscle length, in spite of the fact that the ability of the gluteus medius to abduct the leg improves as a consequence of improving the direction of the pull of the muscle. The strength output of the abduction movement can also be increased if it is performed with the thigh flexed (91).

The potential for the development of adduction strength is substantial, since the muscles contributing to the movement are massive as a group. However, adduction is not the primary contributor to many movements or sport activities and consequently is minimally loaded or strengthened through activity. Adduction strength values are greater from a position of slight abduction as a stretch is placed on the muscle group.

The strength of the external rotators is 60% greater than that of the internal rotators except in hip flexion, when the internal rotators are slightly stronger (91). The strength output of both the internal and external rotators is greater with the person seated than supine.

Forces generated by the muscles combine with those created by the body weight to produce substantial loads

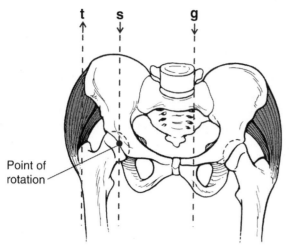

FIGURE 6-11 This diagram shows the frontal view of an individual balancing on the right limb. In stance, the force of gravity pulls the pelvis down (*arrow g*). The rotation of the pelvis downward is counteracted with the creation of an abductor force, t, to counteract the effect of gravity. The result is an increase of the vertical force "s" acting on the right hip joint.

on the hip joint. Standing on two limbs loads the hip joint with a force equivalent to 30% of body weight (91). This force is generated primarily by the body weight above the hip joint and is shared by right and left joints. When a person stands on one limb, the force imposed on the hip joint increases significantly, to approximately 2.5 to 3 times body weight (85,91). This is mainly the result of the increase in the amount of body weight previously shared with the other limb and a vigorous muscular contraction of the abductors. This force generation at the hip joint is illustrated in Figure 6-11, showing the effect of gravity, the muscular force of the abductors upward to control the pelvis, and the corresponding forces applied to the hip joint. With increased muscular activity, the loads become even greater.

In stair climbing, forces can reach levels of 3 times body weight; in walking, the forces range from 4 to 7 times body weight; and in running, the forces can be as high as 10 times body weight (69,85,91). Fortunately, the hip joint can withstand 12 to 15 times body weight before fracture or breakdown in the osseous component will occur (85).

CONDITIONING

The muscles surrounding the hip joint receive some form of conditioning during walking, rising from or lowering into a chair, and performing other common daily activities, such as climbing stairs. The hip musculature should be balanced so that the extensors do not overpower the flexors and the abductors are equivalent to the adductors. This will ensure sufficient control over the pelvis.

Since the hip muscles are used in all support activities, it is best to design exercises using a closed kinetic chain.

In this type of activity, the foot or feet are in contact with a surface (i.e., the ground) and forces are applied to the system at the foot or feet. An example of a closed chain exercise is a squat lift in weight training. An example of an open kinetic chain exercise is one using a machine, in which the muscle group moves the limb through a prescribed arc of motion. Finally, many two-joint muscles act at the hip joint; thus, careful attention should be paid to adjacent joint positioning to maximize a stretch or strengthening exercise.

The flexors are best exercised in the supine or hanging position so that the thigh can be raised against gravity. The hip flexors are minimally used in a lowering activity, such as a squat, when there is flexion of the thigh, because the extensors control the movement eccentrically. Since the hip flexors attach on the trunk and across the knee joint, their contribution to flexion can be enhanced with the trunk extended. Flexion at the knee will also enhance thigh flexion. It is easy to stretch the flexors with both trunk and thigh placed in hyperextension. The rectus femoris can be placed in a very strenuous stretch with thigh hyperextension and maximal knee flexion. Examples of stretching and strengthening of the flexor muscle group are presented in Figure 6-12.

A sampling of conditioning exercises for the extensors is presented in Figure 6-13. The success of conditioning the extensors will depend on trunk and knee joint positioning. The greater the knee flexion, the less the hamstrings will contribute to extension, requiring a greater contribution from the gluteus maximus. For example, in a quarter-squat activity with the extensors used eccentrically to lower the body and concentrically to raise the body, the hamstrings are the most active contributors. However, in a deep squat, with the amount of knee flexion increased to 90° and beyond, the gluteus maximus will be used more, since the hamstrings are incapacitated by their reduced length.

Trunk positioning is also important, and the activity of the hamstrings is enhanced with trunk flexion, because trunk flexion increases the length of both the hamstrings and the gluteus maximus. The extensors are best exercised in a standing, weight-supported position, since they are used in this position in most cases and are one of the propulsive muscle groups in the lower extremity.

The extensors can be stretched to maximum levels with hip flexion accompanied by full extension at the knee. The stretch on the gluteus maximus can be increased with thigh internal rotation and adduction.

The abductors and adductors are difficult to condition because they influence balance and pelvic position so significantly. Some exercises are presented in Figure 6-14. In a standing position, the thigh can be abducted against gravity, but it will shift the pelvis dramatically so that the person loses balance. The adductors present an even greater problem. It is very difficult to place the adductors so that they work against gravity, since the abductors are responsible for lowering the limb to the side after abducting it.

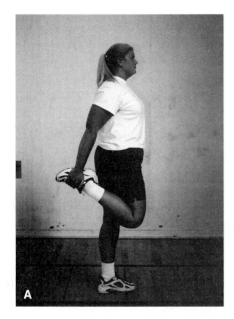

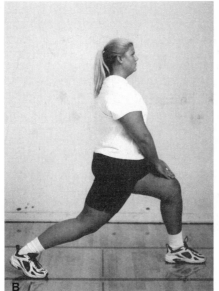

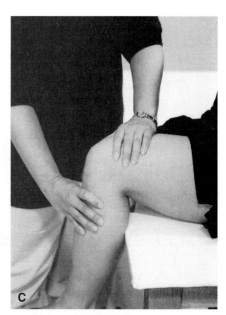

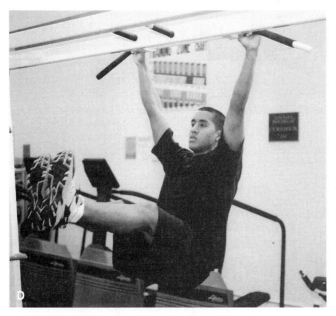

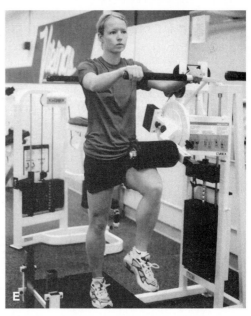

FIGURE 6-12 Flexibility, manual resistance, and weight-training exercises for the flexors. The hip flexors can be stretched by pulling the leg toward the buttock while allowing the pelvis to tilt anteriorly **(A)** or by performing a lunge movement **(B)**. Manual resistance can be applied on top of the thigh as the individual pulls upward **(C)**. Weight-training exercises for the hip flexors include hanging leg lifts **(D)** or flexion on a hip machine **(E)**.

Consequently, the supine position is best for strengthening and stretching the abductors and adductors. Resistance can be offered manually or through an exercise machine with external resistance to the movement.

The abductors and adductors can be exercised from the side-lying position so that they can work against gravity. However, this position requires stabilization of the pelvis and low back. It is hard to exercise the abductors or adductors on one side without working the other side as well; both sides will be affected equally because of the action of the pelvis. For example, 20° of abduction at the right hip joint will result in 20° of abduction at the left

hip joint because of the pelvic tilt accompanying the movement.

The rotators of the thigh are the most challenging in terms of conditioning because it is so difficult to apply resistance to the rotation. Some exercises are presented in Figure 6-15. The seated position is recommended for strengthening the rotators, since the rotators are strong in this position and resistance to the rotation can easily be applied to the leg either with surgical tubing or manually. Since the internal rotators lose effectiveness in the extended supine position, they definitely should be exercised with the person seated. Both muscle groups can be stretched in the same

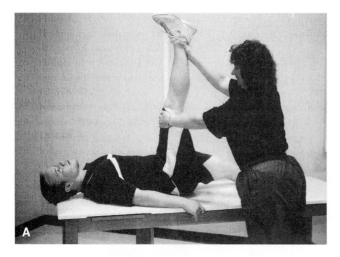

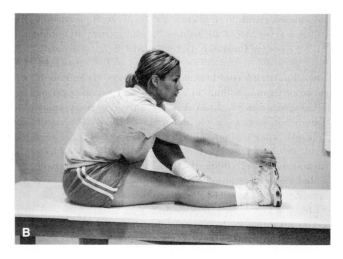

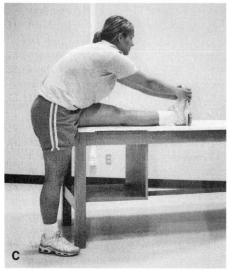

FIGURE 6-13 Flexibility (A to C), Manual Resistance (D and E), and Weight Training (F and G). Thigh extensors are stretched maximally with the hip flexed and the knee extended. Examples of flexibility exercises are the passive straight-leg raise **(A)**; a toe-touch from a seated position **(B)**; and a toe-touch with the contralateral leg stabilized on the floor **(C)**. Manual resistance exercises are done from the prone position and include applying resistance to a straight leg that is extending **(D)**. The gluteus maximus can be somewhat isolated if the same exercise is performed with the knee flexed **(E)**. Weight-training exercises for the extensors include the leg curl **(F)** and the squat **(G)**.

way they are strengthened, using the opposite joint action for the stretch. However, these exercises may be contraindicated for individuals with knee pain, in particular patellofemoral pain.

CONTRIBUTION TO SPORT SKILLS OR MOVEMENTS

Locomotion

Several terms are used in gait studies to describe the timing of the key events. This terminology is necessary to understand the actions of the lower extremity in walking and running. In locomotion studies, a walking or running cycle is generally defined as the period from the contact of one foot on the ground to the next contact of the same foot. A gait cycle is broken down into two phases, referred to as the stance or support phase and the swing phase. In the stance or support phase, the foot is in contact with the ground. The support phase is also broken down into two subphases, referred to as braking or weight acceptance and propelling. These subphases are defined based on the mechanics of the activity and are discussed in greater detail in Chapter 10. The swing or noncontact phase is the

period when the foot is not in contact with the ground. Essentially, this phase represents the recovery of the limb in preparation for the next contact with the ground.

The initiation of a locomotor cycle is foot strike, foot contact, or heel strike and thus is also the initiation of the stance or support phase. This event is also the start of the braking portion of the support phase. The braking subphase ends at midsupport or midstance. This event is also defined based on the mechanics of gait and will be discussed in much detail in Chapter 10. Midstance begins the propelling portion of the support phase that ends at toe-off. Toe-off occurs when the foot leaves the ground. At this point in the cycle, the swing phase begins. Swing phase and the locomotor cycle end when the foot contacts the ground. These events are illustrated in Figures 6-16 (walking) and 6-17 (running).

During walking, the muscles around the pelvis and the hip joint contribute minimally to the actual propulsion in walking and are more involved with control of the pelvis (53). The muscular contribution of the lower extremity muscles active in walking are summarized in Figure 6-16.

At heel strike, moderate activity in the gluteus medius of the weight-bearing limb keeps the pelvis balanced

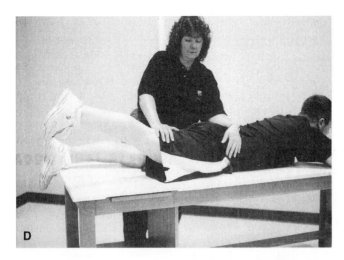

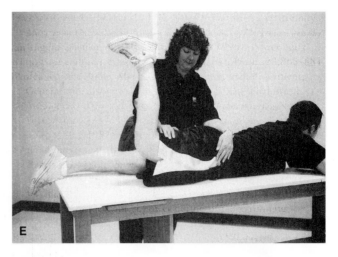

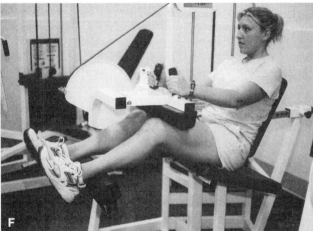

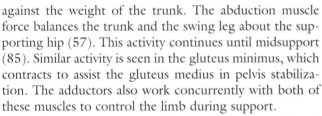

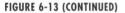

FIGURE 6-13 (CONTINUED)

against the weight of the trunk. The abduction muscle force balances the trunk and the swing leg about the supporting hip (57). This activity continues until midsupport (85). Similar activity is seen in the gluteus minimus, which contracts to assist the gluteus medius in pelvis stabilization. The adductors also work concurrently with both of these muscles to control the limb during support.

The hamstrings contract at heel strike to control both hip flexion and trunk flexion eccentrically. Shortly after heel strike, the activity of the hamstrings becomes less. The gluteus maximus is also active at heel strike to assist with the movement of the body over the leg. Finally, the tensor fascia latae is active from heel strike to midsupport to assist with frontal plane control of the pelvis (85).

Late in the propulsive portion of the support phase, the thigh begins to abduct and activity in the gluteus medius increases, with support contributions from the adductors of the opposite limb. Both the gluteus maximus and the hamstrings are also active at the end of the propulsive phase (85). As the toe begins to leave the ground, the thigh begins to rotate internally and flex, and the activity of the tensor fascia latae increases.

At the beginning of the swing phase, the limb must be swung forward rapidly. This movement is initiated by a vigorous contraction of the iliopsoas, sartorius, and tensor fascia latae. The thigh adducts in the middle of the swing phase and internally rotates just after toe-off. The adductors are active at the beginning of the swing phase and continue into the stance phase. At the end of the swing phase, activity from the hamstrings and the gluteus maximus decelerates the limb (85).

If one graduated to a brisk race-walking technique, the muscular activity would change. Since the race walk creates an exaggerated gait pattern in the frontal plane in which the pelvis tilts away from the straight support limb, greater activity from the abductors is required (13). This technique of exaggerated pelvic shift is necessary because it moderates the rise of the center of gravity created by the straight leg and increases the ability to produce a greater force on the ground. There is also greater hip flexion activity halfway into the swing phase and a more rapid extension by the extensors to propel the body forward quickly (13).

In running, the motions at the hip joint occur over a greater range of motion than in walking. The exception is hyperextension, which is greater in walking because of the increased stance time. The muscular activity in running, however, is similar to that seen in walking (Fig. 6-17). In

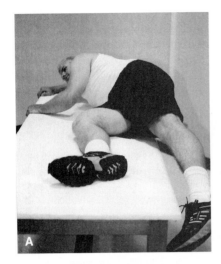

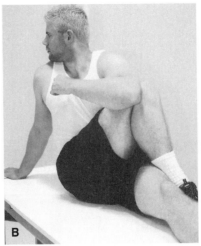

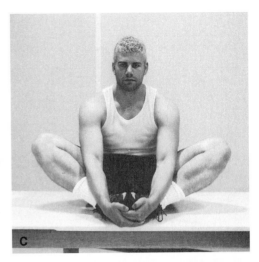

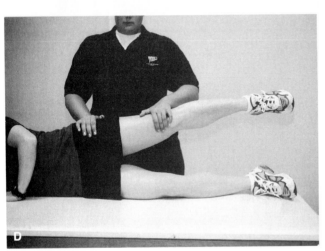

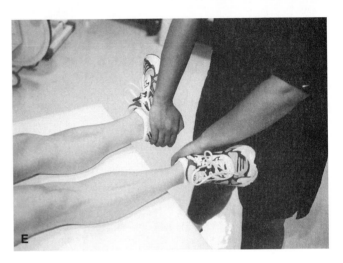

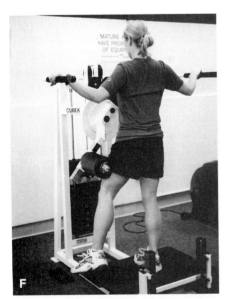

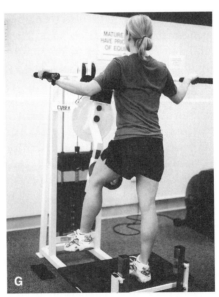

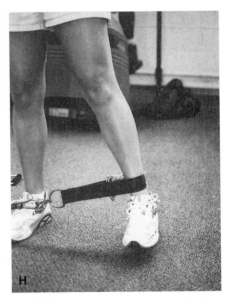

FIGURE 6-14 Flexibility (A to C), Manual Resistance (D and E), and Weight Training (F to H). Thigh abductor and adductor muscles can be best exercised from the side-lying or supine position. Flexibility exercises include side-lying with the leg hanging over the table to stretch the abductors **(A)**, a cross-over sit to stretch the abductors **(B)**, and the adductor stretch with the feet together **(C)**. Manual resistance exercise of the abductors can be administered from the side-lying position with resistance applied to the thigh as the limb is abducted (it is important not to roll forward or backward to compensate with the hip extensors or flexors respectively) **(D)**. Resistance can be applied to the inside of the ankles to resist the adduction movement **(E)**. Weight-training exercises for the abductors **(F)** and adductors **(G)** can be accomplished with a special hip machine **(F)**, or cable **(H)**.

running, there are 800 to 2000 foot contacts with the ground per mile, and 2 to 3 times the body weight is absorbed by the foot, leg, thigh, pelvis, and spine (9).

At heel strike, the force acting at the hip joint is approximately 4 times body weight because of the absorption of the force coming from the ground, the support of the body weight, and the muscular contraction of the abductors. This force increases to approximately 7 times body weight just before toe-off, again because of increases in the activity of the abductors (69).

During the swing phase, when no external forces are acting on the limb, the load on the hip joint is reduced to about body weight. This load is generated by contraction of the extensors. All of these forces are less in women because of their wider pelvises, making the abductors more effective so they do not have to generate as high a force output (69).

In the support phase of running, the gluteus medius and the tensor fascia latae are active just prior to contact and in the initial braking portion of the support phase. These muscles control the pelvis to keep it from tilting to the opposite side. As the speed of the run increases, the activity of the gluteus medius and gluteus minimus will decrease slightly (56).

Also active in the initial portion of the support phase are the gluteus maximus and the hamstrings, which act eccentrically to control the limb in flexion. The hamstrings become more active in the support phase as the speed increases, whereas the gluteus maximus becomes less active at this point (56).

During the propulsive portion of the support phase in running, the hamstrings are very active as the thigh extends. The gluteus maximus also contributes to extension during late stance while also generating external rotation until toe-off.

Once the foot leaves the ground to begin the swing phase, the limb is brought forward by the iliopsoas and rectus femoris, slowing the thigh in hyperextension and moving the thigh forward into flexion. The rectus femoris is the most important muscle for forward propulsion of the body, since it accounts for the large range of motion in the lower extremity. It initiates the flexion movement so vigorously that the iliopsoas action also contributes to knee extension. The iliopsoas is active for more than 50% of the swing phase in running (56). In the early part of the swing phase, there is activity in the adductors, which, as in walking, are working with the abductors to control the pelvis.

At the end of the swing phase, there is a great amount of eccentric muscular activity in the gluteus maximus and the hamstrings as they begin to decelerate the rapidly flexing thigh. As the speed of the run increases, the activity of the gluteus maximus increases as it assumes more of the responsibility for slowing the thigh in preparation for foot contact in descent. Also, in the later portion of the swing phase, the abductors will become active again as they lower the thigh eccentrically to produce adduction.

Pelvic activity in both running and walking is controlled by the arms, the trunk position, and the abductor muscles. Pelvic rotation to the left occurs as the right thigh swings forward. This rotation is countered by swing of the contralateral arm in the opposite direction. If the arm swing is excessive or insufficient in its control of the leg swing, the pelvis will rotate too much, thus placing stress on muscular attachments on the iliac crest.

Pelvic activity in right and left lateral tilt is controlled by the action of the abductors. As the pelvis tilts down to the unsupported limb, the abductors of the support limb stabilize the pelvis so it does not tilt to the opposite side. If the abductors cannot control the pelvic action in the frontal plane, **Trendelenburg gait**, in which the pelvis will drop to the unsupported side, occurs. An illustration of the Trendelenburg gait is presented in Figure 6-18. Excessive tilting in the frontal plane generates shear forces at the pubic symphysis (91).

The pelvis moves very little in anterior and posterior tilt as the leg flexes and extends. However, position of the trunk can greatly influence anterior and posterior tilt of the pelvis during running and walking. In uphill running or walking, the trunk is flexed, creating anterior tilt of the pelvis. The opposite occurs in downhill walking or running, when the trunk hyperextends and creates a posterior tilt of the pelvis.

Stair Ascent and Descent

In stair climbing, a cycle constitutes the movement of the body from one step up or down to the next. A cycle begins with both feet on a stair and begins when one foot is lifted or pulled off the surface of the step. In stair ascent, the initial phase, termed limb lift, ends when the foot is placed securely on the next step. At this point in the cycle, pull-up begins. This phase involves the forceful extension of the limb on the next step to elevate the body from the original step. The phase ends when the foot of the limb on the original step contacts the subsequent step. In stair descent, the events are similarly named, although the actions are different. These events are illustrated in Figure 6-19.

Stair ascent and descent have similar patterns to those described for walking and running. However, the hip muscles generally contribute less than the muscles acting on the knee and ankle joints. A review of the muscles contributing to ascent and descent is presented in Figure 6-19. Going upstairs, or ascent, is first initiated with a limb lift via vigorous contraction of the iliopsoas, which pulls the limb up against gravity to the next stair (58). The rectus femoris becomes active in this phase as it assists in the thigh flexion and eccentrically slows the knee flexion.

Next, the foot is placed on the next step. At this point, there is activity in the hamstrings, primarily working to slow down the extension at the knee joint (58). As the foot makes contact with the next step, weight acceptance involves some activity in the extensors of the thigh.

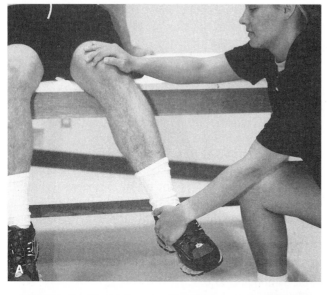

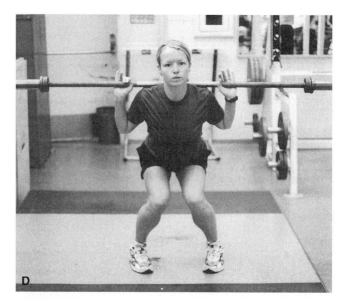

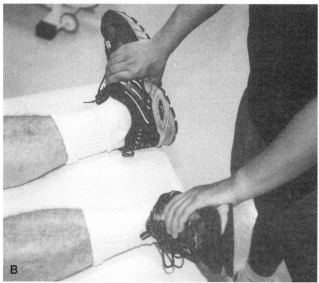

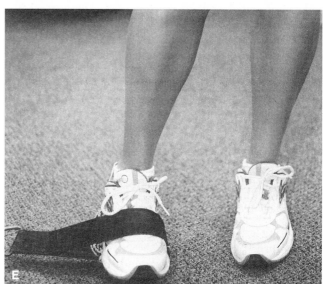

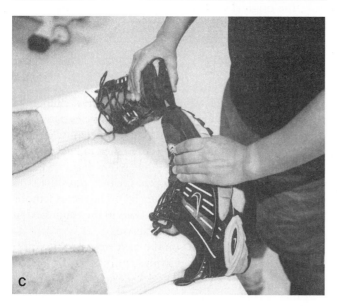

FIGURE 6-15 Flexibility (A), Manual Resistance (B and C), and Weight Training (D and E). The rotators can be easily stretched by using the opposite movement. However, strengthening these muscles requires creativity and attention to stabilization of adjacent body parts. To stretch the rotators, the individual should be placed in a seated position and the leg pulled out to stretch the external rotators and pushed in to stretch the internal rotators **(A)**. Manual resistance to rotation can be applied to the inside of the foot as the individual internally rotates **(B)** or to the outside of the foot during external rotation **(C)**. Weight-training exercises for the rotators include a squat with the toes pointing in (this exercise may be difficult for an individual with patellofemoral pain) **(D)** or cable exercises **(E)**.

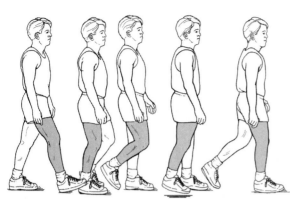

Foot strike Midsupport Toe-off Forward swing Deceleration

Walking

Muscles	Footstrike	Midsupport	Toe-off	Forward Swing	Deceleration
				Support	Swing
Dorsiflexors	***	**	**	**	**
Intrinsic Foot Muscles			***		
Gluteus Maximus	*	**	***		*
Gluteus Medius	**	***	**	*	
Gluteus Minimus	**	***	**	*	
Hamstrings	***	**	**	*	**
Iliopsoas				***	
Plantar Flexors		*	**		
Quadriceps	*	***	**		*
Sartorius				**	*
Tensor Fascia Latae	*	**	*	***	
Thigh Adductors	**	**	*	**	*

* = low activity
** = moderate activity
*** = high activity

FIGURE 6-16 The contribution to walking of the right lower extremity muscles is presented with indications of level of activity. During right foot strike, there is a high level of activity in the dorsiflexors and hamstrings; in midsupport, the gluteus minimus, gluteus medius, and quadriceps femoris group are most active; at right toe-off, the intrinsic foot muscles and gluteus maximus are most active; in the forward swing of the right limb, the iliopsoas and tensor fascia latae are active; at the end of the swing phase, the activity extensors is low to moderate. (Adapted from Mann, R. A., et al. [1986]. Comparative electromyography of the lower extremity in jogging, running, and sprinting. *American Journal of Sports Medicine*, 14:501–510.)

The next phase is pull-up, in which the limb placed on the upper step is extended to bring the body up to that step. Most of the extension is generated at the knee joint. There is minimal contribution from the hip other than contraction by the gluteus medius to pull the trunk up over the limb (58). Finally, in the forward propelling stage in which the limb on the lower step pushes up to the next step, there is minimal activity at the hip, with the ankle joint generating the most of the force.

Going downstairs, or descent, requires minimal hip muscular activity. In the limb pull phase, the hip flexors are active, followed by hamstring activity in the foot placement phase, when the limb is lowered to the step surface (58). As the limb makes contact with the next step in weight acceptance, the hip is minimally involved, as most of the weight is eccentrically absorbed at the knee and ankle joints. The muscles acting at the knee joint are primarily responsible for generating the forces in the forward propelling phase.

In the final phase of support, the controlled lowering phase, the body is lowered onto the step primarily through eccentric muscle activity at the knee joint. There

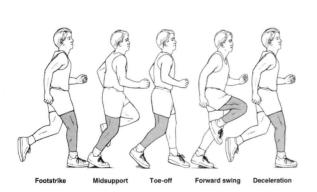

Footstrike Midsupport Toe-off Forward swing Deceleration

Running

Muscles	Footstrike	Midsupport	Toe-off	Forward Swing	Deceleration
				Support	Swing
Dorsiflexors	*	**	**	**	**
Intrinsic Foot Muscles			***		
Gluteus Maximus	**	**	***		*
Gluteus Medius	**	***	**	*	
Gluteus Minimus	**	***	**	*	
Hamstrings	***	**	***	*	**
Iliopsoas				***	
Plantar Flexors	**	*	**		
Quadriceps	**	***	***		*
Sartorius				**	*
Tensor Fascia Latae	**	**	*	***	
Thigh Adductors	**	**	*	**	*

* = low activity
** = moderate activity
*** = high activity

FIGURE 6-17 The events presented here are for the right lower extremity. In running, there is high level of muscular activity in the hamstrings, gluteus minimus, gluteus maximus, the quadriceps femoris group and the intrinsic muscles of the foot, during the right support phase of the activity. During the swing phase, there is substantial activity in the iliopsoas and the tensor fascia latae (Adapted from Mann, R. A. et al. [1986]. Comparative electromyography of the lower extremity in jogging, running, and sprinting. *American Journal of Sports Medicine,* 14:501–510.)

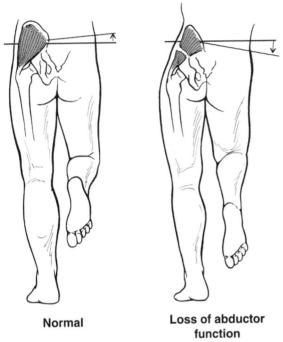

Normal   **Loss of abductor function**

FIGURE 6-18 If the hip abductors lack the strength to control the pelvis in the frontal plane (lateral tilt), a Trendelenburg gait will result. This type of gait is characterized by a drop to the unsupported side during walking or running.

is a minimum amount of hip extensor activity at the end of this phase.

In stair climbing, it is the limb on the higher step that produces the greatest effort for both ascent and descent. The knee joint is more active in ascent than descent and the hip joint activity is small in both, being almost negligible in the descent phase (58).

Cycling

In cycling, the key events are determined from the rotation of the crank of the bicycle. The motion of the crank forms a circle. A cycle is one revolution of this circle with 0° at the 12 o'clock position, 90° at 3 o'clock, 180° at 6 o'clock and 270° at 9 o'clock. The end of the cycle occurs at 360° (or 0°), back at the 12 o'clock position. The 12 o'clock position is also referred to as top dead center, while the 6 o'clock position is referred to as bottom dead center. These events are presented in Figure 6-20.

As shown in Figure 6-20, the muscles of the thigh can contribute significantly to the generation of force in cycling. The muscles active in the top half of the cycle, from 270 to 90°, are the sartorius and tensor fascia latae. These two muscles are active through 270 to 360° to pull the thigh up. They work with the gracilis through the initial 90° of the cycle to assist with the thigh flexion action (25).

Both the gluteus medius and the gluteus maximus become active after about 30° into the cycle and continue through approximately 150° as the thigh is extended. As the activity from the gluteus medius and gluteus maximus begins to decline, the activity of the hamstrings increases and continues from approximately 130° to 250° as they work both the hip and knee (25).

Finally, it is necessary to mention the contribution of the hip joint to movements commonly seen in dance and gymnastics. Excessive hip joint movements are required

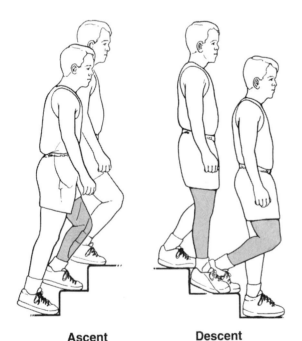

Ascent   **Descent**

FIGURE 6-19 In stair ascent with the left limb leading, there is significant contribution from the quadriceps, with assistance from the plantar flexors and the iliopsoas. In descent with the right limb leading, the same muscles control the movement eccentrically. For stair climbing as a whole, there is less contribution from the hip muscles than in walking or running (Adapted from McFadyen, B. J., Winter, D. A. [1988]. An integrated biomechanical analysis of normal stair ascent and descent. *Journal of Biomechanics*, 21:733–744.)

Stair Climbing

	Phases	
Muscles	Ascent	Descent
Dorsiflexors	*	*
Gluteus Medius	**	*
Hamstrings	*	*
Illiopsoas	**	*
Plantar Flexors	**	**
Quadriceps	***	**

* = low activity
** = moderate activity
*** = high activity

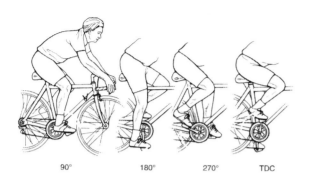

Cycling

Muscles	TDC-90	90–180	180–270	270-TDC
Biceps Femoris	*	***	*	*
Gastrocnemius	**	***	**	*
Gluteus Maximus	***	**	*	*
Gracilis	**	*	*	
Rectus Femoris	**	**	*	***
Sartorius	*	*	*	*
Semimembranosus	**	***	**	*
Tensor Fascia Latae	*	*	*	*
Tibialis Anterior	**	**	**	***
Vastus Lateralis	***	**	*	**
Vastus Medialis	***	**	*	**

* = low activity
** =moderate activity
*** =high activity

FIGURE 6-20 In the first 90° of the cycling stroke, from top dead center to a crank position parallel to the ground, there is high activity in the quadriceps femoris group and the gluteus maximus. From 90 to 180°, the gastrocnemius and hamstrings are more active. In the upswing of the cycle, from 180 to 270°, there is some activity from the hamstrings, the dorsiflexors, and the gastrocnemius. In the last phase of the cycle, 270° to top dead center, there is high activity in the rectus femoris and the tibialis anterior. (Adapted from Jorge, M., and Hull, M. L. [1986]. Analysis of EMG measurements during bicycle pedalling. *Journal of Biomechanics*, 19:683–694.)

in these activities, often with 180° of turnout required at the hip joint to perform specific skills. Turnout at the hip through this range of motion stresses the rotators and the adductors. Inability to generate maximal external rotation of the hip joint often leads to overuse injury of one form or another in the lower extremity as other adjustments are made to accommodate the lack of motion at the hip joint.

INJURY POTENTIAL IN THE PELVIC AND HIP COMPLEX

Injuries to the pelvis and hip joint are a small percentage of injuries in the lower extremity. In fact, overuse injuries to this area account for only 5% of the total for the whole body (76). This may be attributable to the strong ligamentous support, significant muscular support, and solid structural characteristics of the region.

Injuries to the pelvis primarily occur in response to some abnormal function that excessively loads areas of the pelvis. **Iliac apophysitis** is an example of such an injury, in which excessive arm swing in gait causes excessive rotation of the pelvis, creating stress on the attachment site of the gluteus medius and tensor fascia latae on the iliac crest (76). **Apophysitis**, an inflammation of an apophysis, or bony outgrowth, can also develop into a **stress fracture**.

Another site in the pelvis subjected to apophysitis or stress fracture is the anterior superior iliac spine where the sartorius attaches (63). At the anterior inferior iliac spine, the rectus femoris can produce the same type of injury. The iliac crest can also undergo an avulsion fracture from a strong pull by the abdominal attachments (63).

A stress fracture in the pubic rami can be produced by strong contractions from the adductors, often associated with overstriding in a run (94). Finally, the hamstrings can exert enough force to create an avulsion fracture on the ischial tuberosity. All of these injuries are most common in activities such as sprinting, jumping, soccer, football, basketball, and figure skating, in which sudden bursts of motion are required (63).

The sacrum and the sacroiliac joint can dysfunction as a result of injury or poor posture. If one assumes a round-shouldered forward-head posture, the center of gravity of the body moves forward. This increase in the curvature of the lumbar spine produces a ligamentous laxity in the dorsal sacroiliac ligaments and stress on the anterior ligaments (22). Also, any skeletal asymmetry, such as a short leg, will produce a ligament laxity in the sacroiliac joint (77).

With excessive mobility, large forces are transferred to the sacroiliac joint, producing an inflammation of the joint known as **sacroiliitis**. Inflammation of the joint may occur in an activity such as long jumping, in which the landing is absorbed with the leg extended at the knee. At the same time, the hip is flexed or there is extreme flexion of the trunk combined with lateral flexion (77). The sacroiliac joint also becomes very mobile in pregnant women, making them more susceptible to sacroiliac **sprain** (32).

The functional positions of the sacrum and the pelvis are also important for maintaining an injury-free lower extremity. A functional short leg can be created by posterior rotation of the ipsilateral ilium, anterior ilium rotation of the opposite side, superior ilium movement on the same side, forward or backward sacral torsion to the same side, or sacral flexion of the opposite side (77). A functional short leg requires adjustments in the whole limb, creating stress at the sacroiliac joint, the knee, and the foot.

The hip joint, although not susceptible to high rates of injury, does incur some age-related conditions that must be considered when working with children or older adults.

In children 3 to 12 years old, the condition known as **Legg-Calvé-Perthes disease** may appear (85). In this condition, also called **coxa plana**, the femoral head degenerates and the proximal femoral epiphysis is damaged. This disorder strikes males four times more frequently than females and usually occurs to only one limb. It is caused by trauma to the joint, synovitis or inflammation to the capsule, or some vascular condition that limits blood supply to the area.

Slipped capital femoral epiphysitis is another disorder striking children aged 10 to 17. It is usually caused by some traumatic event that forces the femoral neck into external rotation. This tilts the femoral head back and medially and tilts the growth plate forward and vertically, producing a nagging pain on the front of the thigh. An individual with this disorder will also walk with an externally rotated gait and have limited internal rotation with the thigh flexed and abducted (85). Such slippage may occur in the baseball player who rounds a base with the left foot fixed in internal rotation while the trunk and pelvis rotate in the opposite direction.

The final major childhood disorder to the hip joint is **congenital hip dislocation**, a disorder striking females more often than males (85). Usually this condition is diagnosed early, as the infant assumes weight on the lower extremity. The hip joint subluxates or dislocates for no apparent reason. The thigh cannot abduct; the limb shortens; and a limp is usually present. Fortunately, this condition is easily corrected with an abduction orthotic.

An age-related disorder of the hip joint seen commonly in the elderly is **osteoarthritis**. This condition results in degeneration of the joint cartilage and the underlying subchondral bone, narrowing of the joint space, and the growth of osteophytes in and around the joint. This affliction strikes millions of elderly people, creating a significant amount of pain and discomfort during weight support and gait activities. To reduce the pain in the joint, individuals often assume a position of flexion, adduction, and external rotation or whichever position results in the least tension for the hip.

More than 60% of injuries to the hip occur in the soft tissue (51). Of these injuries, 62% will occur in running; 62% are associated with a varum alignment in the lower extremity; and 30% are associated with a leg length discrepancy (51). These types of injuries are usually muscle strains, **tendinitis** of the muscle insertions, or **bursitis**.

The most common soft tissue injury to the hip region is gluteus medius tendinitis, which occurs more frequently in women as a result of excessive pull by the gluteus medius during running (51). A hamstring strain is also common and is seen in activities such as hurdling, in which the lower limb is placed in a position of maximum hip flexion and knee extension. It can also occur with speed or hill running and in individuals performing with poor flexibility or conditioning in this muscle group.

Iliopsoas strain can occur in activities such as sprinting, in which a rapid forceful flexion taxes the muscle or the muscle is used eccentrically to slow a rapid extension at the hip. The adductors are often strained in an activity such as soccer, in which the lower extremity is rapidly abducted and externally rotated in preparation for contact with the ball. Strain to the rectus femoris can occur in a rapid forceful flexion of the thigh, such as is seen in sprinting, or in a vigorous hyperextension of the thigh, such as in the preparatory phase of a kick.

A piriformis strain may be caused by excessive external rotation and abduction when the thigh is being flexed. This creates pain in adduction, flexion, and internal rotation of the thigh. A piriformis syndrome can develop. This is an impingement of the sciatic nerve aggravated by internal and external rotation movement of the thigh during walking (51). The syndrome can also be created by a functional short leg that lengthens the piriformis and then stretches it as the pelvis drops to the shorter leg. The irritation of the sciatic nerve causes pain in the buttock area that can travel down the posterior surface of the thigh and leg.

Other soft tissue injuries to the hip region are seen in the bursae. The most common of these is greater trochanteric bursitis, caused by hyperadduction of the thigh. This can be produced by running with too much leg cross-over in each stride, imbalance between the abductors and adductors, running on banked surfaces, having a leg length difference, or remaining on the outside of the foot during the support phase of a walk or run (9,76). It is especially prevalent in runners with a wide pelvis, a large Q-angle, and an imbalance between the abductors and adductors (9,76).

Since the right hip adductors work with the left hip abductors and vice versa, any imbalance causes asymmetrical posture. For example, a weak right abductor would create a lateral pelvic tilt, with the right side high and the left side low. This places stress on the lateral hip, setting up the conditions for bursitis. Pain on the outside of the hip is accentuated with trochanteric bursitis when the legs are crossed.

Ischial bursitis can develop with prolonged sitting and is aggravated by walking, stair climbing and flexion of the thigh. Finally, iliopectineal bursitis may develop in reaction to a tight iliopsoas muscle or osteoarthritis of the hip (85).

Two remaining soft tissue injuries seen in dancers and distance runners are lateral hip pain created by **iliotibial band syndrome** and **snapping hip syndrome**. The strain to the iliotibial band is created because dancers warm up with the hip abducted and externally rotated. They have very few flexion and extension routines in warmup and dance routines. The stress to the iliotibial band occurs with thigh adduction and internal rotation, movements that are extremely limited in dancers by technique (80). Iliotibial band syndrome can also be caused by excess tension in the tensor fascia latae in abducting the hip in single-stance weight bearing. The snapping hip also commonly produces a click as the hip capsule moves or the iliopsoas tendon snaps over a bony surface.

The bony or osseous injuries to the hip are usually a result of a strong muscular contraction creating an avulsion fracture. The abductors can create an avulsion fracture on the greater trochanter, and the iliopsoas can pull hard enough to produce an avulsion fracture at the **lesser trochanter** (85). Stress fractures can also appear in the femoral neck. It is believed that these stress fractures may be related to some type of vascular necrosis in which the blood supply is limited or to some hormonal deficiency that reduces the bone density in the neck (51). Stress fracture at this site produces pain in the groin area.

 The Knee Joint

The knee joint is a double condyloid joint with 2 df. In this joint, flexion and extension occur much like flexion and extension at the elbow joint. However, in the knee joint, flexion is accompanied by a small but significant amount of rotation (88). The joint is vulnerable to injury because of the mechanical demands upon it and the reliance on soft tissue for support.

The knee joint supports the weight of the body and transmits forces from the ground while allowing a great deal of movement between the femur and the tibia. In the extended position, the knee joint is stable because of its vertical alignment, the congruency of the joint surfaces, and the effect of gravity. In any flexed position, the knee joint is mobile and requires special stabilization from the powerful capsule, ligaments, and muscles surrounding the joint (88).

The ligaments surrounding the knee support the joint passively as they are loaded in tension only. The muscles support the joint actively and are also loaded in tension, and bone offers support and resistance to compressive loads (60). Functional stability of the joint is derived from the passive restraint of the ligaments, joint geometry, the active muscles, and the compressive forces pushing the bones together.

ANATOMICAL AND FUNCTIONAL CHARACTERISTICS OF THE JOINT

There are three articulations in the region known as the knee joint: the **tibiofemoral joint**, the **patellofemoral joint**, and the superior **tibiofibular joint** (96). The structure of the knee joint is illustrated in Figure 6-21.

The tibiofemoral joint, commonly referred to as the actual knee joint, is the articulation between the two longest and strongest bones in the body, the femur and the tibia. At the end of the femur are two large convex surfaces, the medial and lateral **condyles**, separated by the **intercondylar notch** in the posterior and the patellar, or trochlear, groove in the anterior (88).

It is important to review the anatomical characteristics of these two condyles because their differences and the corresponding differences on the tibia account for the rotation in the knee joint. The lateral condyle is flatter, has a larger surface area, is more prominent anteriorly to hold the **patella** in place, and is basically aligned with the femur (96). The medial condyle projects more longitudinally and medially, is longer in the anteroposterior direction,

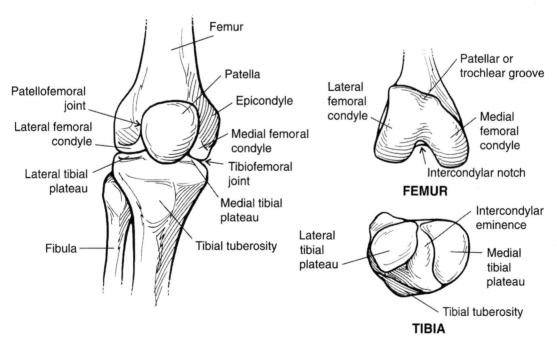

FIGURE 6-21 The knee is a condyloid joint allowing movement in two directions, flexion–extension and rotation. Movements at the knee joint are complex because of the structural differences in the medial and lateral compartments of the joint.

angles away from the femur in the rear, and is aligned with the tibia (96). Above the condyles on both sides are the **epicondyles**, which are the sites of capsule, ligament, and muscular attachment.

The condyles rest on the condyle **facet** or **tibial plateau**, a medial and lateral surface separated by a ridge of bone termed the **intercondylar eminence**. This ridge of bone serves as an attachment site for ligaments, centers the joint, and stabilizes the bones in weight bearing (96). The medial surface of the plateau is oval, longer in the anteroposterior direction, and concave to accept the convex condyle of the femur. The lateral tibial plateau is circular and slightly convex (96). Consequently, the medial tibia and femur fit fairly snugly together, but the lateral tibia and femur do not fit together well because both surfaces are convex (88). This structural difference is one of the determinants of rotation, as the lateral condyle has a greater excursion with flexion and extension at the knee.

Two separate fibrocartilage menisci lie between the tibia and the femur. As shown in Figure 6-22, the lateral **meniscus** is oval, with attachments at the anterior and posterior horns (28,96). It also receives attachments from the quadriceps femoris anteriorly and the popliteus muscle

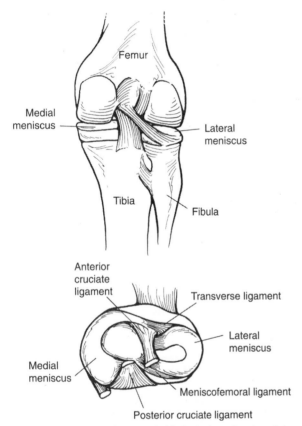

FIGURE 6-22 Two fibrocartilage menisci lie in the lateral and medial compartments of the knee. The medial meniscus is crescent-shaped and the lateral meniscus is oval, to match the surfaces of the tibial plateau and the differences in the shape of the femoral condyles. Both menisci serve important roles in the knee joint by offering shock absorption, stability, and lubrication and by increasing the contact area between the tibia and the femur.

and the **posterior cruciate ligament** posteriorly. The lateral meniscus occupies a larger percentage of the area in the lateral compartment than the medial meniscus in the medial compartment. Also, the lateral meniscus is more mobile, capable of moving more than twice the distance of the medial meniscus in the anteroposterior direction (96).

The medial meniscus is more crescent-shaped, with a wide base of attachment on both the anterior and posterior horns via the coronary ligaments (Fig. 6-22). It is connected to the quadriceps femoris and the anterior cruciate ligament anteriorly, the tibial collateral ligament laterally, and the semimembranosus muscle posteriorly (96).

The menisci are connected to each other at the anterior horns by a **transverse ligament**. The menisci are avascular, having no blood supply to the inner portion of the fibrocartilage. Thus, if a tear occurs, healing is almost impossible. There is some blood supply to the fibrocartilage on the outer portion of the menisci, making healing of that structure possible.

The menisci are important in the knee joint. The menisci enhance stability in the joint by deepening the contact surface on the tibia. They participate in shock absorption by transmitting half of the weight-bearing load in full extension and a significant portion of the load in flexion (100). In flexion, the lateral meniscus carries the greater portion of the load. By absorbing some of the load, the menisci protect the underlying articular cartilage and subchondral bone. The menisci transmit the load across the surface of the joint, reducing the load per unit of area on the tibiofemoral contact sites (28). The contact area in the joint is reduced by two-thirds when the menisci are absent. This increases the pressure on the contacting surfaces and increases the susceptibility to injury (67). During low-load situations, the contact is primarily on the menisci, while in high-load situations, the contact area increases, with 70% of the load still on the menisci (28). The lateral meniscus carries a significantly greater percentage of the load.

The menisci also enhance lubrication of the joint. By acting as a space-filling mechanism, they allow dispersal of more synovial fluid to the surface of the tibia and the femur. It has been demonstrated that a 20% increase in friction within the joint will occur with the removal of the meniscus (100).

Finally, the menisci limit motion between the tibia and femur. In flexion and extension, the menisci move with the femoral condyles. As the leg flexes, the menisci move posteriorly because of the rolling of the femur and muscular action of the popliteus and semimembranosus muscles (100). At the end of the flexion movement, the menisci fill up the posterior portion of the joint, acting as a space-filling buffer. The reverse occurs in extension. The quadriceps femoris and the patella assist in moving the menisci forward on the surface. Additionally, the menisci follow the tibia during rotation.

The tibiofemoral joint is supported by four main ligaments, two collateral and two cruciate. These ligaments assist in maintaining the relative position of the tibia and femur so that contact is appropriate and at the right time. See Appendix A for insertions, actions, and illustration of these ligaments. They are the passive load-carrying structures of the joint and serve as a backup to the muscles (60).

On the sides of the joint are the collateral ligaments. The **medial collateral ligament** (MCL) supports the knee against any **valgus** force (a medially directed force acting on the lateral side of the knee) and offers some resistance to both internal and external rotation (68). It is taut in extension and reduces in length by approximately 17% in full flexion (97). The MCL offers 78% of the total valgus restraint at 25° of knee flexion (70).

The **lateral collateral ligament** (LCL) is thinner and rounder than the MCL. It offers the main resistance to varus force (a lateral force acting on the medial side) at the knee. This ligament is also taut in extension and reduces its length by approximately 25% in full flexion (97). The LCL offers 69% of the varus restraint at 25° of knee flexion (70). The LCL is not affected by rotation at the knee joint (97).

In full extension, the collateral ligaments are assisted by tightening of the posteromedial and posterolateral capsules, thus making the extended position the most stable. There is a deep layer of ligaments under the collaterals that have been considered a branch of the collaterals and termed capsular ligaments (59).

The cruciate ligaments are intrinsic, lying inside the joint in the intercondylar space. These ligaments control both anteroposterior and rotational motion in the joint. The **anterior cruciate ligament** (ACL) provides the primary restraint for anterior movement of the tibia relative to the femur. It accounts for 85% of the total restraint in this direction (70). The ACL is 40% longer than its counterpart, the posterior cruciate ligament. It elongates by about 7% as the knee moves from extension to 90° of flexion and maintains the same length up through maximum flexion (97). If the joint is internally rotated, the insertion of the ACL moves anteriorly, elongating the ligament slightly more. With the joint externally rotated, the ACL does not elongate up through 90° of knee flexion but elongates up to 10% from 90° to full flexion (97). Different parts of the ACL are taut in different knee positions. The anterior fibers are taut in extension, the middle fibers taut in internal rotation, and the posterior fibers taut in flexion. The ACL as a whole is considered to be taut in the extended position (Fig. 6-23).

The posterior cruciate ligament (PCL) offers the primary restraint to posterior movement of the tibia on the femur, accounting for 95% of the total resistance to this movement (70). This ligament decreases in length and slackens by 10% at 30° of knee flexion and then maintains that length throughout flexion (97). The PCL increases in length by about 5% with internal rotation of the joint up to 60° of flexion and then decreases in length by 5 to 10% as flexion continues. The PCL is not affected by external rotation in the joint, maintaining a fairly constant length.

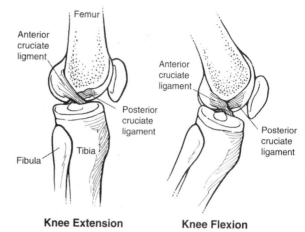

Knee Extension   **Knee Flexion**

FIGURE 6-23 The anterior cruciate ligament provides anterior restraint of the movement of the tibia relative to the femur. It is taut in knee extension. The posterior cruciate ligament offers restraint to posterior movement of the tibia relative to the femur. It is taut in flexion. Both sets of cruciate ligaments limit rotation at the knee joint.

It is maximally strained through 45 to 60° of flexion (97) (Fig. 6-23). As with the ACL, the fibers of the PCL participate in different functions. The posterior fibers are taut in extension, the anterior fibers taut in midflexion, and the posterior fibers taut in full flexion.

Both the cruciate ligaments stabilize, limit rotation, and cause sliding of the condyles over the tibia in flexion. In a standing posture, with the tibial shaft vertical, the femur is aligned with the tibia and tends to slide posteriorly. A hyperextended position to 9° of flexion is unstable, since the femur tilts posteriorly and is minimally restricted (60). At a 9° tilt of the tibia, the femur slides anteriorly to a position where it is more stable and supported by the patella and the quadriceps femoris.

Another important support structure surrounding the knee is the joint capsule. One of the largest capsules in the body, it is reinforced by numerous ligaments and muscles, including the MCL, the cruciate ligaments, and the arcuate complex (96). In the front, the capsule forms a substantial pocket that offers a large patellar area and is filled with the infrapatellar fat pad and the **infrapatellar bursa**. The fat pad offers a stopgap in the anterior compartment of the knee.

The capsule is lined with the largest synovial membrane in the body, which forms embryonically from three separate pouches (6). In 20 to 60% of the population, a permanent fold, called **plica**, remains in the synovial membrane (7). The common location of plica is medial and superior to the patella. It is soft and pliant and passes over the femoral condyle in flexion and extension. If injured, it can become fibrous and create both resistance and pain in motion (7). There are also more than 20 bursae in and around the knee, reducing friction between muscle, tendon, and bone (96).

The second joint in the region of the knee is the patellofemoral joint, consisting of the articulation of the

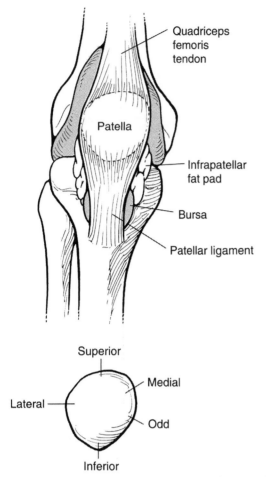

FIGURE 6-24 The patella increases the mechanical advantage of the quadriceps femoris muscle group. The patella has five facets, or articulating surfaces: the superior, inferior, medial, lateral and odd facet.

patella with the trochlear groove on the femur. The patella is a triangular sesamoid bone encased by the tendons of the quadriceps femoris. The primary role of the patella is to increase the mechanical advantage of the quadriceps femoris (6).

The posterior articulating surface of the patella is covered with the thickest cartilage found in any joint in the body (88). A vertical ridge of bone separates the underside of the patella into medial and lateral facets, each of which can be further divided into superior, middle, and inferior facets. A seventh facet, the odd facet, lies on the far medial side of the patella (96). The structure of the patella and the location of these facets are presented in Figure 6-24. During normal flexion and extension, typically five of these facets make contact with the femur.

The patella is connected to the tibial tuberosity via the strong **patellar ligament**. It is connected to the femur and tibia by small patellofemoral and patellotibial ligaments that are actually thickenings in the extensor retinaculum surrounding the joint (6).

Positioning of the patella and alignment of the lower extremity in the frontal plane is determined by measuring the Q-angle. Illustrated in Figure 6-25, the Q-angle is formed by drawing one line from the anterior superior spine of the ilium to the middle of the patella and a second line from the middle of the patella to the tibial tuberosity. The most efficient Q-angle for quadriceps femoris function is one close to 10° (54). Males typically have Q-angles averaging 10° to 14° while females average 15° to 17°, primarily because of their wider pelvic basins (54).

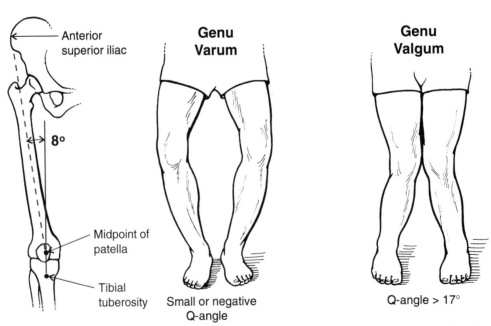

FIGURE 6-25 The Q-angle is measured between a line from the anterior superior iliac spine to the middle of the patella and the projection of a line from the middle of the patella to the tibial tuberosity. Q-angles range from 10 to 14° for males and 15 to 17° for females. Very small Q-angles create a condition known as genu varum, or bowleggedness. Large Q-angles create genu valgrum, or knock-kneed position.

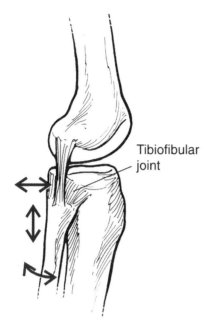

FIGURE 6-26 The tibiofibular joint is a small joint between the head of the fibula and the tibial condyle. It moves anteroposteriorly, superiorly, and inferiorly and rotates in response to movements of the tibia or the foot.

The Q-angle represents the valgus stress acting on the knee, and if it is excessive, many patellofemoral problems can develop. Any Q-angle over 17° is considered to be excessive and might be termed **genu valgum**, or knock-knees (54). A very small Q-angle constitutes bowleggedness, or **genu varum**.

The third and final articulation is the small, superior tibiofibular joint, shown in Figure 6-26. This joint consists of the articulation between the head of the fibula and the posterolateral and inferior aspect of the tibial condyle.

It is a gliding joint moving anteroposteriorly, superiorly, and inferiorly and rotating in response to rotation of the tibia and the foot (78). The fibula externally rotates and moves externally and superiorly with **dorsiflexion** of the foot and accepts approximately 16% of the static load applied to the leg (78).

The primary functions of the superior tibiofibular joint are to dissipate the torsional stresses applied by the movements of the foot and to attenuate lateral tibial bending. Both the tibiofibular joint and the fibula absorb and control tensile rather than compressive loads applied to the lower extremity. The middle part of the fibula has more ability to withstand tensile forces than any other part of the skeleton (78).

The function of the knee is complex because of its asymmetrical medial and lateral articulations and the patellar mechanics on the front. The knee flexes through approximately 145° with the thigh flexed and 120° with the thigh hyperextended (42). This difference in range is due to the length–tension relationship in the hamstring muscle group.

When flexion is initiated, the femur rolls on the tibia with the medial condyle rolling 10° and the lateral condyle rolling 15° (42). After the initial rolling is complete, the femur rotates, translates, and finishes off in maximal flexion by just sliding anteriorly. These movements are illustrated in Figure 6-27.

Accompanying flexion is internal rotation of the tibia on the femur. This rotation is created in part by the greater movement of the lateral condyle on the tibia through almost twice the distance. Rotation can occur only with the joint in some amount of flexion. Thus there is no rotation in the extended, locked position. There is 6 to 30° of internal rotation through 90° of flexion at the joint around an axis passing through the medial intercondylar tubercle of

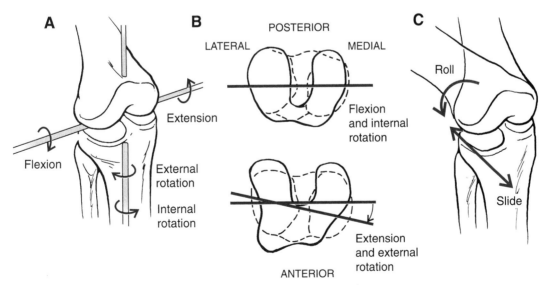

FIGURE 6-27 A. The movements at the knee joint are flexion and extension and internal and external rotation. **B.** When the knee flexes, there is an accompanying internal rotation of the tibia on the femur (non–weight bearing). In extension, the tibia externally rotates on the femur. **C.** There are also translatory movements of the femur on the tibial plateau surface. In flexion, the femur rolls and slides posteriorly.

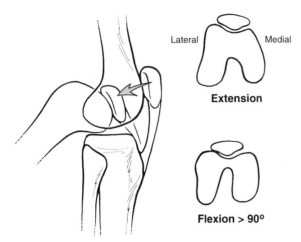

FIGURE 6-28 When the knee flexes, the patella moves inferiorly and posteriorly over two times its length. The patella sits in the groove and is held in place by the lateral condyle of the femur. If the knee continues into flexion past 90°, the patella will move laterally over the condyle until at approximately 135° of flexion, contact is made with the odd facet.

the tibial plateau (43,69). Internal tibial rotation also occurs with dorsiflexion and pronation at the foot. Roughly 6° of subtalar motion results in roughly 10° of internal rotation (83).

When the knee flexes, the patella moves down a distance more than twice its length, entering the intercondylar notch on the femur (42) (Fig. 6-28). The movement of the patella is most affected by the joint surface and the length of the patellar tendon and minimally affected by the quadriceps femoris. In the first 20°, the tibia internally rotates and the patella is drawn from its lateral position down into the groove, where first contact is made with the inferior facets (96). In the first 20° of flexion, stability offered by the lateral condyle is most important, since most subluxations and dislocations of the patella occur in this early range of motion.

The patella follows the groove to 90° of flexion, at which point contact is made with the superior facets of the patella (Fig. 6-28). At that time, the patella again moves laterally over the medial condyle. If flexion continues to 135°, contact will be made with the odd facet (96). In flexion, the linear and translatory movements of the patella are posterior and inferior, but the patella also has some angular movements affecting its position. During knee flexion, the patella also flexes, abducts, and externally rotates. The movements of the patella for one leg cycle in walking are presented in Figure 6-29.

Flexion of the patella occurs about a mediolateral axis running through a fixed axis in the distal femur, with flexion representing the upward tilt about this axis. Likewise, patellar abduction involves movement of the patella away from the midline in the frontal plane, and external rotation is rotation of the patella outward about a longitudinal axis (46).

In extension, the reverse movements to flexion occur. The extension range of motion is usually terminated at

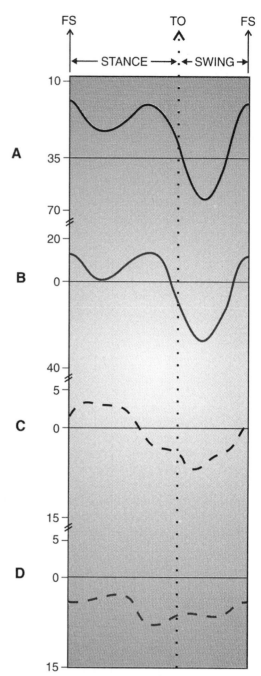

FIGURE 6-29 The angular movements of the patella are shown for one walking cycle. The top graph **(A)** represents the tibiofemoral flexion and extension pattern in walking shown with the accompanying patellar movements of **(B)** flexion and extension, **(C)** abduction and adduction and **(D)** rotation. (Redrawn from Lafortune, M. A., and Cavanagh, P. R. [1985]. Three-dimensional kinematics of the patella during walking. pp. 337–341 In B. Jonsson [Ed.]. *Biomechanics X*. Champaign, IL: Human Kinetics.)

approximately 10° of hyperextension. The contact point in the tibiofemoral joint moves anteriorly on the tibial plateau as the femur slides, rolls, and slides and then rolls in the last few degrees of extension. Through 120° of extension, the anterior movement is 40% of the length of the tibial plateau (96).

With extension is accompanying external rotation that terminates in the locking action at the end of extension and is termed the **screw home mechanism**. The screw home mechanism is the point at which the medial and lateral condyles are locked to form the close-packed position for the knee joint. This occurs during the last 20° of extension. The screw home mechanism moves the tibial tuberosity laterally and produces a medial shift at the knee. Some of the speculative causes of the screw home movement are that the lateral condyle surface is covered first and a rotation occurs to accommodate the larger surface of the medial condyle or that the ACL becomes taut just before rotation, forcing rotation of the femur on the tibia (89). Finally, it is speculated that the cruciate ligaments become taut in early extension and pull the condyles in opposite directions, causing the rotation.

The screw home mechanism is disrupted with injury to the ACL because the tibia moves more anteriorly on the femur. It is not significantly disrupted with loss of the PCL, indicating that the ACL is the main controller (89).

External rotation of the tibia is possible through approximately 45° (42). External rotation of the tibia also accompanies **plantarflexion** and **supination** of the foot. With 34° of supination, there will be a corresponding 58° of external rotation (83).

In extension, the patella returns to its resting position high and lateral on the femur, where it is above the trochlear groove and resting on the suprapatellar fat pad. The linear movement is reversed as it moves anteriorly and up in the groove. The angular movements of the patella are extension, adduction, and internal rotation (11,47).

There is medial and lateral translatory motion at the knee joint as the knee flexes. This motion is varus or abduction and valgus or adduction. No active varus or valgus motion can take place while the knee joint is extended, even though it is maintained in a valgus position. The valgus motion is maximum with the knee flexed and internally rotated, while the varus motion is maximum as the joint is nearing maximal extension and external rotation.

During walking, the foot strikes the ground with the knee joint almost extended (5° to 8° flexion), externally rotated, and in a maximal varus position (93). During the support phase, the knee undergoes 17 to 20° of flexion, 5 to 7° of internal rotation, 7 to 14° of external rotation, and 3 to 7° of varus movement (43,47,93). During the support phase, the knee joint moves from slight flexion at heel strike to extension at toe-off, internal rotation to external rotation and valgus to varus. During the swing phase, there is 60° to 88° of knee flexion, 12° to 17° of rotation, and 8° to 11° of valgus (43,93).

The knee joint moves from a position of maximum flexion after toe-off to maximum extension, from internal rotation to external rotation, and from valgus to varus. Maximum extension and maximum external rotation occur just before heel strike, maximum varus at heel strike, and maximum valgus in the swing phase (43,93).

The patella moves through a total of 41° of flexion and extension, 9.5° of abduction and adduction, and 5° of rotation during walking (46). There is lateral movement of the patella from foot strike until maximum flexion in the swing phase. When the foot strikes, the patella also moves posteriorly. As the knee extends prior to foot strike, there is a rapid medial shift of the patella.

During running, there is 80 and 36° of knee flexion in the swing and support phases, respectively. There is 11 and 8° of rotation and 19 and 8° of varus and valgus motion for the swing and support phases, respectively (29). A sample of the knee joint motions in running is presented in Figure 6-30.

Running on a cambered road or track requires greater knee flexion and external rotation and less internal rotation of the knee joint of the downhill limb. This is the case because greater force is directed medially. The uphill foot is also forced into pronation and the downhill foot into supination (29).

Going upstairs requires approximately 83° of flexion, 17° of abduction and adduction, and 16° of rotation (49). Going downstairs uses approximately 83° of flexion, 14° of abduction and adduction, and 15° of rotation. Sitting down in a chair requires the use of approximately 93° of flexion, 15° of abduction and adduction, and 14° of rotation. Tying a shoe while seated uses the greatest range of

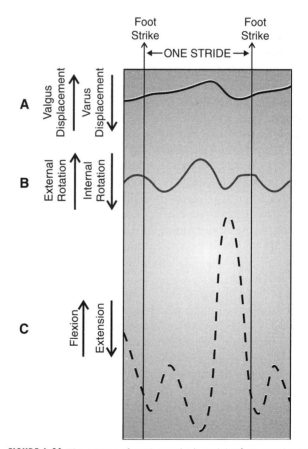

FIGURE 6-30 The pattern of motion at the knee joint for a running stride is presented. The knee joint makes three movements: **A.** linear movement. **B.** Rotation. **C.** Flexion and extension. (Reprinted with permission from Taunton, J. E., et al. [1985]. A triplanar electrogoniometer investigation of running mechanics in runners with compensatory overpronation. *Canadian Journal of Applied Sports Science*, 10:104–115.)

motion at the knee joint, approximately 106° of flexion, 20° of abduction and adduction, and 18° of rotation (49). Any osteoarthritic degeneration of the knee joint can greatly impair function, resulting in a 30 to 50% loss of knee flexion in daily activities (8).

MUSCULAR ACTIONS

Knee extension is a very important contributor to the generation of power in the lower extremity for any form of human projection or translation. The musculature producing extension is also used frequently to contract eccentrically and decelerate a rapidly flexing knee joint. Fortunately, the quadriceps femoris muscle group, the producer of extension at the knee, is one of the strongest muscle groups in the body; it may be as much as three times stronger than its antagonistic muscle group, the hamstrings, because of its involvement in negatively accelerating the leg and continuously contracting against gravity (42).

The quadriceps femoris is a muscle group consisting of the rectus femoris and vastus intermedius forming the middle part of the muscle group, the vastus lateralis on the lateral side, and the vastus medialis on the medial side (7). The specific insertions, actions, and nerve supply are presented in Appendix B.

The quadriceps femoris connect to the tibial tuberosity via the patellar tendon and contribute somewhat to the stability of the patella. As a muscle group, they also pull the menisci anteriorly in extension via the meniscopatellar ligament. When they contract, they also reduce the strain in the MCL and work with the PCL to prevent posterior displacement of the tibia. They are antagonistic to the ACL.

The largest and strongest of the quadriceps femoris is the vastus lateralis, a muscle applying lateral force to the patella. Pulling medially is the vastus medialis. The lower portion of the vastus medialis is referred to as the vastus medialis oblique. This portion of the vastus medialis attaches to the tendon of the adductor magnus tendon. It has more horizontal fibers than the superior portion of the vastus medialis and is a medial stabilizer of the patella (96).

It has been noted in the literature that the vastus medialis was selectively activated in the last few degrees of extension. However, this has been proved not to be true. There is no selective activation of the vastus medialis muscles in the last degrees of extension, and the two muscles contract equally throughout the range of motion (50).

The only two-joint muscle of the quadriceps femoris group, the rectus femoris, does not significantly contribute to knee extension force unless the hip joint is in a favorable position. It is limited as an extensor of the knee if the hip is flexed and is facilitated as a knee extensor if the hip joint is extended, lengthening the rectus femoris. In walking and running, the rectus femoris will contribute to the extension force in the toe-off phase when the thigh is extended. Likewise, in kicking, rectus femoris

activity is maximized in the preparatory phase as the thigh is brought back into hyperextension with the leg in flexion.

Flexion of the leg at the knee joint occurs during support, when the body lowers toward the ground; however, this downward movement is controlled by the extensors so that buckling does not occur. The flexor muscles are very active with the limb off the ground, working frequently to slow a rapidly extending leg.

The major muscle group contributing to knee flexion is the hamstrings, consisting of the lateral biceps femoris and the medial semimembranosus and semitendinosus (see Appendix B). The action of the hamstrings can be quite complex because they are two-joint muscles working to extend the hip. They are also rotators of the knee joint because of their insertions on the sides of the knee. As flexors, the hamstrings can generate the greatest force from a flexion position of 90° (71).

Flexion strength diminishes with extension because of an acute tendon angle that reduces the mechanical advantage. At full extension, flexion strength is reduced by 50% compared to 90° of flexion (71).

The lateral hamstring, the biceps femoris, has two heads connecting on the lateral side of the knee and offering lateral support to the joint. The biceps femoris also produces external rotation of the lower leg. Additionally, the lateral quadriceps femoris works with the ACL to stabilize the knee joint.

The semimembranosus bolsters the posterior and medial capsule and works with the ACL to prevent anterior displacement of the tibia. In flexion, it pulls the meniscus posteriorly (96). This medial hamstring also contributes to the production of internal rotation in the joint. The other medial hamstring, the semitendinosus, is part of the **pes anserinus** muscular attachment on the medial surface of the tibia. It is the most effective flexor of the pes anserinus muscle group, contributing 47% to the flexion force (96). The semitendinosus works with both the ACL and the MCL in supporting the knee joint. It also contributes to the generation of internal rotation.

The hamstrings operate most effectively as knee flexors from a position of hip flexion by increasing the length and tension in the muscle group. If the hamstrings become tight, they offer greater resistance to extension of the knee joint by the quadriceps femoris. This imposes a greater workload on the quadriceps femoris muscle group.

The two remaining pes anserinus muscles, the sartorius and the gracilis, also contribute 19% and 34% to the flexion strength, respectively (71). The popliteus is a weak flexor supporting the PCL in deep flexion and drawing the meniscus posteriorly. Finally, the two-joint gastrocnemius contributes to knee flexion, especially when the foot is in the neutral or dorsiflexed position.

Internal rotation of the tibia is produced by the medial muscles: sartorius, gracilis, semitendinosus, semimembranosus, and popliteus (see Appendix B). Internal rotation force is greatest at 90° of knee flexion and decreases by

59% at full extension (72,73). The internal rotation force can be increased by 50% if it is preceded by 15° of external rotation. Of the three pes anserinus muscles, the sartorius and the gracilis are the most effective rotators, accounting for 34% and 40% of the pes anserinus force in rotation (71). The semitendinosus contributes 26% of the pes anserinus rotation force. Only one muscle, the biceps femoris, contributes significantly to the generation of external rotation of the tibia. Both internal and external rotation are necessary movements associated with function of the knee joint.

STRENGTH AND FORCE AT THE KNEE JOINT

The extensors at the knee joint are usually stronger than the flexors throughout the range of motion. Peak extension strength is achieved at 50 to 70° of knee flexion (67). The position of maximum strength will vary with the speed of movement. For example, if the movement is slow, peak extension strength occurs in the first 20° of knee extension from the 90° flexed position. Flexion strength is greatest in the first 20 to 30° of flexion from the extended position (74). This position will also fluctuate with the speed of movement. Greater knee flexion torques can be obtained if the hips are flexed, since the hamstring length–tension relationship is improved.

It is quite common in sports medicine to evaluate the isokinetic strength of the quadriceps femoris and the hamstrings to construct a hamstring-to-quadriceps ratio. A generally acceptable ratio is 0.5, with the hamstrings at least half as strong as the quadriceps femoris. It has been suggested that anything below this ratio indicates a strength imbalance between the quadriceps femoris and the hamstrings that predisposes one to injury. Caution must be observed when using this ratio, as it applies only to slow isokinetic testing speeds.

At faster testing speeds, when the limbs move through 200 to 300°/second, the ratio approaches 1 because the efficiency of the quadriceps femoris drops at higher speeds. Even at the isometric testing level, the hamstring-to-quadriceps ratio is 0.7. Thus, a ratio of 0.5 between the hamstrings and the quadriceps femoris would not be acceptable at fast speeds and would indicate a strength imbalance between the two groups, whereas at a slower speed, it would not (66).

Internal and external rotation torques are both greatest with the knee flexed to 90°, because a greater range of rotation motion can be achieved in that position. Internal rotation strength will increase by 50% from 45° of knee flexion to 90° (73). The position of the hip joint will also influence internal rotation torque, with the greatest strength developed at 120° of hip flexion, at which point the gracilis and the hamstrings are most efficient (72). At low hip flexion angles and in the neutral position, the sartorius is the most effective lateral rotator. Peak rotation torques occur in the first 5 to 10° of rotation. The internal rotation torque is greater than the external rotation torque (73).

The knee is subject to very high forces during most activities, whether generated in response to gravity, as a result of the absorption of the force coming up from the ground, or as a consequence of muscular contraction. The muscles generate considerable force, with the quadriceps femoris tension force being as high as 1 to 3 times body weight in walking, 4 times body weight in stair climbing, 3.4 times body weight in climbing, and 5 times body weight in the squat (11).

The tibiofemoral compression force can also be quite high in specific activities. For example, muscle forces applied against a low resistance (40 Nm [newton-meters]) can create tibiofemoral compression forces of 1100 N during knee extension acting through knee angles of 30 to 120°. This force increases to 1230 N when extension occurs from the fully extended position (67). Tibiofemoral compression force in the extended position is greater, partly because the quadriceps femoris group loses mechanical advantage at the terminal range of motion and thus has to exert a greater muscular force to compensate for the loss in leverage.

The tibiofemoral shear force is maximum in the last few degrees of extension. The direction of the shear force changes with the amount of flexion in the joint, changing direction between 50 and 90° of flexion. Operating against the same 40-Nm resistance in extension, there is posterior shear of 200 N at 120° of flexion and 600 N of anterior shear in extension (67). This is partially because when nearing extension, the patellar tendon pulls the tibia anteriorly relative to the femur, while in flexion, it pulls the tibia posteriorly.

The anterior force in the last 30° of extension places a great deal of stress on the ACL, which takes up 86% of the anterior shear force. By moving the contact pad closer to the knee in an extension exercise, the shear force can be directed posteriorly, taking the strain off of the ACL (67).

Even though tibiofemoral compression forces are greater in the extended position, the contact area is large, which reduces the pressure. There is 50% more contact area at the extended position than in 90° of flexion. Thus, in the extended position, the compression forces are high, but the pressure is less by 25% (67). The forces for women are 20% higher because of a decreased mechanical advantage associated with shorter moment arm. Since females also have less contact area in the joint, greater pressure is created, accounting for the higher rate of osteoarthritis in the knees of women, an occurrence not seen in the hip.

The patellofemoral compressive force approximates 0.5 to 1.5 times body weight in walking, 3 to 4 times body weight in climbing, and 7 to 8 times body weight in a squat exercise (67). The patellofemoral joint absorbs compressive forces from the femur and transforms them into tensile forces in the quadriceps tendon and the patellar ligament. In vigorous activities, in which there are large negative acceleration forces, the patellofemoral force is also large. This force increases with flexion because the angle between the quadriceps femoris and the patella decreases, requiring greater quadriceps femoris force to resist the flexion or produce an extension.

The patellofemoral compressive force is maximum at 50° of flexion and declines at extension, approaching zero as the patella almost comes off the femur. The largest area of contact with the patella is at 60 to 90° of knee flexion. Of the patellar surface, 13 to 38% bears the force in joint loading (67). Fortunately, there is a large contact area when the patellofemoral compressive forces are large, which reduces the pressure. In fact, there is considerable pressure in the extended position even though the patellofemoral force is low because the contact area is small.

Activities using more pronounced knee flexion angles usually involve large patellofemoral compressive forces. These include descending stairs (4000 N), maximal isometric extension (6100 N), kicking (6800 N), the parallel squat (14,900 N), isokinetic knee extension (8300 N), rising from a chair (3800 N), and jogging (5000 N) (67). In activities using lesser amounts of knee flexion, the force is much less. Examples include ascending stairs (1400 N), walking (840–850 N) and bicycling (880 N) (67). The activities with high patellofemoral forces should be limited or avoided by individuals with patellofemoral pain.

The patellofemoral compressive force and the quadriceps femoris force both increase at the same rate with knee flexion in weight bearing. If the leg extends against a resistance, such as in a leg extension machine or weight boot, the quadriceps femoris force will increase, but the patellofemoral force will decrease from flexion to extension. Since the function in a weight-lifting extension exercise is opposite to that in daily activities that use flexion in the weight-bearing position, the use of a weight-bearing closed kinetic chain activity is preferable. At knee flexion angles greater than 60°, the patellar tendon force is only half to two-thirds that of the quadriceps tendon force (67).

Those with pain in the patellar region should avoid exercising at angles greater than 30° to avoid large flexing moments and patellofemoral compression forces. However, in extension, when the patellofemoral force is low, the anterior shear force is high, making terminal extension activities contraindicated for any ACL injury (67). There is a reversal at 50° of flexion, when the shear force is low and the patellofemoral compression force is high.

CONDITIONING

The extensors of the leg are easy to exercise because they are commonly used both to lower and to raise the body. Examples of stretching and strengthening exercises for the extensors are presented in Figure 6-31.

The squat is used to strengthen the quadriceps femoris. When one lowers into a squat, the force coming through the joint, directed vertically in the standing position, is now partially directed across the joint, creating a shear force. This shear force increases as knee flexion increases. Thus, in a deep squat position, most of the original compressive force is directed posteriorly, creating a shear force. With the ligaments and muscles unable to offer much protection in the posterior direction at the full squat position, this is considered a vulnerable position. This position of maximum knee flexion is contraindicated for the beginner or unconditioned lifter.

An experienced and conditioned lifter who has strong musculature and uses good technique at the bottom of the lift will most likely avoid any injury when in this position. Good technique involves control over the speed of descent and proper segmental positioning. For example, if the trunk is in too much flexion, the low back will be excessively loaded and the hamstrings will perform more of the work and the quadriceps femoris less, focusing control on the posterior side.

The quadriceps femoris group may also be exercised in an open-chain activity, as in a leg extension machine. Starting from 90° of flexion, one can exert considerable force, since the quadriceps femoris muscles are very efficient throughout the early parts of the extension action. Near full extension, the quadriceps femoris muscles become inefficient and must exert greater force to move the same load.

The terminal extension exercise is good for individuals having patellar pain because the quadriceps femores are working hard with minimal patellofemoral compression force. It should be avoided, however, in early rehabilitation of an ACL injury, since the anterior shear force is so large in this position. No knee extension exercise should be used at any angle less than 64°, to minimize the stress on the ACL (99). Any knee extension exercise for individuals with ACL injuries should be done from a position of considerable knee flexion. A closed-chain squat exercise is preferable for ACL injuries, since it minimizes the stress to the ligament and passive structures around the joint (99).

The flexors of the knee are not actively recruited in the performance of a flexion action with gravity because the quadriceps femoris muscles control the flexion action via eccentric muscle activity. Fortunately, the hamstrings are extensors of the hip as well as flexors of the knee joint. Thus, they are active during a squat exercise by virtue of their influence at the hip, since hip flexion in lowering is controlled eccentrically by the hip extensors. If it were not for the hamstrings' role as extensors at the hip, the hamstrings group would be considerably weaker than the quadriceps femoris.

The knee flexors are best isolated and exercised in a seated position using a leg curl apparatus. The seated position places the hip in flexion, thus optimizing their performance. The knee flexors, especially the hamstrings and the pes anserinus muscles, are important for knee stability, since they control much of the rotation at the knee. As presented earlier in this chapter, the hamstrings should be half as strong as the quadriceps femoris groups for slow speeds and should be as strong as the quadriceps femoris group at fast speeds. It is also important to maintain

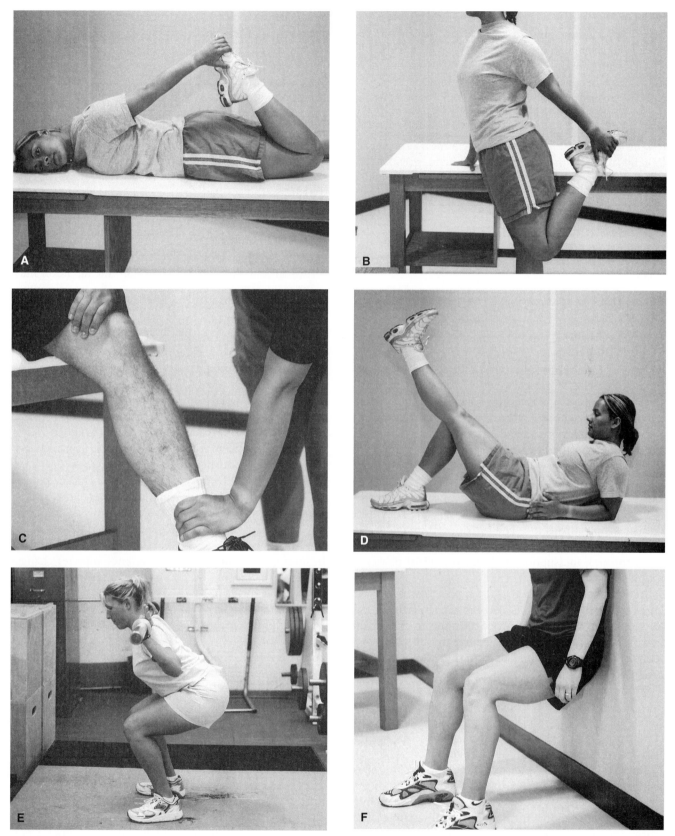

FIGURE 6-31 Exercises for the knee extensors are presented. The extensors can be stretched from the prone or standing position by pulling the leg up to the buttocks **(A and B)**. They can be exercised manually by applying resistance to the leg during extension **(C)**. A low-resistance exercise for the extensors is a simple leg extension from the hook lying position **(D)**. A common weight-training exercise for the knee extensors includes the squat **(E)**. A wall sit will also strengthen the quads to same degree **(F)**.

flexibility in the hamstrings, because if they are tight, the quadriceps femoris muscles must work harder and the pelvis will develop an irregular posture and function.

The rotators of the knee, since they are all flexor muscles, will be exercised along with the flexion movements. If the rotators are to be selectively stretched or strengthened as they perform the rotation, it is best to do the exercise from a seated position with the knee flexed to 90° and the rotators in a position of maximum effectiveness. Toeing the foot in contracts the internal rotators and stretches the external rotators. Different levels of resistance can be added to this exercise through the use of elastic bands or cables.

CONTRIBUTION TO SPORT SKILLS OR MOVEMENTS

Locomotion

Walking uses the musculature around the knee joint to propel and stabilize the body and to absorb significant forces applied to the body. Refer to Figure 6-16 for a review and summary of the lower extremity muscles used in walking.

As the heel strikes the ground to begin the braking portion of the support phase of walking, the hamstrings reach their peak of muscular activity as they attempt to arrest movement at the hip joint. The quadriceps femores then begin to contract to control the load (i.e., weight) being imposed on the knee joint by the body and the reaction force coming up from the ground. The knee is also moving into flexion eccentrically controlled by the quadriceps femoris. A cocontraction of the hamstrings and the quadriceps femoris continues until the foot is flat on the ground, at which time the activity of the hamstrings drops off. The activity of the quadriceps femoris diminishes at approximately 30% of stance and is silent through midsupport and into the initial phases of propulsion.

In the propelling portion of the support phase of walking, the quadriceps femoris become active again around 85 to 90% of stance, when they are used to propel the body upward and forward. The hamstrings become active at approximately the same time to add to the forward propulsion.

In the swing phase, the hamstrings are active after toe-off and again at the end of the swing just prior to foot contact (Fig. 6-16). Similar activity is seen in the quadriceps femoris, which slow knee flexion after toe-off and initiate knee extension prior to heel strike.

Running employs greater muscular activity at the knee joint to control the vigorous actions that running requires. Refer to Figure 6-17 for a review of the lower extremity muscular contributions to running. At the instant of heel strike in running, a brief concentric contraction of the hamstrings flexes the knee to decrease the horizontal or braking force being absorbed at impact. This is followed by activation of the quadriceps femores. Initially, the quadriceps femores act eccentrically to slow the negative vertical of the body velocity. This action lasts until midsupport. The

quadriceps femoris then act concentrically to produce positive vertical velocity of the body. The hamstrings are also active with the quadriceps femoris to generate extension at the hip (57). The period from heel strike to midsupport represents more than half of the energy costs in running.

In the propelling portion of support, the quadriceps femoris are eccentrically active as the heel lifts off and then become concentrically active up through toe-off. The hamstrings are also concentrically active at toe-off.

During the initial portion of the swing phase, the quadriceps femoris is active eccentrically to slow rapid knee flexion. In the later part of the swing phase, the hamstrings become active to both limit knee extension and hip flexion (56).

For both walking and running, the concentric knee flexor activity increases as the speed increases to lessen the vertical ground reaction force and assist the hip flexor musculature in reducing the hip vertical velocity at contact. Eccentric activity from the quadriceps femoris also increases with an increase in speed to slow the knee flexion and stop the negative vertical velocity of the body. Finally, the quadriceps femoris increases its activity with speed to contribute to the propelling force through increased extension activity at the knee. Knee extension is more related to sprint speed than any other joint movement or muscle action.

Stair Ascent and Descent

In stair ascent, there is a significant peak of musculature activity from the vastus medialis, vastus lateralis, and rectus femoris at 20% into the stance and a smaller peak at 80% of stance (51). A review of the muscular contributions to stair climbing is presented in Figure 6-19.

Lifting

In lifting, the contribution of the knee muscles changes with the posture. The muscular contribution to a straight-leg lift is presented in Figure 6-32. Lifting an object with straight knees and the trunk flexed demonstrates high quadriceps femoris activity at the beginning and end of the lift (18). Overall, for the total lift, the quadriceps femoris activity is lower than one might think. Moderate use of the hamstrings occurs in the middle third of the lift. While this example demonstrates the change in the contribution of the muscles that cross the knee joint, this type of lift is extremely bad for the low back and should not be used.

If the same lift is performed with the knees flexed, the flexion moment at the beginning of the lift changes to an extension moment (Fig. 6-33). Unlike the straight-leg lift, the quadriceps femoris activity is moderate to high in this lift. The hamstring activity is low, and a cocontraction takes place in the lift (67). In flexed-knee working postures, there is medium to high activity in the vastus lateralis, less activity in the rectus femoris, and low to medium activities in the biceps femoris.

In straight-knee postures, a working height of 1 m from the ground produces the lowest extensor moment at

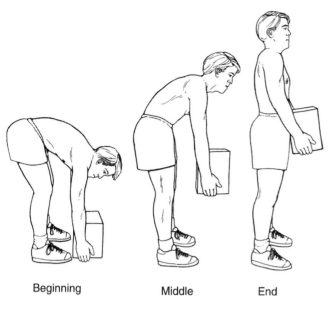

Lifting with Knees Straight

Muscles	Beginning	Phases Middle	End
Quadriceps	***	*	***
Hamstrings	*	**	*

* = low activity
** = moderate activity
*** = high activity

FIGURE 6-32 The contribution of the knee muscles to lifting depends on the posture used. In a straight-leg lift, the quadriceps femoris muscle group contributes significantly at the beginning and the end of the lift. The hamstrings are moderately active during the middle of the lift. This type of lift is not recommended. (Adapted with permission from Nisell, R. [1985]. Mechanics of the knee: A study of joint and muscle load with clinical applications. *Acta Orthopaedica Scandinavica*, 56:1–42.)

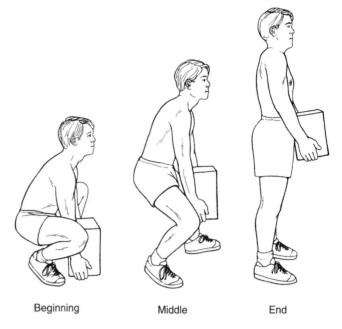

Lifting with Knees Flexed

Muscles	Beginning	Phases Middle	End
Quadriceps	***	***	***
Hamstrings	*	*	*

* = low activity
*** = high activity

FIGURE 6-33 A lift starting from a position of flexed knees uses more of the quadriceps femoris group than the straight-leg lift. The quadriceps femoris group is active throughout the lift. A cocontraction of the hamstrings accompanies the quadriceps femoris activity. (Adapted with permission from Nisell, R. [1985]. Mechanics of the knee: A study of joint and muscle load with clinical applications. *Acta Orthopaedica Scandinavica*, 56:1–42.)

the knee (18). The horizontal distance from the workstation is also important, because as one assumes a work posture or stance farther from the station, the knee extensors must work harder.

Cycling

In cycling, the knee musculature is responsible for a significant portion of power production. As shown in Figure 6-20, power in the cycling stroke is generated through 25 to 160° (78). At the top of the crank cycle, from 0 to 90°, the quadriceps femoris is very active. The rectus femoris is active through the arc of 200° to 130° of the next cycle. The vastus medialis is active from 300 to 135°, and the vastus lateralis is active from 315° through 130° of the next cycle (78).

In the middle of the cycle, from 90 to 270°, the hamstrings contribute more to power production, with the biceps femoris active from 5 to 265° and the semimembranosus active from 10 to 265° (78). There is cocontraction of the quadriceps femoris and the hamstrings through the early portions of the cycle. In the last portion of the cycle, from 270 to 360°, the rectus femoris is actively involved as the leg is brought back up into the top position.

INJURY POTENTIAL IN THE KNEE JOINT

The knee joint is a frequently injured area of the body, depending on the sport, accounting for 25 to 70% of reported injuries. Approximately 97% of these injuries are associated with athletics or some form of vigorous activity. Only 22% of knee injuries occur as a result of contact (65).

Often the cause of an injury to the knee can be related to poor conditioning or training or to an alignment problem in the lower extremity. Injuries in the knee have been attributable to **hindfoot** and forefoot varus or valgus, tibial or femoral varus or valgus, limb length differences, deficits in flexibility, strength imbalances between agonists and antagonists, and improper technique or training.

A number of knee injuries are associated with running or jogging, because the knee and the lower extremity are subjected to a force equivalent to approximately 3 times body weight at every foot contact. It is clear that if 1500 foot contacts are made per mile of running, the potential for injury is high.

The traumatic injuries to the knee usually involve the ligaments. Ligaments are injured as a result of application of a force causing a twisting action of the knee. High-friction or uneven surfaces are usually associated with increased ligamentous injury. Any movement fixing the foot while the body continues to move forward, such as often occurs in skiing, will likely produce a ligament sprain or tear. Simply, any turn on a weight-bearing limb leaves the knee vulnerable to ligamentous injury.

The ACL is the most common site of ligament injuries, which are usually caused by a twisting action while the knee is flexed, internally rotated, and in a valgus position while supporting weight. If the trunk and thigh rotate over a lower extremity while supporting the body's weight, the ACL can be sprained or torn because the lateral femoral condyle moves posteriorly in external rotation (33). Examples from sport in which this ligament is often injured are skiers catching the edge of the ski, a football player being blocked from the side, a basketball player landing off-balance from a jump, and a gymnast landing off-balance from a dismount (72).

Loss of the ACL creates valgus laxity and single-plane or rotatory instability (15). The planar instability is usually anterior, while rotatory instabilities can occur in a variety of directions, depending on the other structures injured (9). Instability created by an inefficient or missing ACL will place added stress on the secondary stabilizers of the knee, such as the capsule, collateral ligaments, and iliotibial band. There is an accompanying deficit in quadriceps femoris musculature. The "side effects" of the ACL injury are often more debilitating in the long run.

Injury to the PCL is less common than to the ACL. The PCL is injured by receiving an anterior blow to a flexed or hyperextended knee or by forcing the knee into external rotation when it is flexed and supporting weight. Damage to the PCL results in anterior or posterior planar instability.

The collateral ligaments on the side are injured upon receipt of a force applied to the side of the joint. The MCL, torn in an application of force in the direction of the medial side of the joint, can also sprain or tear with a violent external rotation or tibial varus (19,90). The MCL is typically injured when the foot is fixed and slightly flexed. A change in direction with the person moving away from the support limb, as when running the bases in baseball, is a common event leading to an MCL injury.

The LCL is injured upon receipt of a lateral that is usually applied when the foot is fixed and the knee is in slight flexion (19). Injury to the MCL or LCL creates medial or lateral planar instabilities, respectively. A forceful varus or valgus force can also create a **distal femoral epiphysitis** as the collateral ligaments forcefully pull on their attachment site (48).

Rotatory instabilities created by injury to the ligaments or capsule are usually one of three types. An anteromedial rotatory instability is generated with external rotation of the tibia with a fixed foot, flexed knee, and abducted thigh. These actions damage the middle third of the capsule, the semimembranosus attachment, the **posterior oblique ligament**, and the middle part of the ACL (19).

An anterolateral rotatory instability is associated with an injury in which a lateral force is applied while the foot is fixed and the knee slightly flexed. This damages the middle third of the lateral capsule, the arcuate complex, the posterior lateral capsule, and the anterior portion of the ACL (19).

The third instability is the posterolateral rotatory instability created by a blow to the front of the tibia with the leg externally rotated and in a varus position (19). This damages the posterior third of the lateral capsule, the arcuate complex, and the posterior portion of the ACL.

Damage to the menisci occurs much the same way as ligament damage. The menisci can be torn through compression associated with a twisting action in a weight-bearing position. They can also be torn in kicking and other violent extension actions. Tearing the meniscus by compression is a result of the femur grinding into the tibia and ripping the menisci. A meniscal tear in rapid extension is a result of the meniscus getting caught and torn as the femur moves rapidly forward on the tibia.

Tears to the medial meniscus are usually incurred during moves incorporating valgus, knee flexion, and external rotation in the supported limb or when the knee is hyperflexed (88). The lateral meniscus tear has been associated with a forced axial movement in the flexed position; a forced lateral movement with impact on the knee in extension; a forceful rotational movement; a movement incorporating varus, flexion, and internal rotation of the support limb; and the hyperflexed position (88).

Many injuries to the knee are a result of less traumatic noncontact forces. Muscle strains to the quadriceps femoris or the hamstrings muscle groups occur frequently. Strain to the quadriceps femoris usually involves the rectus femoris, since it can be placed in a very lengthened position with hip hyperextension and knee flexion. It is injured commonly in a kicking action, especially if the kick is mistimed. A hamstring strain is usually associated with inflexibility in the hamstrings or a stronger quadriceps femoris that pulls the hamstrings into a lengthened position. Sprinting, when the runner is not in condition to handle the stresses of sprinting, can lead to a hamstring strain.

On the lateral side of the knee is the iliotibial band, which is frequently irritated as the band moves over the lateral epicondyle of the femur in flexion and extension. Iliotibial band syndrome is seen in individuals who run on crowned roads, specifically affecting the downhill limb. It has also been identified with individuals who run more than 5 miles per session, in stair climbing and downhill running, and in individuals who have a varum alignment in the lower extremity (31). Medial knee pain can be associated with many structures, such as tendinitis of the pes anserinus muscle attachment and irritation of the semimembranosus, parapatellar, or pes bursae (31).

Posterior knee pain is likely associated with popliteus tendinitis, which causes posterior lateral pain. This is often brought on by hill running. Posterior pain can also be associated with strain or tendinitis of the gastrocnemius muscle insertion.

Anterior knee pain accounts for most overuse injuries to the knee, especially in women. **Patellofemoral pain syndrome** is pain around the patella and is often seen in individuals exhibiting valgum alignments or femoral anteversion in the extremity (18).

The stress on the patella is associated with the Q-angle, because a greater Q-angle may increase stress on the patella. Patellar injury may be caused by abnormal tracking, which in addition to an increased Q-angle can be created by a functional short leg, tight hamstrings, tight gastrocnemius, a long patellar tendon (termed **patella alta**), a short patellar tendon (termed **patella baja**), tight lateral retinaculum or iliotibial band, or excessive pronation at the foot.

Some patellofemoral pain syndromes are associated with cartilage destruction, in which the cartilage underneath the patella becomes soft and fibrillated. This condition is known as **chondromalacia patellae**. Patellar pain similar to that of patellar pain syndrome or chondromalacia patellae is also seen with medial retinaculitis, in which the medial retinaculum is irritated in running (96).

A subluxated or dislocated patella is common in individuals having predisposing factors. These are patella alta, ligamentous laxity, a small Q-angle with out-facing patella, external tibial torsion, and an enlarged fat pad with patella alta (96). Dislocation of the patella may be congenital. The dislocation occurs in flexion as a result of a faulty knee extension mechanism.

The attachment site of the quadriceps femoris to the tibia at the tibial tuberosity is also a site for injury and the development of anterior pain. The tensile force of the quadriceps femoris can create tendinitis at this insertion site. This is commonly seen in athletes who do vigorous jumping, such as in volleyball, basketball, and track and field (64). In children aged 8 to 15 years, a tibial tubercle epiphysitis can develop. This is referred to as **Osgood-Schlatter disease**. This disease is an avulsion fracture of the growing tibial tuberosity that can also avulse the epiphysis. Bony growths can develop on the site. The cause of both of these conditions is overuse of the extensor mechanism (64).

Overuse of the extensor mechanism can also cause irritation of the plica. Plica injury can also result from a direct blow, a valgus rotary force applied to the knee, or weakness in the vastus medialis oblique. The plica become thick, inelastic, and fibrous with injury, making it difficult to sit for long periods and creating pain on the superior knee (7). The medial patella may snap and catch during flexion and extension with injury to the plica.

The Ankle and Foot

The foot and the ankle make up a complex anatomical structure consisting of 26 irregularly shaped bones, 30 synovial joints, more than 100 ligaments, and 30 muscles acting on the segments. All of these joints must interact harmoniously and in combination to achieve a smooth motion. Most of the motion in the foot occurs at three of the synovial joints: the talocrural, the subtalar, and the **midtarsal joints** (62). The foot moves in three planes, with most of the motion occurring in the rear foot.

The foot contributes significantly to the function of the whole lower limb. The foot supports the weight of the body in both standing and locomotion. The foot must be a loose adapter to uneven surfaces at contact. Also, upon contact with the ground, it serves as a shock absorber, attenuating the large forces resulting from ground contact. Late in the support phase, it must be a rigid lever for effective propulsion. Finally, when the foot is fixed during stance, it must absorb the rotation of the lower extremity. These functions of the foot all occur during a closed kinetic chain as it is receiving frictional and reaction forces from the ground or another surface (62).

ANATOMICAL AND FUNCTIONAL CHARACTERISTICS OF THE JOINTS

Talocrural Joint

The proximal joint of the foot is the **talocrural joint**, or ankle joint (Fig. 6-34). It is a uniaxial hinge joint formed by the tibia and fibula (tibiofibular joint) and the tibia and talus (**tibiotalar joint**). This joint is designed for stability rather than mobility. The ankle is stable when large forces are absorbed through the limb, when stopping and turning, and in many of the lower limb movements one performs on a daily basis. However, if any of the anatomical

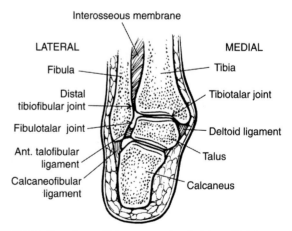

FIGURE 6-34 The talocrural joint, commonly called the ankle joint, consists of the articulations between the tibia and the talus (tibiotalar joint) and the tibia and the fibula (tibiofibular joint). The tibia and fibula create a mortise, making the joint very stable unless the mortise is altered through injury.

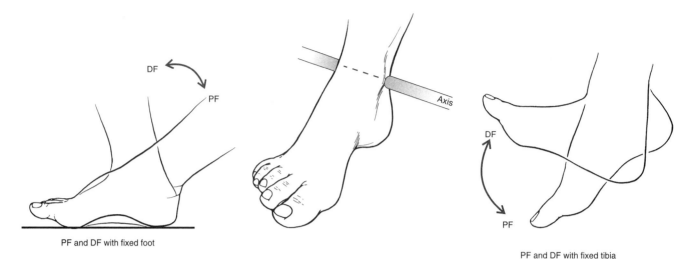

FIGURE 6-35 Plantarflexion and dorsiflexion occur about a mediolateral axis running through the ankle joint. The range of motion for plantar flexion and dorsiflexion is approximately 50° and 20°, respectively. Plantarflexion and dorsiflexion can be produced with the foot moving on a fixed tibia or with the tibia moving on a fixed foot.

support structures around the ankle joint are injured, it can become very unstable (33).

The tibia and fibula form a deep socket for the trochlea of the talus, creating a mortise. The medial side of the mortise is the inner side of the medial malleolus, a projection on the distal end of the tibia. On the lateral side is the inner surface of the lateral malleolus, a distal projection on the fibula. The lateral malleolus projects more inferiorly than the medial malleolus and protects the medial ligaments of the ankle. It also acts as a bulwark against any lateral displacement. Because the lateral malleolus projects more inferiorly, it is also more susceptible to fracture with an **inversion** sprain to the lateral ankle.

The tibia and fibula fit snugly over the trochlea of the talus, a bone wider anteriorly than posteriorly (42). The difference in width of the talus allows for some abduction and adduction of the foot. The close-packed position for the ankle is the dorsiflexed position when the talus is wedged in at its widest spot.

The ankle has excellent ligamentous support on the medial and lateral sides. The location and actions of the ligaments are presented in Appendix A. The ligaments surrounding the ankle limit plantarflexion and dorsiflexion, anterior and posterior movement of the foot, tilting of the talus, and inversion and eversion (92).

The stability of the ankle depends on the orientation of the ligaments, the type of loading, and the position of the ankle at the time of stress. The lateral side of the ankle joint is more susceptible to injury, accounting for 85% of ankle sprains (92).

The axis of rotation for the ankle joint is a line between the two malleoli, running oblique to the tibia and not in line with the body (17). Dorsiflexion occurs at the ankle joint as the foot moves toward the leg (e.g., when lifting the toes and forefoot off the floor) or as the leg moves toward the foot (e.g., in lowering down with the foot flat on the floor). These actions are illustrated in Figure 6-35.

The range of motion in dorsiflexion is limited by the bony contact between the neck of the talus and the tibia, the capsule and ligaments, and the plantar flexor muscles. The average range of dorsiflexion is 20°, although approximately 10° of dorsiflexion is required for efficient gait (10). Healthy elderly individuals typically exhibit less passive dorsiflexion range of motion but more dorsiflexion in gait than their younger counterparts.

Any arthritic condition in the ankle also reduces passive and increases active dorsiflexion range of motion. The increase in dorsiflexion in the arthritic joint is primarily due to a decrease in flexibility in the gastrocnemius or a weakness in the soleus. With the maintenance of the knee flexion angle during the support period of gait, a collapse into greater dorsiflexion is observed (52). With increased dorsiflexion and knee flexion, more weight is maintained on the heel.

Plantarflexion is movement of the foot away from the leg (e.g., rising up on the toes) or moving the leg away from the foot (such as in leaning back, away from the front of the foot) (Fig. 6-35). Plantarflexion is limited by the talus and the tibia, the ligaments and the capsule, and the dorsiflexor muscles. The average range of motion for plantarflexion is 50°, with 20° to 25° of plantarflexion used in gait (10).

In the arthritic or pathological gait, plantarflexion range of motion is less for both passive and active measurements. The reduction of plantarflexion in gait is substantial because of weak calf muscles. Healthy elderly people do not demonstrate substantial loss in either passive or active plantarflexion range of motion (52).

During gait, there is 20 to 40° of total plantarflexion and dorsiflexion movement (14,65). The foot strikes the ground with the ankle at 90° and moves through approximately 10° of plantarflexion to lower the foot to the ground

(75). Through midstance, the foot moves into approximately 5° of dorsiflexion, increasing to approximately 10° in late support. At push-off, the ankle rapidly plantar flexes 20° to unload the limb and begin the swing phase (75). In the swing phase of gait, the ankle dorsiflexes to move back to the neutral position. Dorsiflexion during the swing phase prevents the toes from contacting the ground and tripping the individual and prepares the foot for heel strike (98).

In running, there is approximately 10° of dorsiflexion prior to contact and as much as 50° of dorsiflexion through 50% of stance. Rapid plantarflexion of approximately 25° is observed at toe-off. As speed increases, the amount of plantarflexion decreases (93).

Subtalar Joint

Moving distally from the talocrural joint is the subtalar, or talocalcaneal, joint, which consists of the articulation between the talus and the calcaneus. All of the joints in the foot, including the subtalar joint, are shown in Figure 6-36. The talus and the calcaneus are the largest of the weight-bearing bones in the foot and form the hindfoot. The talus links the tibia and fibula to the foot and is called the keystone of the foot. No muscles attach to the talus.

The talus articulates with the calcaneus at three sites, anteriorly, posteriorly, and medially, where the convex surface of the talus fits into a concave surface on the calcaneus. The subtalar joint is supported by five short and powerful ligaments that resist severe stresses in lower extremity movements. The location and action of these

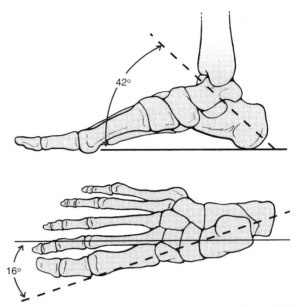

FIGURE 6-37 The axis of rotation for the subtalar joint runs diagonally from the posterolateral plantar surface to the anteromedial dorsal surface. The axis is approximately 42° in the sagittal plane (*top*) and 16° in the transverse plane. The solid line bisects the posterior surface of the calcaneus and the distal anteromedial corner of the calcaneus; the broken line bisects the talus.

ligaments are presented in Appendix A. The ligaments supporting the talus limit the motions of the subtalar joint.

The axis of rotation for the subtalar joint runs obliquely from the posterior lateral plantar surface to the anterior dorsal medial surface of the talus (Fig. 6-37). It is tilted vertically, 41 to 45° from the horizontal axis in the sagittal plane and is slanted 16 to 23° medially from the longitudinal axis of the tibia in the frontal plane (91). Because the axis of the subtalar joint is oblique through the sagittal, frontal, and transverse planes of the foot, triplanar motion can occur.

The triplanar movements at the subtalar joint are termed pronation and supination. Pronation, occurring in an open-chain system with the foot off the ground, consists of calcaneal eversion, abduction, and dorsiflexion (86). **Eversion** is the movement in the frontal plane in which the lateral border of the foot moves toward the leg in non–weight bearing or the leg moves toward the foot in weight bearing (Fig. 6-38). The transverse plane movement is abduction, or pointing the toes out. It occurs with external rotation of the foot on the leg and lateral movement of the calcaneus in the non–weight bearing position or internal rotation of the leg with respect to the calcaneus and medial movement of the talus in weight bearing. The sagittal plane movement of dorsiflexion occurs as the calcaneus moves up on the talus in non–weight bearing or as the talus moves down on the calcaneus in weight bearing. An illustration of differences in subtalar movements between open-chain and closed-chain positioning is shown in Figure 6-38.

Supination is just the opposite of pronation, with calcaneal inversion, adduction, and plantarflexion in the

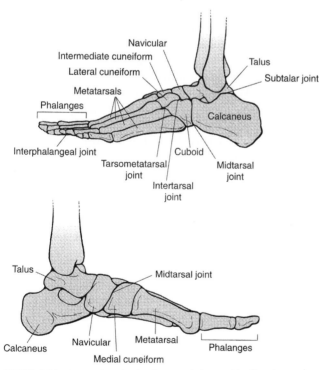

FIGURE 6-36 Thirty joints in the foot work in combination to produce the movements of the rear foot, midfoot and forefoot. The subtalar and midtarsal joints contribute to pronation and supination. The intertarsal, tarsometatarsal, metatarsophalangeal, and interphalangeal joints contribute to movements of the forefoot and the toes.

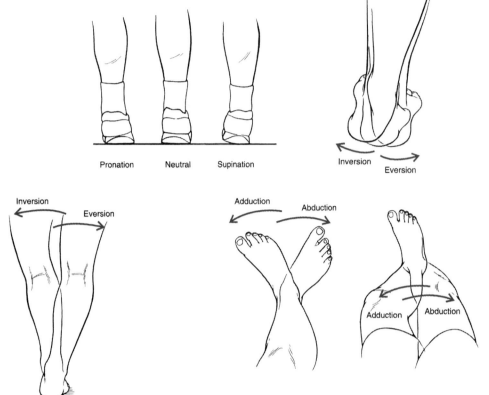

Pronation   Neutral   Supination

Inversion   Eversion

Inversion   Eversion

Adduction   Abduction

Adduction   Abduction

FIGURE 6-38 Using the right leg and foot, combinations of movements at the subtalar joint are termed pronation and supination. With the foot off the ground, the foot moves on a fixed tibia, and the subtalar movement of pronation is produced by eversion, abduction, and dorsiflexion. Supination in the open chain is produced by inversion, adduction, and plantarflexion. In a closed kinetic chain with the foot on the ground, much of the pronation and supination is produced by the weight of the body acting on the talus. In this weight-bearing position, the tibia moves on the talus to produce pronation and supination.

non–weight-bearing position and calcaneal inversion and talar abduction and dorsiflexion in the weight-bearing position (61). The frontal plane movement of inversion occurs as the medial border of the foot moves toward the medial leg in non–weight bearing or as the medial aspect of the leg moves toward the medial foot in weight bearing, as the calcaneus lies on the lateral surface. In the transverse plane, adduction, or toeing-in, occurs as the foot internally rotates on the leg in non–weight bearing and the calcaneus moves medially or the leg externally rotates on the foot in weight bearing and the talus moves laterally. The plantarflexion movements in the sagittal plane occur as the calcaneus moves distally while non–weight bearing or as the talus moves proximally while weight bearing.

The prime function of the subtalar joint is to absorb the rotation of the lower extremity during the support phase of gait. With the foot fixed on the surface and the femur and tibia rotating internally at the beginning of stance and externally at the end of stance, the subtalar joint absorbs the rotation through the opposite actions of pronation and supination (39). Pronation is a combination of dorsiflexion, abduction, and eversion, while supination is a combination of plantarflexion, adduction, and inversion.

A second function of the subtalar joint is shock absorption. This may also be accomplished by pronation. The subtalar movements also allow the tibia to rotate internally faster than the femur, facilitating unlocking at the knee joint.

Calcaneal movements are the same, regardless of weight bearing. This makes calcaneal inversion and eversion measurements very useful in determining subtalar motion (Fig. 6-38). Passive calcaneal inversion is possible through 20° of motion in young healthy individuals and 18° in healthy elderly individuals (52). Calcaneal varus or inversion is greatly reduced in individuals with osteoarthritis in the ankle joint. Calcaneal eversion, measured passively, averages 5 and 4° for healthy young and elderly individuals, respectively (52). In 84% of arthritic patients, excessive calcaneal eversion creates what is known as a hindfoot valgus deformity.

In gait, approximately 4° of calcaneal inversion and 6 to 7° of calcaneal eversion are used by healthy individuals. Motion of the foot during running is shown in Figure 6-39 for one leg cycle. Calcaneal inversion, maximum at toe-off, is usually not present in the gait of individuals with arthritis of the ankle. Calcaneal eversion, maximum at midstance, is usually excessive, ranging from 11 to 21° in arthritic gait (52).

The dynamic range of motion for pronation and supination is 20 to 62°, with supination about double the range of pronation (20,61). During the support phase of gait, pronation and supination should correspond with rotation of the tibia and femur. At heel strike, the foot typically makes contact with the ground in a slightly supinated position (2–3°) and the foot is lowered to the ground in plantarflexion (21). The subtalar joint begins immediately to pronate, accompanying internal rotation of both the tibia and the femur (34).

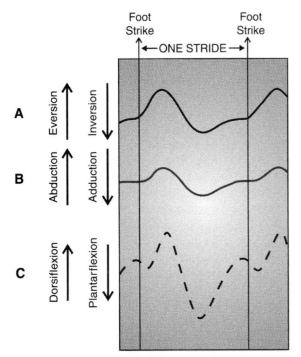

FIGURE 6-39 The pattern of motion of the foot during one running stride is presented. The foot **(A)** everts and inverts, **(B)** abducts and adducts, and **(C)** plantar flexes and dorsiflexes in the running stride. (Adapted with permission from Taunton, J. E., et al. [1985]. A triplanar electrogoniometer investigation of running mechanics in runners with compensatory overpronation. *Canadian Journal of Applied Sports Science*, 10:104–115.)

The talus rotates medially on the calcaneus, initiating pronation as a result of lateral heel strike and putting stress on the medial side (82). Pronation continues until it reaches a maximum at approximately 35 to 45% of the stance phase (4). In walking, maximum pronation is in the range of 3 to 10° and in running, 8 to 15° (3,16,93). More than 19° of pronation is considered excessive, although there is no clinical definition of excessive pronation.

At the stage of foot flat in stance, the tibia begins to rotate externally, and since the forefoot is still fixed on the ground, this external rotation is transmitted to the talus (34). The subtalar joint should begin to supinate in response to the external rotation. Approximately 3 to 10° of supination should occur up until heel-off.

Many injuries of the lower extremity are thought to be associated with excessive pronation. This association involves not just the maximum degree of pronation but also the percentage of support in which pronation is present and the timing of the pronation. Pronation can be present for as much as 55 to 85% of stance, creating problems when the lower limb moves into external rotation as the subtalar joint is still pronating (63). This is discussed later in this chapter.

Midtarsal Joint

Of the remaining articulations in the foot, the midtarsal, or transverse tarsal, joint has the greatest functional significance (Fig. 6-36). It actually consists of two joints, the **calca-**

neocuboid joint on the lateral side and the **talonavicular joint** on the medial side of the foot. In combination, they form an S-shaped joint with two axes, oblique and longitudinal (91). Five ligaments support this region of the foot (see Appendix A).

Movement at the midtarsal joint depends on the subtalar joint position. When the subtalar joint is in pronation, the two axes of the midtarsal joint are parallel, which unlocks the joint, creating hypermobility in the foot (69). This allows the foot to be very mobile in absorbing the shock of contact with the ground and also in adapting to uneven surfaces. When the axes are parallel, the forefoot is also allowed to flex freely and extend with respect to the **rear foot**. The motion at the midtarsal joint is unrestricted from heel strike to foot flat, as the foot bends toward the surface.

During supination of the subtalar joint, the two axes run through the midtarsal joint converge. This locks the joint in, creating rigidity in the foot necessary for efficient force application during the later stages of stance (69). The midtarsal joint becomes rigid and more stable from foot flat to toe-off in gait as the foot supinates. It is usually stabilized, creating a rigid lever, at 70% of the stance phase (61). At this time there is also a greater load on the midtarsal joint, making the articulation between the talus and the navicular more stable. Figure 6-40 contains an illustration of these actions.

Other Articulations of the Foot

The other articulations in the **midfoot**, the intertarsal articulations, between the cuneiforms and the navicular and cuboid and intercuneiform, are gliding joints (Fig. 6-36). At the articulation between the cuneiforms and the navicular and cuboid, small amounts of gliding and rotation are allowed (42).

At the intercuneiform articulations, a small vertical movement takes place, thus altering the shape of the **transverse**

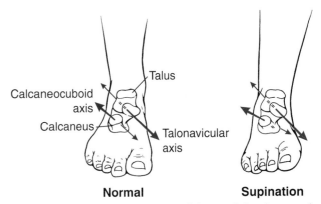

FIGURE 6-40 The midtarsal joints consist of the articulations between the calcaneus and the cuboid (calcaneocuboid joint) and the talus and the navicular (talonavicular joint). Each joint has an axis of rotation that runs obliquely across the joint. When the two axes are parallel to each other, the foot is flexible and can freely move. If the axes do not run parallel to each other, the foot is locked in a rigid position. This occurs with supination.

arch in the foot (20). These joints are supported by strong **interosseous ligaments**.

The forefoot comprises the metatarsals and the phalanges and the joints between them. The function of the forefoot is to maintain the transverse metatarsal arch, maintain the medial **longitudinal arch**, and maintain the flexibility in the first metatarsal. The plane of the forefoot at the metatarsal head is formed by the second, third, and fourth metatarsals. This plane is perpendicular to the vertical axis of the heel in normal forefoot alignment. This is the neutral position for the forefoot (Fig. 6-41). If the plane is tilted so that the medial side lifts, it is termed forefoot supination or varus (40). If the medial side drops below the neutral plane, it is termed forefoot pronation or valgus. **Forefoot valgus** is not as common as **forefoot varus** (Fig. 6-41). Also, if the first metatarsal is below the plane of the adjacent metatarsal heads, it is considered to be a **plantarflexed first ray** and is commonly associated with high-arched feet (40).

The base of the metatarsals is wedge-shaped, forming a mediolateral or transverse arch across the foot. The tarsometatarsal articulations are gliding or planar joints allowing limited motion between the cuneiforms and the first, second, and third metatarsals and the cuboid and the fourth and fifth metatarsals (42).

The **tarsometatarsal joint** movements change the shape of the arch. When the first metatarsal flexes and abducts as the fifth metatarsal flexes and adducts, the arch deepens, or increases in curvature. Likewise, if the first metatarsal extends and adducts and the fifth metatarsal extends and abducts, the arch will flatten.

Flexion and extension at the tarsometatarsal articulations also contribute to inversion and eversion of the foot. Greater movement is allowed between the first metatarsal and the first cuneiform than between the second metatarsal and the cuneiforms (61). Mobility is an important factor in the first metatarsal, since it is significantly involved in weight bearing and propulsion. The limited mobility at the second metatarsal is also significant, since it is the peak of the plantar arch and a continuation of the long axis of the foot. The tarsometatarsal joints are supported by the medial and lateral dorsal ligaments.

The **metatarsophalangeal joints** are biaxial, allowing both flexion and extension and abduction and adduction (Fig. 6-36). These joints are loaded during the propulsive phase of gait after heel-off and the initiation of plantarflexion and phalangeal flexion (33). Two sesamoid bones lie under the first metatarsal and reduce the load on one of the hallucis muscles in the propulsive phase. The movements at the metatarsophalangeal joints are similar to those seen in the same joints in the hand except that greater extension occurs in the foot as a result of requirements for the propulsive phase of gait.

The **interphalangeal joints** are similar to those found in the hand (Fig. 6-36). These uniaxial hinge joints allow for flexion and extension of the toes. The toes are much smaller than the fingers. They are also less developed, probably because of continual wearing of shoes (42). The toes are less functional than the fingers because they lack an opposable structure like the thumb.

Arches of the Foot

The tarsals and metatarsals of the foot form three arches, two running longitudinally and one running transversely across the foot. This creates an elastic shock-absorbing system. In standing, half of the weight is borne by the heel and half by the metatarsals. One-third of the weight borne by the metatarsals is on the first metatarsal, while the remaining load is on the other metatarsal heads (33). The arches form a concave surface that is a quarter of a sphere (42). The arches are shown in Figure 6-42.

The lateral longitudinal arch is formed by the calcaneus, cuboid, and fourth and fifth metatarsals. It is relatively flat and limited in mobility (33). Since it is lower than the medial arch, it may make contact with the ground and bear some of the weight in locomotion, thus playing a support role in the foot.

The more dynamic medial longitudinal arch runs across the calcaneus to the talus, navicular, cuneiforms, and first three metatarsals. It is much more flexible and mobile than the lateral arch and plays a significant role in shock absorption upon contact with the ground. At heel strike, part of the initial force is attenuated by compression of a fat pad positioned on the inferior surface of the calcaneus. This is followed by a rapid elongation of the medial arch that continues to maximum elongation at toe contact with the ground. The medial arch shortens at midsupport, then slightly elongates and again rapidly shortens at toe-off (33).

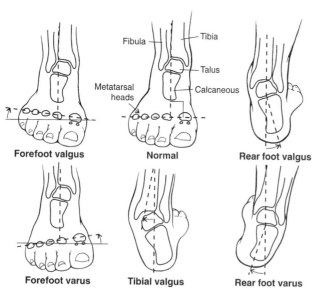

FIGURE 6-41 The metatarsal head should be perpendicular to the heel in a normal alignment in the foot. There are many variations in this alignment, including forefoot valgus, in which the medial side of the forefoot drops below the neutral plane; forefoot varus, in which the medial side lifts; rear foot valgus, in which the calcaneus is everted; and rear foot varus, in which the calcaneus is inverted. There can also be tibial and subtalar varum or valgus, in which the tibia or talus moves laterally or medially, respectively.

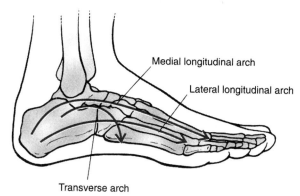

FIGURE 6-42 Three arches are formed by the tarsals and metatarsals: the lateral longitudinal arch, which participates in a support role function during weight bearing; the medial longitudinal arch, which dynamically contributes to shock absorption; and the transverse arch, which supports a significant portion of the body weight during weight bearing.

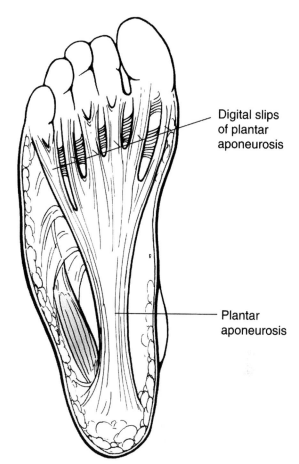

FIGURE 6-43 The plantar fascia is a strong fibrous aponeurosis that runs from the calcaneus to the base of the phalanges. It supports the arches and protects structures in the foot.

Flexion at the transverse tarsal and tarsometatarsal joints increases the height of the longitudinal arch as the metatarsophalangeal joints extend at push-off (87). The movement of the medial arch is important, for it dampens impact by transmitting the vertical load through deflection of the arch.

Even though the medial arch is very adjustable, it usually does not make contact with the ground unless a person has functional flat feet. The medial arch is supported by the keystone navicular bone, the **calcaneonavicular ligament**, the long plantar ligament, and the **plantar fascia** (20,34).

The plantar fascia, illustrated in Figure 6-43, is a strong, fibrous plantar aponeurosis running from the calcaneus to the metatarsophalangeal articulation. It supports both arches and protects the underlying neurovascular bundles. The plantar fascia can be irritated as a result of ankle motion through extreme ranges of motion, since the arch is flattened in dorsiflexion and increased in plantarflexion. These actions place a wide range of tensions on the fascial attachments (20). Also, if the plantar fascia is short, the arch is likely to be higher.

The transverse arch is formed by the wedging of the tarsals and the base of the metatarsals. The bones act as beams for support of this arch, which flattens with weight bearing and can support 3 to 4 times body weight (91). The flattening of this arch causes the forefoot to spread considerably in a shoe, indicating the importance of sufficient room in the shoe to allow for this spread.

Individuals can be classified according to the height of the medial arch into foot types that are normal, high-arched or **pes cavus**, and flat-footed or **pes planus**. They can be further classified as being rigid or flexible. The midfoot of the high-arched rigid foot does not make any contact with the ground and usually has little or no inversion or eversion in stance. It is a foot type that has poor shock absorption. The flat foot, on the other hand, is usually hypermobile, with most of the plantar surface making contact in stance. This weakens the medial side. It is a foot type usually asso-ciated with excessive pronation throughout the support phase of gait.

Foot Function

Foot function can be altered significantly with any variation in alignment in the lower extremity or as a result of abnormal motion in the lower extremity linkage. Typically, any varum alignment in the lower extremity will increase the pronation at the subtalar joint in stance (37). A Q-angle at the knee greater than 20°, tibial varum greater than 5°, rear foot varum greater than 2°, and forefoot varum greater than 3° are all deemed to be significant enough to produce an increase in subtalar pronation (52).

Rear foot varus is usually a combination of subtalar varus and tibial varum in which the calcaneus inverts and the lower third of the tibia deviates in the direction of inversion. Forefoot varus, the most common cause of excessive pronation, is the inversion of the forefoot on the rear foot with the subtalar joint in the neutral position (10). It is caused by the inability of the talus to derotate, leaving the foot pronated at heel lift and preventing any supination. This shifts the body weight to the medial side of the foot, creating a hypermobile midtarsal joint and an unstable first metatarsal.

Both rear foot and forefoot varus will double the amount of pronation in midstance as compared to normal foot function and will continue pronation into late stance (37). In some cases, the pronation will continue until the very end of the support period. This is a major injury-producing mechanism because the continued pronation is contrary to the external rotation being produced in the leg. It is the primary cause of discomfort and dysfunction in the foot and leg. The transverse rotation being produced by the hypermobile foot, still in pronation late in stance, is absorbed at the knee joint and can create lateral hip pain through an anterior tilt of the pelvis or strain the invertor muscles (21).

A plantarflexed first ray can also produce excessive pronation (37). The first ray is usually plantarflexed by the pull of the peroneus longus muscle and is commonly seen in both rear foot and forefoot varus alignments. This alignment causes the medial side of the foot to load prematurely, with greater than normal loads limiting forefoot inversion and creating supination in midstance. However, sudden pronation is generated at heel-off, developing high shear forces across the forefoot, especially at the first and fifth metatarsals (37).

Hypermobility of the first ray is generated because the peroneus longus muscle cannot stabilize the first metatarsal. During pronation, the medial side is hypermobile, placing a large load and shear force on the second metatarsal. This is a common etiology for stress fracture of the second metatarsal and subluxation of the first metatarsophalangeal joint (1,10).

Although it is not common, a person may have a forefoot valgus alignment. This may be caused by a bony deformity in which the plantar surface of the metatarsals evert relative to the calcaneus with the subtalar joint in the neutral position (10). Forefoot valgus causes the forefoot to be prematurely loaded in gait, creating supination at the subtalar joint. This alignment is typically seen in the high-arched foot.

Foot type, as mentioned previously, can also affect the amount of pronation or supination. In the normal foot with a subtalar axis of 42 to 45°, the internal rotation of the leg is equal to the internal rotation of the foot (39). In a high-arched foot, the axis of the subtalar joint is more vertical and is greater than 45°, so that for any given internal rotation of the leg, there is less internal rotation of the foot, creating less pronation for any given leg rotation.

In the flat foot, the subtalar joint axis is less than 45°, that is, closer to the horizontal. This has the opposite effect to an axis that is greater than 45°. Thus, for any given internal rotation of the leg, there will be greater internal rotation of the foot, creating greater pronation (39).

A final alignment consideration is the equine foot, in which the Achilles tendon is short, creating a significant limitation of dorsiflexion in gait. The **equinus** deviation can be reproduced with a tight and inflexible gastrocnemius and soleus. Since the tibia is unable to move forward on the talus in midsupport, the talus moves anteriorly and pronates excessively to compensate (21). An early heel rise and toe walking are symptoms of this disorder.

MUSCLE ACTIONS

There are 23 muscles acting on the ankle and the foot, 12 originating outside the foot and 11 inside the foot. All of the 12 extrinsic muscles, except for the gastrocnemius, soleus, and plantaris, act across both the subtalar and midtarsal joints (26). The insertion, actions, and nerve supply of all of these muscles are presented in Appendix B.

The muscles of the foot play an important role in sustaining impacts of very high magnitude. They also generate and absorb energy during movement. The ligaments and tendons of the muscles store some of the energy for later return. For example, the Achilles tendon can store 37 joules (J) of elastic energy, and the ligaments of the arch can store 17 J as the foot absorbs the forces and body weight (84).

Plantarflexion is used to propel the body forward and upward, contributing significantly to the other propelling forces generated in heel-off and toe-off. Plantar flexor muscles are also used eccentrically to slow down a rapidly dorsiflexing foot or to assist in the control of the forward movement of the body, specifically the forward rotation of the tibia over the foot.

Plantarflexion is a powerful action created by muscles that insert posterior to the transverse axis running through the ankle joint. The majority of the plantarflexion force is produced by the gastrocnemius and the soleus, which together are referred to as the triceps surae muscle group. Since the gastrocnemius also crosses the knee joint and can act as a knee flexor, it is more effective as a plantar flexor with the knee extended and the quadriceps femoris activated.

In the sprint racing start, the gastrocnemius is maximally activated with the knee extended and the foot placed in full dorsiflexion. The soleus, termed the workhorse of plantarflexion, is flatter than the gastrocnemius (20). It is also the predominant plantar flexor during a standing posture. A tight soleus can create a functional short leg, often seen in the left leg of people who drive a car a great deal. As explained in an earlier section, an inflexible or tight soleus limits dorsiflexion and facilitates compensatory pronation that creates the functionally shorter limb.

The action of these plantar flexor muscles is mediated through a stiff subtalar joint, allowing for an efficient transfer of the muscular force. The gastrocnemius and possibly the soleus have also been shown to produce supination when the forefoot is on the floor during the later stages of the stance phase of gait. Plantarflexion is usually accompanied by both supination and adduction.

The other plantar flexor muscles produce only 7% of the remaining plantar flexor force (20). Of these, the peroneus longus and the peroneus brevis are the most significant, with minimal plantar flexor contribution from the plantaris, the flexor hallucis longus, the flexor digitorum longus, and the tibialis posterior. The plantaris is an interesting muscle, similar to the palmaris longus in the hand, in that it is absent in some individuals, very small in others, and well developed in yet others. Overall, its contribution is usually insignificant.

Dorsiflexion at the ankle is actively used in the swing phase of gait to help the foot clear the ground and in the stance phase of gait to control lowering of the foot to the floor after heel strike. Dorsiflexion is also present in the middle part of the stance phase as the body lowers and the tibia travels over the foot, but this action is controlled eccentrically by the plantar flexor muscles (24). The dorsiflexor muscles are those that insert anterior to the transverse axis running through the ankle (26) (see Appendix B).

The most medial dorsiflexor is the tibialis anterior, whose tendon is farthest from the joint, thus giving it a significant mechanical advantage and making it the most powerful dorsiflexor (20). The tibialis anterior has a long tendon that begins halfway down the leg. Assisting the tibialis anterior in dorsiflexion are the extensor digitorum longus and the extensor hallucis longus. These muscles pull the toes up in extension. The peroneus tertius also contributes minimally to the dorsiflexion force.

Pronation is created primarily by the peroneal muscle group. These muscles lie lateral to the long axis of the tibia. They are known as pronators in the non–weight-bearing position because they evert the calcaneus and abduct the **forefoot**. The peroneus longus is an everter and abductor that is also responsible for controlling the pressure on the first metatarsal and some of the finer movements of the first metatarsal and big toe, or hallux.

The lack of stabilization of the first metatarsal by the peroneus longus leads to hypermobility of the medial side of the foot. The peroneus brevis also contributes through the production of eversion and abduction, while the peroneus tertius contributes through dorsiflexion and eversion. Both the peroneus tertius and peroneus brevis stabilize the lateral aspect of the foot. Pronation in the weight-bearing position is primarily generated by weight bearing on the lateral side of the foot in heel strike. This drives the talus medially, producing pronation. Figure 6-44 shows how pronation is produced through weight bearing.

The supinators of the foot are the muscles lying medial to the long axis of the tibia. These muscles generate inversion of the calcaneus and adduction of the forefoot (20). Inversion is created primarily by the tibialis anterior and the tibialis posterior, with assistance from the toe flexors, the flexor digitorum longus, and the flexor hallucis longus. The extensor hallucis longus works with the flexor hallucis longus to adduct the forefoot during supination.

The intrinsic muscles of the foot work as a group and are very active in the support phase of stance. They basically follow supination and are more active in the later

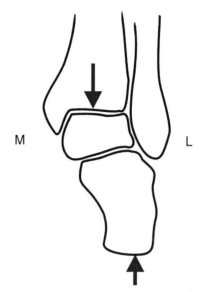

FIGURE 6-44 When the heel strikes the ground on the lateral aspect, a vertical force is directed on the outside of the foot. The force of body weight is acting down through the ankle joint. Since these two forces do not line up, the talus is driven medially, producing the pronation movement.

portions of stance to stabilize the foot in propulsion (39). In a foot that excessively pronates, they are also more active as they work to stabilize the midtarsal and subtalar joints. There are 11 intrinsic muscles, and 10 of these are on the plantar surface arranged in four layers. Appendix B has a full listing of these muscles.

STRENGTH AND FORCES OF THE ANKLE AND FOOT

The strongest movement at the ankle or foot is plantarflexion. This is because of the larger muscle mass contributing to the movement. However, it is also related to the fact that the plantar flexors are used more to work against gravity and maintain an upright posture, control lowering to the ground, and add to propulsion. Even standing, the plantar flexors, specifically the soleus, contract to control dorsiflexion in the standing posture.

Plantarflexion strength is greatest from a position of slight dorsiflexion. A starting dorsiflexion angle of 105° will increase plantarflexion strength by 16% from the neutral 90° position. Plantarflexion strength measured from 75 and 60° of plantarflexion is reduced by 27 and 42%, respectively, compared to strength measured in the neutral position (91). Additionally, plantarflexion strength can be increased if the knee is maintained in an extended position, placing the gastrocnemius at a more advantageous muscle length.

Dorsiflexion is incapable of generating a large force because of its reduced muscle mass and because it is minimally used in daily activities. The strength of the dorsiflexor muscles is only about one-fourth that of the plantar flexor muscles (91). Dorsiflexion strength can be enhanced by placing the foot in a few degrees of plantarflexion before initiating dorsiflexion.

The ankle and foot are subjected to significant compressive and shear forces in both walking and running. In walking, a vertical force 0.8 to 1.1 times body weight comes at heel strike. The magnitude of this force drops to about 0.8 times body weight in the midstance to 1.3 times body weight at toe-off (17,82). This force, along with the contraction force of the plantar flexors, creates a compression force in the ankle.

In walking, the compression force in the ankle joint can be as high as 3 times body weight at heel strike and 5 times body weight at toe-off. A shear force of 0.45 to 0.8 times body weight is also present, primarily as a result of the shear forces absorbed from the ground and the position of the foot relative to the body (12,17). In running, the peak ankle joint forces are predicted to range from 9 to 13.3 times body weight. The peak Achilles tendon force can be in the range of 5.3 to 10 times body weight (12). The ankle joint is subjected to forces similar to those in the hip and knee joints. Amazingly, the ankle joint has very little incidence of osteoarthritis. This may be due in part to the large weight-bearing surface in the ankle, which lowers the pressure on the joint.

The subtalar joint is subjected to forces equivalent to 2.4 times body weight, with the anterior articulation between the talus, calcaneus, and navicular recording forces as high as 2.8 times body weight (17,82). Large loads on the talus must be expected, since it is the keystone of the foot. Loads travel into the foot from the talus to the calcaneus and then forward to the navicular and cuneiforms.

During locomotion, forces applied to the foot from the ground are usually applied to the lateral aspect of the heel, travel laterally to the cuboid, and then transfer to the second metatarsal and the hallux at toe-off. In Figure 6-45, the path of the forces across the plantar surface of the foot is shown. The greatest percentage of support time is spent in contact with the forefoot and the first and second metatarsal. If the contact time of the second metatarsal is longer than that of the first metatarsal, a condition known as **Morton's toe** develops and the pressure on the head of the second metatarsal is greatly increased (82). This pattern of foot strike and transfer of the forces across the foot depends on a variety of factors and can vary with speed, foot type, and the foot contact patterns of individuals.

Forces in running are two times greater than those seen in walking. At foot strike, the forces received from the ground create a vertical force of 2.2 times body weight and 0.5 times body weight shear force. A vertical force of 2.8 times body weight and a shear force of 0.5 times body weight are produced at toe-off (17,82). With the addition of the muscular forces, the compressive forces can be as high as 8 to 13 times body weight in running. The anterior shear forces can be in the range of 3.3 to 5.5 times body weight, the medial shear force in the range of 0.8 times body weight, and lateral shear force in the range of 0.5 times body weight (17). Forces are large because the foot must transmit them between the body and the foot as well

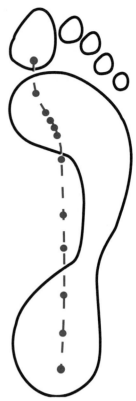

FIGURE 6-45 Forces applied to the plantar surface of the foot during gait normally travel a path from the lateral heel to the cuboid and across to the first and second metatarsal.

as the ground and the body. Given the injury record for the ankle and the foot, the foot is resilient and adaptable to the forces it must control with each step in walking or running.

CONDITIONING

The plantar flexor muscles are exercised to a great extent in daily living activities, being used to walk, get out of chairs, go up stairs or even drive the car. Strengthening the plantar flexors by using resistive exercises is also relatively easy. Any heel-raising exercise offers a significant amount of resistance because body weight is lifted by this muscle group. With the weight centered over the foot, the leverage of the plantar flexors is very efficient for handling large loads; thus, a heel-raise activity with weight on the shoulders can usually be done with a considerable amount of weight. This exercise is perfect for the gastrocnemius, since the strength of this muscle is enhanced with the knee extended and the quadriceps femoris contracting.

To specifically strengthen the soleus, a seated position is best. This position flexes the knee and reduces the contribution of the gastrocnemius significantly. Weight or resistance can be placed on the thigh as plantarflexion is produced.

It is important to maintain flexibility in the plantar flexors because any inflexibility in this muscle group can create an early heel raise and excessive pronation in gait. Inflexibility in the plantar flexors is common in women who wear high heels much of the time (42). In fact, both men and women are susceptible to strain in the plantar flexors when going from a higher heel to a lower heel in either exercise or activities of daily living. It is better to maintain the flexibility in the muscle group through stretching with the knee extended and the ankle in maximum dorsiflexion.

Flexibility in the gastrocnemius and the soleus can be somewhat isolated. Flexibility of the gastrocnemius can

best be tested with the knee extended, while flexibility of the soleus is best tested with the knees flexed to 35°. Both stretching and strengthening exercises for the plantar flexors are shown in Figure 6-46.

The strength of the dorsiflexors is limited, but it should be maintained so that fatigue does not set in during a long walk or run. Fatigue in the muscle group would lead to foot drop in swing and slapping of the foot on the surface following

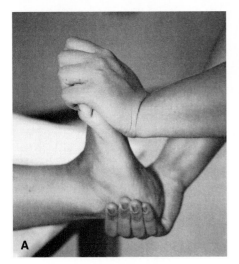

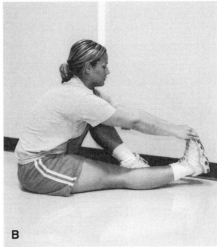

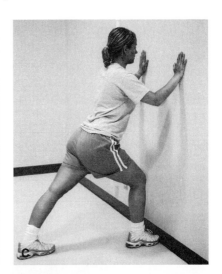

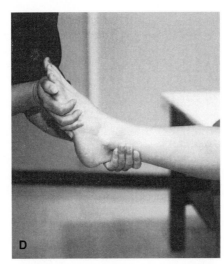

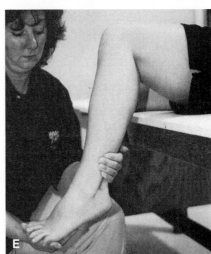

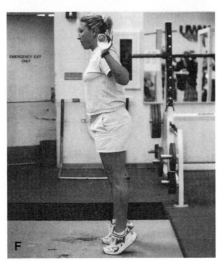

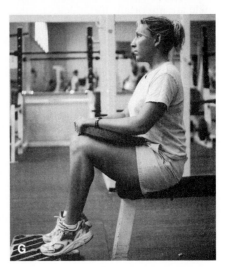

FIGURE 6-46 The plantar flexors are easy both to stretch and to strengthen. Flexibility exercises include a passive stretch into dorsiflexion **(A)**, a stretch on the plantar flexors from a straight leg position **(B)**, and a wall stretch **(C)**. Manual resistance can be applied across the toes with the knee extended **(D)** or flexed **(E)**, isolating the gastrocnemius and soleus, respectively. The plantar flexors can be strengthened in weight training with a heel-raise lift **(F)**. To isolate the soleus more, a seated heel raise exercise with weights on the thigh is used **(G)**.

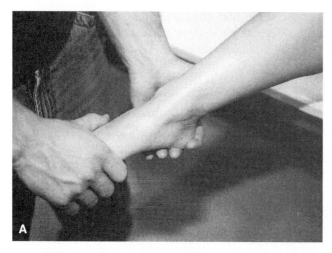

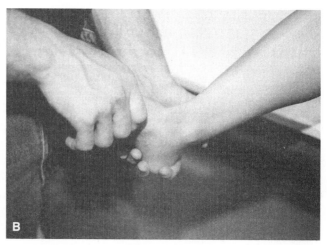

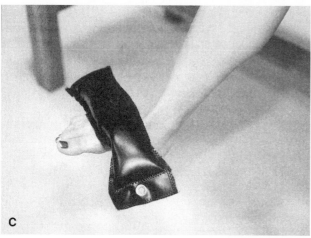

FIGURE 6-47 To stretch the dorsiflexors, the foot is moved slowly into maximum plantar flexion **(A)**. From the same position, manual resistance is applied to the top of the foot as the foot is pulled into dorsiflexion **(B)**. Weight-training exercises for the dorsiflexors is limited, but weight can be added by sandbag weights or cables as the foot is dorsiflexed **(C)**.

heel strike. To strengthen the muscle group, a seated position works best so that resistance can be applied below the foot with sandbags, weights, or surgical tubing (Fig. 6-47). There are also ankle machines allowing a full range of dorsiflexion and high-resistance training of this movement. Flexibility of dorsiflexion can also be best achieved in the seated position through maximum plantarflexion activities.

Strength and flexibility of the inverters and everters of the ankle are important for athletes participating in activities in which ankle injuries are common. This includes basketball, volleyball, football, soccer, tennis, and a wide variety of other activities. Stretching and strengthening the inversion and eversion muscles can be done with the foot flat on the floor on a towel or attached to surgical tubing. Weight can be put on the towel, which can then be pulled toward the foot in either inversion or eversion depending on which side of the weights the foot is placed. Circumduction and figure-eight tracing are good flexibility exercises. Figure 6-48 demonstrates some exercises for the muscles creating inversion, eversion, abduction, and adduction of the foot. These exercises should be a part of a sports conditioning program to add a preventative measure for ankle sprains. These exercises may be intensified and expanded for individuals with chronic ankle problems.

The intrinsic muscles of the foot are usually atrophied and weak because we regularly wear shoes. Since the intrinsic muscles support the arch of the foot and stabilize the foot during the propulsive phase of gait, it is worthwhile to give them some conditioning. The best way to exercise the intrinsic muscle group as a whole would be to forego shoes and go barefoot. The movement potential of the foot is best illustrated by individuals who have upper extremity disabilities and must use their feet to perform daily functions. These individuals can become very versatile and adept at using the foot to perform a wide range of functions.

During walking or running, impact is the same either with shoes or barefoot; it is the manner in which the forces are absorbed that is different between the two. With a shoe, the foot is more rigid during the shock absorption phase of support and depends on the shoe for support and protection. During shock absorption in barefoot gait, the foot is more mobile, with more arch deflection upon loading (81). This does not necessarily mean that shoes should not be worn, since the injury rate in barefoot running would be initially high because of the significant change imposed by removing the shoes. There is also a danger associated with barefoot activity and the possibility of injury from sharp

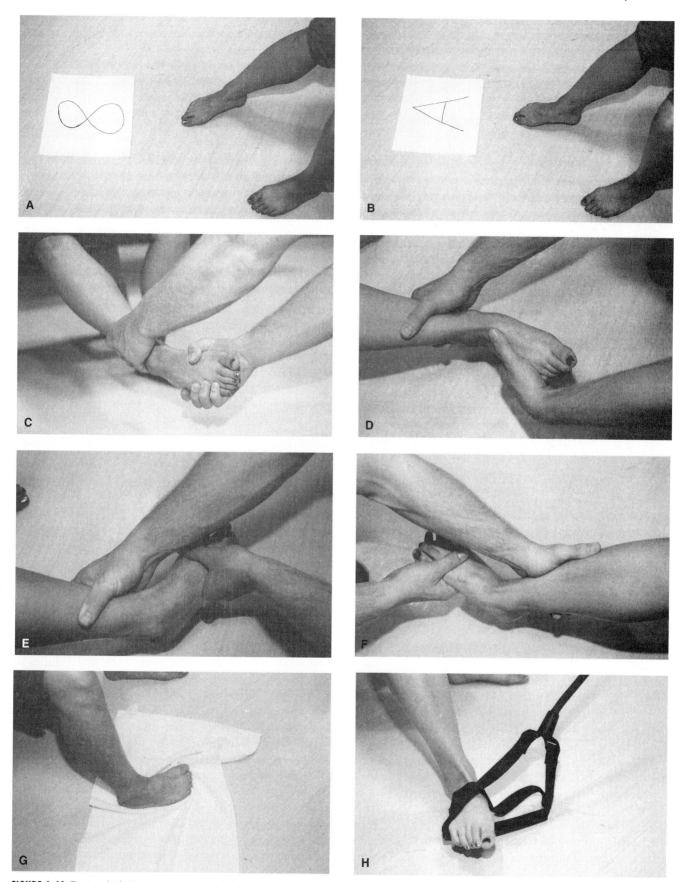

FIGURE 6-48 To stretch the inverters, everters, abductors, and adductors, simple exercises such as drawing a figure eight **(A)** or letters of the alphabet **(B)** are beneficial. Exercises using manual resistance include applying resistance to the inside or outside of the foot **(C)** during inversion or **(D)** eversion. Foot adduction and abduction can also be resisted by applying force on the outside **(E)** or inside **(F)** respectively. Higher-resistance exercises include placing weights on a towel as it is pulled toward or away **(G)** and using surgical tubing or cables **(H)**.

objects. However, going barefoot in the summer is one way of improving the condition of the intrinsic muscles.

A point attesting to the benefits of barefoot activity is the low injury rate in populations that remain largely barefoot. The incidence of injury to barefoot runners is much less than among the shod population (81). Finally, the intrinsic musculature in a person with a flat mobile foot will be much more developed than in a person with a high-arched, rigid foot because of the difference in movement characteristics in loading of the foot.

CONTRIBUTION TO SPORT SKILLS OR MOVEMENTS

Locomotion

The ankle and foot muscles are active in walking, as they control the foot on the ground and generate a significant portion of the propulsive force. Figure 6-16 provides a summary of the muscles contributing to walking.

At heel strike in walking, there is maximum activity in the dorsiflexor muscles during the attempt to eccentrically control the lowering of the foot to the ground in plantarflexion. The most muscle activity is seen in the tibialis anterior, extensor digitorum longus, and extensor hallucis longus (88). The activity in this muscle group drops but maintains activity throughout the total stance phase.

There is little activity in the gastrocnemius and soleus at heel strike. They begin to activate after foot flat and continue into the propulsive phase as they control the movement of the tibia over the foot and generate propelling forces. The intrinsic muscles of the foot are inactive in this portion of stance.

In the propelling portion of support, the dorsiflexor muscles are still active, generating a second peak in the stance phase right before toe-off. The gastrocnemius and soleus reach a peak of muscular activity just prior to toe-off. The intrinsic muscles of the foot are active in the propelling phase of stance as they work to make the foot rigid and stable and control depression of the arch. Activity in the gastrocnemius, soleus, and intrinsic muscles ceases at toe-off.

During the swing phase, the dorsiflexor muscles generate the only significant muscular activity in the ankle and foot. They hold the foot in a dorsiflexed position so that the foot clears the ground while the limb is swinging through.

In running, the plantar flexor muscles become much more active than in walking, even though the amount of plantarflexion range of motion is diminished. Plantar flexor activity increases sharply after heel strike and dominates through the total stance period (56) (Fig. 6-17). In the braking portion of stance, the plantar flexor muscles work not at the ankle but to eccentrically halt the vertical descent of the body over the foot. This continues into the propelling portion of support, when the plantar flexors shift to a concentric contraction, adding to the driving force of the run (56).

Stair Ascent and Descent

In stair climbing, the ankle musculature does contribute to the action, even though the quadriceps femoris is the main muscle group. During the pull-up phase of ascent, the leg moves posteriorly via plantarflexion at the ankle to increase the vertical position (Fig. 6-19). The primary ankle muscle producing this motion is the soleus, with some contribution from the gastrocnemius. The greatest ankle power is generated in the forward continuance phase of ascent as the individual continues on to the next step. At this point, the ankle pushes off, with the plantar flexors active as the body is pushed up to the next step (58).

During descent, the plantar flexor muscles act eccentrically to absorb foot–surface contact (27,60). There is also cocontraction of the soleus and the tibialis anterior muscles early in the absorption phase to stabilize the ankle joint. As the person steps down, there is a small eccentric muscular activity in the soleus muscle as it contributes to the controlled drop and forward movement of the body.

Cycling

The ankle musculature is also a major contributor to propulsion in cycling, even though the ankle undergoes very little angular change in motion during the 360° cycle (25,41). As shown in Figure 6-20, the gastrocnemius contributes through most of the power portion of the cycle, being active from 30 to 270° in the revolution. When the activity of the gastrocnemius ceases, the tibialis anterior becomes active from 280° until slightly past top dead center, thus contributing to the lift of the pedal. Again, when the tibialis anterior activity ceases, the gastrocnemius becomes active. Unlike the knee and hip, the ankle does not cocontract.

INJURY POTENTIAL IN THE ANKLE AND FOOT

Injuries to the foot and ankle account for a large portion of the injuries to the lower extremity. In some sports or activities, such as basketball, the ankle joint is the most frequently injured part of the lower extremity. Injuries to the hindfoot usually occur as a result of vertical compression, while injuries to the midfoot occur with excessive lateral movement or range of motion in the foot (20). Injuries to the forefoot occur similarly to injuries in long bones elsewhere in the body. In this area of the foot, both compressive and tensile forces create the injury.

Most injuries to the ankle joint and the foot occur as a result of overtraining or an excessive training bout. The ankle joint is injured frequently in activities such as running, during which the foot is loaded suddenly and repeatedly (81). Foot and ankle injuries are also associated with anatomical factors; a greater incidence of injury is seen in individuals who overpronate and in those with cavus alignment in the lower extremity.

One of the most common injuries to the foot is ankle sprain. Sprains most commonly occur in the lateral complex

by the quadriceps tendon and the patellar ligament. The patella fits into the trochlear groove of the femur, which also offers stabilization to the patella.

An important alignment feature at the knee joint is the Q-angle, the angle representing the position of the patella with respect to the femur. An increase in this angle will increase the valgus stress on the knee joint. High Q-angles are most common in females because of their wider pelvic girdles.

Flexion at the knee joint occurs through approximately 120 to 145° and is produced by the hamstrings, the biceps femoris, the semimembranosus, and the semitendinosus. Accompanying flexion is internal rotation of the tibia, which is produced by the sartorius, popliteus, gracilis, semimembranosus, and semitendinosus. As the knee joint flexes and internally rotates, the patella also moves down in the groove and then moves laterally.

Extension at the knee joint is produced by the powerful quadriceps femoris muscle group, which includes the vastus lateralis, vastus medialis, rectus femoris, and vastus intermedius. When the knee extends, the tibia externally rotates via action by the biceps femoris. At the end of extension, the knee joint locks into the terminal position by a screw home movement in which the condyles rotate into their final positions. In extension, the patella moves up in the groove and terminates in a resting position that is high and lateral on the femur.

The strength of the muscles around the knee joint is substantial, with the extensors being one of the strongest muscle groups in the body. The extensors are stronger than the flexors in all joint positions but not necessarily at all joint speeds. The flexors should not be significantly weaker than the extensors, or the injury potential around the joint will increase.

The knee joint can handle high loads and commonly absorbs 1 to 5 times body weight in activities such as walking, running, and weight lifting. A maximum flexion position should be evaluated for safety, given the high shear forces that are present in the position. Patellofemoral forces can also be high, in the range of 0.5 to 8 times body weight, in daily living activities. The patellofemoral force is high in positions of maximum knee flexion.

Conditioning of the knee extensors is an easy task, since these muscles control simple lowering and rising movements. Closed-chain exercises are also very beneficial for the extensors because of their relation to daily living activities. The flexors are also exercised during a squat movement because of their action at the hip joint but can best be isolated and exercised in a seated position.

The knee joint muscles contribute significantly to a wide variety of movements and sport activities. The quadriceps femoris serves as a shock absorption mechanism and a power producer for walking, running, and stair climbing. In cycling, the quadriceps femoris is responsible for a significant amount of power production.

The knee is the most frequently injured joint in the body. Traumatic injuries damage the ligaments or menisci,

and numerous chronic injuries result in tendinitis, iliotibial band syndrome, and general knee pain. Muscle strains to the quadriceps femoris and hamstrings are also common. The patella is a site for injuries such as subluxation and dislocation and other patellar pain syndromes, such as chondromalacia patella.

The foot and ankle consist of 26 bones articulating at 30 synovial joints, supported by more than 100 ligaments and 30 muscles. The ankle, or talocrural joint, has two main articulations, the tibiotalar and tibiofibular joints. The tibia and fibula form a mortise over the talus defined on the medial and lateral sides by the malleoli. Both sides of the joint are strongly reinforced by ligaments, making the ankle very stable.

The foot moves at the tibiotalar joint in two directions, plantarflexion and dorsiflexion. Plantarflexion can occur through a range of motion of approximately 50° and is produced by the gastrocnemius and soleus with some assistance from the peroneal muscles and the toe flexors. Dorsiflexion range of motion is approximately 20°, and the movement is created by the tibialis anterior and the toe extensors.

Another important joint in the foot is the subtalar or talocalcaneal joint, in which pronation and supination occur. It is at this joint that the rotation of the lower extremity and forces of impact are absorbed. Pronation at the subtalar articulation is a triplane movement consisting of calcaneal eversion, abduction, and dorsiflexion with the foot off the ground and calcaneal eversion, talar adduction, and plantarflexion with the foot on the ground in a closed chain. Muscles responsible for creating eversion are the peroneals, consisting of the peroneus longus, peroneus brevis, and peroneus tertius. Supination, the reverse movement, is created in the open chain through calcaneal inversion, talar adduction, and plantarflexion and in the closed chain through calcaneal inversion, talar abduction, and dorsiflexion. Muscles responsible for producing inversion are the tibialis anterior, tibialis posterior, and hallux flexors and extensors. The range of motion for pronation and supination is 20 to 62°.

The midtarsal joint also contributes to pronation and supination of the foot. These two joints, the calcaneocuboid and the talonavicular, allow the foot great mobility if the axes of the two joints lie parallel to each other. This is beneficial in the early portion of support, when the body is absorbing forces of contact. When these axes are not parallel, the foot becomes rigid. This is beneficial in the later portion of support, when the foot is propelling the body up and forward. Numerous other articulations in the foot, such as the intertarsal, tarsometatarsal, metatarsophalangeal, and interphalangeal joints, influence both total foot and toe motion.

The foot has two longitudinal arches that provide both shock absorption and support. The medial arch is higher and more dynamic than the lateral arch. The longitudinal arches are supported by the plantar fascia running along the plantar surface of the foot. Transverse arches running across the foot depress and spread in weight bearing. The shape of the arches and the bony arrangement determine foot type, which can be normal, flat, or high arched and flexible or rigid. An extremely flat foot is termed pes planus and a high-arched foot is called pes cavus. Other foot alignments include forefoot and rear foot varus and valgus, a plantarflexed first ray, and equinus positions that influence function of the foot.

Plantarflexion of the foot is a very strong joint action and is a major contributor to the development of a propulsion force. Dorsiflexion is weak and not capable of generating high muscle forces. The foot and ankle can handle high loads, and the forces in the ankle joint range from 0.5 to 13 times body weight in walking and running. The subtalar joint also handles forces in the magnitude of 2 to 3 times body weight.

The muscles of the foot and ankle receive a considerable amount of conditioning in daily living activities such as walking. Specific muscles can be isolated through exercises. For example, the gastrocnemius can be strengthened in a standing heel raise and the soleus in a seated heel raise. The intrinsic muscles of the foot can be exercised by drawing the alphabet or drawing figure-eights with the foot or by just going barefoot.

The foot and ankle muscles contribute to a variety of activities, generally serving as a major source of propulsion. Thus, the gastrocnemius and soleus are important contributors to walking, running, stair climbing, and cycling.

The foot and ankle are frequently injured in sports and physical activity. Common injuries are ankle sprains; Achilles tendinitis; posterior, lateral, or medial tibial syndrome; plantar fasciitis; bursitis; metatarsalgia; and stress fractures.

REVIEW QUESTIONS

True or False

1. ____ Because of the extreme mobility of the hip joint, each of the lower limbs effectively has complete independence of the other.

2. ____ Because of the stresses of childbirth, the female pelvis is wider and heavier than the male pelvis.

3. ____ Mobility in the female sacroiliac joint fluctuates with hormonal cycles.

4. ____ The sacrum is three fused vertebrae.

5. ____ All of the pelvic bones join at the acetabulum.

6. ____ The cartilage on the underside of the acetabulum is some of the thickest in the body.

7. ____ Coxa valga will increase leg length and decrease the effectiveness of the abductors.

8. ____ Contribution from the rectus femoris as a hip flexor depends on knee position.

9. ____ Impairment of gluteus maximus function will result in significant loss of thigh extension strength.

10. ____ During running, forces in the hip joint are highest at midsupport.

11. ____ The knee is a hinge joint with 1 degree of freedom.

12. ____ Leg rotation accompanies knee flexion primarily because of the actions of the semitendinosus and semimembranosus muscles.

13. ____ The medial collateral ligament supports the knee against valgus forces.

14. ____ The lateral collateral ligament is not affected by rotation at the knee joint.

15. ____ The fibula primarily controls tensile forces.

16. ____ The axis of rotation of the ankle joint is in line with the body and at a right angle to the tibia.

17. ____ The cuboid is also known as the keystone of the foot.

18. ____ The primary function of the subtalar joint is to limit tibial rotation.

19. ____ Movement at the subtalar joint can facilitate unlocking of the knee.

20. ____ Three of the twelve extrinsic ankle and foot muscles act across the subtalar and midtarsal joints.

21. ____ The tibialis anterior is termed the workhorse of plantarflexion.

22. ____ If the plantar fascia are short, the rigidity is likely to be low.

23. ____ Pronation is said to be excessive when the rear foot angle is greater than 14°.

24. ____ Stress fractures are generally traumatic injuries.

25. ____ A vigorous contraction of the posterior tibialis is one cause of Achilles tendon rupture.

Multiple Choice

1. The pelvic girdle serves as a site of muscular attachment for ____ trunk and thigh muscles.
   a. 10
   b. 18
   c. 24
   d. 28

2. ____ of the 28 muscles that attach to the pelvic girdle act independently.
   a. Two
   b. Three
   c. Seven
   d. None of the above

3. The pubic symphysis is a ____ joint.
   a. Synovial
   b. Cartilaginous
   c. Epiphysial
   d. A and c

4. ____ ligaments maintain the relationship between the sacrum and the ilium.
   a. Six
   b. Eight
   c. Ten
   d. None of the above

5. ___ of 10 males have fused sacroiliac joints.
   a. Two
   b. Three
   c. Four
   d. Five

6. When the base (the widest part) of the sacrum moves ___, it is termed sacral flexion.
   a. Anteriorly
   b. Posteriorly
   c. Laterally
   d. A or b

7. Anterior pelvic tilt accompanies ___.
   a. Trunk flexion or thigh extension
   b. Trunk flexion or thigh flexion
   c. Trunk extension or thigh extension
   d. Trunk extension or thigh flexion

8. The capsule surrounding the hip joint is more dense on the ___ and ___ where the stresses are greatest.
   a. Front, top
   b. Front, bottom
   c. Front, back
   d. Top, bottom

9. The angle of inclination of the neck of the femur is approximately ___.
   a. 110°
   b. 125°
   c. 140°
   d. None of the above

10. Coxa varus will ___ the leg and ___ the effectiveness of the abductors.
   a. Shorten, increase
   b. Shorten, decrease
   c. Lengthen, increase
   d. Lengthen, decrease

11. Anteversion in excess of 14° will cause a person to ___ while walking.
   a. Toe in
   b. Toe out
   c. Supinate
   d. B and c

12. The tensor fascia latae is put on stretch in a position of knee ___.
   a. Flexion
   b. Extension
   c. External rotation
   d. The tensor fascia latae does not cross the knee

13. The sartorius is a ___ joint muscle, and it crosses the knee on the ___ side.
   a. 1, lateral
   b. 1, medial
   c. 2, lateral
   d. 2, medial

14. Tight hamstrings can create ___ pelvic tilt that can result in postural problems.
   a. Anterior
   b. Posterior
   c. Lateral
   d. None of the above

15. The gluteus maximus ___ rotates and ___ the thigh.
   a. Internally, extends
   b. Internally, flexes
   c. Externally, extends
   d. Externally, flexes

16. When a person stands on one limb, the force imposed on the hip joint increases to ___ times body weight.
   a. 1–1.5
   b. 1.5–2
   c. 2–2.5
   d. 2.5–3

17. In running, forces in the hip joint can be as high as ___ times body weight.
   a. 3
   b. 5
   c. 10
   d. 15

18. Excessive or insufficient arm counterrotation during gait can result in stress on the muscular attachments on the ___.
   a. Iliac crest
   b. Pubic symphysis
   c. Lumbar vertebrae
   d. Greater trochanter

19. The ___ joint is commonly referred to as the actual knee joint.
   a. Tibiofibular
   b. Tibiofemoral
   c. Patellofemoral
   d. All of the above

20. A plica is ___.
   a. A fat pad
   b. A tear in the meniscus
   c. A type of bursa
   d. None of the above

21. Males typically have Q-angles ranging from ___, while those of females average from ___.
   a. 3–6°, 10–12°
   b. 10–14°, 3–6°
   c. 10–14°, 15–17°
   d. 15–17°, 20–23°

22. Loss of the anterior cruciate ligament of the knee creates ___.
   a. Valgus laxity
   b. Rotary instability
   c. Single-plane instability
   d. Any of the above

23. The close-packed position for the ankle is the ___ position.
   a. Plantarflexed
   b. Dorsiflexed
   c. Inverted
   d. Everted

24. In terms of the ankle joint, leaning backward is described as ___.
   a. Pronation
   b. Supination
   c. Dorsiflexion
   d. Plantarflexion

25. The ___ plane movements at the subtalar joint are termed pronation and supination.
- a. Uni
- b. Bi
- c. Tri
- d. Pronation and supination do not occur at the subtalar joint

REFERENCES

1. Adelaar, R. (1986). The practical biomechanics of running. *American Journal of Sports Medicine,* 14:497–500.
2. Apkarian, J., et al. (1989). Three-dimensional kinematic and dynamic model of the lower limb. *Journal of Biomechanics,* 22:143–155.
3. Areblad, M., et al. (1990). Three-dimensional measurement of rear foot motion during running. *Journal of Biomechanics,* 23:933–940.
4. Bates, B. (1983). Foot function in running: Researcher to coach. In J. Terauds (Ed.). *Biomechanics in Sports.* Del Mar, CA: Academic Publishers, 293–303.
5. Bazzoli, A., Pollina, F. (1989). Heel pain in recreational runners. *Physician and Sportsmedicine,* 17:55–56.
6. Blackburn, T. A., Craig, E. (1980). Knee anatomy: A brief review. *Physical Therapy,* 60:1556–1560.
7. Blackburn, T. A., et al. (1982). An introduction to the plica. *Journal of Orthopaedic and Sports Physical Therapy,* 3:171–177.
8. Brinkmann, J. R., Perry, J. (1985). Rate and range of knee motion during ambulation in healthy and arthritic subjects. *Physical Therapy,* 65:1055–1060.
9. Brody, D. M. (1980). Running injuries. *Clinical Symposium,* 32:2–36.
10. Brown, L. P., Yavarsky, P. (1987). Locomotor biomechanics and pathomechanics: A review. *Journal of Orthopaedic and Sports Physical Therapy,* 9:3–10.
11. Buchbinder, M. R., et al. (1979). The relationship of abnormal pronation to chondromalacia of the patella in distance runners. *Podiatric Sports Medicine,* 69:159–162.
12. Burdett, R. G. (1982). Forces predicted at the ankle during running. *Medicine and Science in Sports and Exercise,* 14:308–316.
13. Cairnes, M. A., et al. (1986). A biomechanical analysis of racewalking gait. *Medicine and Science in Sports and Exercise,* 18:446–453.
14. Cerny, K., et al. (1990). Effect of an unrestricted knee-ankle-foot orthosis on the stance phase gait in healthy persons. *Orthopedics,* 13:1121–1127.
15. Chesworth, B. M., et al. (1989). Validation of outcome measures in patients with patellofemoral syndrome. *Journal of Sports Physical Therapy,* 10(8):302–308.
16. Clark, T. E., et al. (1983). The effects of shoe design parameters on rearfoot control in running. *Medicine and Science in Sports and Exercise,* 5:376–381.
17. Czerniecki, J. M. (1988). Foot and ankle biomechanics in walking and running. *American Journal of Physical Medicine and Rehabilitation,* 67:246–252.
18. Davies, G. J., et al. (1980). Knee examination. *Physical Therapy,* 60:1565–1574.
19. Davies, G. J., et al. (1980). Mechanism of selected knee injuries. *Physical Therapy,* 60:1590–1595.
20. DiStefano, V. (1981). Anatomy and biomechanics of the ankle and foot. *Athletic Training,* 16:43–47.
21. Donatelli, R. (1987). Abnormal biomechanics of the foot and ankle. *Journal of Orthopaedic and Sports Physical Therapy,* 9:11–15.
22. DonTigny, R. L. (1985). Function and pathomechanics of the sacroiliac joint: A review. *Physical Therapy,* 65:35–43.
23. Drez, D. Jr., et al. (1982). Nonoperative treatment of double lateral ligament tears of the ankle. *American Journal of Sports Medicine,* 10:197–200.
24. Engsberg, J. R., Andrews, J. G. (1987). Kinematic analysis of the talocalcaneal/talocrural joint during running support. *Medicine and Science in Sports and Exercise,* 19:275–284.
25. Erickson, M. O., et al. (1986). Power output and work in different muscle groups during ergometer cycling. *European Journal of Applied Physiology,* 55:229–235.
26. Fiore, R. D., Leard, J. S. (1980). A functional approach in the rehabilitation of the ankle and rearfoot. *Athletic Training,* 15:231–235.
27. Freedman, W., et al. (1976). EMG patterns and forces developed during step-down. *American Journal of Physical Medicine,* 55:275–290.
28. Fukubayashi, T., Kurosawa,H. (1980). The contact area and pressure distribution pattern of the knee: A study of normal and osteoarthritic knee joints. *Acta Orthopaedica Scandinavica,* 51:871–879.
29. Gehlsen, G. M ., et al. (1989). Knee kinematics: The effects of running on cambers. *Medicine and Science in Sports and Exercise,* 21:463–466.
30. Godges, J. J., et al. (1989). The effects of two stretching procedures on hip range of motion and gait economy. *Journal of Orthopaedic and Sports Physical Therapy,* 10(9):350–357.
31. Grana, W. A., Coniglione, T. C. (1985). Knee disorders in runners. *Physician and Sportsmedicine,* 13:127–133.
32. Grieve, G. P. (1976). The sacroiliac joint. *Journal of Anatomy,* 58:384–399.
33. Hamilton, J. J., Ziemer, L. K. (1981). Functional anatomy of the human ankle and foot. In R. H. Kiene, K. A. Johnson (Eds.). *Proceedings of the AAOS Symposium on the Foot and Ankle.* St. Louis: Mosby, 1–14.
34. Halbach, J. (1981). Pronated foot disorders. *Athletic Training,* 16:53–55.
35. Hodge, W. A., et al. (1987). The influence of hip arthroplasty on stair climbing and rising from a chair. In J. L. Stein (Ed.). *Biomechanics of Normal and Prosthetic Gait.* New York: American Society of Mechanical Engineers, 65–67.
36. Hole, J. W. (1990). *Human Anatomy and Physiology* (5th Ed.). Dubuque, IA: William C. Brown.
37. Hunt, G. C. (1985). Examination of lower extremity dysfunction. In J. Gould, G. J. Davies (Eds.). *Orthopaedic and Sports Physical Therapy.* St. Louis: Mosby, 408–436.
38. Hutson, M. A., Jackson, J. P. (1982). Injuries to the lateral ligament of the ankle: Assessment and treatment. *British Journal of Sports Medicine,* 4:245–249.
39. Inman, V. T. (1959). The influence of the foot-ankle complex on the proximal skeletal structures. *Artificial Limbs,* 13:59–65.
40. James, S. L., et al. (1978). Injuries to runners. *American Journal of Sports Medicine,* 6:40–50.
41. Jorge, M., Hull, M. L. (1986). Analysis of EMG measurements during bicycle pedalling. *Journal of Biomechanics,* 19:683–694.
42. Kapandji, I. A. (1970). *The Physiology of the Joints* (Vol. 2). Edinburgh: Churchill Livingstone.

43. Kettlecamp, D. H., et al. (1970). An electrogoniometric study of knee motion in normal gait. *Journal of Bone and Joint Surgery*, 52-A:775–790.

44. Kempson, G. E., et al. (1971). Patterns of cartilage stiffness on the normal and degenerative human femoral head. *Journal of Biomechanics*, 4:597–609.

45. Kosmahl, E., Kosmahl, H. (1987). Painful plantar heel, plantar fasciitis, and calcaneal spur: Etiology and treatment. *Journal of Orthopaedic and Sports Physical Therapy*, 9:17–24.

46. Lafortune, M. A., Cavanagh, P.R. (1985). Three-dimensional kinematics of the patella during walking. In B. Jonsson (Ed.). *Biomechanics X-A*. Champaign, IL: Human Kinetics, 337–341.

47. Lafortune, M. A., et al. (1992). Three-dimensional kinematics of the human knee during walking. *Journal of Biomechanics*, 25:347–357.

48. Larson, R. L. (1973). Epiphyseal injuries in the adolescent athlete. *Orthopedic Clinics of North America*, 4:839–851.

49. Laubenthal, K. N., et al. (1972). A quantitative analysis of knee motion during activities of daily living. *Physical Therapy*, 52:34–42.

50. Leib, F. J., Perry, J. (1971). Quadriceps function: An electromyographic study under isometric conditions. *Journal of Bone and Joint Surgery*, 53-A:749–758.

51. Lloyd-Smith, R., et al. (1985). A survey of overuse and traumatic hip and pelvic injuries in athletes. *Physician and Sports Medicine*, 13(10):131–141.

52. Locke, M., et al. (1984). Ankle and subtalar motion during gait in arthritic patients. *Physical Therapy*, 64:504–509.

53. Lovejoy, C. O. (1988). Evolution of human walking. *Scientific American*, 259(5):118–125.

54. Lyon, K. K., et al. (1988). Q-Angle: A factor in peak torque occurrence in isokinetic knee extension. *Journal of Orthopaedic and Sports Physical Therapy*, 9:250–253.

55. Markhede, G., Stener, G. (1981). Function after removal of various hip and thigh muscles for extirpation of tumors. *Acta Orthopaedica Scandinavica*, 52:373–395.

56. Mann, R. A., et al. (1986). Comparative electromyography of the lower extremity in jogging, running, and sprinting. *American Journal of Sports Medicine*, 14:501–510.

57. MacKinnon, C. D., Winter, D. A. (1993). Control of whole body balance in the frontal plane during human walking. *Journal of Biomechanics*, 26:633–644.

58. McFadyen, B. J., Winter, D. A. (1988). An integrated biomechanical analysis of normal stair ascent and descent. *Journal of Biomechanics*, 21:733–744.

59. McClusky, G., Blackburn, T. A. (1980). Classification of knee ligament instabilities. *Physical Therapy*, 60:1575–1577.

60. McLeod, W. D., Hunter, S. (1980). Biomechanical analysis of the knee: Primary functions as elucidated by anatomy. *Physical Therapy*, 60:1561–1564.

61. McPoil, T., Brocato, R. S. (1985). The foot and ankle: Biomechanical evaluation and treatment. In J. A. Gould, G. J. Davies (Eds.). *Orthopaedic and Sports Physical Therapy*. St. Louis: Mosby, 313–341.

62. McPoil, T., Knecht, H. (1987). Biomechanics of the foot in walking: A functional approach. *Journal of Orthopedic and Sports Physical Therapy*, 7:69–72.

63. Metzmaker, J. N., Pappas, A. M. (1985). Avulsion fractures of the pelvis. *American Journal of Sports Medicine*, 13:349–358.

64. Mital, M. A., et al. (1980). The so-called unresolved Osgood-Schlatter lesion: A concept based on fifteen surgically treated lesions. *Journal of Bone and Joint Surgery*, 62-A:732–739.

65. Murray, M. P., et al. (1964). Walking patterns of normal men. *Journal of Bone and Joint Surgery*, 46A(2):335–360.

66. Murray, S. M., et al. (1984). Torque-velocity relationships of the knee extensor and flexor muscles in individuals sustaining injuries of the anterior cruciate ligament. *American Journal of Sports Medicine*, 12:436–439.

67. Nisell, R. (1985). Mechanics of the knee: A study of joint and muscle load with clinical applications. *Acta Orthopaedica Scandinavica*, 56:1–42.

68. Nissan, M. (1979). Review of some basic assumptions in knee biomechanics. *Journal of Biomechanics*, 13:375–381.

69. Nordin, M., Frankel, V. H. (1989). Biomechanics of the Hip. In M. Nordin & V. H. Frankel (Eds.). *Basic Biomechanics of the Musculoskeletal System*. Philadelphia: Lea & Febiger, 135–152.

70. Noyes, F. R., et al. (1980). Knee ligament tests: What do they really mean? *Physical Therapy*, 60:1578–1581.

71. Noyes, F. R., Sonstegard, D. A. (1973). Biomechanical function of the pes anserinus at the knee and the effect of its transplantation. *Journal of Bone and Joint Surgery*, 35-A:1225–1240.

72. Oshimo, T. A., et al. (1983). The effect of varied hip angles on the generation of internal tibial rotary torque. *Medicine and Science in Sports and Exercise*, 15:529–534.

73. Osternig, L. R., et al. (1979). Knee rotary torque patterns in healthy subjects. In J. Terauds (Ed.). *Science in Sports*. Del Mar, CA: Academic, 37–43.

74. Osternig, L. R., et al. (1981). Relationships between tibial rotary torque and knee flexion/extension after tendon transplant surgery. *Archives of Physical and Medical Rehabilitation*, 62:381–385.

75. Perry, J. (1992). *Gait Analysis: Normal and Pathological Function*. Thorofare, NJ: Slack.

76. Polisson, R. P. (1986). Sports medicine for the internist. *Medical Clinics of North America*, 70:469–474.

77. Porterfield, J. A. (1985). The sacroiliac joint. In J. A. Gould, G. J. Davies (Eds.). *Orthopedic and Sports Physical Therapy*. St. Louis: Mosby, 550–579.

78. Radakovich, M., Malone, T. (1980). The superior tibiofibular joint: The forgotten joint. *Journal of Orthopaedic and Sports Physical Therapy*, 3:129–132.

79. Radin, E. L. (1980). Biomechanics of the human hip. *Clinical Orthopaedics*, 152:28–34.

80. Reid, D. C., et al. (1987). Lower extremity flexibility patterns in classical ballet dancers and their correlation to lateral hip and knee injuries. *American Journal of Sports Medicine*, 15(4):347–352.

81. Robbins, S. E., Hanna, A. M. (1987). Running-related injury prevention through barefoot adaptations. *Medicine and Science in Sports and Exercise*, 19:148–156.

82. Rodgers, M. (1988). Dynamic biomechanics of the normal foot and ankle during walking and running. *Physical Therapy*, 68:1822–1830.

83. Rubin, G. (1971). Tibial rotation. *Bulletin of Prosthetics Research*, 10(15):95–101.

84. Salathe, E. P. Jr., et al. (1990). The foot as a shock absorber. *Journal of Biomechanics*, 23:655–659.

85. Saudek, C. E. (1985). The hip. In J. Gould, G. J. Davies (Eds.). *Orthopaedic and Sports Physical Therapy*. St. Louis: Mosby, 365–407.

86. Scott, S. H., Winter, D. A. (1991). Talocrural and talocalcaneal joint kinematics and kinetics during the stance phase of walking. *Journal of Biomechanics*, 24:734–752.

87. Scott, S. H., Winter, D. A. (1993). Biomechanical model of the human foot: Kinematics and kinetics during the stance phase of walking. *Journal of Biomechanics*, 26:1091–1104.

88. Segal, P., Jacob, M. (1973). *The Knee*. Chicago: Year Book Medical.

89. Shaw, J. A., et al. (1973). The longitudinal axis of the knee and the role of the cruciate ligaments in controlling transverse rotation. *Journal of Bone and Joint Surgery*, 56-A:1603–1609.

90. Slocum, D. B., Larson, R. L. (1963). Pes anserinus transplantation: A surgical procedure for control of rotatory instability of the knee. *Journal of Bone and Joint Surgery*, 50-A:226–242.

91. Soderberg, G. L. (1986). *Kinesiology: Application to Pathological Motion*. Baltimore: Williams & Wilkins, 243–266.

92. Stormont, D. M., et al. (1985). Stability of the loaded ankle. Relation between articular restraint and primary and secondary static restraints. *American Journal of Sports Medicine*, 13:295–300.

93. Taunton, J. E., et al. (1985). A triplanar electrogoniometer investigation of running mechanics in runners with compensatory overpronation. *Canadian Journal of Applied Sports Science*, 10:104–115.

94. Tehranzadeh, J., et al. (1982). Combined pelvic stress fracture and avulsion of the adductor longus in a middle distance runner. *American Journal of Sports Medicine*, 10:108–111.

95. Vleeming, A., et al. (1990). Relation between form and function in the sacroiliac joint: Part I. Clinical anatomical aspects. *Spine*, 15:130–132.

96. Wallace, L. A., et al. (1985). The knee. In J. Gould, G. J. Davies (Eds.). *Orthopaedic and Sports Physical Therapy*. St. Louis: Mosby, 342–364.

97. Wang, C., et al. (1973). The effects of flexion and rotation on the length patterns of the ligaments of the knee. *Journal of Biomechanics*, 6:587–596.

98. Wright, D., et al. (1964). Action of the subtalar and ankle-joint complex during the stance phase of walking. *Journal of Bone and Joint Surgery*, 46-A:361–383.

99. Yack, H. J., et al. (1993). Comparison of closed and open kinetic chain exercise in the anterior cruciate ligament-deficient knee. *American Journal of Sports Medicine*, 21:49–53.

100. Yates, J. W., Jackson, D. W. (1984). Current status of meniscus surgery. *Physician and Sports Medicine*, 12:51–56.

ADDITIONAL READING

Alexander, M. J. L. (1989). The relationship between muscle strength and sprint kinematics in elite sprinters. *Canadian Journal of Sports Science*, 14:148–157.

Allard, P., et al. (1985). Application of steriophotogrammetry and mathematical modelling in the study of ankle kinematics. In B. Jonsson (Ed.). *Biomechanics X-B*. Champaign, IL: Human Kinetics, 1111–1115.

Andrews, J. R. (1980). Posterolateral rotatory instability of the knee: Surgery for acute and chronic problems. *Physical Therapy*, 60:1637–1639.

Andrews, J. R., et al. (1985). Surgical treatment of anterolateral rotatory instability. *American Journal of Sports Medicine*, 13:112–119.

Arno, S. A. (1990). The A-angle: A quantitative measurement of patella alignment and realignment. *Journal of Orthopaedic and Sports Physical Therapy*, 12:237–242.

Bates, B., et al. (1979). Functional variability of the lower extremity during the support phase of running. *Medicine and Science in Sports and Exercise*, 11:328–331.

Bobbert, M. F., Van Ingen Schenau, G. J. (1990). Mechanical output about the ankle joint in isokinetic plantar flexion and jumping. *Medicine and Science in Sports and Exercise*, 22:660–668.

Borzov, V. (1978). The optimal starting position in sprinting. *Legkaya Atletika*, 4:173–174.

Bose, K., et al. (1980). Vastus medialis oblique: An anatomic and physiologic study. *Orthopedics*, 3:880–883.

Brand, R. A., et al. (1982). A model of lower extremity muscular anatomy. *Transactions of the ACSM*, 104:304–310.

Briner, W. W., et al. (1989). Anteroinferior tibiofibular ligament injury: Not just another ankle sprain. *Physician and Sports Medicine*, 17:63–69.

Brooke, R. (1924). The sacroiliac joint. *Journal of Anatomy*, 58:299–305.

Cavanagh, P., Lafortune, M. (1980). Ground reaction forces in distance running. *Journal of Biomechanics*, 13:397–406.

Caylor, D., et al. (1993). The relationship between quadriceps angle and anterior knee pain syndrome. *Journal of Sports Physical Therapy*, 17:11–15.

Cibulka, M. T., et al. (1986). Hamstring muscle strain treated by mobilizing the sacroiliac joint. *Physical Therapy*, 66:1220–1224.

Clancy, W. G. (1980). Runners' injuries. Part two: Evaluation and treatment of specific injuries. *American Journal of Sports Medicine*, 8:287–289.

Clark, J. M., Jaynor, D. R. (1987). Anatomy of the abductor muscles of the hip as studied by computer tomography. *Journal of Bone and Joint Surgery*, 69-A:1021–1031.

Colville, M. R., et al. (1990). Strain measurement in lateral ankle ligaments. *American Journal of Sports Medicine*, 18:196–200.

Conteduca, F., et al. (1991). Chondromalacia and chronic anterior instabilities of the knee. *American Journal of Sports Medicine*, 9:119–123.

Coplan, J. A. (1989). Rotational motion of the knee: A comparison of normal and pronating subjects. *Journal of Orthopaedic and Sports Physical Therapy*, 10:366–369.

Crowninshield, R. D., et al. (1978). A biomechanical investigation of the human hip. *Journal of Biomechanics*, 11:75–85.

Czerniecki, J. M., et al. (1988). A biomechanical evaluation of tibiofemoral rotation in anterior cruciate deficient knees during walking and running. *American Journal of Sports Medicine*, 16:327–331.

Donatelli, R. (1985). Normal biomechanics of the foot and ankle. *Journal of Orthopaedic and Sports Physical Therapy*, 7:91–95.

DonTigny, R. L. (1990). Anterior dysfunction of the sacroiliac joint as a major factor in the etiology of low back pain syndrome. *Physical Therapy*, 70:250–262.

Dostal, W. F., Andrews, J. G. (1981). A three-dimensional biomechanical model of hip musculature. *Journal of Biomechanics*, 14:803–812.

Doxey, G. (1987). Calcaneal pain: A review of various disorders. *Journal of Orthopaedic and Sports Physical Therapy*, 9:25–32.

Ellison, J. B., et al. (1990). Patterns of hip rotation range of motion between healthy subjects and patients with low back pain. *Physical Therapy*, 70:537–541.

Falkel, J. (1978). Plantar flexor strength testing using the Cybex isokinetic dynamometer. *Physical Therapy*, 58:847–850.

Ferkel, R. D., et al. (1981). An analysis of roller skating injuries. *American Journal of Sports Medicine*, 10:24–30.

Fischer, R. L. (1972). An epidemiological study of Legg-Perthes disease. *Journal of Bone and Joint Surgery*, 54-A, 769–777.

Goodfellow, J., et al. (1976). Patellofemoral joint mechanics and pathology: 1. Functional anatomy of the patellofemoral joint. *Journal of Bone and Joint Surgery*, 58-B:287–290.

Gross, T. S., Nelson, R. C. (1988). The shock attenuation role of the ankle during landing from a vertical jump. *Medicine and Science in Sports and Exercise*, 20:506–514.

Hajak, M. R., Noble, H. B. (1982). Stress fractures of the femoral neck in joggers. *American Journal of Sports Medicine*, 10:112–116.

Hontas, M. J., et al. (1986). Conditions of the talus in the runner. *American Journal of Sports Medicine*, 14:486–490.

Houtz, S. J., Fischer, F. J. (1959). An analysis of muscle action and joint excursion during exercise on a stationary bicycle. *Journal of Bone and Joint Surgery*, 41-A:123–131.

Hughes, L. Y. (1985). Biomechanical analysis of the foot and ankle for predisposition to developing stress fractures. *Journal of Orthopaedic and Sports Physical Therapy*, 7:96–101.

Illingworth, C. M. (1978). 128 limping children with no fracture, sprain, or obvious cause. *Clinical Pediatrics*, 17:139–142.

Insall, J. (1982). Current concepts review: Patellar pain. *Journal of Bone and Joint Surgery*, 64-A:147–152.

Jones, A. L. (1982). Rehabilitation for anterior instability of the knee: Preliminary report. *Journal of Orthopaedic and Sports Physical Therapy*, 3:121–127.

Jorgensen, U. (1985). Achillodynia and loss of heel pad shock absorbency. *American Journal of Sports Medicine*, 13:128–132.

Kannus, P. (1990). Relationships between peak torque, peak angular impulse, and average power in the thigh muscles of subjects with knee damage. *Research Quarterly for Exercise and Sport*, 61:141–145.

Klampner, S. L., Wissinger, A. (1972). Anterior slipping of the capital femoral epiphysis. *Journal of Bone and Joint Surgery*, 54-A:1531–1537.

Leib, F. J., Perry, J. (1968). Quadriceps function: An anatomical and mechanical study using amputated limbs. *Journal of Bone and Joint Surgery*, 50-A:749–758.

Lentell, G. L., et al. (1990). The relationship between muscle function and ankle stability. *Journal of Orthopaedic and Sports Physical Therapy*, 11:605–611.

Mann, R., Inman, V. (1964). Phasic activity of intrinsic muscles of the foot. *Journal of Bone and Joint Surgery*, 46-A:469–481.

Mann, R., Sprague, P. (1980). A kinetic analysis of the ground leg during sprint running. *Research Quarterly for Exercise and Sport*, 51:334–348.

Marquet, P. (1979). Mechanics and osteoarthritis of the patellofemoral joint. *Clinical Orthopaedics and Related Research*, 144:70–73.

Martens, M., et al. (1980). The mechanical characteristics of the long bones of the lower extremity in torsional loading. *Journal of Biomechanics*, 13:667–676.

Massada, J. L. (1991). Ankle overuse injuries in soccer players. *Journal of Sports Medicine and Physical Fitness*, 31:447–451.

Mathews, H. S., et al. (1977). Load-bearing characteristics of the patellofemoral joint. *Acta Orthopaedica Scandinavica*, 48:511–516.

McBride, I. D., Reid, J. G. (1988). Biomechanical considerations of the menisci of the knee. *Canadian Journal of Sports Science*, 13:175–187.

McLeish, R. D., Charnley, J. (1970). Abduction forces in the one-legged stance. *Journal of Biomechanics*, 3:191–209.

Mero, A., Komi, P. V. (1986). Force-, EMG-, and elasticity-velocity relationships at submaximal, maximal, and supramaximal running speeds in sprinters. *European Journal of Applied Physiology*, 55:553–561.

Messier, S., Pittala, K. (1988). Etiologic factors associated with selected running injuries. *Medicine and Science in Sports and Exercise*, 20:501–505.

Neumann, D. A., et al. (1988). Comparison of maximum isometric hip abductor muscle torques between hip sides. *Physical Therapy*, 68:496–502.

Noyes, F. R., et al. (1991). An analysis of the pivot shift phenomenon. *American Journal of Sports Medicine*, 19:148–155.

Nuber, G. W. (1988). Biomechanics of the foot and ankle during gait. *Clinics in Sports Medicine*, 7:1–13.

Offuerski, C. M., Macnab, I. (1983). Hip-spine syndrome. *Spine*, 8:316–321.

Reilly, D. T., Martens, M. (1972). Experimental analysis of the quadriceps muscle force and patellofemoral joint reaction force for various activities. *Acta Orthopaedica Scandinavica*, 43:126–137.

Roy, S. (1983). How I manage plantar fasciitis. *Physician and Sports Medicine*, 11:127–131.

Takai, S., et al. (1985). Rotational alignment of the lower limb in osteoarthritis of the knee. *International Orthopaedics (SICOT)*, 9:209–216.

Thorstensson, A. (1986). How is the normal locomotor program modified to produce backward walking? *Experimental Brain Research*, 61:664–668.

Vagenas, G., Hoshizaki, B. (1988). Evaluation of rearfoot asymmetries in running with worn and new running shoes. *International Journal of Sport Biomechanics*, 4:220–230.

Vaz, M. D., et al. (1993). Isometric hip abductor strength following total hip replacement and its relationship to functional assessments. *Journal of Sports Physical Therapy*, 18:526–531.

Vleeming, A., et al. (1990). Relation between form and function in the sacroiliac joint. Part II: Biomechanical aspects. *Spine*, 15:133–135.

Vrahas, M. S., et al. (1990). Contribution of passive tissues to the intersegmental moments at the hip. *Journal of Biomechanics*, 23:357–362.

Wang, C., Walker, P. S. (1974). Rotatory laxity of the human knee joint. *Journal of Bone and Joint Surgery*, 56-A:161–170.

Warren, B. Anatomical factors associated with predicting plantar fasciitis in long-distance runners. Medicine and Science in Sports and Exercise 16:60–63, 1984.

Winter, D. A., et al. (1990). Biomechanical walking pattern changes in the fit and healthy elderly. *Physical Therapy* 70:340–347.

Yoshioka, Y., et al. (1987). The anatomy and functional axes of the femur. *Journal of Bone and Joint Surgery* 69-A:873–879.

GLOSSARY

Abduction: Sideways movement of the segment away from the midline or sagittal plane.

Acetabular Labrum: Rim of fibrocartilage that encircles the acetabulum, deepening the socket.

Acetabulum: The concave, cup-shaped cavity on the lateral, inferior, anterior surface of the pelvis.

Adduction: Sideways movement of a segment toward the midline or sagittal plane.

Angle of Anteversion: Angle of the femoral neck in the transverse plane; anterior inclination of the femoral neck.

Angle of Inclination: Angle formed by the neck of the femur in the frontal plane.

Angle of Retroversion: Reversal of the angle of anteversion in which the femoral neck is angled posteriorly in the transverse plane.

Anterior Compartment Syndrome: Nerve and vascular compression due to hypertrophy of the anterior tibial muscles in a small muscular compartment.

Anterior Cruciate Ligament: Ligament inserting on the anterior intercondylar area and medial surface of the lateral condyle; prevents anterior displacement of the tibia and restrains knee extension, flexion, and internal rotation.

Anterior Tilt: Pelvic movement; superior portion of the ilium moves anteriorly.

Apophysitis: Inflammation of the apophysis, or bony outgrowth.

Arcuate Ligament: Ligament inserting on the lateral condyle of the femur and head of the fibula; reinforces the posterior capsule of the knee.

Bursitis: Inflammation of the bursae.

Calcaneal Apophysitis: Inflammation at the epiphysis on the calcaneus.

Calcaneocuboid Joint: The articulation between the calcaneus and the cuboid bones; part of the midtarsal joint.

Calcaneofibular Ligament: Ligament inserting on the lateral malleolus and outer calcaneus; limits backward movement of the foot and restrains inversion.

Calcaneonavicular Ligament: Ligament inserting on the calcaneus and the navicular; supports the arch and limits abduction of the foot.

Chondromalacia Patellae: Cartilage destruction on the underside of the patella; soft and fibrillated cartilage.

Condyle: A rounded projection on a bone.

Congenital Hip Dislocation: A condition existing at birth in which the hip joint subluxates or dislocates for no apparent reason.

Counternutation: See sacral extension.

Coxa Plana: Degeneration and recalcification (osteochondritis) of the capitular epiphysis (head) of the femur; also called Legg-Calvé-Perthes disease.

Coxa Valga: An increase in the angle of inclination of the femoral neck (greater than 125°).

Coxa Vara: A decrease in the angle of inclination of the femoral neck (less than 125°).

Deltoid Ligament: Ligament inserting on the medial malleolus, talus, navicular, and calcaneus; resists valgus forces and restrains plantarflexion, dorsiflexion, eversion, and abduction of the foot.

Distal Femoral Epiphysitis: Inflammation of the epiphysis at the attachment of the collateral ligaments at the knee.

Dorsiflexion: Movement of the foot up in the sagittal plane; movement toward the leg.

Epicondyle: Eminence on a bone above the condyle.

Equinus: A limitation in dorsiflexion caused by a short Achilles tendon or tight gastrocnemius and soleus muscles.

Eversion: Lifting of the lateral border of the foot.

Extension: Movement of a segment away from an adjacent segment so that the angle between the two segments is increased.

External Rotation: Movement of the anterior surface of a segment away from the midline; also termed lateral rotation.

Facet: A small plane surface on a bone where it articulates with another structure.

Flexion: Movement of a segment toward an adjacent segment so that the angle between the two is decreased.

Forefoot: Region of the foot that includes the metatarsals and phalanges.

Forefoot Valgus: Eversion of the forefoot on the rear foot, with the subtalar joint in neutral position.

Forefoot Varus: Inversion of the forefoot on the rear foot with subtalar in the neutral position.

Genu Valgum: A condition in which the knees are abnormally close together with the space between the ankles increased; knock-knees.

Genu Varum: A condition in which the knees are abnormally far apart with the space between the ankles decreased; bowlegs.

Hamstring: A group of muscles on the posterior thigh consisting of the semimembranosus, semitendinosus, and biceps femoris.

Head of Femur: The proximal end of the femur, a large round structure.

Hindfoot: Region of foot that includes the talus and calcaneus; also called rear foot.

Hyperextension: Continuation of extension past the neutral position.

Iliac Apophysitis: Inflammation of the attachment sites of the gluteus medius and tensor fascia latae on the iliac crest.

Iliofemoral Ligament: Ligament inserting on the anterosuperior spine of the ilium and intertrochanteric line of the femur; supports the anterior hip joint and offers restraint in extension and internal and external rotation.

Iliotibial Band: A fibrous band of fascia running from the ilium to the lateral condyle of the tibia.

Iliotibial Band Syndrome: Inflammation of the iliotibial band caused by thigh adduction and internal rotation.

Ilium: The superior bone of the pelvic girdle.

Infrapatellar Bursa: A bursa between the patellar ligament and the tibia.

Intercondylar Eminence: Ridge of bone on the tibial plateau that separates the surface into medial and lateral compartments.

Intercondylar Notch: Convex surface on the distal posterior surface of the femur.

Internal Rotation: Movement of the anterior surface of a segment toward the midline; also termed medial rotation.

Interosseous Ligament: Ligament connecting adjacent tarsals; supports the arch and the intertarsal joints.

Interphalangeal Joint: Articulation between adjacent phalanges of the fingers and toes.

Intertarsal Joint: Articulation between adjacent tarsal bones.

Inversion: Lifting of the medial border of the foot.

Ischiofemoral Ligament: Ligament inserting on the posterior acetabulum and iliofemoral ligament; restrains adduction and internal rotation of the thigh.

Ischium: The inferoposterior bone of the pelvic girdle.

Lateral Collateral Ligament: Ligament inserting on the lateral epicondyle of the femur and head of the fibula; resists varus forces and is taut in extension.

Lateral Tibial Syndrome: Pain on the lateral anterior leg caused by tendinitis of the tibialis anterior or irritation to the interosseous membrane.

Legg-Calvé-Perthes Disease: Degeneration and recalcification (osteochondritis) of the capitular epiphysis (head) of the femur; also called coxa plana.

Longitudinal Arch: Two arches (medial and lateral) formed by the tarsals and metatarsals, which run the length of the foot and participate in both shock absorption and support while the foot is bearing weight.

Medial Collateral Ligament: Ligament inserting on the medial epicondyle of the femur, medial condyle of the tibia, and medial meniscus; resists valgus forces and restrains the knee joint in internal and external rotation; taut in extension.

Medial Tibial Syndrome: Pain above the medial malleolus caused by tendinitis of the tibialis posterior or irritation of the interosseous membrane or periosteum; previously called shin splints.

Meniscus: A crescent-shaped fibrocartilage on the articular surface of the knee joint.

Metatarsalgia: Strain of the ligaments supporting the metatarsals.

Metatarsophalangeal Joints: Articulations between the metatarsals and the phalanges in the foot.

Midfoot: Region of the foot that includes all of the tarsals except the talus and calcaneus.

Midtarsal Joint: Two articulations: the calcaneocuboid and the talonavicular joints; also called the transverse tarsal joint.

Morton's Toe: A condition in which the second metatarsal is longer than the first metatarsal.

Neck of Femur: Column of bone connecting the head of the femur to the shaft.

Nutation: See sacral flexion.

Osgood-Schlatter Disease: Irritation of the epiphysis at the tibial tuberosity, caused by overuse of the quadriceps femoris muscle group.

Osteoarthritis: Degenerative joint disease characterized by breakdown in the cartilage and underlying subchondral bone, narrowing of the joint space, and osteophyte formation.

Osteochondral Fracture: Fracture at the bone and cartilage junction.

Osteochondritis Dissecans: Inflammation of bone and cartilage, resulting in splitting of pieces of cartilage into the joint.

Patella: Triangular sesamoid bone on the anterior knee joint; encased by the tendons of the quadriceps femoris muscle group.

Patella Alta: Long patellar tendon.

Patella Baja: Short patellar tendon.

Patellar Groove: The convex surface on the distal anterior surface of the femur; accommodates the patella; also called the trochlear groove.

Patellar Ligament: Ligament inserting on the inferior patella and the tibial tuberosity; transfers the quadriceps femoris muscle force to the tibia.

Patellofemoral Joint: Articulation between the posterior surface of the patella and the patellar groove on the femur.

Patellofemoral Pain Syndrome: Pain around the patella.

Pelvic Girdle: A complete ring of bones composed of two coxal bones anteriorly and laterally and the sacrum and coccyx posteriorly.

Periostitis: Inflammation of the periosteum, marked by tenderness and swelling on the bone.

Pes Anserinus: The combined insertion of the tendinous expansions from the sartorius, gracilis, and semitendinosus muscles.

Pes Cavus: High-arched foot.

Pes Planus: Flat foot.

Plantar Fascia: Fibrous band of fascia running along the plantar surface of the foot from the calcaneus to the metatarsophalangeal articulation.

Plantar Fasciitis: Inflammation of the plantar fascia.

Plantar-Flexed First Ray: Position of the first metatarsal below the plane of the adjacent metatarsal heads.

Plantarflexion: Movement of the foot downward in the sagittal plane; movement away from the leg.

Plica: Ridge or fold in the synovial membrane.

Posterior Cruciate Ligament: Ligament inserting on the posterior spine of the tibia and the inner condyle of the femur; resists posterior movement of the tibia on the femur and restrains flexion and rotation of the knee.

Posterior Oblique Ligament: Ligament inserting on the semimembranosus muscle; supports the posterior medial capsule of the knee joint.

Posterior Tilt: Pelvic movement designated by posterior movement of the superior portion of the ilium.

Pronation: A triplanar movement at the subtalar and midtarsal joints that includes calcaneal eversion, abduction, and dorsiflexion.

Pubic Ligament: Ligament inserting on the bodies of the right and left pubic bones; maintains the relationship between right and left pubic bones.

Pubic Symphysis: A cartilaginous joint connecting the pubic bones of the right and left coxal bones of the pelvis.

Pubis: The anterior inferior bone of the pelvic girdle.

Pubofemoral Ligament: Ligament inserting on the pubic part of the acetabulum, superior rami, and intertrochanteric line; restrains hip abduction and external rotation.

Q-Angle: The angle formed by the longitudinal axis of the femur and the line of pull of the patellar ligament.

Quadriceps Femoris: A combination of muscles on the anterior thigh, including vastus lateralis, vastus intermedius, vastus medialis, and rectus femoris.

Rear Foot: Region of foot that includes the talus and calcaneus; also called hindfoot.

Rear Foot Varus: Inversion of the calcaneus with deviation of the tibia in the same direction.

Retrocalcaneal Bursitis: Inflammation of the bursa between the Achilles tendon and the calcaneus.

Sacral Extension: Posterior movement of the top of the sacrum.

Sacral Flexion: Anterior movement of the top of the sacrum.

Sacral Rotation: Rotation of the sacrum about an axis running diagonally through the bone; right rotation occurs as the anterior surface of the sacrum faces right.

Sacroiliac Joint: A strong synovial joint between the sacrum and the ilium.

Sacroiliitis: Inflammation at the sacroiliac joint.

Sacrum: A triangular bone below the lumbar vertebrae that consists of five fused vertebrae.

Screw Home Mechanism: The locking action at the end of knee extension; external rotation of the tibia on the femur caused by incongruent joint surfaces.

Slipped Capital Femoral Epiphysitis: Displacement of the capital femoral epiphysis of the femur caused by external forces that drive the femoral head back and medial to tilt the growth plate.

Snapping Hip Syndrome: A clicking sound that accompanies thigh movements; caused by the hip capsule or iliopsoas tendon moving on a bony surface.

Sprain: An injury to a ligament surrounding a joint; rupture of fibers of a ligament.

Strain: Injury to the muscle, tendon, or muscle–tendon junction due to overstretching or excessive tension on the muscle; tearing and rupture of the muscle or tendon fibers.

Stress Fracture: Microfracture of the bones developed through repetitive force application exceeding the structural strength of the bone or the rate of remodeling in the body tissue.

Subtalar Joint: The articulation of the talus with the calcaneus; also called the talocalcaneal joint.

Supination: Triplane movement at the subtalar and midtarsal joints that includes calcaneal inversion, adduction, and plantarflexion.

Talocalcaneal Ligament: Ligament inserting on the talus and calcaneus; supports the subtalar joint.

Talocrural Joint: The articulation of the tibia and fibula with the talus; the ankle joint.

Talofibular Ligament: Ligament inserting on the lateral malleolus and the posterior talus; limits plantarflexion and inversion; supports the lateral ankle.

Talonavicular Joint: Articulation between the talus and the navicular bones; part of the midtarsal joint.

Talonavicular Ligament: Ligament inserting on the neck of the talus and navicular; limits inversion and stabilizes the talonavicular joint.

Talotibial Ligament: Ligament inserting on the tibia and talus; limits plantarflexion and supports the medial ankle.

Tarsometatarsal Joint: Articulation between the tarsals and metatarsals.

Tarsometatarsal Ligaments: Ligaments inserting on the tarsals and metatarsals; supports the arch and maintains stability between the tarsals and metatarsals.

Tendinitis: Inflammation of a tendon.

Tibial Plateau: A level area on the proximal end of the tibia.

Tibiofemoral Joint: Articulation between the tibia and the femur; the knee joint.

Tibiofibular Joint (inferior): Articulation between the distal end of the fibula and the distal end of the tibia.

Tibiofibular Joint (superior): Articulation between the head of the fibula and the posterolateral inferior aspect of the tibial condyle.

Tibiotalar Joint: Articulation between the tibia and the talus.

Transverse Arch: An arch formed by the tarsals and metatarsals; runs across the foot, contributing to shock absorption in weight bearing.

Transverse Ligament: Ligament inserting on the medial and lateral meniscus; connects the menisci to each other.

Trendelenburg Gait: Alteration in a walking or running gait caused by inefficiency in the abductors of the thigh, causing a drop in the pelvis to the unsupported side.

Trochanteric Bursa: A fibrous, fluid-filled sac between the gluteus maximus and the greater trochanter.

Valgus: Segment angle bowed medially; medial force.

Varus: Segment angle bowed laterally; lateral force.

7

Functional Anatomy of the Trunk

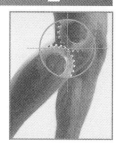

OBJECTIVES

After reading this chapter, the student will be able to:

1. Identify the four curves of the spine and discuss the factors contributing to the formation of each curve.

2. Describe the structure and motion characteristics of the cervical, thoracic, and lumbar vertebrae.

3. Describe the movement relationship between the pelvis and the lumbar vertebrae for the full range of trunk movements.

4. Compare the differences in strength for the various trunk movements.

5. Describe specific strength and flexibility exercises for all of the movements of the trunk.

6. Explain how loads are absorbed by the vertebrae and describe some of the typical loads imposed upon the vertebrae for specific movements or activities.

7. Describe some of the common injuries to the cervical, thoracic, and lumbar vertebrae.

8. Identify the muscular contributions of the trunk to walking and running.

9. Discuss the causes and source of pain for the low back.

10. Evaluate common trunk exercises for their effectiveness and safety.

11. Discuss the influence of aging on trunk structure and function.

The vertebral column acts as a modified elastic rod, providing rigid support and flexibility (36). There are 33 vertebrae in the vertebral column, 24 of which are movable and contribute to trunk movements. The vertebrae are arranged into four curves that facilitate support of the column by offering a springlike response to loading (26). These curves provide balance and strengthen the spine.

Seven cervical vertebrae form a convex curve to the anterior side of the body. This curve develops as an infant begins to lift its head; it supports the head and assumes its curvature in response to head position. The 12 thoracic vertebrae form a curve that is convex to the posterior side of the body. The curvature in the thoracic spine is present at birth. Five lumbar vertebrae form a curve convex to the anterior side, which develops in response to weight bearing and is influenced by pelvic and lower extremity positioning. The last curve is the sacrococcygeal curve, formed by five fused sacral vertebrae and the four or five fused vertebrae of the coccyx. Fig. 7-1 presents the curvature of the whole spine as seen from the side and the rear.

The junction where one curve ends and the next one begins is usually a site of great mobility, which is also vulnerable to injury. These junctions are the cervicothoracic, the thoracolumbar, and the lumbosacral regions. Additionally, if the curves of the spine are exaggerated, the column will be more mobile, and if the curves are flat, the spine will be more rigid. The cervical and lumbar regions of the spinal column are the most mobile, and the thoracic and pelvic regions are more rigid (26).

Besides offering support and flexibility to the trunk, the vertebral column has the main responsibility of protecting the spinal cord. As illustrated in Fig. 7-2, the cord runs down through the vertebrae in a canal formed by the

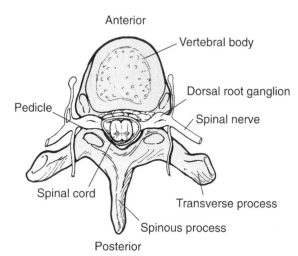

FIGURE 7-2 The vertebral column protects the spinal cord, which runs down the posterior aspect of the column through the vertebral foramen or canal. Spinal nerves exit at each vertebral level.

body, pedicles, and pillars of the vertebrae, the disc, and a ligament, the ligamentum flavum. Peripheral nerves exit through the intervertebral foramen on the lateral side of the vertebrae, forming aggregates of nerve fibers resulting in segmental innervations throughout the body.

The trunk, as the largest segment of the body, plays an integral role in both upper and lower extremity function, since its position can significantly alter the function of the extremities. Trunk movement or position can be examined as a whole, or it can be examined by observing the movements or position of the different regions of the vertebral column or movement at the individual vertebral level. This chapter examines both the movement of the trunk as a whole and the movements and function within each region of the spine. The structural characteristics of the vertebral column are presented first, followed by an examination of the differences between the three regions of the spine: the cervical, thoracic, and lumbar.

The Vertebral Column

ANATOMICAL AND FUNCTIONAL CHARACTERISTICS OF THE JOINTS

The functional unit of the vertebral column, the motion segment, is similar in structure throughout the spinal column, except for the first two cervical vertebrae, which have unique structure. The motion segment consists of two adjacent vertebrae and a disc that separates them (Fig. 7-3). The segment can be further broken down into anterior and posterior portions, each playing a different role in vertebral function.

Motion Segment: Anterior Portion

The anterior portion of the motion segment contains the two bodies of the vertebrae, the intervertebral disc, and the anterior and posterior longitudinal ligaments. The two

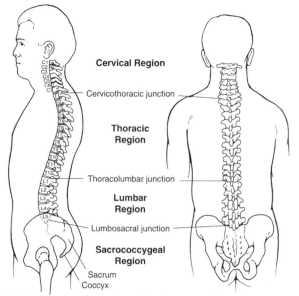

FIGURE 7-1 The vertebral column is both strong and flexible as a result of the four alternating curves. We are born with the thoracic and sacrococcygeal curves. The cervical and lumbar curves form in response to weight bearing and muscular stresses imposed upon them during infancy.

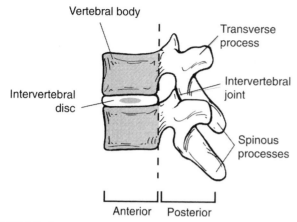

FIGURE 7-3 The vertebral motion segment can be divided into anterior and posterior portions. The anterior portion contains the vertebral bodies, intervertebral disc, and ligaments. The posterior portion contains the vertebral foramen, neural arches, intervertebral joints, transverse and spinous processes, and ligaments.

bodies and the disc separating them form a cartilaginous joint that is not found at any other site in the body.

Each vertebral body is tube-shaped and thicker on the front side (10), where it absorbs large amounts of compressive forces. It consists of cancellous tissue surrounded by a hard cortical layer and has a raised rim that facilitates attachment of the disc, muscles, and ligaments. Also, the surface of the body is covered with hyaline cartilage, forming articular end plates into which the disc attaches.

Separating the two adjacent bodies is the intervertebral disc, a structure binding the vertebrae together while permitting movement between adjacent vertebrae. The disc is capable of withstanding compressive forces as well as torsional and bending forces applied to the column. The roles of the disc are to bear and distribute loads in the vertebral column and to restrain excessive motion in the vertebral segment. The load transmitted via the intervertebral discs distributes stress uniformly over the vertebral end plates and is also responsible for most of the mobility in the spine (22). A lateral, superior, and cross-sectional view of the disc is presented in Fig. 7-4.

Each disc consists of the nucleus pulposus and the annulus fibrosus. The nucleus pulposus is a gel-like spherical mass in the central portion of the cervical and thoracic discs and toward the posterior in the lumbar discs. The nucleus pulposus is 80 to 90% water and 15 to 20% collagen (9), creating a fluid mass that is always under pressure and exerting a preload to the disc. The nucleus pulposus is well suited for withstanding compressive forces applied to the motion segment.

During the day, the water content of the disc is reduced, with compressive forces applied during daily activities, resulting in a shortening of the column by about 15 to 25 mm (1). The height and volume of the discs are reduced by about 20%, causing the disc to bulge radially outward and increase the axial loading on the posterior joints (1). However, at night, the nucleus pulposus imbibes water,

restoring height to the disc. In the elderly, the total water content of the disc is less (approximately 70%) and the ability to imbibe water is reduced, leaving a shorter vertebral column.

The nucleus pulposus is surrounded by rings of fibrous tissue and fibrocartilage, the annulus fibrosus. The fibers of the annulus fibrosus run parallel in concentric layers but are oriented diagonally at 45 to 65° to the vertebral bodies (28,70). Each alternate layer of fibers runs perpendicular to the previous layer, creating a criss-cross pattern similar to that seen in a radial tire (25). When rotation is applied to the disc, half of the fibers will tighten, while the fibers running in the other direction will be loose.

The fibers making up the annulus fibrosus consist of 50 to 60% collagen, providing the tensile strength in the disc (9). As a result of aging and maturation, the collagen is remodeled in the disc in response to changes in loading. This results in thicker annular fibers with higher concentrations of collagen fibers in the anterior disc area and thinner annular fibers in the lateral posterior portion of the disc because the fibers are less abundant. Fibers from the annulus fibrosus attach to the end plates of the adjacent vertebral bodies in the center of the segment and attach to the actual osseous material at the periphery of the disc (65). The fiber directions in the annulus fibrosus limit rotational and shearing motion between the vertebrae. The pressure on the tissue of the peripheral layer maintains the interspace between the end plates of the adjoining vertebrae (22). Tension is maintained in the annulus fibrosus by the end plates and by pressure exerted outward from the nucleus pulposus. The pressure tightens the outer layer and prevents radial bulging of the disc. Loss of disc tissue, such as occurs in aging, may impair spine function because of an increase in radial bulging, compression of the joints, or a reduction in space for the nerve tissue in the foramen (22).

The disc is both avascular and aneural, except for some sensory input from the outer layers of the annulus fibrosus.

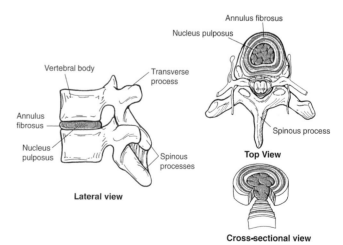

FIGURE 7-4 The intervertebral disc bears and distributes loads on the vertebral column. The disc consists of a gel-like central portion, the nucleus pulposus, which is surrounded by rings of fibrous tissue, the annulus fibrosus.

Because of this, healing of a damaged disc is unpredictable and not very promising.

The intervertebral disc functions hydrostatically when it is healthy, responding with flexibility under low loads and stiffly when subjected to high loads. When the disc is loaded in compression, the nucleus pulposus uniformly distributes pressure through the disc and acts as a cushion. The disc flattens and widens and the nucleus pulposus bulges laterally as the disc loses fluid. This places tension on the annulus fibers and converts vertical compression force to tensile stress in the annulus fibers. The tensile stress absorbed by the annulus fibers is 4 to 5 times the applied axial load (44). Examples of typical loads on the third lumbar vertebra for a 70-kg individual are presented in Table 7-1. The loads on the disc created by activities such as sitting, coughing, and laughing are larger than those measured in standing, walking, or twisting.

There are two weak points where disc injury is likely when subjected to high loads. First, the cartilage end plates, to which the disc is attached, is supported only by a thin layer of bone and thus is subject to fracture. Second, the posterior annulus is thinner and not attached as firmly as other portions of the disc, making it more vulnerable to injury (70).

The pressure in the disc increases linearly with increased compressive loads, with the pressure 30 to 50% greater than the applied load per unit area (10). The greatest change in disc pressure occurs with compression. During compression, the disc loses fluid and the fiber angle increases (28). The disc is very resilient to the effects of a compressive force and rarely fails under compression. The cancellous bone of the vertebral body will yield and fracture before the disc is damaged (28).

Movements such as flexion, extension, and lateral flexion generate a bending force that causes both compression and tension. With this asymmetrical loading, the vertebral

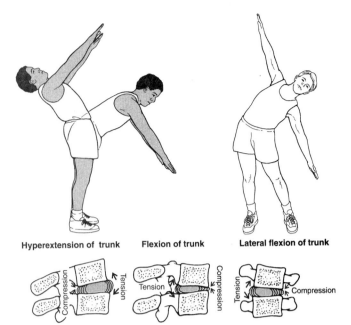

FIGURE 7-5 When the trunk flexes, extends, or laterally flexes, compressive force develops to the side of the bend and tension force develops on the opposite side.

body translates toward the loaded side, where compression develops, and the fibers are stretched on the other side, resulting in tension force.

In flexion, the vertebrae tilt anteriorly, forcing the nucleus pulposus posteriorly, creating a compression load on the anterior portion of the disc and a tension load on the posterior annulus. In extension the opposite occurs, as the upper vertebrae tilt posteriorly, driving the nucleus pulposus anteriorly and placing tensile pressure on the anterior fibers of the annulus.

In lateral flexion, the upper vertebrae tilt to the side of flexion, generating compression on that side and tension on the opposite side. Fig. 7-5 illustrates disc behavior in flexion, extension, and lateral flexion.

As the trunk rotates, both tension and shear develop in the annulus fibrosus of the disc (Fig. 7-6). The half of the annulus fibers that are oriented in the direction of the rotation become taut, and the rest, which are oriented in the opposite direction, slacken. This raises the intradiscal pressure, narrows the joint space, and creates a shear force in the horizontal plane of rotation and tension in fibers oriented in the direction of the rotation. The peripheral fibers of the annulus fibrosus are subjected to the greatest stress during rotation (65).

The final structures of the anterior portion of the vertebral segment are the longitudinal ligaments running along the spine from the base of the occiput to the sacrum. The anterior longitudinal ligament is a very dense, powerful ligament that attaches to both the anterior disc and the vertebral bodies of the motion segment. This ligament limits hyperextension of the spine and restrains forward movement of one vertebra over another. It also maintains a constant load on the vertebral column and supports the anterior portion of the disc in lifting (25).

TABLE 7-1 Loads on L3 Disc in 70-Kg Person

Activity	Load on Disc (N)
Supine	294
Standing	686
Walking	833
Twisting	882
Bend Sideways	931
Upright Sitting	980
Coughing	1078
Jumping	1078
Straining	1176
Laughing	1176
Lifting 20 kg, back straight, knees bent	2058
Lifting 20 kg, back bent, knees straight	3332

Adapted from Nachemson, A. (1976). Lumbar intradiscal pressure. In M. Jayson (Ed.). *The Lumbar Spine and Back Pain*. Kent: Pitman Medical.

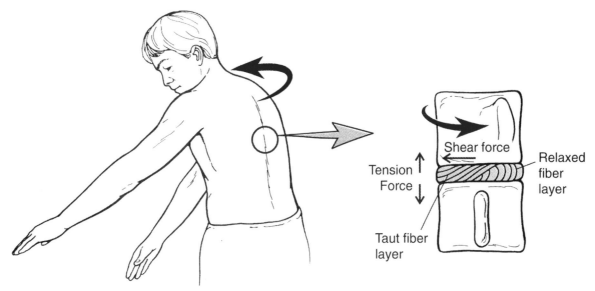

FIGURE 7-6 When the trunk rotates, half of the fibers of the annulus fibrosus become taut and the rest relax. This creates tension force in the fibers running in the direction of the rotation and shear force across the plane of rotation.

The posterior longitudinal ligament runs down the posterior surface of the vertebral bodies inside the spinal canal and connects to the rim of the vertebral bodies and the center of the disc. The posterolateral aspect of the segment is not covered by this ligament, adding to the vulnerability of this site for disc protrusion. It is broad in the cervical region and narrow in the lumbar region. This ligament offers resistance in flexion of the spine. The location and function of all of the spinal ligaments are presented in Appendix A.

Motion Segment: Posterior Portion

The posterior portion of the vertebral motion segment includes the neural arches, the intervertebral joints, the transverse and spinous processes, and ligaments (Fig. 7-7 and Appendix A). The neural arch is formed by the two pedicles and two laminae, and together with the posterior side of the vertebral body, they form the vertebral foramen, in which the spinal cord travels. The bone in the pedicles and laminae is very hard, providing good resistance to the large tensile forces that must be accommodated. Notches above and below each pedicle form the intervertebral foramen, through which the spinal nerves leave the canal.

Projecting sideways at the union of the laminae and the pedicles are the transverse processes, and projecting posteriorly from the junction of the two laminae is the spinous process. The spinous and transverse processes serve as attachment sites for the spinal muscles running the length of the column.

The two synovial joints, termed the apophyseal joints, are formed by articulating facets on the upper and lower border of each laminae. The superior articulating facet is concave and fits into the convex inferior facet of the adjacent vertebra, forming a joint on each side of the vertebrae. The articulating facets are oriented at different angles in the cervical, thoracic, and lumbar regions of the spine, accounting for most of the functional differences between regions. These differences are discussed more specifically in a later section of this chapter.

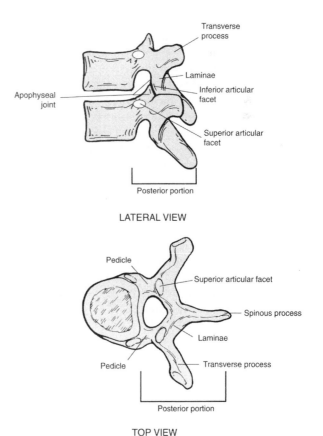

LATERAL VIEW

TOP VIEW

FIGURE 7-7 The posterior portion of the spinal motion segment is responsible for a significant amount of spinal support and restriction owing to its ligaments and structure. The posterior portion contains the only synovial joint in the spine, the apophyseal joint, which joins the superior and inferior facets of each vertebra.

The apophyseal joints are enclosed within a joint capsule and have all of the other characteristics of a typical synovial joint. Depending on the orientation of the facet joints, these joints can prevent the forward displacement of one vertebra over another and also participate in load bearing. In the hyperextended position, these joints bear 30% of the load (36). They also bear a significant portion of the load when the spine is flexed and rotated (20). Highest pressures in the facet joints occur with combined torsion, flexion, and compression of the vertebrae (8). The apophyseal joints protect the discs from excessive shear and rotation (1).

Five ligaments support the posterior portion of the vertebral segment. These ligaments are presented in Appendix A. The ligamentum flavum connects adjacent vertebral arches longitudinally, attaching laminae to laminae. It is a ligament having elastic qualities, allowing it to deform and return to its original length. It elongates with flexion of the trunk and contracts in extension. In the neutral position it is under constant tension, imposing continual tension on the disc.

The supraspinous and the interspinous ligaments both run from spinous process to spinous process and resist both shear and forward bending of the spine. Finally, the intertransverse ligaments, connecting transverse process to transverse process, resist lateral bending of the trunk. The role of all of the intervertebral ligaments is to prevent excessive bending (1).

Movements of the Total Spine

Motion in the spinal column is very small between each vertebra, but as a whole the spine is capable of considerable range of motion. Motion is restricted by the discs and the arrangement of the facets, but motion can occur in three planes via active muscular initiation and control (68).

The movement characteristics of the total spine are presented in Fig. 7-8. For the total spinal column, flexion and extension occur through approximately 110 to 140°, with free movement in the cervical and lumbar regions and limited flexion and extension in the thoracic region. The axis of rotation for flexion and extension lies in the disc unless there is considerable disc degeneration, which can move the axis of rotation out of the disc. Flexion of the whole trunk occurs primarily in the lumbar vertebrae through the first 50 to 60° and is then moved into more flexion by forward tilt of the pelvis (21). Extension occurs through a reverse movement in which first the pelvis tilts posteriorly and then the lumbar spine extends.

When flexion begins, the top vertebra slides forward on the bottom vertebra and the vertebra tilts, placing compressive force on the anterior portion of the disc. Both ligaments and the annulus fibers absorb the compressive forces.

On the back side, the superior portions of the apophyseal joints slide up on the lower facets, creating compression force between the facets and shear force across the face of the facets. These forces are controlled by the posterior ligaments, the capsules surrounding the apophyseal joints, the posterior muscles, the fascia, and the posterior annulus fibers (65). The full flexion position is maintained

and supported by the apophyseal capsular ligaments, the intervertebral discs, the supraspinous and interspinous ligaments, the ligamentum flavum, and passive resistance from the back muscles, in that order (3).

Lateral flexion range of motion is about 75 to 85°, mainly in the cervical and lumbar regions (Fig. 7-8). During lateral flexion, there is a slight movement of the vertebrae sideways, with disc compression to the side of the bend. Lateral flexion is often accompanied by rotation. In a relaxed stance, the accompanying rotation is to the opposite side of lateral flexion, that is, left rotation accompanying right lateral flexion.

If the vertebra is in full flexion, the accompanying rotation will occur to the same side, that is, right rotation accompanying right lateral flexion. However, this can vary by region of the spine. Also, an inflexible person will usually perform some lateral flexion to obtain flexion in the trunk (2).

Rotation occurs through 90°, is free in the cervical region, and occurs in the thoracic and lumbar regions in combination with lateral flexion (Fig. 7-8). Generally, rotation is limited in the lumbar region. Right rotation in the thoracic or lumbar region will be accompanied by some left lateral flexion.

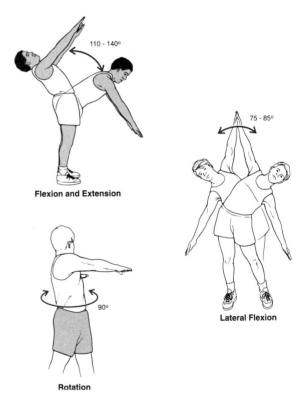

Flexion and Extension

110 - 140°

75 - 85°

Lateral Flexion

90°

Rotation

FIGURE 7-8 The range of motion at the individual motion segment level is small, but in combination, the trunk is capable of moving through a significant motion range. Flexion and extension occur through approximately 110 to 140°, primarily in the cervical and lumbar region, with a very limited contribution from the thoracic region. The trunk rotates through 90°, with movement occurring freely in the cervical region, and with accompanying lateral flexion in the thoracic and lumbar regions. The trunk laterally flexes through 75 to 85°.

The apophyseal joints are in a close-packed position in spinal extension, except for the top two cervical vertebrae, which are in a close-packed position in flexion. The total spine is in a close-packed position and rigid during the military salute posture with the head up, shoulders back, and the trunk vertically aligned (25).

The flexibility of the regions of the trunk varies and is determined by the intervertebral discs and the angle of articulation of the facet joints. As pointed out earlier, mobility is highest at the junction of the regions. Mobility will also increase in a region in response to restriction or rigidity elsewhere in the vertebral column.

Cervical Region

The cervical region has two vertebrae, the atlas (C1) and the axis (C2), that have structures unlike those of any other vertebra (Fig. 7-9). The atlas has no vertebral body and is shaped like a ring with an anterior and a posterior arch. The atlas has large transverse processes with transverse foramen through which blood supply travels. The

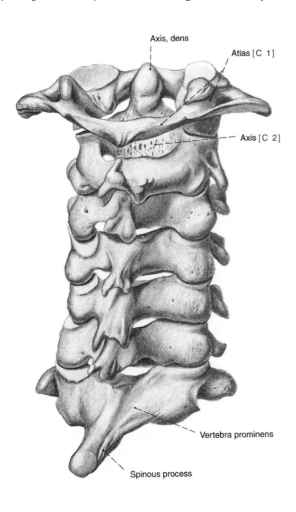

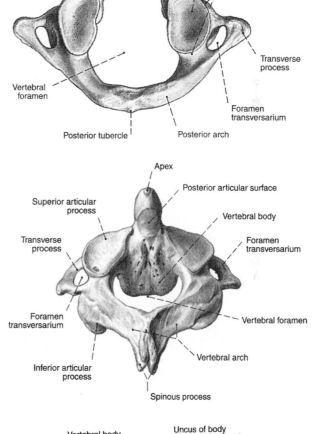

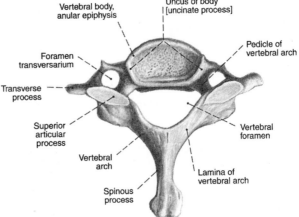

FIGURE 7-9 The cervical vertebrae (left) have two unique vertebrae, the atlas (top right) and the axis (middle right), that are very different from a typical vertebra (bottom right) and have specialized functions of supporting the head. (Reprinted with permission from Sobotta [2001]. R Putz, R. Pabst [Eds.]. *Atlas of Human Anatomy, Vol. 2, Trunk, Viscera, Lower Limb.* Philadelphia: Lippincott Williams & Wilkins, Figs. 720, 723, 725, 727.)

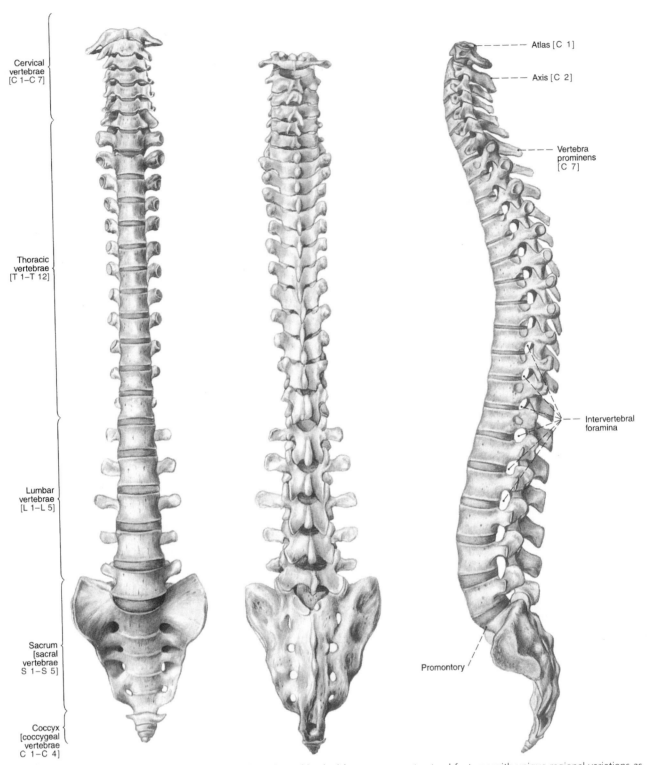

FIGURE 7-10 The vertebrae in each region (cervical, thoracic, and lumbar) have common structural features with unique regional variations as seen here in the anterior (left), posterior (middle), and lateral (left) views. (Reprinted with permission from Sobotta [2001]. R Putz, R. Pabst [Eds.]. *Atlas of Human Anatomy, Vol. 2, Trunk, Viscera, Lower Limb.* Philadelphia: Lippincott Williams & Wilkins, Figs. 708–710.)

atlas has no spinous process. Superiorly, it has a fovea, or dishlike depression, that holds the occiput of the skull.

The articulation of the atlas with the skull is called the atlanto-occipital joint. It is at this joint that the head nods on the spine, for it allows free sagittal plane movements.

This joint allows approximately 10 to 15° of flexion and extension, 8° of lateral flexion, and no rotation (72).

The axis has a modified body with no articulating process on the superior aspect of the body and pedicles. Instead, the articulation with the atlas occurs via a pillar projecting from the superior surface of the axis that fits into the atlas and locks the atlas into a swivel or pivoting joint. The pillar is referred to as the odontoid process or dens.

The articulation between the atlas and the axis is known as the atlantoaxial joint and is the most mobile of the cervical joints, allowing approximately 10° of flexion and extension, 47° of rotation, and no lateral flexion (72). This joint allows us to turn our head and look from one side to the other. In fact, this articulation accounts for 50% of the rotation in the cervical vertebrae (72).

The remainder of the cervical vertebrae have structures in the anterior and posterior compartments similar to those of the typical vertebrae. The bodies of the cervical vertebrae

are small and about half as wide side to side as they are front to back. The cervical vertebrae also have short pedicles, bulky articulating processes, and short spinous processes. The transverse processes of the cervical vertebrae have a foramen where the arteries pass through. This is not found in other regions of the vertebral column. Fig. 7-10 illustrates size, shape, and orientation differences across the regions of the spinal cord. A closer examination of structural differences between the cervical, thoracic, and lumbar vertebrae is presented in Fig. 7-11.

The articulating facets in the cervical vertebrae face 45° to the transverse plane and lie parallel to the frontal plane (63), with the superior articulating process facing posterior

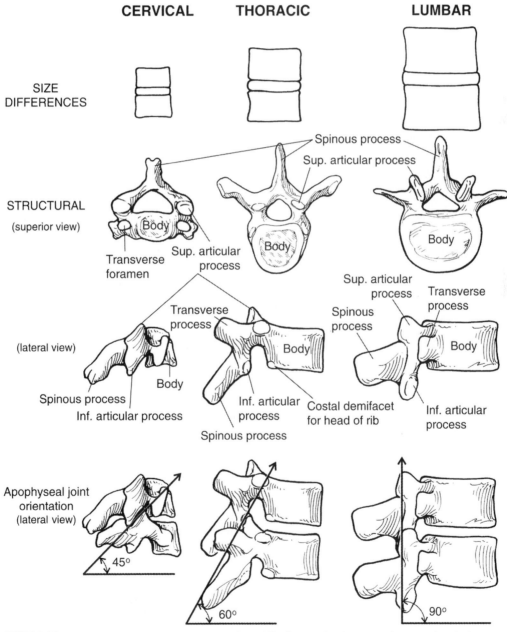

FIGURE 7-11 The cervical, thoracic, and lumbar vertebrae differ from each other. From the cervical to the lumbar region the bodies of the vertebrae become larger, and the transverse processes, spinous processes, and apophyseal joints all change their orientation.

and up and the inferior articulating processes facing anterior and down. In contrast to other regions of the vertebral column, the intervertebral discs are smaller laterally than the bodies of the vertebrae. The cervical discs are thicker ventrally than dorsally, producing a wedge shape and contributing to the lordotic curvature in the cervical region.

Because of the short spinous processes, the shape of the discs, and the backward and downward orientation of the articulating facets, movement in the cervical region is greater than in any other region of the vertebral column. The cervical vertebrae can rotate through approximately 90°, flex 47° to each side, flex through 40°, and extend through 24° (72). Maximum rotation in the cervical vertebrae occurs at C1–C2, maximum lateral flexion at C2–C4, and maximum flexion and extension at C1–C3 and C7–T1. Also, all cervical vertebrae move simultaneously in flexion.

In addition to the ligaments supporting the whole vertebral column, some specialized ligaments are found in the cervical region. The location and action of these ligaments are presented in Appendix A.

Thoracic Region

One of the most restricted regions of the vertebral column is the thoracic vertebrae. Moving down the spinal column, the individual vertebrae increase in size; thus, the 12th thoracic vertebra is larger than the 1st thoracic. The bodies become taller, and the thoracic vertebrae have longer pedicles than the cervical vertebrae (Fig. 7-11). The transverse processes on the thoracic vertebrae are long, and they angle backward, with the tips of the transverse processes posterior to the articulating facets. On the back of the thoracic vertebrae are long spinous processes overlapping the vertebrae and directed downward rather than posteriorly, as in other regions of the spine.

The connection of the thoracic vertebrae to the ribs is illustrated in Fig. 7-12. The thoracic vertebrae articulate with the ribs via articulating facets on the body of each vertebrae. Full facets are located on the bodies of the 1st

and 10th to 12th thoracic vertebrae, while demifacets are located on the 2nd to 9th thoracic vertebrae to connect with the ribs. The thoracic vertebrae are supported by the ligaments presented earlier, along with four others that support the attachment between the ribs and the vertebral body and transverse processes. These ligaments are presented in Appendix A.

The apophyseal joints between adjacent thoracic vertebrae are angled at 60° to the transverse plane and 20° to the frontal plane, with the superior facets facing posterior and a little up and laterally, and the inferior facets facing anteriorly, down, and medially (Fig. 7-11). In comparison to the cervical vertebrae, the thoracic intervertebral joints are oriented more in the vertical plane.

The movements in the thoracic region are limited primarily by the connection with the ribs, the orientation of the facets, and the long spinous processes that overlap in the back. Range of motion in the thoracic region for flexion and extension combined is 3 to 12°, with very limited motion in the upper thoracic (2–4°) that increases in the lower thoracic to 20° at the thoracolumbar junction (8,72).

Lateral flexion is also limited in the thoracic vertebrae, ranging from 2 to 9°, and again increasing as one progresses down through the thoracic vertebrae. In the upper thoracic, lateral flexion is limited to 2 to 4°, while in the lower thoracic it may be as high as 9° (8,72).

Rotation in the thoracic vertebrae ranges from 2 to 9°. Rotation range of motion is opposite to that of flexion and lateral flexion, for it is maximum at the upper levels (9°) and is reduced at the lower levels (2°) (8,72).

The intervertebral discs in the thoracic region have a greater ratio of disc diameter to height of the disc than any other region of the spine. This reduces the tensile stress imposed upon the vertebrae in compression by reducing the stress on the outside of the disc (44). Thus, disc injuries in the thoracic region are not as common as in other regions of the column.

Lumbar Region

The large lumbar vertebra is the most highly loaded structure in the skeletal system. Figure 7-11 illustrates the characteristics of the lumbar vertebrae. The lumbar vertebrae are large, with wider bodies side to side than front to back. They also are wider vertically in the front than in the back. The pedicles of the lumbar vertebrae are short, the spinous processes broad, and small transverse processes project posteriorly, upward, and laterally. The discs in the lumbar region are thick; as in the cervical region, they are thicker ventrally than dorsally, contributing to an increase in the anterior concavity in the region. Frobin et al. (22) reported that the ventral disc height of the lumbar vertebrae remains fairly constant in the age range of 16 to 57 years, but there are gender differences and different disc heights at different levels of the vertebrae. The lumbar vertebrae typically higher in males. Also, the highest disc height is found at L4–L5 and L5–S1.

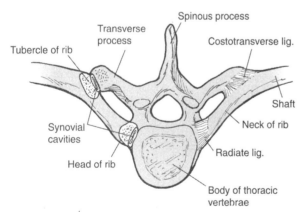

FIGURE 7-12 The thoracic region is restricted in movement because of its connection to the ribs, which connect to a demifacet on the body of the thoracic vertebrae and a facet on the transverse process.

The apophyseal joints in the lumbar region lie in the sagittal plane, as the articulating facets are at right angles to the transverse plane and 45° to the frontal plane (72). The superior facets face medially, and the inferior facets face laterally. This changes at the lumbosacral junction, where the apophyseal joint moves into the frontal plane and the inferior facet on L5 faces front. This change in orientation keeps the vertebral column from sliding forward on the sacrum.

The lumbar region is supported by the ligaments that run the full length of the spine and by one other, the iliolumbar ligament (see Appendix A). Another important support structure in the region is the thoracolumbar fascia, which runs from the sacrum and iliac crest up to the thoracic cage. This fascia offers resistance and support in full flexion of the trunk. The elastic tension in this fascia also assists with initiating trunk extension (25).

The range of motion in the lumbar region is large in flexion and extension, ranging from 8 to 20° at the various levels of the vertebrae (8,72). Lateral flexion at the various levels of the lumbar vertebrae is limited, ranging from 3 to 6°, and there is very little rotation (1 to 2°) at all levels of the lumbar vertebrae (8,72). A review of the range of motion at each level of the vertebral column is presented in Fig. 7-13.

The lumbosacral joint is the most mobile of the lumbar joints, accounting for a large proportion of the flexion and extension in the region. Of the flexion and extension in the lumbar vertebrae, 75% may occur at this joint, with 20% of the remaining flexion at L4–L5 and 5% at the other lumbar levels (59).

COMBINED MOVEMENTS OF THE PELVIS AND TRUNK

The relationship of the movements of the pelvis to the movements of the trunk is discussed in Chapter 6. The movement synchronization between the pelvis and the trunk is referred to as the lumbopelvic rhythm. As shown in Fig. 7-14, the lumbar curve reverses itself, flattens out, and curves in the opposite direction as trunk flexion progresses. This continues to a point at which the low back is

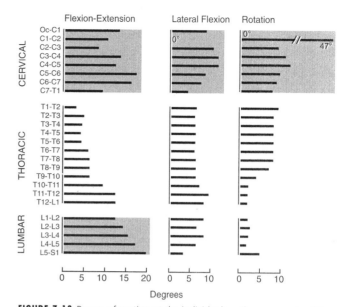

FIGURE 7-13 Range of motion at the individual motion segments of the spine is shown. The cervical vertebrae can produce the most range of motion at the individual motion segments. (Redrawn from White, A. A., Panjabi, M.M. [1978]. Clinical biomechanics of the spine. Philadelphia: Lippincott.)

rounded in full flexion of the trunk. Accompanying the movements in the lumbar vertebrae are flexion of the sacrum, anterior tilt of the pelvis, and finally, extension of the sacrum. The pelvis also moves backward as weight is shifted over the hips.

As discussed earlier in this chapter, lumbar activity is maximum through the first 50 to 60° of flexion, after which pelvic rotation becomes the predominant factor increasing trunk flexion. On the return extension movement, pelvic posterior tilt dominates the initial stages of the extension, and lumbar activity reverses itself, dominating the later stages of trunk extension. The pelvis also moves forward as weight is shifted.

Movement relationships between the pelvis and the trunk during trunk rotation or lateral flexion are not as clear-cut as in flexion and extension, because of restrictions to the movement introduced by the lower extremity. The pelvis will move with the trunk in rotation and rotate

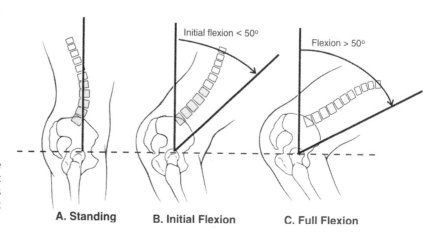

FIGURE 7-14 **A.** In the normal standing posture, there is slight curvature in the lumbar region. **B.** The first 50° of flexion takes place in the lumbar vertebrae as they flatten. **C.** The continuation of flexion is a result of an anterior tilt of the pelvis.

right with trunk right rotation unless the lower extremity is forcing a rotation of the pelvis in the opposite direction. In this case, the pelvis may remain in the neutral position or rotate to the side exerting greater force.

Similarly, in lateral flexion of the trunk, the pelvis will lower to the side of the lateral flexion unless resistance is offered by the lower extremity. The accompanying pelvic movements will be determined by the trunk movement and the unilateral or bilateral positioning of the lower extremity.

MUSCULAR ACTIONS

Trunk extension is an important movement used to raise the trunk and to maintain an upright posture. The muscles actively used to extend the trunk also play dominant roles in trunk flexion; thus it seems logical to review the extensors first.

Trunk Extension

The spinal extensors are graphically presented, and insertion, action, and nerve supply information are provided in Appendix B.

Numerous small muscles constitute the extensor muscle group; however, they can be classified into two groups, the erector spinae (iliocostalis, longissimus, spinalis) and the deep posterior, or paravertebral, muscles (intertransversarii, interspinales, rotatores, multifidus). These muscles run up and down the spinal column in pairs and create extension if activated as a pair or rotation or lateral flexion if activated unilaterally. There is also a superficial layer of muscle that includes the trapezius and the latissimus dorsi. While both the trapezius and the latissimus dorsi can influence trunk motion, they are not discussed in the present chapter.

The three erector spinae muscles constitute the largest mass of muscles contributing to trunk extension. Extension is also produced by contributions from the deep vertebral muscles and other muscles specific to the region. These deep muscles contribute to trunk extension and other trunk movements, and they support the vertebral column, maintain rigidity in the column, and produce some of the finer movements in the motion segment (65).

There are some other muscles besides the erector spinae and the deep posterior muscle groups specific to each region. Appendix B has a full description of these muscles.

The erector spinae muscles are thickest in the cervical and lumbar regions, where most of the extension in the spine occurs. The multifidus is also thickest in the cervical and lumbar regions, adding to the muscle mass for generation of a trunk extension force.

The erector spinae and the multifidus muscles are 57 to 62% Type I muscle fibers but also have both Type IIa and Type IIb fibers, making them functionally versatile so they can generate rapid, forceful movements while still resisting fatigue for the maintenance of postures over long periods (67). In addition to providing the muscle force for extension of the trunk, these muscles provide posterior stability to the vertebral column, counteract gravity in the mainte-

nance of an upright posture, and are important in the control of forward flexion (54).

Trunk Flexion

Flexion of the trunk is free in the cervical region, limited in the thoracic region, and free again in the lumbar region. Unlike the posterior extensor muscles, the anterior flexors do not run the length of the column. Flexion of the lumbar spine is created by the abdominals, with assistance from the psoas major and minor. The flexion force of the abdominals also creates what little flexion there is in the thoracic vertebrae. The abdominals consist of four muscles: the rectus abdominus, the internal oblique, the external oblique, and the transverse abdominus (see Appendix B).

Besides flexing the trunk, the abdominals increase intra-abdominal pressure when they contract. This decreases the compressive force on the spine and reduces the activity of the erector spinae muscles (54,64). As the trunk flexes, the intra-abdominal pressure can assist in flexion by playing a supportive role. This is done by increasing pressure in the trunk cavities, which produces an extension effect, thereby reducing the extensor muscular forces needed to counteract the resistance produced in trunk flexion (7). The transverse abdominus plays a greater role in increasing intra-abdominal pressure than the obliques (64).

Additionally, the internal and external oblique muscles and the transverse abdominus attach into the thoracolumbar fascia covering the posterior region of the trunk. When they contract, they place tension on the fascia, supporting the low back and reducing the strain on the posterior erector spinae muscles (54). The obliques are active in erect posture and in sitting, possibly stabilizing the base of the spine (64). The activity of the obliques drops off in a stooped standing posture as the load is transferred to other structures (64).

The abdominals consist of 55 to 58% Type I fibers, 15 to 23% Type IIa fibers, and 21 to 22% Type IIb fibers (67). This fiber makeup, similar to that in the erector spinae muscles, allows for the same type of versatility in the production of short, rapid movements or prolonged movements of the trunk.

Two other muscles contribute to flexion in the lumbar region. First is the powerful flexor acting at the hip, the iliopsoas muscle, which attaches to the anterior bodies of the lumbar vertebrae and the inside of the ilium. The iliopsoas can initiate trunk flexion and pull the pelvis forward, creating lordotic posture in the lumbar vertebrae. Additionally, if this muscle is tight, an exaggerated anterior tilt of the pelvis may develop. If the tilt is not counteracted by the abdominals, lordosis increases, compressive stress on the facet joints develops, and the intervertebral disc is pushed posteriorly.

The second muscle found in the lumbar region is the quadratus lumborum, which forms the lateral wall of the abdomen and runs from the iliac crest to the last rib (see Appendix B). Although positioned to be more of a lateral flexor, the quadratus lumborum will contribute to the flexion movement. It is also responsible for maintaining pelvic position on the swing side in gait (25).

When a person is standing or sitting upright, there is intermittent activity in both the erector spinae muscles and the internal and external obliques. The iliopsoas, on the other hand, is continuously active in the upright posture, while the rectus abdominus is inactive (62).

Movement into the fully flexed position from a standing posture is initiated by the abdominals and the iliopsoas muscles. Once the movement begins, it is continued by the force of gravity acting on the trunk and controlled by the eccentric action of the erector spinae muscles. There is a gradual increase in the level of activity in the erector spinae muscles up to 50 to 60° of flexion as the trunk flexes at the lumbar vertebrae (4).

As the lumbar vertebrae discontinue their contribution to trunk flexion, the movement continues as a result of the contribution of anterior pelvic tilt. The posterior hip muscles, the hamstrings, and the gluteus maximus eccentrically work to control this forward tilt of the pelvis. As the trunk moves deeper into flexion, the activity in the erector spinae diminishes to total inactivity in the fully flexed position. In this position, the posterior ligaments and the passive resistance of the elongated erector spinae muscles are controlling and resisting the trunk flexion (36). The load on the ligaments in this fully flexed position is close to their failure strength (21), placing additional importance on loads sustained by the thoracolumbar fascia and the lumbar apophyseal joints.

As the trunk rises back to the standing position through extension, the movement is initiated by a contraction of the posterior hip muscles, the gluteus maximus, and the hamstrings, which flex and rotate the pelvis posteriorly. The erector spinae are active initially but are most active through the last 45 to 50° of the extension movement (54).

The erector spinae muscles are more active in the raising than in the lowering phase, being very active in the initial parts of the movements and again at the end of the extension movement, with some diminished activity in the middle of the movement. The abdominals can also be active in the return movement as they serve to control the extension movement (36).

Flexion in the thoracic region, which is limited, is developed by the muscles of the lumbar and cervical regions. In the cervical region are five pairs of muscles producing flexion, if both muscles in the pair are contracting. If only one of the muscles in the pair contracts, the result will be motion in all three directions, including flexion, rotation, and lateral flexion (65). The insertion, action, and nerve supply of these muscles are presented in Appendix B.

Trunk Lateral Flexion

Lateral flexion of the spine is created by contraction of muscles on both sides of the vertebral column, with most activity on the side to which the lateral flexion occurs. The most activity in lateral flexion of the trunk occurs in the lumbar erector spinae muscles and the deep intertransversarii and interspinales muscles on the contralateral side. The multifidus muscle is inactive during lateral flexion. If load is held in the arm during lateral flexion, there is also an increase in the thoracic erector spinae muscles on the opposite side.

The quadratus lumborum and the abdominals also contribute to lateral flexion. The quadratus lumborum on the side of the bend is in a position to make a significant contribution to lateral flexion. The abdominals will also contract as the lateral flexion is initiated and will remain active to modify the lateral flexion movement.

In the cervical spine, lateral flexion is further facilitated by unilateral contractions of the sternocleidomastoid, the scalenes, and the deep anterior muscles. Lateral flexion is quite free in the cervical region.

Trunk Rotation

The rotation of the trunk is more complicated in terms of muscle actions because it is produced by muscle actions on both sides of the vertebral column. In the lumbar region, the multifidus muscles on the side to which the rotation occurs are active, as are the longissimus and iliocostalis on the other side (6). The abdominals exhibit a similar pattern, as the internal oblique on the side of the rotation is active, and the external oblique on the opposite side of the rotation is also active.

STRENGTH AND FORCES AT THE VERTEBRAL JOINTS

Strength

The greatest strength output in the trunk can be developed in extension, averaging values of 210 Nm (newton-meters) for males (41). Reported trunk flexion strength was 150 Nm, or approximately 70% of the strength of the extensors. Lateral flexion was 145 Nm, or 69% of the extensor strength, and rotation strength was 90 Nm, or 43% of the extensor values (41). Female strength values were approximately 60% of the values recorded for males. In fact, other studies have shown women to be capable of generating only 50% of the lifting force of men for lifts low to the ground and 33% of the male lifting force for lifts high off the ground (74).

Taking into consideration all things such as forces generated by intra-abdominal pressure, ligaments, and other structures, the total extensor moment is slightly greater than the flexor moment (55). The abdominals contribute to one-third of the flexor moments and the erector spinae contribute half of the extensor moments. In rotation, the abdominals dominate, with some contribution by the small posterior muscles (55).

Trunk position plays a significant role in the development of strength output in the various movements. Trunk flexion strength, measured isometrically, has been shown to improve by approximately 9% when measured from a position of 20° of hyperextension (65). Isometric trunk extension strength, measured from a position of 20° of trunk flexion, was 22% greater as compared to a 20° trunk flexion position (65). Higher trunk flexion and extension strength values can also be achieved if the measurement is made with the person seated rather than supine or prone.

The strength of the trunk is significantly altered in a dynamic situation. There is a reported 15 to 70% increase in trunk moments during dynamic exertions accompanied by increases in antagonist and agonist muscle activity, an increase in intra-abdominal pressure, an increase in spinal load, and a reduction in the capacity of the muscles to respond to external loads (15). Because of higher levels of coactivity, there is greater loading on the spinal structures without contributing to the ability to offset external moments. It is suggested that trunk velocity and acceleration, especially in multiple directions, may be more accurate discriminators of low-back disorders than just range of motion because of the diminished strength and functional capacity that accompany the coactivation in faster dynamic movements (15).

Strength output while lifting an object using the trunk extensors will also diminish when there is greater horizontal distance between the feet and the hands placed on the object (23). In fact, the forces applied vertically to an object held away from the body are about half those of a lift completed with the object close to the body. Additionally, an increase in the width of a box will decrease lifting capacity, while an increase in the length of a box has been shown to have no influence (23).

Lifting an object by pulling up at an angle reduces the load at the elbow, shoulder, lumbar, and hip regions, but increases it at the knees and ankles. This type of lift decreases the compressive force on the lumbar vertebrae 9 to 15% (24). Also, 16% more weight can be lifted by a more freestyle lift than the traditional straight-back, bent-knee lift (24).

Loads Acting on the Vertebrae

Loads applied to the vertebral column are produced by body weight, muscular force acting on each motion segment, prestress forces due to the disc and ligament forces, and external loads being handled or applied (36). The discs, apophyseal joints, and intervertebral ligaments are the load-bearing structures. Compressive forces are applied perpendicular to the disc; thus the line of action varies with the orientation of the disc. For example, in the lumbar vertebrae, only at the L3–L4 level is the compressive force vertical in upright standing (17). Compression forces are primarily resisted by the disc unless there is disc narrowing, where the resistance is offered by the apophyseal joints (17). For flexion bending moments, 70% of the moment is resisted by the intervertebral ligaments and 30% by the discs and in extension, and two-thirds of the moment is resisted by the apophyseal joints and the neural arch and a third by the discs (17). Lateral bending moments are resisted by the discs, and rotation is resisted by the discs and bony contact at the apophyseal joints (17).

The lumbar vertebrae handle the largest load, primarily because of their positioning, the position of the center of

mass relative to the lumbar region, and greater body weight acting at the lumbar region than other regions of the spine. Of the compressional load carried by the lumbar vertebrae, 18% is a result of the weight of the head and trunk (42). The other source of substantial compression is muscle activity. Muscle forces protect the spine from excessive bending and torsion but subject the spine to high compressive forces. The compressive forces are increased with more lumbar flexion, and it is fairly common to see substantial increases in lumbar flexion with actions such as crossing legs (+35–53%), squatting on the heels (+70–75%), lifting weights from the ground (+70–100%), and rapid lunging movements (+100–110%) (17).

The axial load on the lumbar vertebrae in standing is 700 N. This can quickly increase to values greater than 3000 N when a heavy load is lifted from the ground and can be reduced by almost half in the supine position (300 N) (10). Fortunately, the lumbar spine can resist approximately 9800 N of vertical load before fracturing (45).

The intradiscal pressure in the nucleus at the L3–L4 level for a variety of postures and movements is presented in Table 7-2. Basically, the load on the lumbar vertebrae is more affected by distance of the load from the body than the actual posture of lifting (45). For example, the magnitude of the compressive force acting on the lumbar vertebrae in a half squat is 6 to 10 times body weight (13). If the weight is taken farther as a result of flexion, compressive loads will increase, even with postural adjustments such as flattening the lumbar curve (19).

Loads acting at the lumbar vertebrae can be as high as 2 to 2.5 times body weight in an activity such as walking (12). These loads are maximum at toe-off and increase with an increase in walking speed. Loads on the vertebrae in an activity such as walking are a result of muscle activity in the extensors and the amount of trunk lean in the walker (36).

The direction of the force or load acting on the vertebrae is influenced by positioning. In a standing posture with the sacrum inclined 30° to the vertical, there is a

TABLE 7-2 L3 to L4 Intradiscal Pressure and Compressive Forces

Activity	Intradiscal Pressure (kPA)	Spinal Compressive Force (N)
Standing	270	380
Flexion (414 Nm)	710	990
Extension (28 Nm)	720	1010
Lateral flex (43 Nm)	620	870
Twisting (28 Nm)	480	670
Flexion to 30°, 4 kg in each hand	1620	2270

Adapted from Nachemson, A., Morris, J. M. (1964). In vivo measurements of intradiscal pressure: Discometry, a method for the determination of pressure in the lower lumbar discs. *Journal of Bone and Joint Surgery*, 46-A:1077–1092.

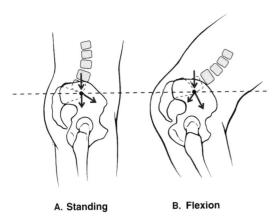

A. Standing   **B. Flexion**

FIGURE 7-15 A. The shear force across the lumbosacral joint in standing is approximately 50% of the body weight. **B.** If one flexes to where the sacral angle increases to 50°, the shear force can increase to as much as 75% of the body weight above the joint.

shear force acting across the lumbosacral joint that is approximately 50% of the body weight above the joint (Fig. 7-15). If the sacral angle increases to 40°, the shear force increases to 65% of the body weight, and with a 50° sacral inclination, the force acting across the joint is 75% of the body weight above the joint (59).

Lumbosacral loads are also high in exercises such as the squat, in which maximum forces are generated at the so-called sticking point of the ascent. These loads are higher than loads recorded at either the knee or the hip for the same activity (48).

Loads are applied to the lumbar vertebrae even in a relaxed supine position of repose. The loads are significantly reduced because of the loss of the body weight forces but still present as a result of muscular and ligamentous forces. In fact, the straight-leg lying position imposes load on the lumbar vertebrae because of the pull of the psoas muscle. Flexing the thigh by placing a pillow under the knees can reduce this load.

Loads imposed upon the vertebrae are carried by the various structural elements of the segment. The articulating facets carry large loads in the lumbar vertebrae during extension, torsion, and lateral bending but no loads in flexion (60). Facet loads in extension have been shown to be as high as 30 to 50% of the total spine load, and in the arthritic joint, the percentage can be higher (27). The posterior and anterior ligaments carry loads in flexion and extension, respectively, but carry little load in lateral bending and torsion. The intervertebral discs absorb and distribute a great proportion of the load imposed upon the vertebrae. The intradiscal pressure is 1.3 to 1.5 times the compressional load applied per unit area of disc (45,61), and the pressure increases linearly with loads up to 2000 N (44). The load on the third lumbar vertebra in standing is approximately 60% of total body weight (46).

Pressures in sitting are 40% more than those in standing, though standing interdiscal pressures can be reduced by placing one foot in front of the other and elevating it (65). In standing, the natural curvature of the lumbar spine is increased, whereas in sitting, the curvature is reduced. The increased curvature reduces the pressure in the nucleus pulposus, while at the same time it increases loading of the apophyseal joints and increases compression on the posterior annulus fibrosus fibers (1). Pressures within the disc are large with flexion and lateral flexion movements of the trunk and small with extension and rotation (47). The pressure increases can be attributed to tension generated in the ligaments, which can increase intradiscal pressure by 100% or more in full flexion (1). The lateral bend produces larger pressures than flexion and even more pressure if rotation added to the side bend causes asymmetrical bending and compression (6).

Intervertebral discs have been shown to withstand compressive loads in the range of 2500 to 7650 N (52). In older individuals, the range is much smaller, and in individuals younger than 40, the range is much larger (52).

The posterior elements of the spinal segment assist with load bearing. When the spine is under compression, the load is supported partially by the pedicles and pars interarticularis and somewhat by the apophyseal joints. When compression and bending loads are applied to the spine, 25% of the load is carried by the apophyseal joints. Only 16% of the loads imposed by compressive and shear forces are carried by the apophyseal joints (42). Any extension of the spine is accompanied by an increase in the compressive strain on the pedicles, an increase in both compressive and tensile strain in the pars articularis, and an increase in the compressive force acting at the apophyseal joints (31).

In full trunk flexion, the loads are maintained and absorbed by the apophyseal capsular ligaments, the intervertebral disc, the supraspinous and interspinous ligaments, and the ligamentum flavum, in that order (3). The erector spinae muscles also offer some resistance passively.

In compression, most of the load is carried by the disc and the vertebral body. The vertebral body is susceptible to injury before the disc and will fail at compressive loads of only 3700 N in the elderly and 13,000 in a young, healthy adult (35). In rotation, during which torsional forces are applied, the apophyseal joints are more susceptible to injury, and during a forward bend movement, the disc and the apophyseal joints are at risk for injury because of compressive forces on the anterior motion segment and tensile forces on the posterior elements.

Loads in the cervical region of the spine are lower than in the thoracic or lumbar region and vary with position of the head, becoming significant in extreme positions of flexion and extension (63). Loads on the lumbar disc have been calculated using a miniaturized pressure transducer (45). Approximate loads for various postures and exercises are presented in Fig. 7-16 although the researchers recommend caution about the interpretation of absolute values and direct more attention to the relative values (45). Recent studies have demonstrated that the compressive load on the low back can be greater than 3000 N in exercises such as sit-ups, and a sit-up with the feet fixed results

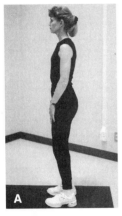
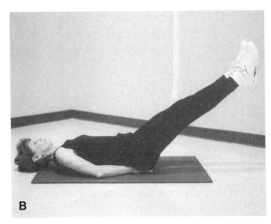
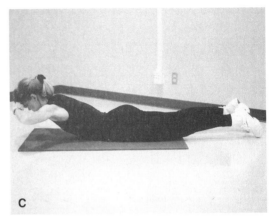

LOWEST

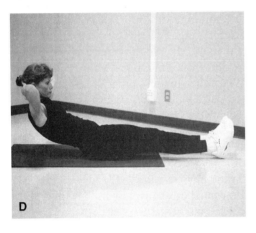
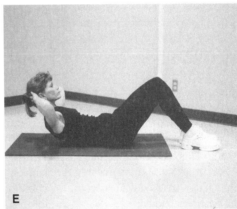
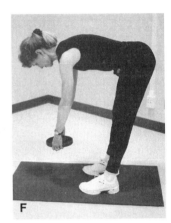

HIGHEST

FIGURE 7-16 The representative postures or movements are shown in order of calculated load on the lumbar vertebrae using a miniaturized pressure transducer. The standing posture imposed the least amount of load (686 N) **(A)**, followed by the double straight-leg raise (1176 N) **(B)**, back hyperextension (1470 N) **(C)**, sit-ups with knees straight (1715 N) **(D)**, sit-ups with knees bent (1764 N) **(E)**, and bending forward with weight in the hands (1813 N) **(F)**. (Adapted with permission from Nachemson, A. [1976]. Lumbar intradiscal pressure. In M. Jayson [Ed.]. *The Lumbar Spine and Back Pain*. Kent: Pitman Medical.)

in similar loads whether the bent-knee or straight-leg technique is used (38).

POSTURE

Efficiency of motion and stresses imposed upon the spine are very much determined by the posture maintained in the trunk. Positioning of the vertebral segments is so important that a special section on posture is warranted.

Standing Posture

To maintain an upright posture in standing, the S-shaped spine acts as an elastic rod in supporting the weight. A continuous forward bending action is imposed upon the trunk in standing, since the center of gravity lies in front of the spine. As a result of the forward bending action on the trunk, the posterior muscles and ligaments must control and maintain the standing posture.

There is more erector spinae activity in an erect posture than in a slouched posture. In the slouched posture, most of the responsibility for maintaining the posture is passed

on to the ligaments and capsules. Any disruption in the standing posture or any postural swaying is controlled and brought back into alignment by the erector spinae, the abdominals, and the psoas muscles (50). All of these muscles are slightly active in standing, with more activity in the thoracic region than the other two regions (6).

Sitting Posture

Posture in the sitting position requires less energy expenditure and imposes less load on the lower extremity than standing. However, prolonged sitting can have deleterious effects on the lumbar spine (65). Unsupported sitting is similar to standing, such that there is high muscle activity in the thoracic regions of the trunk with accompanying low levels of activity in the abdominals and the psoas muscles (5).

The unsupported sitting position places more load on the lumbar spine than standing because it creates a backward tilt, a flattening of the low back, and a corresponding forward shift in the center of gravity (36). This places load on the discs and the posterior structures of the vertebral segment. Sitting long in the flexed position may increase the resting length of the erector spinae muscles (54) and overstretch the posterior ligamentous structures.

Continuous flexion positions are a cause of both lumbar and cervical flexion injuries in the workplace. These postures can be eliminated by raising the height of the work station so that no more than 20° of flexion is present (65). The use of a footrest can also relieve strain. A fully flexed spine should be avoided in any lift because of the changes imposed on the major lumbar extensors. The fully flexed spine reduces the moment arms for the extensor muscles, decreases the tolerance to compressive loads, and transfers load from the muscles to the passive tissues (39). The workplace also has a high incidence of twisting, in which the spine undergoes combined flexion and lateral bending. This posture maximally stretches the posterolateral structures, particularly the annulus (53). Twisting in the upright posture is limited by contact at the facet joints, while twisting in a flexed posture disengages the facet joints and shifts the resistance to the annulus fibrosus (37).

In supported sitting, the load on the lumbar vertebrae is lessened. A chair back reclined slightly backward and including lumbar support creates a seated posture that produces the least load on the lumbar region of the spine. Both the intradiscal pressure and the muscle activity in the trunk are decreased in this position (62).

Postural Deviations

Postural deviations in the trunk are common in the general population (Fig. 7-17). In the cervical region, the curve is concave to the anterior side. This curve should be small and lie over the shoulder girdle. The head should be above the shoulder girdle. When the cervical curve is accentuated to the anterior side, lordosis is said to be present. Thus, cervical lordosis is an increase in the curve in the cervical region, often concomitant with exaggerated curves in other regions of the spine.

In the thoracic region, the curvature is concave to the posterior side. A rounded-shoulder posture may cause thoracic kyphosis, a common postural disorder in this region. The kyphotic thoracic region is also associated with osteoporosis and several other disorders.

The lumbar region, curving anteriorly, is subjected to forces that may be created by an exaggerated lumbar curve, termed lumbar lordosis or hyperlordosis. This accentuated swayback position is often created by anterior positioning of the pelvis or by weak abdominals. In the lumbar region, it is also not uncommon to have a flat back with decreased lumbar curve. This has been associated with a pelvis that is inclined upward at the front or with muscle tightness and rigidity in the spine.

The most serious of the postural disorders affecting the spine is scoliosis, a lateral deviation of the spine. The curve can be C-shaped or S-shaped depending on the direction and the beginning and ending segments. C-shaped scoliosis is designated when the deviation occurs in one region only. For example, a convex curve to the left in the cervical region would be termed a left cervical C-shaped curve. In an S-shaped curve, the lateral deviation occurs in different regions and in opposite directions, as with a right thoracic, left lumbar convexity. Rotation can accompany the lateral deviation, creating a very complex postural malalignment. The cause of scoliosis is unknown, and it is more prevalent in females than in males.

CONDITIONING

The muscles around the trunk are active during most activities as they stabilize the trunk, move the trunk into an advantageous position for supplementing force production, or assist limb movement. Since the low back is a common site of injury in sports and in the workplace, special attention should be given to exercises that strengthen and stretch this part of the trunk. Trunk exercises should also be evaluated for negative impact on trunk function and structure.

Exercises creating excessive lordosis or hyperextension of the lumbar vertebrae should be avoided, since they put excessive pressure on the posterior element of the spinal segment and can disrupt the facets or the posterior arch. Examples of such exercises are the double leg raise, double leg raise with scissoring, thigh extension from the prone position, donkey kicks, back bends, and ballet arches. When selecting an exercise for the trunk, pay attention to its risks. The supine position produces the least amount of load on the lumbar vertebrae. However, the load in the supine position increases substantially if the abdominals and the iliopsoas are activated.

Trunk Flexors

The trunk flexors are usually exercised with some form of trunk or thigh flexion exercise from the supine position so that these muscles can work against gravity. Trunk flexion

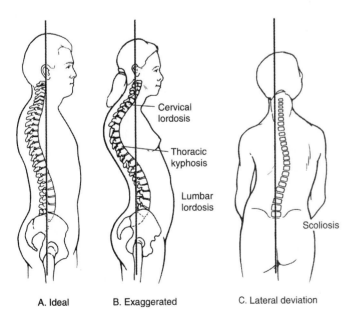

A. Ideal   B. Exaggerated   C. Lateral deviation

FIGURE 7-17 **A.** The ideal posture is one in which the curves are balanced but not exaggerated. **B.** Curves can become exaggerated. **C.** Lateral deviation of the spine, scoliosis, can create serious postural malalignment throughout the whole body.

exercises should be evaluated for their effectiveness and safety. The sit-up has been done for many years. It involves trunk flexion from the supine position with the legs fully extended. Sometimes the feet are secured by a partner or an external support. This exercise is performed by a contraction of both the rectus abdominus and the obliques during the first 37 to 40° of trunk flexion, followed by hip flexor activity that continues the sit-up through the remainder of the motion (54,65). Dynamic sit-ups have been shown not to challenge the abdominals over the length range (38).

The long-lying sit-up position can cause an anterior movement of the fifth lumbar vertebra on the sacrum. Also, the muscular force of the flexors in the midrange of motion may create additional stress on the lumbar vertebrae by increasing the lordosis. However, there is some evidence to suggest that there is very little change in spinal curvature during a sit-up (38), which may discount some of the influence of the psoas. The psoas may in fact stabilize the lumbar spine by creating a compressive force with bilateral loading even though it has the potential to create large anterior shear forces (33).

The curl-up or hook-lying position, with the knees flexed and the feet on the floor close to the buttocks, may reduce the amount of lordosis in the lumbar spine by forcing the pelvis posteriorly. The tradeoff in the reduction of lordosis is an increase in the intervertebral disc pressure over pressures measured in the long-lying sit-up (54). If a trunk raise is performed from this position, the abdominals are still the most active muscles through the initial 30 to 45°, and the hip flexors are active through the remainder of the flexion movement (54,65). The rectus abdominus appears to be more active in the hook-lying curl-up than the long-lying sit-up (65). As in the sit-up, the contribution from the hip flexors is greater if the feet are held.

This exercise is often performed quickly in a predetermined time to measure abdominal endurance and strength. This type of test should be used with caution, especially with individuals having low-back pain, since rapid flexion exercises stress the posterior structures (49). Repeating this exercise quickly forces the hip flexors to become more active as the abdominals fatigue (54).

The double leg raise has also been used to strengthen the abdominals, and it does activate both the rectus abdominus and the external obliques (65). This exercise engages the hip flexors to a greater degree than the other abdominal exercises, creating a great deal of lordosis in the lumbar spine. The strain on the low back is significant enough to label this exercise as contraindicated for those with weak abdominals. The exercise can be modified to a single-leg raise with the contralateral limb flexed at the knee and the foot flat on the floor, as in the hook-lying position.

There is no one single best exercise for all abdominals at once. The best exercise for the rectus abdominus that maximizes activation and minimizes psoas activation is the arm-cross curl, and the best exercise for the obliques is a side-supported position held either isometrically or dynamically (33). Trunk flexion stretching and strengthening exercises are demonstrated in Fig. 7-18.

Trunk Extensors

Extension of the trunk is usually developed through some type of lift using the legs and back. Refer to Fig. 7-19 for examples of extensor exercises for stretching and strengthening these muscles.

Two basic types of lifts will activate the erector spinae: the leg lift and the back lift. The leg lift is the squat or dead-lift exercise in which the back is maintained in an erect or slightly flexed posture and the knees are flexed. This lift has the least amount of erector spinae activity and imposes the lowest shear and compressive forces on the spine (56). The leg lift is begun with posterior tilt of the pelvis initiated by the gluteus maximus and the hamstrings. The erector spinae can be delayed and not involved until later in the leg lift, when the extension is increased. The delay is related to the magnitude of the weight being lifted, and the muscles usually do not become active until the initial acceleration is completed (4). Since there is considerable stress on the ligaments at the beginning of the lift, it is suggested that the erector spinae activity begin at the initial part of the lift to stabilize the back (36).

In the back lift, the person bends over at the waist with the knees straight, as in the good morning exercise. This exercise creates the highest shear and compressive stress on the lumbar vertebrae, but the erector spinae are much more active in this type of exercise (56). In the back lift, the movement is initiated by the hamstrings and the gluteus maximus and then followed up by activity from the erector spinae. Extension of the spine begins approximately a third of the way into the lift (4). In performing the back lift with no load, the erector spinae becomes active after the beginning of the lift, but if the lift is performed with weight, the erector spinae is active before the start of the lift (66).

In comparing leg lifts and back lifts, one must consider both the risks and the gains. The back lift imposes a greater risk of injury to the vertebrae because of the higher forces imposed upon the system. Any stooping posture of the trunk will impose greater compression forces on the spine; consequently, a trunk flexion posture in a lift should be discouraged (14). The disc pressures are much higher in the back lift than in the leg lift, mainly because of the trunk position and distance (46). The erector spinae activity in the back lift is greater than that in the leg lift.

Trunk extensor activity increases with increases in trunk lean, while knee extension activity decreases as trunk lean decreases (40). Maximal erector spinae activity also occurs later in the back lift than the leg lift. Finally, the abdominal activity is lower in the back lift than in the leg lift (66). Consequently, the back is not as well supported in the back lift as it is in the leg lift, creating additional potential for injury.

It is believed that some of the load on the vertebrae in a lifting activity can be partially reduced by intra-abdominal pressure. The intra-abdominal pressure in lifting increases

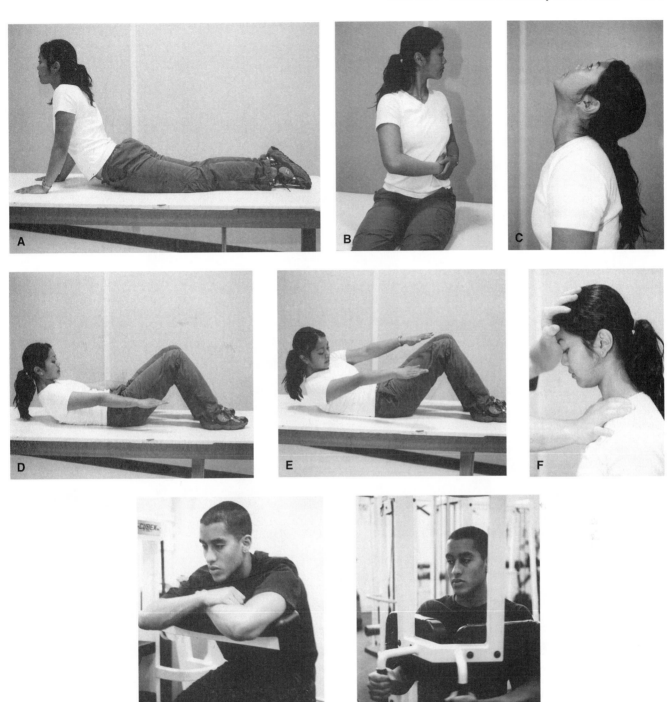

FIGURE 7-18 Flexibility, manual or low resistance, and high resistance exercises are presented for the abdominals: whole group (*left*), the obliques (*middle*), and the cervical vertebrae (*right*). To stretch the flexors, back hyperextension with pelvis maintained on the floor **(A)**, rotation **(B)**, or neck hyperextension exercise **(C)** is used. Low or manual resistance exercises for the flexors include a cross-crunch (rectus abdominus) **(D)**, side bend (static or dynamic) (obliques) **(E)**, and manual resistance applied to the forehead during neck flexion (cervical) **(F)**. Higher-resistance weight-training exercises include flexion **(G)** and rotation **(H)** on a trunk machine. Weight training for cervical flexion is also available on a neck machine but not usually recommended.

with an increase in the weight being lifted, is greater in dynamic lifting than in static lifting, and increases with forward bending of the trunk (4). It is also greater in leg lifting than in back lifting (14). This may be due to the increased activity in the abdominals seen in the leg lift or to the greater

pressure developed in the push movement of the leg lift as compared to the pull movement of the back lift (14).

Maximal intra-abdominal pressure occurs at the bottom of the lift and is increased if one uses a weight belt. The hypothesized effect of greater intra-abdominal pressure is

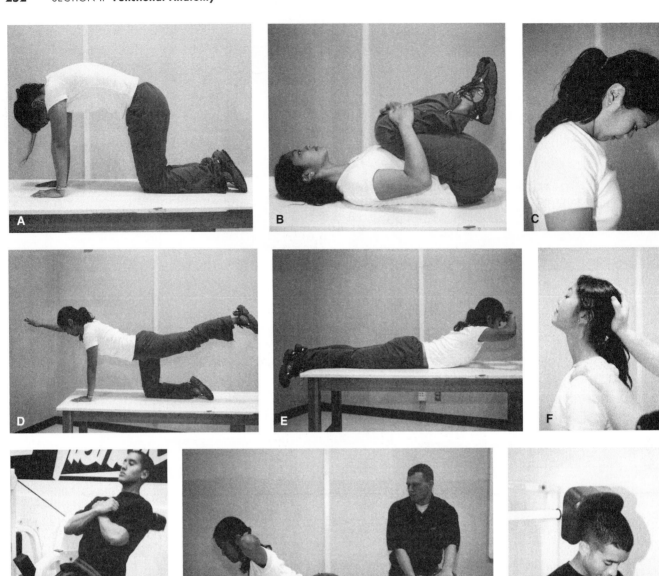

FIGURE 7-19 Flexibility, manual or low resistance, and high-resistance or weight-training exercises are presented for the low back and for the cervical regions of the trunk. The low back can be stretched with back rounding **(A)** or a knee tuck **(B)**, and the neck can be stretched with a simple flexion movement **(C)**. Manual or low-resistance exercises include a diagonal leg and arm lift **(D)**, back hyperextensions **(E)**, and manual resistance during neck hyperextension **(F)**. High-resistance or weight-training exercises for the extensors include exercises on a trunk machine **(G)** and back hyperextensions with the feet supported **(H)**. High-resistance exercises for the trunk extensors **(I)** are contraindicated for individuals with low back problems. High-resistance weight training for the cervical region is usually avoided except when athletes need to develop strong neck muscles.

that it creates an extensor moment that reduces some of the load from the erector spinae muscles. The net effect is smaller forces on the lumbosacral joint (35).

To work the extensors from the standing position by hyperextending the trunk requires an initial contribution from the erector spinae. This activity drops off and then picks up again later in the hyperextension movement (51). If resistance to the movement is offered, the activity in the lumbar erector spinae movement increases dramatically (32).

Trunk Rotators and Lateral Flexors

The rotation and lateral flexion movements of the trunk are not usually emphasized in an exercise program. Some examples of rotation and lateral bending exercises are provided in Fig. 7-20. There is some benefit to including some of these exercises in a training routine, since rotation is an important component of many movement patterns. Likewise, lateral flexion is an important component of activities such as throwing, diving, and gymnastics.

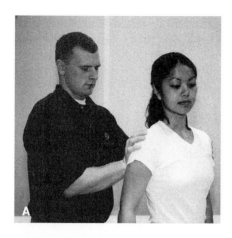

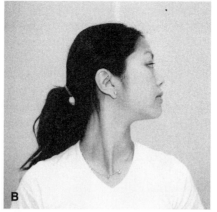

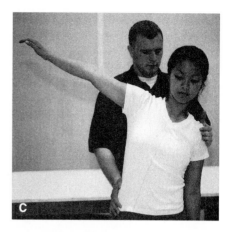

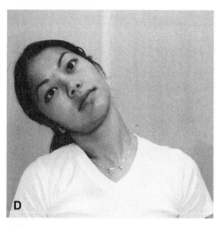

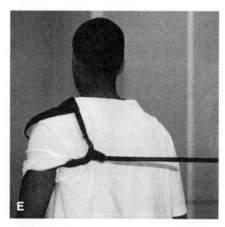

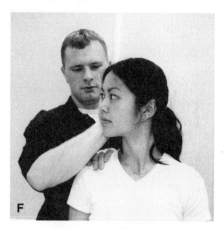

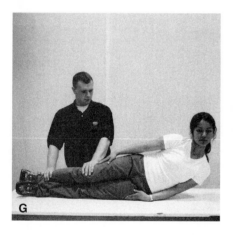

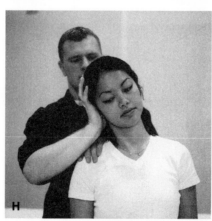

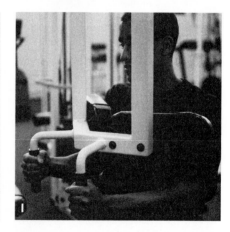

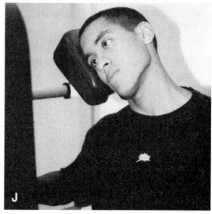

FIGURE 7-20 Flexibility exercises are provided for the trunk rotators, cervical rotators, trunk lateral flexors, and cervical lateral flexors. The trunk rotators can be stretched by applying a passive force to rotate the trunk **(A)** or by moving through maximum trunk or head rotation **(B)**. Likewise, the trunk and neck can be stretched in lateral flexion either passively **(C)** or through an active movement **(D)** sideways with the head or trunk. Manual or low-resistance exercises for the rotators and lateral flexors include the use of surgical tubing **(E)**, manual resistance to the side of the head during a rotation or lateral flexion movement **(F and H)**, and lateral raise of the trunk with the feet stabilized **(G)**. High-resistance or weight-training exercises for the rotators or lateral flexors are usually done on specialized machines, such as the trunk machine **(I and J)**.

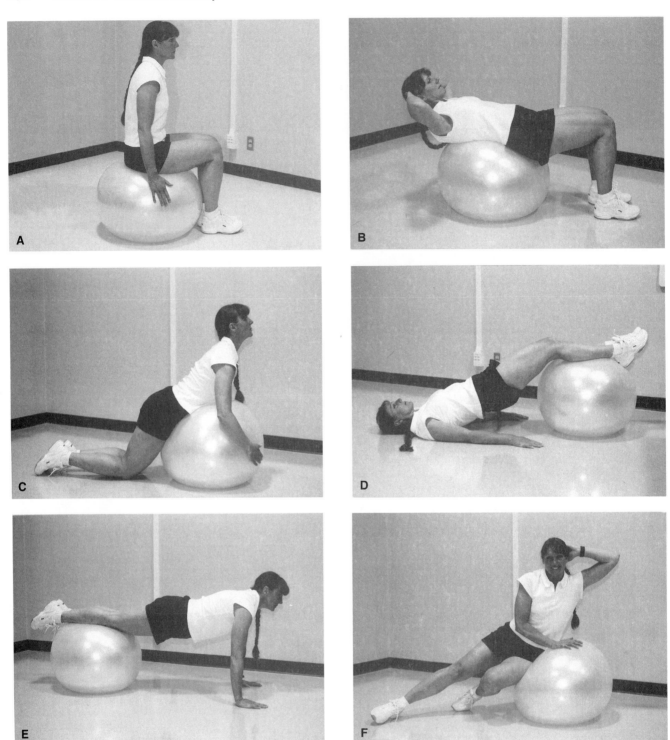

FIGURE 7-21 Ball exercises. **A.** Balancing in an upright sitting position is good for overall posture using both flexors and extensors. **B.** The flexors can specifically be exercised by curling the upper trunk while lying on the ball. Trunk extensors can be exercised in isolation **(C)** or in conjunction with hamstrings and the gluteus maximus **(D and E)**. **F.** Ball exercises can be made progressively more difficult by increasing the distance of the ball from the body. Lateral flexors can be similarly exercised.

Some individuals try to isolate the obliques by performing trunk rotation exercises against external resistance. The obliques are not isolated in this type of exercise, since the erector spinae muscles are also actively involved. If a rotation exercise is added to an exercise set, caution should be used. No combined exercises should be performed in which the trunk is flexed or extended and then rotated. This loads the vertebrae excessively and unnecessarily. If rotation is to be included, it should be done in isolation. The same holds true for lateral flexion exercises that can be performed against a resistance from a stand or from the side-lying position.

Many strength routines for the trunk incorporate the use of an exercise ball. The advantage of exercises using the ball is the improvement in posture because of the ongoing spine stabilization that is required while sitting or balancing on the ball. Exercises can progress from easy to hard depending on the distance of the ball from the body. Fig. 7-21 illustrates some typical ball exercises for the trunk muscles.

Stretching of the trunk muscles is easy and can be done from a standing or lying position. The lying positions offer stabilization of the lower extremity and the pelvis, which will contribute to the movements if the exercise is performed from a stand. All stretching of the trunk muscles should be done through one plane only, since movements through more than one plane at a time will excessively load the vertebral segments.

Use caution in prescribing maximum trunk flexion exercises, such as touching the toes for the stretch of the extensors. Remember, the trunk is supported by the ligaments and the posterior elements of the segment in this position, and the loads on the discs are large, so choose an alternative exercise.

Similarly, the sit–reach test is often used as a measure of both low-back and hamstring flexibility. It has been recently suggested that the sit–reach is primarily an assessment of hamstring, not low-back, flexibility (54). The sit–reach position has also been shown to increase the strain on the low back as a result of exaggerated posterior tilt of the pelvis. It is recommended that the sit–reach stretching exercise be done while maintaining a mild lordotic lumbar curve throughout to avoid the exaggerated curve.

Inflexibility in the trunk or posterior thigh will influence the load and strains incurred during exercise. If the low back is inflexible, the reversal of the lumbar curve is restrained in forward flexion movements. This places an additional strain on the hamstrings. If the hamstrings are inflexible, rotation of the pelvis is restricted, placing additional strain on the low-back muscles and ligaments. Additionally, inhibition of forward rotation of the pelvis will increase the overall compressive stress on the spine (54).

CONTRIBUTION OF TRUNK MUSCLES TO SPORTS SKILLS OR MOVEMENTS

The contribution of the back muscles to lifting has been presented in an earlier discussion. Likewise, the contribution of the abdominals to a sit-up or curl-up exercise was evaluated. The trunk muscles also contribute to activities such as walking and running. A summary of the contributions of the trunk muscles to walking and running is presented in Fig. 7-22.

In walking, the trunk moves side to side as one segment. At touchdown, the trunk flexes toward the side of the limb making contact with the ground. It also moves back, and both of these movements are maximum at the end of the double support phase. After moving into single support, the trunk moves forward while still maintaining

lateral flexion toward the support limb (69). As the speed of walking increases, there is a corresponding increase in lumbar range of motion accompanied by higher muscle activation levels (11).

For running, the movements in the support phase are much the same, with trunk flexion and lateral flexion to the support side. One difference is that in walking, there is trunk extension at touchdown, whereas in running, the trunk will be flexed at touchdown only at fast speeds (68). At slower speeds, the trunk will be extended at touchdown. For a full cycle in both running and walking, the trunk will move forward and backward twice per cycle.

Another difference between walking and running is the amount and duration of lateral flexion in the support

Trunk extensor muscle activity during walking and running.

Muscles	Swing Phase (Ipsilateral)			Support Phase (Ipsilateral)		
WALKING (1.5 m/s)	R	FS	FD	HS	MS	TO
Multifidus						
Ipsilateral	***	*	**	**	*	*
Contralateral	***	*	*	***	**	*
Longissimus						
Ipsilateral	***	*	*	*	*	*
Contralateral	**	*	*	***	*	*

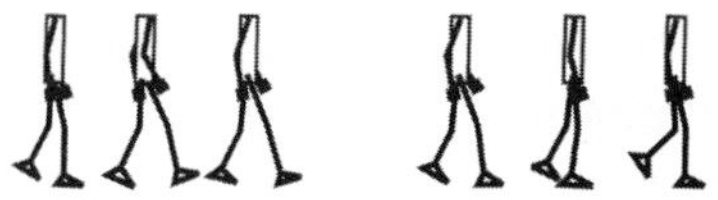

Muscles	Swing Phase (Ipsilateral)			Support Phase (Ipsilateral)		
RUNNING (5 m/s)	R	FS	FD	HS	MS	TO
Multifidus						
Ipsilateral	***	*	**	***	*	**
Contralateral	***	*	*	***	*	**
Longissimus						
Ipsilateral	*	**	**	***	*	**
Contralateral	***	*	*	***	*	**

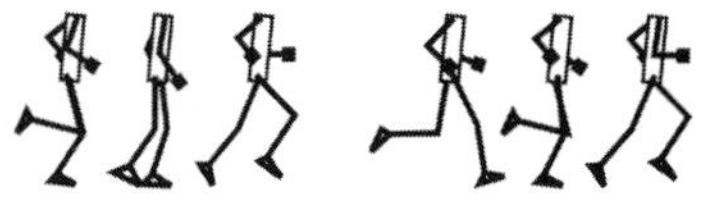

* = low activity
** = moderate activity
*** = high activity

FIGURE 7-22 The trunk extensors are active in both walking and running as they work to control the flexion and lateral flexion of the trunk (Adapted from Thorstensson, et al., 1980; 1982). Trunk extensor muscle activity during walking and running.

phase. In running, the amount of lateral flexion is greater, but lateral flexion is held longer in the maximal position in walking than in running (69). There is one full oscillation of lateral flexion from one side to the other for every walking and running cycle.

As contact is made with the ground in both running and walking, there is a burst of activity in the longissimus and multifidus muscles. This activity can begin just before contact, usually as an ipsilateral contraction to control the lateral bending of the trunk. It is followed up with a contraction of the contralateral erector spinae muscles, so that both sides contract (68).

There is a second burst of activity in these muscles in the middle of the cycle, occurring with contact of the other limb. Here, both the longissimus and the multifidus are again active. In the first burst of activity, the ipsilateral muscles are more active, while in this second burst, the contralateral muscles are more active (68). The activity of the erector spinae muscles coincides with extensor activity at the hip, knee, and ankle joints.

The lumbar muscles serve to restrict locomotion by controlling the lateral flexion and the forward flexion of the trunk (68). Cervical muscles serve to maintain the head in an erect position on the trunk and are not as active as the muscles in other regions of the spine.

INJURY POTENTIAL IN THE TRUNK

The incidence of injury to the trunk is very high, for in the general population, 60 to 80% will have back pain at some time in their lives (8). Low-back pain is a chronic problem for 1 to 5% of the population and recurs in 30 to 70% of those with an initial low-back problem (54). The sexes are affected equally. Low-back pain is most common in the age range of 25 to 60, with the highest incidence of low-back pain at age 40 (54). Back pain is uncommon in children and athletes. Back sprain accounts for only 2 to 3% of the total sprains in the athletic population (16), but it is very debilitating. Back pain is a particular problem in sports that require high levels of bending and rotation, such as golf, gymnastics, and baseball.

Back pain can be caused by compression on the spinal cord or nerve roots from an intervertebral disc protrusion or disc prolapse. Disc protrusions occur most frequently at the intervertebral junctions of C5–C6, C6–C7, L4–L5, and L5–S1 (34). Lumbar disc protrusions occur at a significantly higher rate than in any other region of the trunk. As shown in Fig. 7-23, the disc protrusion may impinge upon the nerve exiting from the cord, causing problems throughout the back and the lower extremity.

A disc injury commonly occurs to a motion segment that is compressed while being flexed slightly more than the normal limits of motion (3). Also, a significant amount of torsion, or rotation, of the trunk has been shown to tear fibers in the annulus fibrosus of the disc. Pure compression to the spine usually injures the vertebral bodies and end plates rather than the disc. Likewise, maximal flexion of the

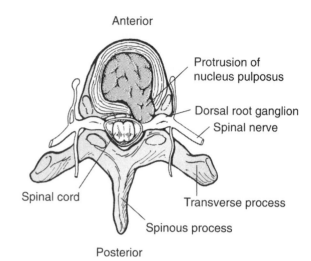

FIGURE 7-23 Injury to a disc can be caused by extreme trunk flexion while the trunk is compressed or loaded. Rotation movements can also tear the disc. When a disc is ruptured, pressure can be put on the spinal nerves.

trunk without compression will injure the posterior ligaments of the arch rather than the disc (3).

In the case of a disc prolapse, the nucleus pulposus extrudes into the annulus fibrosus either laterally or vertically. Vertical prolapse is more common than posterior prolapse, and the result is an anterolateral bulge of the annulus. This causes the bodies to tilt forward and pivot on the apophyseal joints, placing stress on the facets (70). A posterior or posterolateral prolapse of the disc into the spinal canal creates back pain and neurological symptoms via nerve impingement. Schmorl's nodes is a condition in which a vertical prolapse of part of the nucleus pulposus protrudes into an end plate lesion of the adjacent vertebrae (29). Damage to the disc is created through excessive load, failure of the inner posterior annulus fibers, or disc degeneration (8).

Disc degeneration in the early elderly years consists of a gradual process during which splits and tears develop in the disc tissue. The progression of disc degeneration is illustrated in Fig. 7-24. Although the symptoms of disc degeneration may not appear until the early elderly years, the process may begin much earlier in life. It is common for disc degeneration to begin as the posterior muscles and ligaments relax, compressing the anterior portion and putting tension on the posterior portion of the disc. The tears in the disc are usually parallel to the end plates halfway between the end plate and the middle of the disc (70). As these tears get larger, there is potential for separation of the central portion of the disc. The splits and tears usually occur in the posterior and posterolateral portions of the disc along the posterior border of the marginal edges of the vertebral bodies (70). Eventually, the tears may be filled with connective tissue and later with bone. Osteophytes develop on the periphery of the vertebral bodies, and cancellous bone is gradually laid down in the anterior portion of the disc where the pressure is great.

Progression

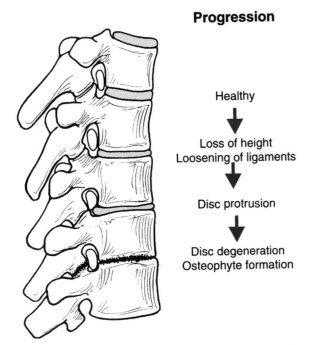

Healthy

Loss of height
Loosening of ligaments

Disc protrusion

Disc degeneration
Osteophyte formation

FIGURE 7-24 Disc degeneration narrows the joint space, causing a shortening of the ligaments, increased pressure on the disc, and stress on the apophyseal joints.

This condition can progress to a point of forming an osseous connection between two vertebral bodies that leads to further necrosis of the disc. Osteoarthritis of the apophyseal joints is also a by-product of disc degeneration as added stress is placed on these joints. A disc that has undergone slight degeneration is also more susceptible to prolapse (3).

There can be fractures of the various osseous components of the vertebrae. The fractures can be in the spinous processes, transverse processes, or laminae, or they can be compressive fractures of the vertebral body itself. Spondylolysis, shown in Fig. 7-25, involves a fatigue fracture of the posterior neural arch at the pars interarticularis. This injury is most common in sports requiring repeated flexion, extension, and rotation, such as gymnastics, weightlifting, football, dance, and wrestling (58). There is a 20.7% incidence of spondylolysis in athletes (30).

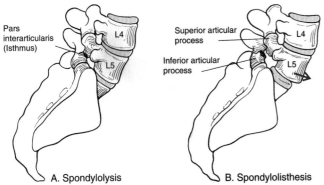

Pars
interarticularis
(Isthmus)

L4
L5

A. Spondylolysis

Superior articular
process

Inferior articular
process

L4
L5

B. Spondylolisthesis

FIGURE 7-25 A. A fatigue fracture to the pars interarticularis is called spondylolysis. **B.** When the fracture occurs bilaterally, spondylolisthesis develops.

A typical example of an athlete who may fracture the neural arch is the football lineman. The lineman assumes a starting position in a three- or four-point stance with the trunk flexed. This flattens the low back, compresses and narrows the anterior portion of the disc, and stresses the transverse arch. When the lineman drives up with trunk extension and makes contact with an opponent, a large shear force across the apophyseal joint is created (58).

Another example of a spondylolysis-causing activity is pole vaulting. The vaulter extends the trunk at the plant and follows with rapid flexion of the trunk (57). The large range of motion occurring with rapid acceleration and deceleration is responsible for the development of the stress fracture. This condition is usually associated with repetitive activities, seldom with a single traumatic event (8).

With spondylolysis on both sides, spondylolisthesis can develop (Fig. 7-25). With a bilateral defect of the neural arch, the motion segment is unstable, and the anterior and posterior elements separate. The top vertebrae slip anteriorly over the bottom vertebrae. This condition is most common in the lumbar vertebrae, especially at the site of L5–S1, where shear forces are often high. The condition worsens with flexion of the spine, which adds to the anterior shear on the motion segment (71).

The cervical, thoracic, and lumbar regions of the trunk are subject to their specific injuries. In the cervical region of the spine, flexion and extension injuries, or whiplash injuries, are common. In whiplash, the head is rapidly flexed, straining the posterior ligaments or even dislocating the posterior apophyseal joints if the force is large (63). The rapid acceleration and deceleration of the head causes both sprain and muscular strain in the cervical region. During a rear-end impact the body is thrown forward and the head is forced into hyperextension. This is followed by a rapid jerk of the head forward into flexion. This forceful whiplash can fracture the vertebral bodies through the wedging action in the flexion movement, which compresses the bodies together. The seventh cervical vertebra is a likely site of fracture in a flexion injury.

Flexion and compression injuries are also common in the cervical vertebrae and seen in sports such as football and diving. The cervical spine straightens with flexion, creating a columnlike structure that lacks flexibility when contact is made. The discs, vertebral bodies, process, and ligaments resist this load, and when capacity is exceeded, vertebral dislocation and spinal cord impingement can result.

Injuries to the cervical vertebrae as a result of forceful extension include rupture of the anterior longitudinal ligament and actual separation of the annulus fibers of the disc from the vertebrae. Forceful hyperextension of the spine can be a part of whiplash injury, usually affecting the sixth cervical vertebra (65).

The cervical vertebrae are susceptible to injury in certain activities that subject the region to repeated forces. In diving, high jumping, and other activities having unusual landing techniques, individuals will be subjected to repeated extension and flexion forces on the cervical vertebrae that may cause an injury (8). Positioning and posture of the cervical vertebrae are important in many of these activities that involve external contact in the region.

The thoracic region of the spine is not injured as frequently as the cervical and lumbar regions, probably because of its stabilization and limited motion as a result of interface with the ribs. The condition called Scheuermann's disease is commonly found in the thoracic region. This disease is an increase in the kyphosis of the thoracic region from wedging of the vertebrae. The cause of Scheuermann's disease is unknown, but it appears to be most prevalent in individuals who handle heavy objects. It is also common among competitive butterfly-stroke swimmers (8).

The lumbar region of the spine is the most injured, primarily because of the magnitude of the loads it carries. Low-back pain can originate in any of a number of sites in the lumbar area. It is believed that in a sudden onset of pain, muscles are usually the problem, irritated through some rapid twisting or reaching movement. If the pain is of the low-grade chronic type, overuse is seen as the culprit (71).

Myofascial pain, common in the low back, involves muscle sheaths and tendons that have been strained as a result of some mechanical trauma or reflex spasm in the muscle (73). Muscle strain in the lumbar region is also related to the high tensions created while lifting from a stooped position.

Muscle spasms over time will produce a dull aching pain in the lumbar region. Likewise, a dull pain can be caused by distorted postures maintained for long periods. The muscles fatigue, the ligaments are stressed, and connective tissue can become inflamed as a result of poor posture.

Irritation of the joints in the lumbar region occurs most often in activities that involve frequent stooping, such as gardening and construction. Abnormal stress on the apophyseal joints is also common in activities such as gymnastics, ballet,

and figure skating (73). Both spondylolysis and spondylolisthesis occur more frequently in the lumbar region than any other region of the trunk.

The intervertebral discs in the lumbar region have a greater incidence of disc prolapse than any other segment of the spinal column. A disc protrusion, as in any other area of the trunk, may impinge upon nerve roots exiting the spinal cord, creating numbness, tingling, or pain in the adjacent body segments. Sciatica is such a condition. In it, the sciatic nerve is compressed, sending pain down the lateral aspect of the lower extremity.

The etiology of low-back pain is not clearly defined because of the multiple risk factors associated with the disorder. Some of these factors are repetitive work, bending and twisting, pushing and pulling, tripping, slipping, and falling, and sitting or static work posture (54). A low-back injury can be created through some uncoordinated or abnormal lift or through repetitive loading over time.

Low-back pain associated with standing postures is related to positions maintaining hyperextension of the knees, hyperlordosis of the lumbar vertebrae, rounded shoulders, or hyperlordosis of the cervical vertebrae. In the seated posture, it is best to avoid crossing the legs at the knees, for this position places stress on the low back. Likewise, positions that maintain the legs in an extended position with the hips flexed should be avoided, since they accentuate lordosis in the low back.

Low-back injuries as a result of lifting are primarily a consequence of the weight of the load and its distance from the body. A correct lifting posture, as mentioned earlier in this chapter, is one with the back erect, knees bent, weight close to the body, and movement through one plane only (Fig. 7-26). This lifting technique will minimize the load imposed on the low back. A stooped lifting posture reduces

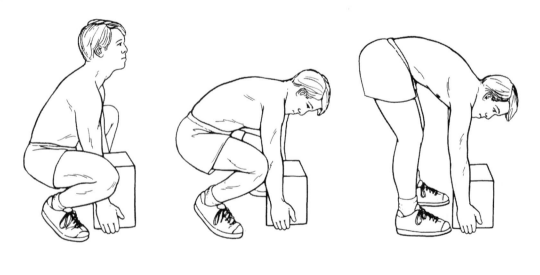

A. Correct   **B. Leg lift**   **C. Back lift**

FIGURE 7-26 Low back injury can be reduced if proper lifting techniques are used. The most important consideration is not whether you use your legs, but where the weight is with respect to your body. Proper lifting technique has the weight close to the body with the head up and the back arched **(A)**. The leg lift technique **(B)** is no better than the back lift **(C)** if the weight is held far from the body. Both B and C should be avoided.

the activity of the trunk extensors, and the forward moment is resisted by passive structures such as the discs, ligaments, and fascia. Lifting with flexed posture can place as much as 16 to 31% of the extensor moment on the passive structures (18), placing them at risk for injury.

Muscle strength and flexibility are also seen as predisposing factors for low-back pain. Tight hamstrings and an inflexible iliotibial band have both been associated with low-back pain (54). Weak abdominals are also related to low-back pain. If the abdominals are weak, control over the pelvis is lacking, and hyperlordosis will prevail. The hyperlordotic position puts undue stress on the posterior apophyseal joints and the intervertebral disc. This is an important consideration in an activity such as a sit-up or curl-up.

Erector spinae muscle activity has also been shown to relate to incidence of low-back pain. Individuals having low-back pain also have increased electrical activity and fatigue in the erector spinae muscle group (54). Even though there are inverse relationships between strength and flexibility and low-back pain, the strength and flexibility of an individual may not predict whether that person will have low-back pain. However, strength, flexibility, and fitness are predictive of the recurrence of low-back pain (54).

EFFECTS OF AGING ON THE TRUNK

The effects of aging on the spine may predispose someone to an injury or painful condition. During the process of aging, the flexibility of the spine decreases to as little as a tenth of that of younger individuals (45). There is also a corresponding loss of strength in the trunk muscles of approximately 1% per year (54). Between ages 30 and 80, the strength in cartilage, bone, and ligaments reduces by approximately 30%, 20%, and 18%, respectively (54).

The shape and length of the spine also change with aging. There is a smaller fluid region in the aging disc that places more stress on the annulus fibrosus (17). The discs may also lose height and create a shorter spine, although it has been reported that the ventral disc height is constant in both males and females in the age range of 16 to 57 years (22). There is also an increase in lateral bending of the trunk, an increase in thoracic kyphosis, and a decrease in lumbar lordosis (43). In the lumbar region specifically, there is a loss of mobility in the L5–S1 segment with an accompanying increase in the mobility of the other segments (29). It is not clear whether these age-related changes are a normal process of aging or are associated with abuse of the trunk or disuse of the trunk or are disease related. It is clear that there is benefit in maintaining strength and flexibility in the trunk well into the elderly years.

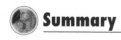 **Summary**

The vertebral column provides both flexibility and stability to the body. The four curves, cervical, thoracic, lumbar, and sacral, form a modified elastic rod. The cervical, thoracic, and lumbar curves are mobile, and the sacral curve is rigid.

Spinal column movement as a whole is created by small movements at each motion segment. Each motion segment consists of two adjacent vertebrae and the disc separating them. The anterior portion of the motion segment includes the vertebral body, the intervertebral disc, and ligaments. Movement is allowed as the disc compresses. Within the disc itself, the gel-like mass in the center, the nucleus pulposus, absorbs the compression and creates tension force in the annulus fibrosus, the concentric layers of fibrous tissue surrounding the pulposus.

The posterior portion of the motion segment includes the neural arches, the intervertebral joints, the transverse and spinous processes, and ligaments. This portion of the motion segment must accommodate large tensile forces.

The range of motion in each motion segment is only a few degrees, but in combination, the trunk is capable of moving through considerable range of motion. Flexion occurs freely in the lumbar region through 50 to 60°. Lateral flexion range of motion is approximately 75 to 85°, mainly in the cervical and lumbar regions, with some contribution from the thoracic region. Rotation occurs through 90° and is free in the cervical region. Rotation takes place in combination with lateral flexion in the thoracic and lumbar region.

Most lumbar spine movements are accompanied by pelvic movements, termed the lumbopelvic rhythm. In trunk flexion, the pelvis tilts anteriorly and moves backward. In trunk extension, the pelvis moves posteriorly and shifts forward. The pelvis will move with the trunk in rotation and lateral flexion.

The extension movement of the trunk is produced by the erector spinae and the deep posterior muscles running in pairs along the spinal column. The extensors also are very active, controlling flexion of the trunk through the first 50 to 60° of a lowering action with gravity. The abdominals produce flexion of the trunk against gravity or resistance. They also produce rotation and lateral flexion of the trunk with assistance from the extensors.

The trunk muscles can generate the greatest amount of strength in the extension movement, but the total extensor moment supplemented by intra-abdominal pressure and ligaments is only slightly greater than flexor moment. The strength output is also influenced by trunk position. In lifting, the extensor contribution will diminish the farther the object is horizontally from the body. The contribution of the various segments and muscles is also influenced by the angle of pull and the width of the object being lifted.

The loads on the vertebrae are substantial in lifting and in different postures. The loads on the lumbar vertebrae can range from 2 to 10 times body weight in activities such as walking and weightlifting. Loads on the actual intervertebral discs are influenced by a change in posture. For example, the pressures on the disc are 40% more in sitting than standing.

Posture is an important consideration in the maintenance of a healthy back. Postures that should be avoided include a slouched standing posture, prolonged sitting, unsupported sitting, and continuous flexion positions.

Postural deviations are common in the general population. Some of the common postural deviations in the trunk are excessive lordosis, excessive kyphosis, and scoliosis. The most serious of these is scoliosis.

Conditioning of the trunk muscles should always include exercises for the low back. Additionally, trunk exercises should be evaluated in terms of safety and effectiveness. For example, the trunk flexors can be strengthened using the long-lying sit-up, the curl-up or hook-lying sit-up, or the double straight leg raise. All of these exercises work the abdominals, but only through the first 30 to 45°, and then the hip flexors take over. A good alternative exercise that does not place undue stress on the low back is the crunch.

Conditioning of the extensors can be done through the use of various lifts. Both the leg lift and the back lift are commonly used to strengthen the extensors. The back lift imposes more stress on the vertebrae and produces more disc pressure than the leg lift.

Stretching of the trunk muscles can be done either standing or lying. The lying position offers more support for the trunk. Toe-touch exercises for flexibility should be avoided because of the strain to the posterior elements of the vertebral column.

The contribution of the muscles of the trunk to sport skills and movements is important for balance and stability. Trunk muscles are active in both walking and running, as the trunk laterally flexes, flexes and extends, and rotates. There is also considerable activity in the cervical region of the trunk as the head and upper body are maintained in an upright position.

The incidence of injury to the trunk is high, and it is predicted that 60 to 80% of the population will have back pain at some time in their lives. Back pain can be caused by disc protrusion or prolapse on a nerve but is more likely to be associated with soft tissue sprain or strain. Disc degeneration occurs with aging and eventually may lead to reduction of the joint space and nerve compression. The spinal column can also undergo fractures in the vertebral body as a result of compressive loading or in the posterior neural arch associated with hyperlordosis (spondylolysis). When the defect occurs on both sides of the neural arch, spondylolisthesis develops: the vertebrae slip anteriorly over each other. Some injuries are specific to regions of the trunk, such as whiplash in the cervical region and Scheuermann's disease in the thoracic vertebrae.

Changes in the spine associated with aging include decreased flexibility, loss of strength, loss of height in the spine, and an increase in lateral bending and thoracic kyphosis. It is not clear whether these changes are a normal consequence of aging or are related to disuse, misuse, or a specific disease process.

REVIEW QUESTIONS

True or False

1. ____ Lateral flexion of the spine is produced by contraction of one side of the pair only.

2. ____ The curvature in the thoracic spine develops as an infant begins to lift the head.

3. ____ The curvature in the lumbar spine develops as a response to loading.

4. ____ The functional unit of the vertebral column is similar in structure throughout the entire column, except for the first three vertebrae.

5. ____ Compressive forces on the intervertebral disc cause it to lose water.

6. ____ When a rotation is applied to the annulus fibrosus, half of the fibers will loosen and the other half will tighten.

7. ____ The posterior longitudinal ligament covers the posterolateral aspect of the vertebral motion segment.

8. ____ The abdominal muscles have a significantly higher percentage of Type II muscle fibers than the erector spinae muscles.

9. ____ The cause of scoliosis has been found to be insufficient prenatal calcium consumption.

10. ____ Trunk rotation against resistance involves activity from the erector spinae and the obliques.

11. ____ Exercises in which the trunk is flexed or extended and then rotated are a safe and effective way of conditioning the trunk.

12. ____ If the curves of the spine are exaggerated, the column will be more rigid.

13. ____ The thoracic and lumbar regions of the spinal column are the most mobile.

14. ____ The spinous process is on the anterior side of the vertebral column.

15. ____ The intervertebral disc is most susceptible to injury during flexion.

16. ____ Right rotation in the thoracic or lumbar region will be accompanied by left lateral flexion.

17. ____ Because they have a greater ratio of disc diameter to height, the discs in the thoracic region of the vertebral column are less prone to injury.

18. ____ In an upright and static stance the iliopsoas muscle is inactive.

19. ____ The sit-and-reach test is primarily a measure of hamstring flexibility.

20. ____ Scheuermann's disease is most commonly found in the sacral region.

21. ____ A sudden onset of low back pain usually indicates disc degeneration.

22. ____ The greatest strength output in the trunk can be developed in the flexion movement.

23. ____ In standing, the center of gravity is usually in the center of the spine.

24. ____ Loads measured at the L3 disc are higher for sitting than walking.

25. ____ The fully flexed position of the spinal column is maintained and supported primarily by the apophyseal ligaments.

Multiple Choice

1. There are ____ vertebrae, ____ of which are movable.
   a. 33, 29
   b. 33, 24
   c. 29, 22
   d. 29, 21

2. The fibers of the annulus fibrosus are approximately ____ collagen.
   a. 10–20%
   b. 30–40%
   c. 50–60%
   d. 70–80%

3. During excessive compressive loading of the vertebral column, the ____ will fail first.
   a. annulus fibrosus
   b. cancellous bone
   c. nucleus pulposus
   d. A and c

4. In trunk flexion, the posterior fibers of the annulus fibrosus are in ____, while the anterior fibers are in ____.
   a. Compression, tension
   b. Compression, compression
   c. Tension, compression
   d. Tension, tension

5. The anterior longitudinal ligament of the spinal column ____.
   a. Limits hyperflexion
   b. Limits hyperextension
   c. Attaches to the disc and vertebral bodies
   d. A and c

6. The ____ serve as attachment points for the spinal muscles running the length of the column.
   a. Pedicles
   b. Transverse processes
   c. Spinous processes
   d. B and c

7. In the hyperextended position, the apophyseal joints carry ____ of the load.
   a. 10%
   b. 30%
   c. 50%
   d. 70%

8. The ligamentum flavum connects ____ to ____ longitudinally.
   a. Spinous process, spinous process
   b. Transverse process, transverse process
   c. Transverse process, spinous process
   d. Laminae, laminae

9. Lateral trunk flexion is in the range of ____ and occurs primarily in the ____ and ____ regions.
   a. 45–50°, thoracic, lumbar
   b. 45–50°, lumbar, cervical
   c. 75–85°, thoracic, cervical
   d. 75–85°, lumbar, cervical

10. The apophyseal joints are in a close packed position in spinal ____.
   a. Flexion
   b. Extension
   c. A, except the top two are b
   d. B, except the top two are a

11. ____ has large transverse processes and no spinous process.
   a. C1
   b. C2
   c. L1
   d. L2

12. The ____ contribute(s) to the lordotic shaped curve in the cervical region of the spinal column.
   a. Difference in ligament length
   b. Articulation angle
   c. Wedge shaped discs
   d. All of the above

13. Because of the shape of the vertebrae, the angle of the articulating facets, and the shape of the discs, the ____ region has more movement than any other region of the spinal column.
   a. Sacral
   b. Lumbar
   c. Thoracic
   d. Cervical

14. ____ of the flexion and extension in the lumbar region occurs at the lumbosacral joint.
   a. 25%
   b. 50%
   c. 75%
   d. 95%

15. If the erector spinae muscles are contracted as a pair, they will create ____ ; if contracted unilaterally, they will create ____.
   a. Extension, rotation
   b. Flexion, lateral flexion
   c. Extension, lateral flexion
   d. A or c

16. Contraction of the abdominals ____.
   a. Increases intra-abdominal pressure
   b. Flexes the trunk
   c. Decreases activity of the erector spinae
   d. All of above

17. Excessive tightness of the iliopsoas can cause the intervertebral discs to ____.
   a. Move anteriorly
   b. Move posteriorly
   c. Rupture
   d. B and c

18. When a person is standing or sitting upright, there is continuous activity in the ____ muscle.
   a. Iliopsoas
   b. Erector spinae
   c. Rectus abdominus
   d. All of above

19. Pressure within the lumbar intervertebral discs while sitting is ____ that of standing.
   a. 50%
   b. 100%
   c. 140%
   d. 200%

20. Pressure within the intervertebral discs is highest during ____.
   a. Flexion with rotation
   b. Extension with rotation
   c. Lateral flexion with rotation
   d. Lateral flexion

21. When the spinal curve in the cervical region is accentuated toward the anterior side, ____ is said to be present.
   a. Lordosis
   b. Kyphosis
   c. Scoliosis
   d. Curvosis

22. ____ of the general population will have low back pain.
   a. 30–40%
   b. 40–60%
   c. 60–80%
   d. 80–100%

23. Disc protrusions occur most frequently at the intervertebral junctions of ____.
   a. L4–L5
   b. L5–S1
   c. T4–T5
   d. A and b

24. Disc prolapse is a condition in which ____.
   a. Tears appear in the annulus fibrosus
   b. The disc slips anteriorly
   c. The nucleus pulposus is extruded
   d. None of the above

25. A bilateral fatigue fracture most commonly found at the ____ site is called spondylolisthesis.
   a. L5, S1
   b. L5, L4
   c. T12, L1
   d. C7, T1

REFERENCES

1. Adams, M. A., Dolan, P. (1995). Recent advances in lumbar spinal mechanics and their clinical significance. *Clinical Biomechanics*, 10(1):3–19.
2. Adams, M. A., Hutton, W. C. (1982). Prolapsed intervertebral disc: A hyperflexion study. *Spine*, 7:184–191.
3. Adams, M. A., et al. (1980). The resistance to flexion of the lumbar intervertebral joint. *Spine*, 5:245–253.
4. Andersson, G. B. J., et al. (1976). Myoelectric back muscle activity in standardized lifting postures. In P. V. Komi (Ed.). *Biomechanics 5-A*. Baltimore: University Park Press, 520–529.
5. Andersson, G. B. J., et al. (1974). Myoelectric activity in individual lumbar erector spinae muscles in sitting. *Scandinavian Journal of Rehabilitative Medicine*, 3:91.
6. Andersson, G. B. J., et al. (1974). Quantitative electromyographic studies of back muscle activity related to posture and loading. *Orthopedic Clinics of North America*, 8:85–96.
7. Andersson, G. B. J., et al. (1977). Intradiscal pressure, intra-abdominal pressure and myoelectric back muscle activity related to posture and loading. *Clinical Orthopaedics*, 129:156–164.
8. Ashton-Miller, J. A., Schultz, A. B. (1988). Biomechanics of the human spine and trunk. In K. B. Pandolf (Ed.). *Exercise and Sport Sciences Reviews*. New York: Macmillan, 169–204.
9. Beard, H. K., Stevens, R. L. (1976). Biochemical changes in the intervertebral disc. In M. Jayson (Ed.). *The Lumbar Spine and Back Pain*. Kent: Pitman Medical Publishing Company Ltd, 407–433.
10. Broberg, K. B. (1983). On the mechanical behavior of intervertebral discs. *Spine*, 8:151–165.
11. Callaghan, J. P., et al. (1999). Low back three-dimensional joint forces, kinematics, and kinetics during walking. *Clinical Biomechanics*, 14:203–216.
12. Capazzo, A. (1984). Compressive loads in the lumbar vertebral column during normal level walking. *Journal of Orthopaedic Research*, 1:292.
13. Capazzo, A., et al. (1985). Lumbar spine loading during half squat exercises. *Medicine and Science in Sports and Exercise*, 17:613–620.
14. Davies, P. R. (1981). The use of intra-abdominal pressure in evaluating stresses on the lumbar spine. *Spine*, 6:90–92.
15. Davis, K.G., Marras, W. S. (2000). The effects of motion on trunk biomechanics. *Clinical Biomechanics*, 15:703–717.
16. Dehaven, K. E., Lintner, D. M. (1986). Athletic injuries: Comparison by age, sport, and gender. *American Journal of Sports Medicine*, 14:218–224.
17. Dolan, P., Adams, M. A. (2001). Recent advances in lumbar spinal mechanics and their significance for modeling. *Clinical Biomechanics*, 16:S8–S16.
18. Dolan, P., et al. (1994). Passive tissues help the back muscles to generate extensor moments during lifting. *Journal of Biomechanics*, 27:1077–1085.
19. Eklund, J. A. E., et al. (1983). A method for measuring the load imposed on the back of a sitting person. *Ergonomics*, 26:1063–1076.
20. El-Bohy, A. A., King, A. I. (1986). Intervertebral disc and facet contact pressure in axial torsion. In S. A. Lantz, A. I. King (Eds.). *Advances in Bioengineering*. New York: American Society of Mechanical Engineers, 26–27.
21. Farfan, H. F. (1975). Muscular mechanism of the lumbar spine and the position of power and efficiency. *Orthopedic Clinics of North America*, 6:135.
22. Frobin, W., et al. (1997). Precision measurement of disc height, vertebral height and sagittal plane displacement from lateral radiographic views of the lumbar spine. *Clinical Biomechanics*, 12:S5–S63.
23. Garg, A. (1980). A comparison of isometric strength and dynamic lifting capability. *Ergonomics*, 23:13–27.
24. Garg, A., et al. (1983). Biomechanical stresses as related to motion trajectory of lifting. *Human Factors*, 25:527–539.
25. Gould, J. A. (1985). The spine. In J. A. Gould and G. J. Davies (Eds.). *Orthopaedic and Sports Physical Therapy*. St. Louis: Mosby, 518–549.
26. Haher, T. R., et al. (1993). Biomechanics of the spine in sports. *Clinics in Sports Medicine*, 12:449–463.
27. Hedman, T. (1992). A new transducer for facet force measurement in the lumbar spine: Benchmark and in vitro test results. *Journal of Biomechanics*, 25:69–80.
28. Hickey, D. S., Hukins, D. W. L. (1980). Relation between the structure of the annulus fibrosus and the function and failure of the intervertebral disc. *Spine*, 5:106–116.
29. Hilton, R. C. (1976). Systematic studies of spinal mobility and Schmorl's nodes. In M. Jayson (Ed.). *The Lumbar Spine and Back Pain*. Kent: Pitman Medical, 115–131.

30. Hoshina, H. (1980). Spondylolysis in athletes. *Physician and Sportsmedicine*, 3:75–78.

31. Jayson, M. I. V. (1983). Compression stresses in the posterior elements and pathologic consequences. *Spine*, 8:338–339.

32. Jonsson, B. (1970). The functions of individual muscles in the lumbar part of the erector spinae muscle. *Electromyography*, 10:5–21.

33. Juker, D., et al. (1998). Quantitative intramuscular myoelectric activity of lumbar portions of psoas and the abdominal wall during a wide variety of tasks. *Medicine and Science in Sports and Exercise*, 30:301–310.

34. Kelsey, J. L., et al. (1984). Acute prolapsed lumbar intervertebral disc: An epidemiological study with special reference to driving automobiles and cigarette smoking. *Spine*, 9:608–613.

35. Lander, J. E., et al. (1990). The effectiveness of weight-belts during the squat exercise. *Medicine and Science in Sports and Exercise*, 22:117–126.

36. Lindh, M. (1989). Biomechanics of the lumbar spine. In M. Nordin, V. H. Frankel (Eds.). *Basic Biomechanics of the Musculoskeletal System*. Philadelphia: Lea & Febiger, 183–208.

37. Marras, W. S., et al. (1998). Trunk muscle activities during asymmetric twisting motions. *Journal of Electromyography and Kinesiology*, 8:247–256.

38. McGill, S. M. (1995). The mechanics of torso flexion: Sit-ups and standing dynamic flexion manoeuvres. *Clinical Biomechanics*, 10:184–192.

39. McGill, S. M., et al. (2000). Changes in lumbar lordosis modify role of the extensor muscles. *Clinical Biomechanics*, 15:777–780.

40. McLaughlin, T. M., et al. (1978). Kinetics of the parallel squat. *Research Quarterly*, 49:175–189.

41. McNeill, T., et al. (1980). Trunk strengths in attempted flexion, extension, and lateral bending in healthy subjects and patients with low-back disorders. *Spine*, 5:529–538.

42. Miller, J. A. A., et al. (1983). Posterior element loads in lumbar motion segments. *Spine*, 8:331–337.

43. Milne, J. S., and Lauder, I. J. (1974). Age effects in kyphosis and lordosis in adults. *Annals of Human Biology*, 1:327–337.

44. Nachemson, A. (1960). Lumbar intradiscal pressure. Experimental studies of post-mortem material. *Acta Orthopaedica Scandinavia*, 43:10–104.

45. Nachemson, A. (1976). Lumbar intradiscal pressure. In M. Jayson (Ed.). *The Lumbar Spine and Back Pain*. Kent: Pitman Medical, 257–269.

46. Nachemson, A., Morris, J. M. (1964). In vivo measurements of intradiscal pressure: Discometry, a method for the determination of pressure in the lower lumbar discs. *Journal of Bone and Joint Surgery*, 46-A:1077–1092.

47. Nachemson, A., et al. (1979). Mechanical properties of human lumbar spine motion segments. Influence of age, sex, disc level and degeneration. *Spine*, 4:1–8.

48. Nisell, R., Ekholm, J. (1986). Joint load during the parallel squat in powerlifting and force analysis of in vivo bilateral quadriceps tendon rupture. *Scandinavian Journal of Sports Science*, 8:63–70.

49. Norris, C. M. (1993). Abdominal muscle training in sport. *British Journal of Sports Medicine*, 27:19–26.

50. Oddsson, L., Thorstensson, A. (1987). Fast voluntary trunk flexion movements in standing: Motor patterns. *Acta Physiologica Scandinavia*, 129:93–106.

51. Pauly, J. E. (1966). An electromyographic analysis of certain movements and exercises. I. Some deep muscles of the back. *Anatomical Record*, 155:223.

52. Perey, O. (1957). Fracture of the vertebral end plates in the lumbar spine. An experimental biomechanical investigation. *Acta Orthopaedica Scandinavia*, 25:1–101.

53. Plamondon, A. et al. (1995). Moments at the L5/S1 joint during asymmetrical lifting: effects of different load trajectories and initial load positions. *Clinical Biomechanics*, 10(3):128–136.

54. Plowman, S. A. (1992). Physical activity, physical fitness, and low-back pain. In J. O. Holloszy (Ed.). *Exercise and Sport Sciences Reviews*. Baltimore: Williams & Wilkins, 221–242.

55. Rab, G. T., et al. (1977). Muscle force analysis of the lumbar spine. *Orthopedic Clinics of North America*, 8:193.

56. Roozbazar, A. (1974). Biomechanics of lifting. In R. C. Nelson, C. A. Morehouse (Eds.). *Biomechanics IV*. Baltimore: University Park Press, 37–43.

57. Rossi, F. (1978). Spondylolysis, spondylolisthesis and sports. *Journal of Sports Medicine and Physical Fitness*, 18:317–340.

58. Saal, J. (1988). Rehabilitation of football players with lumbar spine injury: Part 1. *Physician and Sportsmedicine*, 16:61–67.

59. Saunders, H. D. (1985). *Evaluation, Treatment and Prevention of Musculoskeletal Disorders*. Minneapolis: Viking.

60. Schendel, M. J., et al. (1993). Experimental measurement of ligament force, facet force, and segment motion in the human lumbar spine. *Journal of Biomechanics*, 26:427–438.

61. Schultz, A. B., et al. (1982). Loads on the lumbar spine: Validation of a biomechanical analysis by measurements of intradiscal pressures and myoelectric signals. *Journal of Bone and Joint Surgery*, 64-A:713–720.

62. Shah, J. S. (1976). Structure, morphology, and mechanics of the lumbar spine. In M. Jayson (Ed.). *The Lumbar Spine and Back Pain*. Kent: Pitman Medical, 339–405.

63. Shapiro, I., Frankel, V. H. (1989). Biomechanics of the cervical spine. In M. Nordin, V. H. Frankel (Eds.). *Basic Biomechanics of the Musculoskeletal System*. Philadelphia: Lea & Febiger.

64. Snijders, C. J., et al. (1995). Oblique abdominal muscle activity in standing and in sitting on hard and soft surfaces. *Clinical Biomechanics*, 10:73–78.

65. Soderberg, G. L. (1986). *Kinesiology: Application to Pathological Motion*. Baltimore: Williams & Wilkins.

66. Takala, E., et al. (1987). Electromyographic activity of hip extensor and trunk muscles during stooping and lifting. In B. Jonsson (Ed.). *Biomechanics X-A*. Champaign, IL: Human Kinetics.

67. Thorstensson, A., Carlson, H. (1987). Fiber types in human lumbar back muscles. *Acta Physiologica Scandinavia*, 131:195–202.

68. Thorstensson, A., et al. (1982). Lumbar back muscle activity in relation to trunk movements during locomotion in man. *Acta Physiologica Scandinavia*, 116:13–20.

69. Thorstensson, A., et al. (1984). Trunk movements in human locomotion. *Acta Physiologica Scandinavia*, 121:9–22.

70. Vernon-Roberts, B. (1976). The pathology and interrelation of intervertebral disc lesions, osteoarthrosis of the apophyseal joints, lumbar spondylosis and low-back pain. In M. Jayson (Ed.). *The Lumbar Spine and Back Pain*. Kent: Pitman Medical, 83–113.

71. Weiker, G. G. (1989). Evaluation and treatment of common spine and trunk problems. *Clinics in Sports Medicine*, 8:399–417.

72. White, A. A., Panjabi, M. M. (1978). The basic kinematics of the spine. Spine 3:12–20.

73. Wyke, B. (1976). The neurology of lower back pain. In M. Jayson (Ed.). *The Lumbar Spine and Back Pain*. Kent: Pitman Medical, 266–315.

74. Yates, J. W., et al. (1980). Static lifting strength and maximal isometric voluntary contractions of back, arm, and shoulder muscles. *Ergonomics*, 23:37–47.

ADDITIONAL READING

Adams, M. A., Hutton, W. C. (1983). The effects of posture on the fluid content of lumbar intervertebral discs. *Spine*, 8:665–671.

Adams, M. A., Hutton, W. C. (1983). The mechanical function of the lumbar apophyseal joints. *Spine*, 8:327–329.

Andersson, G. B. (1981). Epidemiologic aspects on low-back pain in industry. *Spine*, 6:53–60.

Andersson, G. B. J., et al. (1977). Quantitative studies of back loads in lifting. *Spine*, 1:178–185.

Andersson, G. B. J., et al. (1980). Analysis and measurement of the loads on the lumbar spine during work at a table. *Journal of Biomechanics*, 13:513–520.

Bartelink, D. L. (1957). The role of abdominal pressure in relieving the pressure on the lumbar intervertebral discs. *Journal of Bone and Joint Surgery*, 39-B:718–725.

Battie, M. C., et al. (1990). The role of spinal flexibility in back pain complaints within industry: A prospective study. *Spine*, 15:768.

Bogduk, N. (1983). The innervation of the lumbar spine. *Spine*, 8:286–293.

Bogduk, N., Mercer, S. (2000). Biomechanics of the cervical spine. I: Normal kinematics. *Clinical Biomechanics*, 15:633–648.

Burton, A. K., et al. (1989). Prediction of low-back trouble frequency in a working population. *Spine*, 14:939–946.

Burton, A. K., et al. (1989). Variation in lumbar sagittal mobility with low-back trouble. *Spine*, 14:584–590.

Cholewicki, J., et al. (1999). Intra-abdominal pressure mechanism for stabilizing the lumbar spine. *Journal of Biomechanics*, 32:13–17.

Dempster, D. W., et al. (1993). Relationships between bone structure in the iliac crest and bone structure and strength in the lumbar spine. *Osteoporosis International*, 3:90–96.

Dolan, P., Adams, M. A. (1993). The relationship between EMG activity and extensor moment generation in the erector spinae muscles during bending and lifting activities. *Journal of Biomechanics*, 26:513–522.

Ekholm, J., et al. (1979). Activation of abdominal muscles during some physiotherapeutic exercises. *Scandinavian Journal of Rehabilitative Medicine*, 11:75–84.

Ekholm, J., et al. (1982). The load of the lumbosacral joint and trunk muscle activity during lifting. *Ergonomics*, 24:145–161.

Farfan, H. F., et al. (1972). Lumbar intervertebral disc degeneration: The influence of geometrical features on the pattern of disc degeneration. *Journal of Bone and Joint Surgery*, 54-A:492–510.

Gatton, M. L., Pearcy, M. J. (1999). Kinematics and movement sequencing during flexion of the lumbar spine. *Clinical Biomechanics*, 14:376–383.

Good, C. J., Mikkelsen, G. B. (1992). Intersegmental sagittal motion in the lower cervical spine and discogenic spondylosis: A preliminary study. *Journal of Manipulative and Physiological Therapeutics*, 15:556–563.

Gracovetsky, S., et al. (1985). The abdominal mechanism. *Spine*, 10:317–324.

Gracovetsky, S., et al. (1990). Analysis of spinal and muscular activity during flexion/extension and free lifts. *Spine*, 15:1333–1339.

Granata, K. P., et al. (1999). Variation in spinal load and trunk dynamics during repeated lifting exertions. *Clinical Biomechanics*, 14:367–375.

Gravetsky, S., et al. (1989). The importance of pelvic tilt in reducing compressive stress in the spine during flexion/extension exercises. *Spine*, 14:412–416.

Gunzburg, R., et al. (1992). A cadaveric study comparing discography, magnetic resonance imaging, histology, and mechanical behavior of the human lumbar disc. *Spine*, 17:417–423.

Haggmark, T., Thorstensson, A. (1979). Fibre types in human abdominal muscles. *Acta Physiologica Scandinavia*, 107:319–325.

Jackson, A. W., Baker, A. A. (1986). The relationship of the sit-and-reach test to criterion measures of hamstring and back flexibility in young females. *Research Quarterly for Exercise and Sport Science*, 57:183–186.

Kalimo, H., et al. (1989). Lumbar muscles: Structure and function. *Annals of Medicine*, 21:353–359.

Kelsey, J. L., et al. (1984). An epidemiologic study of lifting and twisting on the job and risk for acute prolapsed lumbar intervertebral disc. *Journal of Orthopaedic Research*, 2:61–66.

Kraus, D. R., Shapiro, D. (1989). The symptomatic lumbar spine in the athlete. *Clinics in Sports Medicine*, 8:59–69.

Lin, H. S., et al. (1978). Mechanical response of the lumbar intervertebral joint under physiological (complex) loading. *Journal of Bone and Joint Surgery*, 60-A:41.

Marras, W. S., et al. (1999). Variability in spine-loading model performance *Clinical Biomechanics*, 14:505–514.

McCarrol, J., et al. (1986). Lumbar spondylolysis and spondylolisthesis in college football players. *The American Journal of Sportsmedicine*, 14:404–406.

Morris, J. M., et al. (1961). Role of the trunk in stability of the spine. *Journal of Bone and Joint Surgery*, 43:327–351.

Mutoh, Y., et al. (1981). The relationship between sit-up exercises and the occurrence of low-back pain. In H. Matsui, K. Kobahshi (Eds.), *Biomechanics VIII-A*. Champaign, IL: Human Kinetics, 180–185.

Nachemson, A. (1965). The effect of forward leaning on lumbar intradiscal pressure. *Acta Orthopaedica Scandinavia*, 35:314–328.

Nachemson, A. (1966). Electromyographic studies on the vertebral portion of the psoas muscle. *Acta Orthopaedica Scandinavia*, 37:177.

Nachemson, A. L. (1975). Towards a better understanding of low-back pain: A review of the mechanics of the lumbar disc. *Rheumatological Rehabilitation*, 14:129–143.

Nemeth, G. (1984). On hip and lumbar biomechanics: A study of joint load and muscular activity. *Scandinavian Journal of Rehabilitative Medicine*, 10.

Noble, L. (1981). Effects of various types of sit-ups on EMG of the abdominal musculature. *Journal of Human Movement*, 7:124–130.

Oddsson, L., Thorstensson, A. (1986). Fast voluntary trunk flexion movements in standing: Primary movements and associated postural adjustments. *Acta Physiologica Scandinavia*, 128:341–349.

Oddsson, L. I. E., Thorstensson, A. T. (1986). Reaction time and pattern of muscle activation in trunk flexion and extension movements. In B. Johnson (Ed.). *Biomechanics X.* Champaign, IL: Human Kinetics, 1–10.

Ortengren, R., Andersson, G. B. J. (1977). Electromyographic studies of trunk muscles, with special reference to the lumbar spine. *Spine,* 2:44–52.

Ortengren, R., et al. (1978). Lumbar back loads in fired spinal postures during flexion and rotation. In E. Asmussem, K. Jorgerson (Eds.). *Biomechanics VI.* Baltimore: University Park Press, 159–166.

Panjabi, M. M., et al. (1976). Mechanical properties of the human thoracic spine. *Journal of Bone and Joint Surgery,* 58-A:642–652.

Pintar, F. A., et al. (1992). Biomechanical properties of human lumbar spine ligaments. *Journal of Biomechanics,* 25:1351–1356.

Reuber, M., et al. (1982). Bulging of lumbar intervertebral discs. *Journal of Biomechanical Engineering,* 104:187–192.

Ricci, B., et al. (1981). Biomechanics of sit-up exercises. *Medicine and Science in Sports and Exercise,* 13:54–59.

Roy, S. H., et al. (1989). Lumbar muscle fatigue and chronic lower back pain. *Spine,* 14:992–1001.

Roy, S. H., et al. (1990). Fatigue, recovery, and low-back pain in varsity rowers. *Medicine and Science in Sports and Exercise,* 22:463–469.

Shirazi-Adl, A., Dronin, G. (1986). Load-sharing function of lumbar intervertebral disc and facet joints in compression, extension, and flexion. *Advances in Bioengineering,* 2:18–19.

Schultz, A. B., et al. (1979). Mechanical properties of human lumbar spine motion segments: Part 1. Responses in flexion, extension, lateral bending and torsion. *Journal of Biomechanical Engineering,* 101:46–52.

Snijders, C. J., et al. (1991). A biomechanical model for the analysis of the cervical spine in static postures. *Journal of Biomechanics,* 24:783–792.

Stokes, I. A., Abery, J. M. (1980). Influences of the hamstring muscles on lumbar spine curvature in sitting. *Spine,* 5:525–528.

Sullivan, M. (1989). Back support mechanisms during manual lifting. *Physical Therapy,* 69:38–45.

Thorstensson, A., Arvidson, A. (1982). Trunk muscle strength and low-back pain. *Scandinavian Journal of Rehabilitative Medicine,* 14:69–74.

Warwick, D., et al. (1980). Maximum voluntary strengths of male adults in some lifting, pushing and pulling activities. *Ergonomics,* 23:49–54.

Williams, J. G. (1980). Biomechanical factors in spinal injuries. *British Journal of Sports Medicine,* 14:14–17.

GLOSSARY

Abdominals: A combination of muscles, including rectus abdominis, internal oblique, external oblique, and transverse abdominis; flexors and rotators of the trunk.

Annulus Fibrosus: Ring of fibrocartilage that runs in concentric layers around the nucleus pulposus in the intervertebral disc; absorbs tensile stress as the disc is compressed.

Anterior Longitudinal Ligament: Ligament inserting from the sacrum, anterior vertebral body and disc, up to the atlas; limits hyperextension; limits forward sliding of vertebrae.

Apophyseal Joints: Synovial joints between adjacent vertebrae, connected at the superior and inferior facets on the laminae.

Atlantoaxial Joint: Articulation between the atlas and the axis.

Atlanto-occipital Joint: The articulation between the atlas with the occipital bone of the skull.

Atlas: The first cervical vertebra; articulates with the occipital bone.

Axis: The second cervical vertebra.

Cervix: The neck region of the trunk, consisting of seven vertebrae.

Cervicothoracic Junction: The vertebral region where the cervical curve ends and the thoracic curve begins; C7–T1.

Costotransverse Ligament: Ligament inserting on the tubercles of the ribs, transverse process of the vertebrae; supports rib attachment to thoracic vertebrae.

Cruciform Ligament: Ligament inserting on the odontoid bone and arch of the atlas; stabilizes the odontoid and atlas; prevents posterior movement of dens in atlas.

Dens: Toothlike process projecting from the superior surface of the axis; articulating surface with the atlas; also called odontoid process.

Disc Degeneration: Gradual breakdown of the intervertebral disc in which splits and tears develop.

Disc Prolapse: Injury to the intervertebral disc in which the nucleus pulposus extrudes into the annulus fibrosus.

Erector Spinae: A combination of muscles, including iliocostalis, longissimus, and spinalis muscles; extensors of the trunk.

External Oblique: Muscle inserting on ribs 9–12, anterior, superior spine, pubic tubercle, anterior iliac crest; flexes, laterally flexes and rotates the trunk to the opposite side.

Iliocostalis Cervicis: Muscle inserting on ribs 3–6, transverse process of C4–C6; extends, laterally flexes, and rotates the cervical region of the trunk to the same side.

Iliocostalis Lumborum: Muscle inserting on the sacrum, spinous processes of L1–L5, T11, T12, iliac crest, lower six ribs; extends, laterally flexes, and rotates the thoracic region of the trunk to the same side.

Iliocostalis Thoracis: Muscle inserting on the lower six ribs, upper six ribs, transverse process of C7; extends, laterally flexes, and rotates the thoracic region of the trunk of the same side.

Iliolumbar Ligament: Ligament inserting on the transverse process of L5 to the iliac crest; limits lumbar flexion and rotation.

Iliopsoas: Two muscles, the iliacus and the psoas, which insert on the bodies of T12, L1–L5, the transverse processes of L1–L5, and the inner surface of ilium, sacrum, and lesser trochanter; flexes the trunk and thigh.

Internal Oblique: Muscle inserting on the iliac crest, lumbar fascia, ribs 8–10, and linea alba; flexes, laterally flexes, and rotates the trunk to the same side.

Interspinales: Muscle inserting on the spinous processes; extends and hyperextends the trunk.

Interspinous Ligament: Ligament inserting on the spinous processes; limits flexion of trunk; limits shear forces on the vertebrae.

Intertransversarii: Muscles inserting on the transverse processes; extend and laterally flex the trunk.

Intertransverse Ligament: Ligament inserting on the transverse processes; limits lateral flexion of the trunk.

Intervertebral Disc: Layers of fibrocartilage between the adjacent bodies of the vertebrae; a fibrous ring with a pulposus center.

Intervertebral Foramen: A passage through the vertebrae formed by the inferior and superior notches on the pedicles; pathway for spinal nerves.

Kyphosis: Increase in the convexity of the vertebral curve to the posterior.

Lamina: One of the paired dorsal parts of the vertebral arch, connecting to the pedicles.

Ligamentum Flavum: Ligament inserting on the lamina; limits flexion of the trunk, creates extension of the trunk, creates tension in the disc.

Ligamentum Nuchae: Ligament inserting on the lamina; connects with the supraspinous ligament; limits cervical flexion, assists in cervical extension, creates tension in the disc.

Longissimus Capitis: Muscle inserting on the transverse processes of T1–T5, C4–C7, and mastoid process; extends, laterally flexes, and rotates the trunk.

Longissimus Cervicis: Muscle inserting on the transverse processes of T1–T5 and C4–C6; extends, laterally flexes, and rotates the trunk to the same side.

Longissimus Thoracis: Muscle inserting on the transverse processes of L1–L5, thoracolumbar fascia, transverse process of T1–T12; extends, laterally flexes, and rotates the trunk to the same side.

Longus Capitis: Muscle inserting on the transverse processes of C3–C6 and the occipital bone; flexes the head and the cervical region of the trunk, laterally flexes the trunk.

Longus Cervicis, Longus Colli: Muscle inserting on the transverse processes of C3–C5, bodies of T1–T2, bodies of C5–C7, T1–T3, atlas, transverse processes of C5–C6, and bodies of C2–C4; flexes and laterally flexes the cervical region of the trunk.

Lordosis: Increase in the anterior concavity of the vertebral curve.

Lumbar Region: The region of the trunk between the thorax and the pelvis, consisting of five vertebrae.

Lumbar Lordosis: Increase in the lumbar curve; swayback.

Lumbopelvic Rhythm: The movement relationship and synchronization between the pelvis and the lumbar vertebrae.

Lumbosacral Junction: The site on the vertebrae where the lumbar curve ends and the sacral curve begins; L5 and S1.

Multifidus: Muscle inserting on the sacrum, iliac spine, transverse processes of L5–C4, and spinous processes; extends, laterally flexes, and rotates the trunk to the opposite side.

Neural Arch: Protective arch for the spinal cord, formed by the laminae and pedicles; also called the vertebral arch.

Nucleus Pulposus: Spherical gel-like mass in the middle of the intervertebral disc; resists compressive forces applied to the spine.

Odontoid Process: Toothlike process projecting from the superior surface of the axis; articulating surface with the atlas; also called dens.

Pars Interarticularis: A site on the posterior neural arch.

Pedicle: A paired stem that connects the lamina to the vertebral body; part of the vertebral or neural arch.

Posterior Longitudinal Ligament: Ligament inserting on the posterior vertebral bodies and discs of the vertebrae; limits flexion of the trunk.

Quadratus Lumborum: Muscle inserting on the iliac crest, transverse process of L1–L5, and the last rib; laterally flexes the trunk.

Radiate Ligament: Ligament inserting on the head of the ribs and body of the vertebrae; holds the ribs to the vertebrae.

Rotatores: Muscle inserting on the transverse processes and laminae; extends and rotates the trunk to the opposite side.

Scaleni: Muscle inserting on the transverse process of cervical vertebrae and ribs 1 and 2; flexes and laterally flexes the cervical region of the trunk.

Scheuermann's Disease: Necrosis and recalcification of the vertebrae; increase in kyphosis of the thoracic region because of vertebral wedging.

Schmorl's Nodes: Vertical prolapse of part of the nucleus pulposus into an end plate lesion of an adjacent vertebra.

Scoliosis: A lateral curve of the spine.

Semispinalis Capitis: Muscle inserting on the facets of C4–C6, transverse processes of C7 to base of occipital; extends and laterally flexes the trunk.

Semispinalis Cervicis: Muscle inserting on the transverse processes of T1–T6 and spinous processes of C1–C5; extends, laterally flexes, and rotates the trunk.

Semispinales Thoracis: Muscle inserting on the transverse processes of T6–T10, spinous processes of T1–T4, C6, and C7; extends, laterally flexes, and rotates the trunk.

Spinales Thoracis: Muscle inserting on the spinous processes of L1, L2, T11, T12, and spinous processes of T1–T8; extends and laterally flexes the trunk.

Spinales Cervices: Muscle inserting on the spinous process of C7 to the Schmorl's nodes of the axis; extends and laterally flexes the trunk.

Spinous Process: A posterior projection from each vertebra, exiting at the arch.

Splenius Capitis: Muscle inserting on the ligamentum nuchae, spinous processes of C7, T1–T3, mastoid process, and occipital bone; extends, laterally flexes, and rotates the cervical region of the trunk to the same side.

Splenius Cervicis: Muscle inserting on the spinous processes of T3–T6 and the transverse processes of C1–C3; extends, laterally flexes, and rotates the cervical region of the trunk to the same side.

Spondylolisthesis: Forward displacement of one vertebra over another; bilateral defect at the pars interarticularis site.

Spondylolysis: Fatigue fracture of the posterior neural arch of the vertebrae at the pars interarticularis site.

Sternocleidomastoid: Muscle inserting on the sternum, clavicle, and mastoid process; flexes the head and cervical vertebrae, laterally flexes and rotates the cervical region of the trunk to the same side.

Supraspinous Ligament: Ligament inserting on the spinous processes; limits trunk flexion, resists forward shear forces on the spine.

Thorax: The chest or rib area, consisting of 12 vertebrae.

Thoracic Kyphosis: Increase in the thoracic curve; hunchback.

Thoracolumbar Junction: The region of the vertebrae where the thoracic curve ends and the lumbar curve begins; T12 and L1.

Transverse Process: Projection on both sides of each vertebra; projects from the junction of the laminae and the pedicles.

Transverse Abdominus: Muscle inserting on the last six ribs, iliac crest, inguinal ligament, lumbodorsal fascia, linea alba, and pubic crest; increases intra-abdominal pressure.

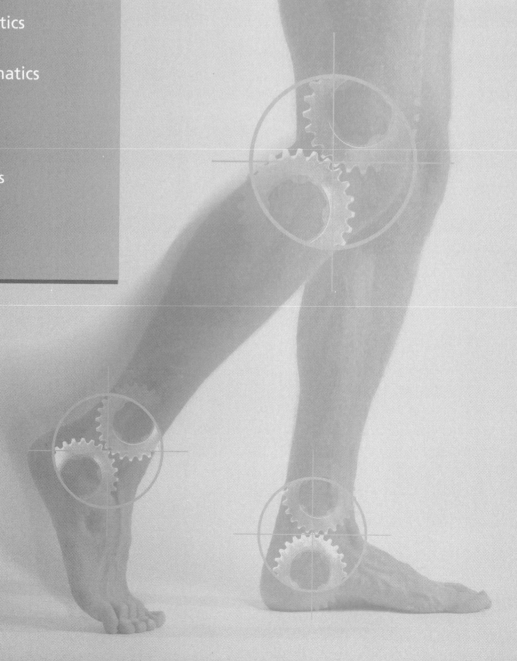

SECTION III

Mechanical Analysis of Human Motion

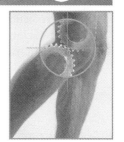

Linear Kinematics

OBJECTIVES

After reading this chapter, the student will be able to:

1. Describe how kinematic data are collected.

2. Distinguish between vectors and scalars.

3. Discuss the relationship among the kinematic parameters of position, displacement, velocity, and acceleration.

4. Distinguish between average and instantaneous quantities.

5. Conduct a numerical calculation of velocity and acceleration using the first central difference method.

6. Conduct a numerical calculation of the area under a parameter–time curve.

7. Sketch the general shape of the derivative of a curve.

8. Discuss various research studies that have used a linear kinematic approach.

9. Demonstrate knowledge of the three equations of constant acceleration.

10. Calculate the range of a projectile using the equations of constant acceleration.

The branch of mechanics that describes the spatial and temporal components of motion is called kinematics. The description involves the position, velocity, and acceleration of a body with no concern for the forces causing the motion. A kinematic analysis of motion may be either qualitative or quantitative. A qualitative kinematic analysis is a nonnumerical description of a movement based on a direct observation. The description can range from a simple dichotomy of performance—good or bad—to a sophisticated identification of the joint actions. The key is that it is nonnumerical and subjective. For example, a coach observing an athlete's performance to correct a flaw in the skill, a clinician making a visual observation of gait after application of a prosthetic limb, or a teacher rating performances in a skill test.

In biomechanics, the primary emphasis is on a quantitative analysis. The word *quantitative* implies a numerical result. In a quantitative analysis, the movement is analyzed numerically based on measurements from data collected during the performance of the movement. Movements may then be described with more precision and can also be compared arithmetically with previous or subsequent performances. With the advent of affordable and sophisticated technology, quantitative systems are now readily available for use by coaches, teachers, and clinicians. Many of these professionals, who relied on qualitative analyses in the past, have joined researchers in the use of quantitative analyses. The advantages of a quantitative analysis are numerous: it provides a thorough, objective, and accurate representation of the movement. For example, podiatrists and physical therapists have at their disposal motion analysis tools that allow them to quantify the range of motion of the foot, movements almost impossible to track with the naked eye. These movements are important in the assessment of lower extremity function during locomotion.

A subset of kinematics that is particular to motion in a straight line is called linear kinematics. Translation or translational motion, referred to as straight-line motion, occurs when all points on a body or an object move the same distance over the same time. In Figure 8-1A, an object undergoes translation. The points A_1 and B_1 move to A_2 and B_2, respectively, in the same time following parallel paths. The distance from A_1 to A_2 and B_1 to B_2 is the same, thus translation. A skater gliding across the ice maintaining a pose is an example of translation. While it appears that translation can occur only in a straight line, linear motion can occur along a curved path. This is known as curvilinear motion (Fig. 8-1*B*). While the object

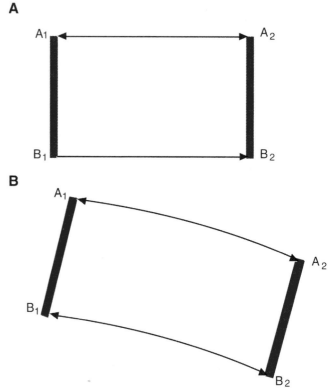

FIGURE 8-1 Types of translational motion. **A.** Straight-line or rectilinear motion. **B.** Curvilinear motion. In both A and B, the motion from A_1 to A_2 and B_1 to B_2 is the same and occurs in the same amount of time.

follows a curved path, the distance from A_1 to A_2 and B_1 to B_2 is the same and is accomplished in the same amount of time. For example, a sky diver falling from an airplane prior to opening the parachute undergoes curvilinear motion.

Collection of Kinematic Data

There are several methods by which kinematic data are collected for use in a quantitative analysis. Biomechanics laboratories, for example, may use accelerometers that measure the accelerations of body segments directly. The most common method of obtaining kinematic data, however, is high-speed video or optoelectric motion capture systems. The data obtained from high-speed video or optoelectric systems report the positions of body segments with respect to time. In the case of high-speed video, these data are acquired from the videotape by means of digitization. In optoelectric motion capture systems, markers on the body are tracked by a camera sensor that scans signals from infrared light emitting diodes (active marker system), or the video capture unit serves as both the source and the recorder of infrared light that reflects from a retroreflective marker (passive marker system). The location of the markers is sequentially fed into a computer, eliminating the digitization used in video systems. In all systems, the cameras are calibrated with a reference frame that allows for conversion between camera coordinates and a set of known actual coordinates of markers in the field of view.

REFERENCE SYSTEMS

Before any analysis, it is necessary to determine a spatial reference system. There are many options for the biomechanist in regard to a reference system; however, most laboratories use a cartesian coordinate system. A cartesian coordinate system is also referred to as a rectangular reference system. This system may either be two-dimensional or three-dimensional.

A two-dimensional reference system has two imaginary axes perpendicular to each other (Fig. 8-2*A*). The two axes (x, y) are usually positioned so that one is vertical (y) and the other is horizontal (x), although they may be oriented in any manner. For example, in certain circumstances, the axes may be reoriented such that one axis (y′) runs along the long axis of a segment. As the segment moves, the y-axis corresponding to the long axis of the segment also moves, with the result that the y-axis may not necessarily be vertical (Fig. 8-2*B*). This local reference system allows for the identification of a point on the body relative to an actual body segment rather than an external reference point.

An ordered pair of numbers is used to designate any point with reference to the axes, with the intersection or origin of the axes designated as (0, 0). This pair of numbers is always designated in the order of the horizontal or x-value followed by the vertical or y-value. Thus, these are referred to as the horizontal and vertical coordinates, respectively. The x-value refers to the distance from the vertical axis, and the y-value refers to the distance from the horizontal axis. The coordinates are usually written as (x, y) and can be used to designate any point on the xy plane. A two-dimensional reference system is used when the motion being described is planar. For example, if the object or body can be seen to move up or down (vertically) and to the right or to the left (horizontally) as viewed from one direction, the movement is planar. A two-dimensional reference system results in four quadrants in which movements to the left of the origin result in negative x-values and movements below the origin result in negative y-values (Fig. 8-3). It is an advantage to place the reference system such that all of the points are within the first quadrant, where both x- and y-values are positive.

If an individual flexed and abducted the thigh while swinging it forward and out to the side, the movement would be not planar but three-dimensional. In any physical space, three pieces of information are required to accurately locate parts of the body or any point of interest because the concept of depth (medial and lateral) must be added to the two-dimensional components of height (up and down) and width (forward and backward).

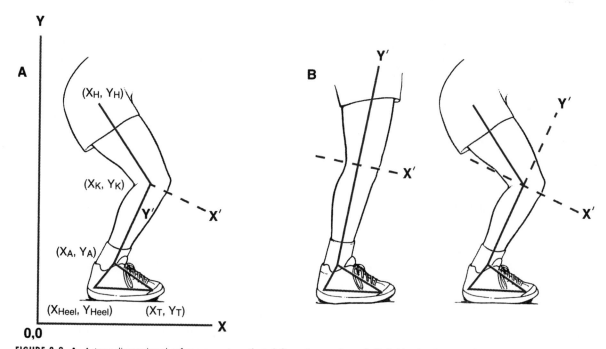

FIGURE 8-2 A. A two-dimensional reference system that defines the motion of all digitized points in a frame. **B.** A two-dimensional reference system placed at the knee joint center with the y-axis defining the long axis of the tibia.

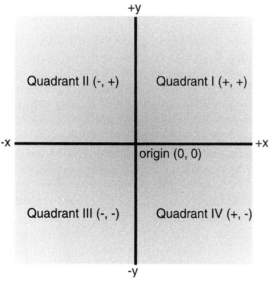

FIGURE 8-3 The quadrants and signs of the coordinates in a two-dimensional coordinate system.

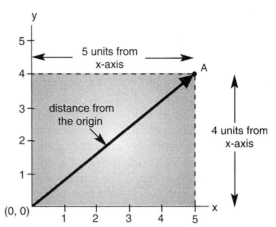

FIGURE 8-5 A two-dimensional coordinate system illustrating the ordered pair of numbers defining a point relative to the origin.

Consequently, a three-dimensional coordinate system must be used to describe the movement in this instance. This reference system has three axes, each perpendicular to the others, to describe a position relative to the horizontal or x-axis, to the vertical or y-axis, and to the mediolateral or z-axis. In a three-dimensional system (Fig. 8-4), the coordinates are written as (x, y, z). The intersection of the axes or the origin is defined as (0, 0, 0) in three-dimensional space. All coordinate values are positive in the first quadrant of the reference system, where the movements are horizontal and to the right (x), vertical and upward (y), and horizontal and forward (z). Correspondingly, negative movements are to the left (−x), downward (−y) and backward (−z). In this system, the coordinates can designate any point on a surface, not just a plane, as in the two-dimensional system. A three-dimensional kinematic analysis of human motion is much

more complicated than a two-dimensional analysis and thus will not be addressed in this book.

Figure 8-5 shows a two-dimensional coordinate system and how a point is referenced in this system. In this figure, point A is 5 units from the y-axis and 4 units from the x-axis. The designation of point A is (5,4). It is important to remember that the number designated as the x-coordinate determines the distance from the y-axis and the y-coordinate determines the distance from the x-axis.

The distance from the origin to the point is called the resultant (r) and can be determined using the Pythagorean theorem as follows:

$$r = \sqrt{x^2 + y^2}$$

In this case:

$$r = \sqrt{5^2 + 4^2}$$
$$= 6.40$$

Prior to recording the movement, the biomechanist usually places markers on the end points of the body segments to be analyzed, allowing for later identification of the position and motion of that segment. For example, if the biomechanist is interested in a sagittal view of walking or running, a typical placement of markers might be the toe, the fifth metatarsal, and the calcaneus of the foot; the lateral malleolus of the ankle; the lateral condyle of the knee; the greater trochanter of the hip; the iliac crest; the acromial process at the shoulder; the lateral epicondyle at the elbow; the styloid process of the wrist; the distal phalanx of the second finger; and the mastoid process of the skull. Figure 8-6 is a single frame of a recording illustrating a sagittal view of a runner using these specific markers. Appendix E presents two-dimensional coordinates for one complete walking cycle using these specific markers.

A global coordinate system is imposed on each frame of data, with the origin at the same location in each frame. In this way, each segment end point location can be referenced according to the same x-y axes and identified in each frame for the duration of the movement.

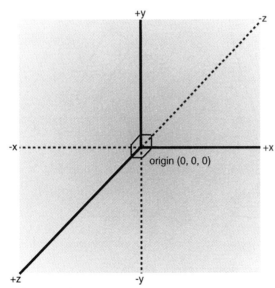

FIGURE 8-4 A three-dimensional coordinate system.

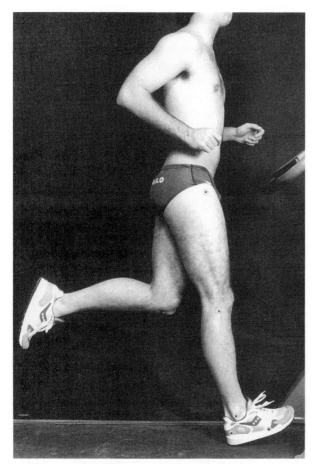

FIGURE 8-6 A runner marked for a sagittal kinematic analysis of the right leg.

Refer to the walking data in Appendix E: Using the first frame, plot the ordered pairs of x, y coordinates for each of the segmental end points and draw lines connecting the segmental end points to create a stick figure.

MOVEMENTS OCCUR OVER TIME

The analysis of the temporal or timing factors in human movement is an initial approach to a biomechanical analysis. In human locomotion, factors such as cadence, stride duration, duration of the stance or support phase (when the body is supported by a limb), duration of swing phase (when the limb is swinging through to prepare for the next ground contact), and the period of nonsupport may be investigated. The knowledge of the temporal patterns of a movement is critical in a kinematic analysis, since changes in position occur over time.

In a kinematic analysis, the time interval between each frame is determined by the sampling or frame rate of the camera or sensor. This forms the basis for timing the movement. Video cameras purchased in electronic stores generally operate at 24 to 30 fields or frames per second (fps). High-speed video cameras or motion capture units typically used in biomechanics can operate at 60, 120, 180, or 200 fps. At 60 fps, the time between each picture or frame is 1/60 s (0.01667 s); it is 1/200 s (0.005 s) at 200 fps.

Usually a key event at the start of the movement is designated as the beginning frame for digitization. For example, in a gait analysis, the first event may be considered to be the ground contact of the heel of the camera-side foot. With camera-side foot contact occurring at time zero, all subsequent events in the movement are timed from this event. The data collected for the walking trial in Appendix E is set up in this fashion, with data presented from time zero with the right-foot heel strike through to 1.15 s later, when the right-foot heel strike next occurs. The time of 1.15 s was computed from the sampling rate of 60 fps; the time between frames is 0.01667 s and 69 frames were collected.

Refer to the walking data in Appendix E: How long after the right foot strikes the ground does the left foot make contact?

UNITS OF MEASUREMENT

If a quantitative analysis is conducted, it is necessary to report the findings in the correct units of measurement. In biomechanics, the metric system is used exclusively in scientific research literature. The metric system is employed for everyday use in most countries. In the United States, however, the English system is still employed. The metric system is based on the Système International d'Unités (SI). Every quantity of a measurement system has a dimension associated with it. The term *dimension* represents the nature of a quantity. In SI the base dimensions are mass, length, time, and temperature. Each dimension has a unit associated with it. The base units of SI are the kilogram (mass), the meter (length), the second (time), and degrees Kelvin (temperature). All other units used in biomechanics are derived from these base units. The SI units and their abbreviations and conversion factors are presented in Appendix C. Since SI units are used most often in biomechanics, they are used in this text.

VECTORS AND SCALARS

Certain quantities, such as mass, distance, and volume, may be described fully by their amount or their magnitude. These are scalar quantities. For example, when one runs a race that is 5 km long, the distance or the magnitude of the race is 5 km. Additional scalar quantities that can be described with a single number include mass, volume, and speed. Other quantities, however, cannot be completely described by their magnitude. These quantities are called vectors and are described by both magnitude and direction. For example, when an object undergoes displacement, the distance and the direction are important. Many of the quantities calculated in kinematic analysis are vectors, so a thorough understanding of vectors is necessary.

In linear kinematics, vectors are represented by an arrow, with the magnitude represented by the length of the line and the arrow pointing in the appropriate direction (Fig. 8-7). Vectors are equal if their magnitudes are equal and they are pointed in the same direction.

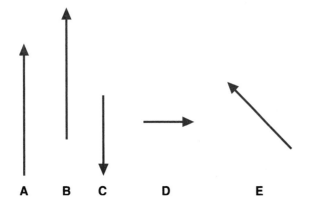

FIGURE 8-7 Vectors. Only vectors A and B are equal, because they are equivalent in magnitude and direction.

Vectors can be added together. Graphically, vectors may be added by placing the tail of one vector at the head of the other vector (Fig. 8-8A). In Figure 8-8B, the vectors are not in the same direction, but the tail of B can still be placed at the head of A. Joining the tail of B to the head of A produces the vector C, which is the sum of A + B, or the resultant of the two vectors. Subtracting vectors is accomplished by adding the negative of one of the vectors. That is:

$$C = A - B$$

or

$$C = A + (-B)$$

This is illustrated in Figure 8-8C.

Vectors may also undergo forms of multiplication that are used mainly in a three-dimensional analysis and is not described in this book. Multiplication by a scalar, however, is discussed. Multiplying a vector by a scalar changes the magnitude of a vector but not its direction. Therefore,

multiplying 3 (a scalar) times the vector A is the same as adding A + A + A (Fig. 8-8D).

A vector may also be resolved, or broken down into its horizontal and vertical components. In Figure 8-9A, the vector a is illustrated with its horizontal and vertical components. The vector may be resolved into these components using the trigonometric functions sine and cosine (see Appendix D). A right triangle can consist of the two components and the vector itself. Consider a right triangle with sides x, y, a, in which a is the hypotenuse of the triangle (Fig. 8-9B). The sine of the angle theta (θ) is defined as:

$$\sin \theta = \frac{\text{length of side opposite } \theta}{\text{hypotenuse}}$$

or

$$\sin \theta = \frac{y}{r}$$

The cosine of the angle θ is defined as:

$$\cos \theta = \frac{\text{length of side adjacent to } \theta}{\text{hypotenuse}}$$

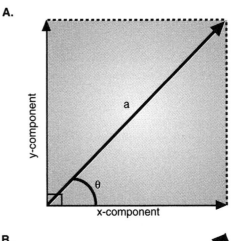

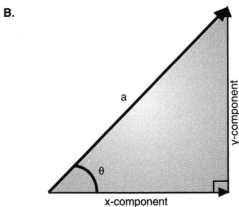

$$\sin \theta = \frac{\text{y-component}}{a} \qquad \cos \theta = \frac{\text{x-component}}{a}$$

FIGURE 8-9 Vector a resolved into its horizontal (x) and vertical (y) components using the trigonometric functions sine and cosine. **A.** Components. **B.** The components and vector form a right triangle.

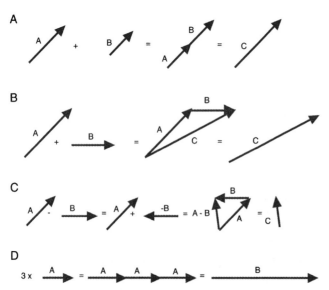

FIGURE 8-8 Vector operations illustrated graphically: **A and B.** Addition. **C.** Subtraction. **D.** Multiplication by a scalar.

or

$$\cos \theta = \frac{x}{r}$$

If the vector components x and y and the resultant r form a right triangle and if the length of the resultant vector and the angle [θ] of the vector with the horizontal are known, the sine and cosine can be used to solve for the components.

If the resultant vector has a length of 7 units and the vector is at an angle of 43°, the horizontal component is found using the definition of the cosine of the angle. That is:

$$\cos 43° = \frac{x}{a}$$

Rearranging this equation to solve for the horizontal component:

$$x = a \cos 43°$$
$$= 7 * 0.7314$$
$$= 5.12$$

where cos 43° is 0.7314 (see Appendix D).

The vertical component is found using the definition of the sine of the angle. That is:

$$\sin 43° = \frac{y}{a}$$

and rearranging this equation to solve for the vertical component y:

$$y = a \sin 43°$$
$$= 7 * 0.6820$$
$$= 4.77$$

where sin 43° is 0.6820 (see Appendix D).

The lengths of the horizontal and vertical components are therefore 5.12 and 4.77, respectively. These two values identify the point relative to the origin of the coordinate system.

Often the vectors will be facing directions relative to the origin that are not in the first quadrant (Fig. 8-3). Take for example the vector illustrated in Figure 8-10. In

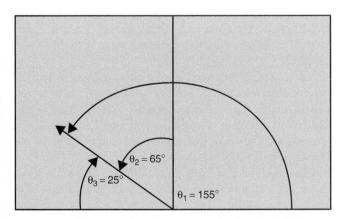

FIGURE 8-10 The orientation of a vector can be described relative to a variety of references, including the right horizontal (θ_1), the vertical (θ_2), and the left horizontal (θ_3).

this case, a vector of length 12 units lies at an angle of 155°, placing it in the second quadrant, where the x values are to the left and negative. Resolution of this vector into horizontal and vertical components can be computed a number of ways, depending on which angle you choose to use. The vertical component of the vector can be computed using:

$$y = a \sin \theta_1$$
$$y = a \sin 155°$$
$$y = 12 * 0.4226$$
$$= 5.07$$

or if you choose to use θ_2

$$y = a \cos \theta_2$$
$$y = a \cos 65°$$
$$y = 12 * 0.4226$$
$$= 5.07$$

or if you 1choose to use θ_3

$$y = a \sin \theta_3$$
$$y = a \sin 25°$$
$$y = 12 * 0.4226$$
$$= 5.07$$

Similarly, the horizontal component of the vector can be computed using the same angles:

$$x = a \cos \theta_1$$
$$x = a \cos 155°$$
$$x = 12 * -0.9063$$
$$= -10.88$$

or if you choose to use θ_2

$$x = a \sin \theta_2$$
$$x = a \sin 65$$
$$x = 12 * 0.9063$$
$$= 10.88$$
$$= -10.88$$

(x is negative in Quadrant II)
or if you choose to use θ_3

$$x = a \cos \theta_3$$
$$x = a \cos 25°$$
$$x = 12 * 0.9063$$
$$= 10.88$$
$$= -10.88$$

It is common to work with multiple vectors that must be combined to evaluate the resultant vector. Vectors can be graphically combined by connecting the vectors head to tail and joining the tail of the first one with the head of the last one to obtain the resultant vector (Fig. 8-8). This can also be done by first resolving each vector into x and y components using the trigonometric technique described earlier and then applying a technique to compose the resultant vector. To illustrate, the two vectors shown in Figure 8-8B will be assigned values of length 10 and $\theta = 45°$ for vector A and length 5 and $\theta = 0°$ for vector B. The first step is to resolve each vector into vertical and horizontal components.

Vector A

$$y = 10 \sin 45°$$
$$y = 10 * 0.7071$$
$$= 7.07$$
$$x = 10 \cos 45°$$
$$x = 10 * 0.7071$$
$$= 7.07$$

Vector B

$$y = 5 \sin 0°$$
$$y = 5 * 0.0$$
$$= 0$$
$$x = 5 \cos 0°$$
$$x = 5 * 1.000$$
$$= 5.00$$

To find the magnitude of the resultant vector, the horizontal and vertical components of each vector are added and resolved using the Pythagorean theorem:

	Horizontal Components	Vertical Components
Vector A	7.07	7.07
Vector B	5.00	0.00
Sum (Σ)	12.07	7.07

$$C = \sqrt{x^2 + y^2}$$
$$C = \sqrt{12.07^2 + 7.07^2}$$
$$= \sqrt{145.69 + 49.99}$$
$$= \sqrt{195.68}$$
$$= 13.99$$

To find the angle of resultant vector, use the trigonometric functions the tangent and the arctangent (see Appendix D). In this example, these functions can be used to calculate the angle between the vectors:

$$\tan \theta = \frac{y\text{-component}}{x\text{-component}}$$
$$\theta = \arctan\left(\frac{7.07}{12.07}\right)$$
$$\theta = \arctan(0.5857)$$
$$= 30.36°$$

The resultant Vector C has a length of 13.99 and an angle of 30.36°, which looks comparable to the vector seen in Figure 8-8B when you add Vector A to Vector B using the graphic method. This composition of multiple vectors can be applied to any number of vectors.

 Position and Displacement

POSITION

The position of an object refers to its location in space relative to some reference. Units of length are used to measure the position of an object from a reference axis. Since the metric system is always used in biomechanics, the most commonly used unit of length is the meter. For example, a platform diver standing on a 10 m tower is 10 m from the surface of the water. The reference is the water surface, and the diver's position is 10 m above the reference. The position of the diver may be determined throughout the dive with a height measured from the water surface. As previously mentioned, the analysis of video or sensor frames determines the position of a body or segment end point relative to two references in a two-dimensional reference system, the x-axis and the y-axis. The walking example in Appendix E has the two-dimensional reference frame originating on the ground in the middle of the experimental area. This makes all y values positive, since they are relative to the ground, and all x values positive or negative depending on whether the body segment is behind ($-$) or in front ($+$) of the origin in the middle of the walking area.

DISPLACEMENT AND DISTANCE

When the diver leaves the platform, motion occurs, as it does whenever an object or body changes position. Objects cannot instantaneously change position, so time is a concern when considering motion. Motion therefore may be thought of as a progressive change of position over time. In this example, the diver underwent a 10 m displacement from the diving board to the water. Displacement is measured in a straight line from one position to the next. Displacement is not to be confused with distance.

The distance an object travels may or may not be a straight line. In Figure 8-11, a runner starts the race, runs to point A, turns right to point B, left to point C, right to point D, and left to the finish. The distance run is the actual length of the path traveled. Displacement, on the other hand, is a straight line between the start and the finish of the race.

Displacement is defined both by how far the object has moved from its starting position and by the direction it moved. Since displacement inherently describes the magnitude and direction of the change in position, it is a vector quantity. Distance, because it refers only to how far an object moved, is a scalar quantity.

The capitalized Greek letter delta (Δ) refers to a change in a parameter; thus Δs means a change in s. If s represents the position of a point, then Δs is the displacement of that point. Subscript f and subscript i refer to the final position and the initial position respectively, with the implication that the final position occurred after the

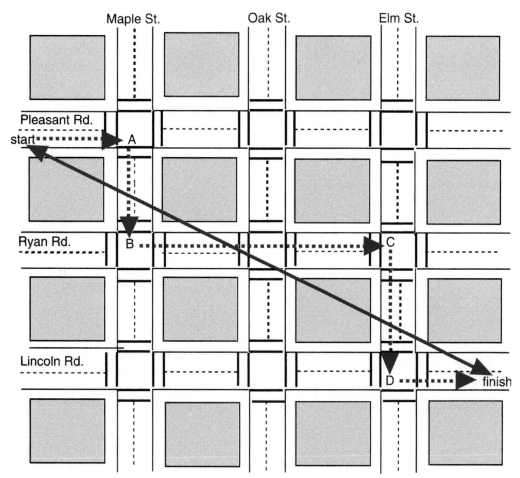

FIGURE 8-11 A runner moves along the path followed by the dotted line. The length of this path is the distance traveled. The length of the solid line is the displacement.

initial position. Mathematically, displacement (Δs) is for the general case:

$$\Delta s = s_f - s_i$$

where s_f is the final position and s_i is the initial position. Displacement for each component of position may also be calculated as follows:

$$\Delta x = x_f - x_i$$

for horizontal displacement and

$$\Delta y = y_f - y_i$$

for vertical displacement.

The resultant displacement may also be calculated by:

For example, if an object is at position A (1,2) at time 0.02 s and position B (7,7) at time 0.04 s (Fig. 8-12*A*), the horizontal and vertical displacements are:

$$\Delta x = 7m - 1m$$
$$= 6m$$

$$\Delta y = 7m - 2m$$
$$= 5m$$

The object is displaced 6 m horizontally and 5 m vertically. The movement may also be described as to the right and upward relative to the origin of the reference system.

The resultant displacement or the length of the vector from A to B may be calculated as:

$$r = \sqrt{6^2\,m + 5^2\,m}$$
$$= 7.81\ m$$

The direction of the displacement of the vector from A to B may be calculated as:

$$\theta = \arctan\left(\frac{5}{6}\right)$$
$$\theta = 0.8333$$
$$= 39.8°$$

The point therefore is displaced 7.81 m up and to the right of the origin at 39.8°.

Refer to the walking data in Appendix E: What is the horizontal, vertical, and resultant displacement of the head between frame 4 (lowest vertical position) and frame 55 (highest vertical position)?

Consider Figure 8-12*B*. In a successive position to B, the object moved to position C (11,3). The displacement is:

$$\Delta x = 11\ m - 7\ m$$
$$= 4\ m$$

A

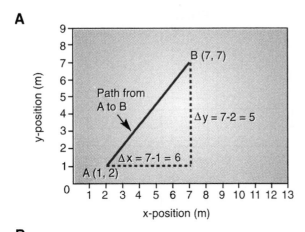

B

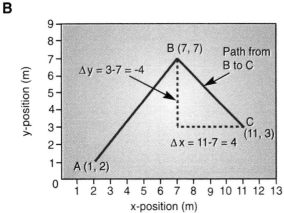

FIGURE 8-12 The horizontal and vertical displacements in a coordinate system of the path from **(A)** A to B and **(B)** B to C.

$$\Delta y = 3 \text{ m} - 7 \text{ m}$$
$$= -4 \text{ m}$$

The object would have been displaced 4 m horizontally and -4 m vertically, or 4 m to the right away from the y-axis and 4 m down toward the x-axis. The resultant displacement between points B and C may be calculated as:

$$r = \sqrt{4^2 \text{ m} + 4^2 \text{ m}}$$
$$= 5.66 \text{ m}$$

The direction of the displacement of the vector from A to B may be calculated as:

$$\theta = \arctan\left(\frac{-4}{4}\right)$$
$$\theta = \arctan(-1)$$
$$= -45°$$

The displacement from point B to C is 5.66 m to the right and down toward the x-axis from point B at an angle of 45° below the horizontal.

Velocity and Speed

Velocity is a vector quantity defined as the time rate of change of position. Speed is a scalar quantity. In automobiles, for example, speed is recorded continuously by the speedometer as one travels from place to place. Speed is defined as the distance traveled divided by the time it took to travel. In the case of the automobile, speed is measured in miles per hour or kilometers per hour. Thus:

$$\text{speed} = \frac{\text{distance}}{\text{time}}$$

In everyday use the terms velocity and speed are interchangeable, but velocity, a vector quantity, describes magnitude and direction, while speed, a scalar quantity, describes only magnitude. In road races, the start is usually close to the finish, and the velocity over the whole race may be quite small. In this case, speed may be more important to the participant.

In biomechanics, however, velocity is generally of more interest than speed. Velocity is usually designated by the lowercase letter v and time by the lower case letter t. Velocity can be determined by:

$$v = \frac{\text{displacement}}{\text{time}}$$

Specifically, velocity is:

$$v = \frac{\text{position}_f - \text{position}_i}{\text{time at final position} - \text{time at initial position}}$$
$$= \frac{\text{change in position}}{\text{change in time}}$$
$$= \frac{\Delta s}{\Delta t}$$

The most commonly used unit of velocity in biomechanics is meters per second (m/s), although any unit of length divided by a unit of time is correct as long as it is appropriate to the situation. A sample of velocity measures are presented in Table 8-1. As you can see, there is a wide

 TABLE 8-1 Sample Linear Velocity Examples

Action	Linear Velocity (m/s)
Golf club head forward velocity at impact (21)	43
High jump approach velocity	7–8
High jump horizontal and vertical velocity at takeoff (8)	4.2, 4
Long jump approach velocity (20)	9.5–10
Pitching, fast ball velocity at release (10)	35.1
Pitching, curve ball velocity at release (10)	28.2
Vertical velocity at takeoff, squat jump and countermovement jump (11)	3.43, 3.8
Hopping vertical velocity (11)	1.52
Walking forward velocity	0.7–3
Race walking	4+
Running, sprinting	4–10
Wheelchair propulsion (28)	1.11–2.22

range of velocities in human movement ranging from the range of 0.7 to 1 m/s for a slow walk to the range of 43 to 50 m/s for a club head in the golf swing. The units for velocity can be determined by using the formula for velocity and dividing the units of length by units of time.

$$\text{Velocity} = \frac{\text{displacement (m)}}{\text{time (seconds)}}$$
$$= \text{m/s or m} \cdot \text{s}^{-1}$$

Consider the position of an object that is at point A (2, 4) at time 1.5 s and moved to point B (4.5, 9) at time 5 s. The horizontal velocity (v_x) is:

$$v_x = \frac{4.5 \text{ m} - 2 \text{ m}}{5 \text{ s} - 1.5 \text{ s}}$$
$$= \frac{2.5 \text{ m}}{3.5 \text{ s}}$$
$$= 0.71 \text{ m/s}$$

The vertical velocity (v_y) could be similarly determined by:

$$v_y = \frac{9 \text{ m} - 4 \text{ m}}{5 \text{ s} - 1.5 \text{ s}}$$
$$= \frac{5 \text{ m}}{3.5 \text{ s}}$$
$$= 1.43 \text{ m/s}$$

The resultant magnitude or overall velocity can be calculated using the Pythagorean relationship as follows:

$$v = \sqrt{0.71^2 + 1.43^2}$$
$$= \sqrt{2.55}$$
$$= 1.60 \text{ m/s}$$

The resultant direction of the velocity is:

$$\tan \theta = \frac{y}{x}$$
$$\theta = \arctan\left(\frac{1.43}{0.71}\right)$$
$$\theta = \arctan(2.04)$$
$$= 63.92°$$

SLOPE

Figure 8-13 is an illustration of the change in horizontal position or position along the x-axis as a function of time. In this graph, the geometric expression describing the change in horizontal position (Δx) is called the rise. The expression that describes the change in time (Δt) is called the run. The slope of a line is:

$$\text{Slope} = \frac{\text{rise}}{\text{run}} = \frac{\Delta x}{\Delta t}$$

The slope of a line indicates the relationship between two parameters, in this case horizontal displacement and time. Therefore, the slope of the line plotted on a displacement–time graph is the relationship between dis-

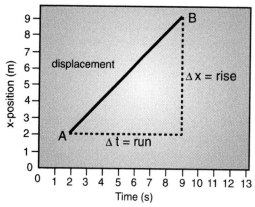

FIGURE 8-13 Horizontal position plotted as a function of time. The slope of the line from A to B is $\frac{\Delta x}{\Delta t}$.

placement and time and represents the average velocity over the time interval.

The steepness of the slope gives a clear picture regarding the velocity. If the slope is very steep, that is, a large number, the position is changing rapidly and the velocity is great. If the slope is zero, the object has not changed position and the velocity is zero. However, since velocity is a vector, it can have both positive and negative slopes. Figure 8-14 shows positive, negative, and zero slopes. Lines a and b have positive slopes, implying that the object was displaced away from the origin of the reference system. However, line a has a steeper slope than b, indicating that the object was displaced a greater distance per unit time. Line c illustrates a negative slope, indicating that the object was moving toward the origin. Line d shows a zero slope, meaning that the object was not displaced either away from or toward the origin over that time. Lines e and f have identical slopes, but e's slope is positive and f's is negative.

FIRST CENTRAL DIFFERENCE METHOD

The kinematic data that are collected in certain biomechanical studies are based on positions of the segment end points generated from each frame of video with a

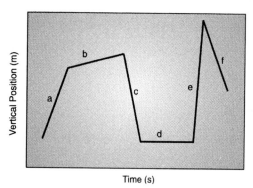

FIGURE 8-14 Different slopes on a vertical position versus time graph. Slopes a, b, and e are positive. Slopes c and f are negative; d has zero slope.

time interval based on the frame rate of the camera. This presents the biomechanist with all of the information that is needed to calculate velocity. However, when velocity over a time interval is calculated, the velocity at either end of the time interval is not generated; that is, the calculated velocity cannot be assumed to occur at the time of the final position nor at the time of the initial position. The position of an object can change over a period less than the interval between video frames. Thus the velocity calculated between two video frames represents an average of the velocities over the whole time interval between frames. An average velocity, therefore, is used to estimate the change in position over the time interval. This is not the velocity at the beginning or end of the time interval. If this is the case, there must be some point in the time interval between frames when the calculated velocity occurs. The best estimate for the occurrence of this velocity is at the midpoint of the time interval. For example, if the velocity is calculated using the data at frames 4 and 5, the calculated velocity would occur at the midpoint of the time interval between frames 4 and 5 (Fig. 8-15*A*).

If data are collected at 60 fps, the positions at video frames 1 to 5 occur at the times 0, 0.0167, 0.0334, 0.0501, and 0.0668 s. The velocities calculated using this method occur at the times 0.0084, 0.0251, 0.0418, and 0.0585 s. This means that after using the general formula for calculating velocity, the positions obtained from the video and velocities calculated are not exactly matched in time. While this problem can be overcome, it may be inconvenient in certain calculations. To overcome this problem, the most often used method for calculating velocity is the first central difference method. This method employs the difference in positions over two frames as the numerator. The denominator in the velocity calculation is the change in time over two time intervals. The formula for this method:

$$v_{xi} = \frac{x_{i+1} - x_{i-1}}{2\Delta t}$$

for the horizontal component and

$$v_{yi} = \frac{y_{i+1} - y_{i-1}}{2\Delta t}$$

for the vertical component.

This means that the velocity at frame i is calculated using the positions at frame i + 1 and frame i − 1. Use of $2\Delta t$ renders the velocity at the same time as frame i, since that is the midpoint of the time interval. For example, if the velocity at frame 5 is calculated, the data at frames 4 and 6 are used. If the time of frame 4 is 0.0501 s and frame 6 is 0.0835 s, the velocity calculated using this method would occur at time 0.0668 s, or at frame 5 (Fig. 8-15*B*).

Similarly, if the velocity at frame 3 is calculated, the positions at frame 2 and frame 4 are used. Since the time interval between the two frames is the same, the change in time would be 2 times the Δt. If the horizontal velocity at the time of frame 13 is calculated, the following equation would be used:

$$v_{x13} = \frac{x_{14} - x_{12}}{t_{14} - t_{12}}$$

The location of the calculated velocity would be at t_{13}, or the same point in time as frame 13. This method of computation exactly aligns in time the position and velocity data. It is assumed that the time intervals between frames of data are constant. As pointed out previously, this usually is the case in biomechanical studies.

The first central difference method uses the data point prior to and after the point where velocity is calculated. One problem is that data will be missing at the beginning and end of the video trial. This means that either the velocity at the beginning and end of the trial are estimated or some other means are used to evaluate the velocity at these points. A simple method is to collect and analyze several frames before and after the movement of interest. For example, if a walking stride was analyzed, the first contact of the right foot on the ground might be picked as the beginning event for the trial. In that case at least one frame prior to that event

A

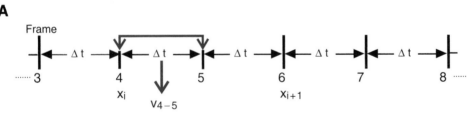

B

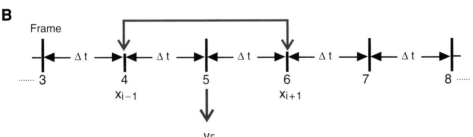

FIGURE 8-15 The location in time of velocity. **A.** Using the traditional method over a single time interval. **B.** Using the first central difference method.

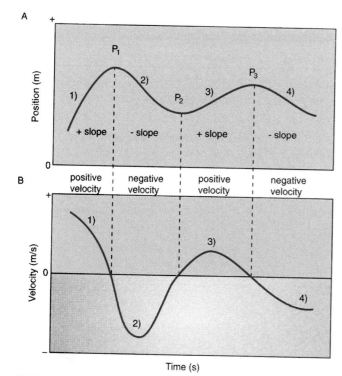

FIGURE 8-19 The position–time curve **(A)** and the respective velocity–time curve **(B)** drawn using the concepts of local extrema and slopes.

zero. In section 2 of the position–time curve, the slope is negative, indicating that the velocity must be negative. The local extrema, P_1 and P_2, however, indicate that the velocity at these points will be zero. Thus, in section 2 the corresponding velocity curve starts at zero, increases negatively, and then becomes less negative, returning to zero at P_2. Similarly, the shape of the velocity curve can be generated for sections 3 and 4 on the position curve (Fig. 8-19B).

 Acceleration

In human motion the velocity of a body or a body segment is rarely constant. The velocity often changes throughout a movement. Even when the velocity is constant, it may be so only when averaged over a large time interval. For example, in a distance race, the runner may run consecutive 300 m distances in 65 s, indicating a constant velocity over each distance. A detailed analysis, however, would reveal that the runner actually increased and decreased velocity, with the average over the 300 m being constant. In fact, it has been shown that runners decrease and then increase velocity during each ground contact with each foot (2). If velocity continually changes, it would appear that these variations in velocity must be described. In addition, the rate at which velocity changes can be related to the forces that cause movement.

The rate of change of velocity with respect to time is called acceleration. In everyday usage, accelerating means

speeding up. In a car, when the accelerator is depressed, the speed of the car increase. When the accelerator is released, the speed of the car decreases. In both instances the direction of the car is not a concern, since speed is a scalar. Acceleration, however, refers to both increasing and decreasing velocities. Since velocity is a vector, acceleration must also be a vector.

Acceleration, usually designated by the lowercase letter a, can be determined thus:

$$a = \frac{\text{change in velocity}}{\text{change in time}}$$

More generally:

$$a = \frac{\text{velocity}_f - \text{velocity}_i}{\text{time at final position} - \text{time at initial position}}$$
$$= \frac{\text{change in velocity}}{\text{change in time}}$$
$$= \frac{\Delta v}{\Delta t}$$

The units of acceleration are the unit of velocity (m/s) divided by the unit of time (second) resulting in meters per second per second (m/s/s), or m/s^2.

$$\text{acceleration} = \frac{\text{velocity (m/s)}}{\text{time (second)}}$$

This is the most common unit of acceleration used in biomechanics.

INSTANTANEOUS ACCELERATION

Since acceleration represents the rate of change of a velocity with respect to time, the concepts regarding velocity also apply to acceleration. Thus, acceleration may be represented as a slope indicating the relationship between velocity and time. On a velocity–time graph, the steepness and direction of the slope will indicate whether the acceleration is positive, negative, or zero. In addition, instantaneous acceleration may be defined in an analogous fashion to instantaneous velocity. Instantaneous acceleration may be defined as the slope of a line tangent to a velocity time graph or as a limit:

$$\lim_{dt -> 0} a_x = \frac{dv_x}{dt}$$

for horizontal acceleration and

$$\lim_{dt -> 0} a_y = \frac{dv_y}{dt}$$

for vertical acceleration.

The term dv refers to a change in velocity. Horizontal acceleration is the limit of v_x as dt approaches zero and vertical acceleration is the limit of v_y as dt approaches zero.

TABLE 8-3 Calculation of Acceleration From a Set of Velocity–Time Data

Frame	Time (s)	Vertical position (y) (m)	Velocity (v_y) (m/s)	Acceleration (a_y) (m/s²)
1	0.0000	0.00	0.00	0.000
2	0.0167	0.15	6.59	$(3.59 - 0.00)(0.0334 - 0.00) = 107.49$
3	0.0334	0.22	3.59	$(2.40 - 6.59)(0.0501 - 0.0167) = -125.45$
4	0.0501	0.27	2.40	$(-2.10 - 3.59)(0.0668 - 0.0334) = -170.36$
5	0.0668	0.30	-2.10	$(-8.98 - 2.40)(0.0835 - 0.0501) = -340.72$
6	0.0835	0.20	-8.98	$(-13.77 - (-2.10))(0.1002 - 0.0668) = -349.40$
7	0.1002	0.00	-13.77	$(-8.98 - (-8.98))(0.1169 - 0.0835) = 0.00$
8	0.1169	-0.26	-8.98	$(1.20 - (-13.77))(0.1336 - 0.1002) = 448.20$
9	0.1336	-0.30	1.20	$(8.98 - (-8.98))(0.1503 - 0.1169) = 537.72$
10	0.1503	-0.22	8.98	$(0.00 - 1.20)(0.1670 - 0.1336) = -35.93$
11	0.1670	0.00	0.00	0.00

The first central difference method is also used to calculate acceleration in many biomechanical studies. The use of this method means that the calculated acceleration is associated with a time in the movement in which a calculated velocity and a digitized point are also associated. The first central difference formula for calculating acceleration is analogous to that for calculating velocity:

$$a_{xi} = \frac{vx_{i+1} - vx_{i-1}}{2\Delta t}$$

for the horizontal component and

$$a_{yi} = \frac{vy_{i+1} - vy_{i-1}}{2\Delta t}$$

for the vertical component.

For example, to calculate the acceleration at frame 7, the velocity values at frames 8 and 6, and 2 times the time interval between individual frames would be used.

NUMERICAL EXAMPLE

The velocity data calculated from Table 8-2 representing the vertical (y) position of an object will be used to illustrate the first central difference method of calculating acceleration. Table 8-3 presents the time at each frame, the vertical position, the vertical velocity, and the calculated vertical acceleration for each frame.

To calculate the acceleration at the time of frame 4:

$$
\begin{aligned}
a_{y4} &= \frac{v_5 - v_3}{t_5 - t_3} \\
&= \frac{-2.10 \text{ m/s} - 3.59 \text{ m/s}}{0.0668 \text{ s} - 0.0334 \text{ s}} \\
&= -170.36 \text{ m/s}^2
\end{aligned}
$$

Figure 8-20 is a graph of the velocity and acceleration profiles of the complete movement. As the velocity increases rapidly, the slope of the acceleration curve becomes

steeper, and as the velocity changes less rapidly, the slope is less steep.

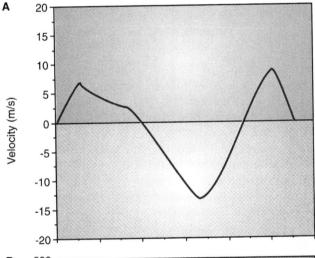

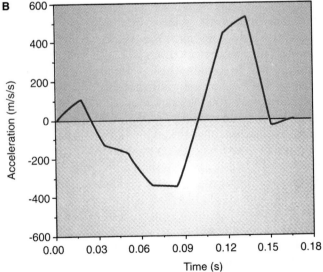

FIGURE 8-20 Velocity–time profile **(A)** and acceleration–time profile **(B)** for Table 8-3.

GRAPHICAL EXAMPLE

Previously, an estimation of the shape of the relationship between position and velocity was graphed using the concepts of slope and local extrema. It is also possible to graph an estimation of the shape of an acceleration curve based on the shape of the velocity–time profile. Once again the two concepts of the slope and the local extrema are used, this time on a velocity–time graph. Figure 8-21*A* represents the horizontal velocity of the data presented in Figure 8-19. The local extrema of the velocity curve, where the curve changes direction, are indicated as v_1 and v_2. At these points the acceleration is zero. Constructing the acceleration curve on the same time line as the velocity curve allows projection of the occurrence of these local extrema from the velocity curve time line to the acceleration time line.

The slopes of each section of the velocity–time curve are (*a*) to v_1, negative; (*b*) v_1 to v_2, positive; and (*c*) beyond v_2, negative. The velocity curve to v_1 has a negative slope, but the curve reaches the local extremum at v_1. The corresponding acceleration curve of this section (Fig. 8-21*B*) is negative, but it becomes zero at the local extremum v_1. Between v_1 and v_2 the velocity curve has a positive slope. The acceleration curve between these points in time will begin with a zero value at the time corresponding to v_1, become more positive, and eventually return to zero at a time corresponding to v_2. Similar logic can be used to describe the construction of the remainder of the acceleration curve.

ACCELERATION AND THE DIRECTION OF MOTION

One complicating factor in understanding the meaning of acceleration relates to the direction of motion of an object. The term *accelerate* is often used to indicate an increase in velocity and the term *decelerate* to describe a decrease in velocity. These terms are satisfactory when the object under consideration is moving in the same direction continually. Even if velocity and therefore acceleration change, the direction in which the object is traveling may not

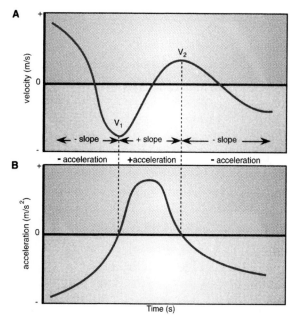

FIGURE 8-21 The relationship between the velocity–time curve and the acceleration–time curve drawn using the concepts of local extrema and slopes.

change. For example, a runner in a 100 m sprint race starts from rest or from a zero velocity. When the race begins, the runner increases velocity up to the 50 m point, and acceleration is positive. After the 50 m mark, the runner's velocity may not change for some of the race; there is zero acceleration. Having crossed the finish line, the runner reduces velocity; this is negative acceleration. Eventually the runner comes to rest, at which point velocity equals zero. Throughout the race, the runner moved in the same direction but had positive, zero, and negative acceleration. Thus it can be seen that acceleration may be considered to be independent of the direction of motion.

Consider an athlete completing a shuttle run that consists of one 10 m run away from a starting position, followed by a 10 m run back to the starting position. The two sections of this run are illustrated in Figure 8-22. The first

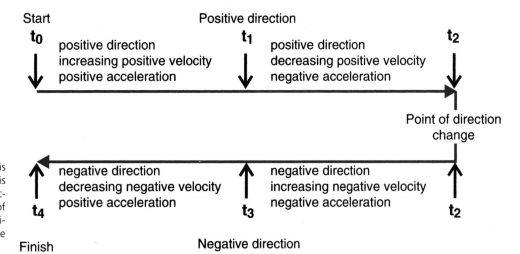

FIGURE 8-22 Motion to the right is regarded as positive and to the left is negative. Positive or negative velocity is based on the direction of motion. Acceleration may be positive, negative, or zero based on the change in velocity.

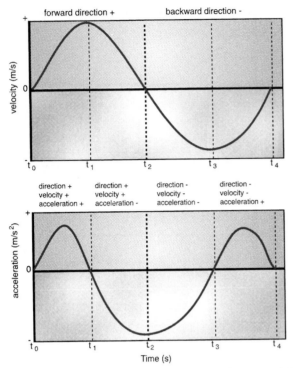

FIGURE 8-23 The graphical relationship between acceleration and direction of motion during a shuttle run (t_2 denotes when the runner changed direction).

10 m section of the run may be considered a run in a positive direction. The runner, running in a positive direction, increases velocity and then, approaching the turn-around point, must decrease positive velocity. Thus the runner has positive acceleration followed by negative acceleration. Figure 8-23 presents an idealized horizontal velocity profile and the corresponding horizontal acceleration for the shuttle run. The 10 meter run in one direction from t_0 to t_2 illustrates that the positive velocity as change in position was constantly away from the y-axis. In addition, the slope of the velocity curve from t_0 to t_1 is positive, indicating positive acceleration when the runner increases velocity, while the slope of the velocity curve from t_1 to t_2 is negative, resulting in negative acceleration as the runner decreases velocity in anticipation of stopping and turning around.

At the turnaround point, the runner, now running in a negative direction, increases negative velocity (Fig. 8-22), resulting in a negative acceleration. Approaching the finish line, the runner must decrease negative velocity to have positive acceleration. This is illustrated graphically in Figure 8-23; from t_2 to t_4, the velocity is negative because the object moved back toward the y-axis or the reference point. The slope of the velocity curve from t_2 to t_3 is negative, indicating negative acceleration. Continuing toward the finish, the runner begins to decrease velocity in the negative direction. This decrease in negative velocity is a positive acceleration and is illustrated in section t_3 to t_4 as the slope of the velocity curve is positive. Thus, since positive and negative accelerations occur in positive and negative directions, it may be seen that acceleration is

independent of the direction of motion. Both positive and negative accelerations can result without the object changing direction. If the final velocity is greater than the initial velocity, the acceleration is positive. For example:

$$
\begin{aligned}
a &= \frac{v_f - v_i}{t_f - t_i} \\
&= \frac{10 \text{ m/s} - 3 \text{ m/s}}{3 \text{ s} - 1 \text{ s}} \\
&= \frac{7 \text{ m/s}}{2 \text{ s}} \\
&= 3.5 \text{ m/s}^2
\end{aligned}
$$

If, however, the final velocity is less than the initial velocity, the acceleration is negative. For example:

$$
\begin{aligned}
a &= \frac{v_f - v_i}{t_f - t_i} \\
&= \frac{4 \text{ m/s} - 10 \text{ m/s}}{5 \text{ s} - 3 \text{ s}} \\
&= \frac{-6 \text{ m/s}}{2 \text{ s}} \\
&= -3 \text{ m/s}^2
\end{aligned}
$$

In the first case it is said that the object is accelerating, and in the latter, decelerating. These terms become confusing, however, when the object actually changes direction. For the sake of easing confusion, it is best that the terms *acceleration* and *deceleration* be avoided and the use of *positive acceleration* and *negative acceleration* is encouraged.

Differentiation and Integration

Discussion thus far is of kinematic analysis based on a process whereby position data are accumulated first. When velocity is calculated from displacement and time or when acceleration is calculated from velocity and time, the mathematics is called differentiation. The solution of the process of differentiation is called a derivative. A derivative is simply the slope of a line, either a secant or tangent, as a function of time. Thus, when velocity is calculated from position and time, differentiation is the method used to calculate the derivative of position. Velocity is called the derivative of displacement and time. Similarly, acceleration is the derivative of velocity and time.

In certain situations, however, acceleration data may be collected. From these data, velocities and positions may be calculated based on a process that is opposite to that of differentiation. This mathematical process is known as integration. Integration is often referred to as antidifferentiation. The result of integration is called the integral. Velocity, then, is the time integral of acceleration. The following equation describes the above statement:

$$
v = \int_{t_1}^{t_2} a \, dt
$$

This expression reads that velocity is the integral of acceleration from time 1 to time 2. The terms t_1 and t_2 define the beginning and end points at which the velocity is evaluated. Likewise, position is the integral of velocity:

$$s = \int_{t_1}^{t_2} v \, dt$$

The meaning of the integral is not quite as obvious as that of the derivative, however. Integration requires calculating the area under a velocity–time curve to determine the average displacement or the area under an acceleration–time curve to determine the average velocity. The integration sign

$$\int_{t_1}^{t_2}$$

is a long s; it indicates summation of areas between time t_1 and time t_2. Figure 8-24 illustrates the concept of the area under the curve. Two rectangles represent a constant acceleration of 3 m/s^2 for 6 s in the first portion of the curve and constant acceleration of 7 m/s^2 for 2 s. The area of a rectangle is length times width. Thus, the area under the first rectangle is 3 m/s^2 times 6 s, or 18 m/s. In the latter rectangle, the area is 7 m/s^2 times 2 s, or 14 m/s. The total area is 32 m/s.

The area under an acceleration–time curve is the change in velocity over the time interval. This can be demonstrated by analysis of the units in calculating the area under the curve. For example, taking the area under an acceleration–time curve involves multiplying an acceleration value by a time value:

$$\text{Area under the curve} = \text{acceleration} * \text{time}$$
$$= \frac{m}{s^2} * s$$
$$= \frac{m}{s * s} * s$$
$$= m/s$$

The area under the curve would have units of velocity. Thus, a measure of velocity is the area under an acceleration–time curve. This area represents the change in velocity over the time interval in question. Similarly, the change in displacement is the area under a velocity–time curve.

Velocity–time or acceleration–time curves do not generally form rectangles as in the previous examples, and thus the computation of the integral is not quite so simple. The technique generally used, a Riemann sum, depends on the size of the time interval, dt. If dt is small enough, and it generally is in a kinematic study, the integral or area under the curve can be calculated by progressively summing the product of each data point along the curve and dt. For example, if the curve to be integrated is a horizontal velocity–time curve, the integral equals the change in position. If the horizontal velocity–time curve is

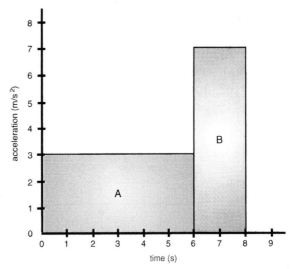

FIGURE 8-24 An idealized acceleration–time curve. Area A equals 3 m/s^2 * 6 s or 18 m/s. This represents the change in velocity over the time interval from 0 to 6 s. The change in velocity for area B is 14 m/s.

made up of 30 data points each 0.005 s apart, the integral would be:

$$\int_{t_1}^{t_{30}} v_{xi} \, dt = ds$$

and to find the area under the curve:

$$ds = \sum_{i=1}^{30} (v_{xi} * dt)$$

The Riemann sum calculation generally gives an excellent estimation of the area under the curve.

Linear Kinematics of Walking and Running

A kinematic analysis describes the positions, velocities, and accelerations of bodies in motion. It is one of the most basic types of analyses that may be conducted, because it is used only to describe the motion, with no reference to the causes of motion. Kinematic data are usually collected using high-speed video cameras or sensors, and positions of the body segments are generated through digitization or other marker recognition techniques. To illustrate kinematic analysis in biomechanics, the study of human gait will be used as an example. The most studied forms of human gait are walking and running.

STRIDE PARAMETERS

In both locomotor forms of movement, the body actions are cyclic, involving sequences in which the body is supported by first one leg and then the other. These sequences are defined by certain parameters. Typical parameters such as the stride and step are presented in

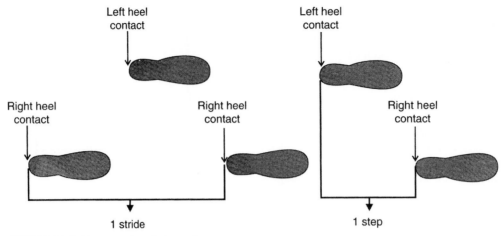

FIGURE 8-25 Stride parameters during gait.

Figure 8-25. A locomotor cycle or stride is defined by events in these sequences. A stride is defined as the interval from one event on one leg until the same event on the same leg in the following contact. Usually an event such as the first instant of foot contact will define the beginning of a stride. For example, a stride could be defined from heel contact of the right limb to subsequent heel contact on the right limb. The stride is subdivided into steps. A step is a portion of the stride from an event occurring on one leg to the same event occurring on the opposite leg. For example, a step could be defined as foot contact on the right limb to foot contact on the left limb. Thus, two steps equal one stride, also called one gait cycle.

Stride length and stride rate are among the most commonly studied linear kinematic parameters. The distance covered by one stride is the stride length, and the number of strides per minute is the stride rate. Running and walking velocity is the result of the relationship between stride rate and stride length. That is:

Running speed = stride length * stride rate

Velocity can be increased by increasing stride length or stride rate or both. Examples of stride characteristics ranging from a slow walk up through a sprint are presented in Table 8-4, which clearly shows adjustments in stride rate and stride length that contribute to the increase in the velocity. The stride can be lengthened only so much; in fact, from walking speeds of 0.75 m/s on, pelvic rotation begins to contribute to the stride lengthening (29). Many studies (9,17,20,26) have shown that in running there is also an increase in both stride rate and stride length with increasing velocity, but the adjustment is not proportional at higher velocities. This is illustrated in Figure 8-26. For velocities up to 7 m/s increases are linear, while at higher speeds there is a smaller increment in stride length and a greater increment in stride rate. This indicates that when sprinting, runners increase their velocity by increasing their stride rate more than their stride length. A runner initially increases velocity by increasing stride length. However, there is a physical limit to how much an individual can increase stride length. To run faster, therefore, the runner must increase stride rate.

Refer to the walking data in Appendix E: Calculate the step length, the step frequency, the stride length, the stride frequency, and the cadence (steps per minute). Calculate the walking velocity.

Each individual has a preferred speed at which he or she opts to start running instead of walking faster. This speed is usually somewhere around 2 m/s. The walking velocity

TABLE 8-4 Stride Characteristic Comparison Between Walking and Running

Variable	Walking (16,23)	Running (20,23)	Sprint
Speed (m/s)	0.67–1.32	1.65–4.00	8.00–9.00
Stride length (m)	1.03–1.35	1.51–3.00	4.60–4.50
Cadence (steps/min)	79.00–118.00	132.00–200.00+	
Stride rate (Hz)	0.65–0.98	1.10–1.38	1.75–2.00
Cycle time (sec)	1.55–1.02	0.91–0.73	0.57–0.50
Stance (% of gait cycle)	66.00–60.00	59.00–30.00	25.00–20.00
Swing (% of gait cycle)	34.00–40.00	41.00–70.00	75.00–80.00

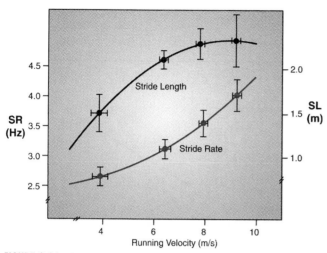

FIGURE 8-26 Changes in stride length and stride rate as a function of running velocity. (After Luhtanen, P., Komi, P. V. [1973]. Mechanical factors influencing running speed. In E. Asmussen, K. Jorgensen (Eds.). *Biomechanics VI-B*. Baltimore: University Park Press.)

at which individuals switch to a run is higher than the running velocity at which they shift back to a walk (18).

Gait parameters are adjusted when physical or environmental conditions offer constraints to the gait cycle. For example, an individual with a limiting physical impairment will usually walk with a slower velocity and cadence by increasing the support phase of the cycle, decreasing the swing phase, and shortening the step length (23). Individuals with cerebral palsy have significant gait restrictions evidenced by slow velocities, short strides, slow cadence, and more time spent in double support. Environmental factors also influence gait; for example, when the walking surface becomes slippery, most individuals reduce the step length. This minimizes the chance of falling by increasing the heel-strike angle with the ground and decreasing the potential for foot displacement on the slippery surface (3).

The running and walking stride can be further subdivided into support, or stance, and nonsupport, or swing, phases. The support or stance phase occurs when the foot is in contact with the ground, that is, from the point of foot contact until the foot leaves the ground. The support phase is often subdivided further into heel strike followed by foot flat, midstance, heel rise, and toe off. The nonsupport or swing phase occurs from the point that the foot leaves the ground until the same foot touches the ground again. The proportional time spent in the stance and swing phases varies considerably between walking and running. In walking the percent of the total stride time spent in support and swing is approximately 60% and 40%, respectively. These ratios change with increased speed in both running and walking (Table 8-4). The absolute time and the relative time (a percent of the total stride time) spent in support decreases as running and walking speeds increase (1,2). Typical changes in relative time of the support phase in running range from 68% at a jogging pace to 54% at a moderate sprint to 47% at a full sprint.

Time spent in the support and the swing phase is just one of the factors that distinguish walking from running. The other factor that determines whether the gait is a walk or a run is whether one foot is always on the ground or not. In walking, there is always one foot on the ground, with a brief period when both feet are on the ground, creating a sequence of alternating single and double support. In running, the person does not always have one foot on the ground; there is an airborne phase followed by alternating single-support phases.

Refer to the walking data in Appendix E: What is the length of time spent in single support and double support during one stride?

VELOCITY CURVE

The linear kinematics of competitive running and walking has also been studied by biomechanists. In several cases, athletes were considered as single points and no consideration was given to the movement of the arms and legs as individual units. Over the years, a number of researchers have tried to measure the velocity curve of a runner during a sprint race (13). A. V. Hill, who later won the Nobel Prize in physiology, proposed a simple mathematical model to represent the velocity curve, and subsequent investigations have confirmed this model (Fig. 8-27). Most sprinters conform relatively closely to this model. At the start of the race the runner's velocity is zero. The velocity increases rapidly at first but then levels off to a constant value. This means that the runner accelerates rapidly at first, but the acceleration decreases toward the end of the run. The sprinter cannot increase velocity indefinitely throughout the race. In fact, the winner of a sprint race is usually the runner whose velocity decreases the least at the end of the race. Figure 8-28 illustrates the displacement, velocity, and acceleration data for the women's 100-m final in the 2000 Olympics. The graphs demonstrate similar characteristics for Marion Jones (Fig. 8-28*A*) and Savatheda Fynes (Fig. 8-28*B*), even though they finished first and seventh, respectively. In a study of female sprinters (6), it was reported that the sprinters reached their maximum velocity between 23 and 37 m

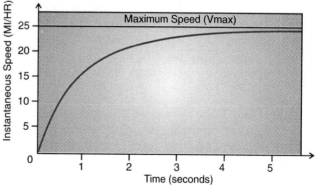

FIGURE 8-27 Hill's proposed mathematical model of a sprint race velocity curve. (After Brancazio, P. J. [1984]. *Sport Science*. New York: Simon & Schuster.)

(A) *Marion Jones*　　　　　　　　　　　　　　　　　**(B)** *Savatheda Fynes*

DISTANCE VS TIME IN 100-METER OLYMPIC FINAL

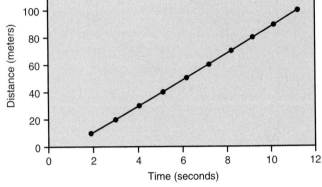

VELOCITY VS TIME IN 100-METER OLYMPIC FINAL

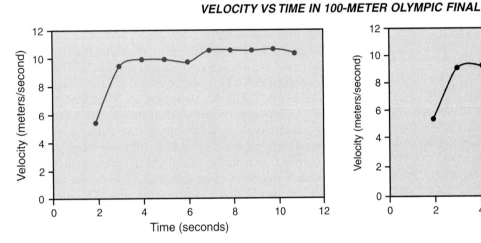
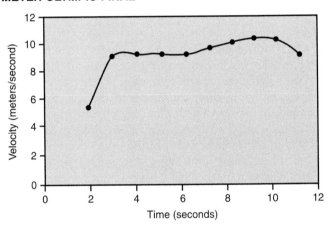

ACCELERATION VS TIME IN 100-METER OLYMPIC FINAL

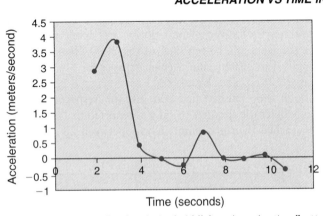
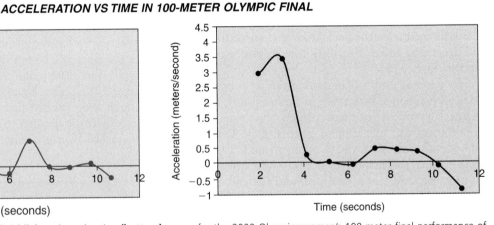

FIGURE 8-28 Distance **(top)**, velocity **(middle)**, and acceleration **(bottom)** curves for the 2000 Olympics women's 100-meter final performance of Marion Jones **(A)** and Savatheda Fynes **(B)**. (Source of split times: http://sydney2000.nbcolympics.com/).

in a 100-m race. It was also reported that these sprinters lost an average of 7.3% from their maximum velocity in the final 10 m of the race. These two trends were also present in the 100-m women's final shown in Figure 8-28.

The fastest instantaneous velocity of a runner during a race has not yet been measured during competition. Average speed can be readily calculated, however. Marion Jones and Maurice Greene, in their gold medal performances at the 2000 Olympic Games, covered 100 m in

10.75 s and 9.87 s, respectively, for an average speed of 9.30 m/s and 10.13 m/s, or speeds equivalent to 20.8 miles/hour and 22.7 miles/hour, respectively.

VARIATION OF VELOCITY DURING SUPPORT

When calculating average velocity over a race, remember that this was not the velocity of the runner at every instant during the race. During a race, a runner contacts

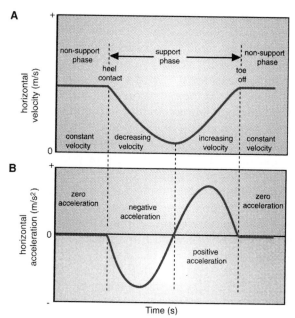

FIGURE 8-29 Changes in velocity **(A)** and acceleration **(B)** during the support phase of a running stride. (After Bates, B. T., et al. [1979]. Variations of velocity within the support phase of running. In J. Terauds and G. Dales (Eds.). *Science in Athletics*. Del Mar: Academic.)

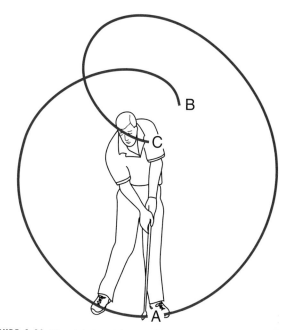

FIGURE 8-30 The club head in a golf swing travels in a curved path through a considerable distance, allowing time to develop velocity in the club head.

the ground numerous times, and it is important to note what occurs to the horizontal velocity during these ground contacts. The horizontal velocity of a runner during the support phase of the running stride from a study by Bates et al. (2) is presented in Figure 8-29*A*. An analysis of runners in this study indicated that the horizontal velocity decreased immediately at foot contact and continued to decrease during the first portion of the support period. As the runner's leg is extending in the latter portion of the support period, the velocity increases. The corresponding acceleration–time graph of a runner during the support phase (Fig. 8-29*B*) shows distinct negative and positive accelerations. It can be seen that the runner instantaneously has zero acceleration during the support phase, representing the transition from negative acceleration to positive acceleration. This results from the runner slowing down during the first portion of support and speeding up in the latter portion. To maintain a constant average velocity, the runner must gain as much speed in the latter portion of the support phase as was lost in the first portion.

 Linear Kinematics of the Golf Swing

SWING CHARACTERISTICS

The purpose of the golf swing is to generate speed in the club head and to control the club head so that it is directed optimally for contact with the ball. While many of the important biomechanical characteristics of the swing are angular, the linear kinematics of the club head ultimately

determine the success of the golf swing. Figure 8-30 shows the path of the club head in the swing. Starting at position A, the golfer brings the club back up behind and in front of the lead shoulder (B) to allow the club head to travel through a longer distance. The purpose of this backswing is to place the appropriate segments in an optimal position for force development and to establish the maximum range of motion for the subsequent downswing. In the downswing, the critical phase in the swing, the club head accelerates at rates greater than 800 m/s² to prepare for contact. Contact is made with the ball at the original starting position (A), where the club head is still accelerating. Peak velocity is obtained shortly after impact. Club head velocities at impact in the range of 40 m/s are very possible; they can be much higher in some golfers. The time to complete the total swing may be in the range of 1000 ms, with the downswing phase accounting for 210 ms, or a little over 20% of the time. Once impact is complete, the follow-through phase decelerates the club until the swing is terminated at C.

VELOCITY AND ACCELERATION OF CLUB

Figure 8-31*A* illustrates the velocity of the club (center of gravity) during the downswing phase (22). The motion of the club was recorded in three dimensions to determine linear kinematic characteristics toward the ball forward or backward (x), up or down (y), and away from or toward the golfer (z). In the initial portion of the downswing, with the club still up behind the head, the velocity in the x direction is backward, away from the ball, in the negative direction as the club is brought from the top of backswing

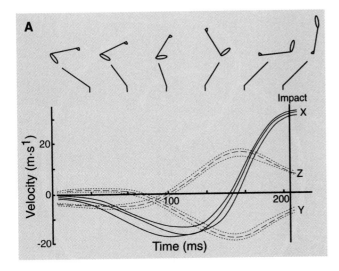

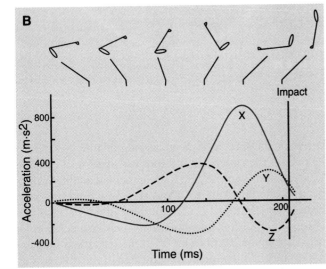

FIGURE 8-31 Velocity–time **(A)** and acceleration–time **(B)** graphs of a driver segment center of gravity toward or away from the ball (X), vertically (Y), and in toward or away from the body (Z). (After Neal, R. J., Wilson, B. D. [1985]. 3D Kinematics and kinetics of the golf swing. *International Journal of Sport Biomechanics*, 1:221–232.)

around the body and toward the ball. In the last half of the downswing, the x velocity climbs sharply and becomes positive as the club comes around and continues toward the ball. The peak forward velocity is achieved after impact.

The z velocity starts out negative, indicating that from the top of the backswing to approaching the halfway point

in the downswing, the club is moving toward the golfer and then shifts positive as the club is swinging away from the golfer. This trend is opposite to that in the vertical direction, where the velocity in the y direction starts out with small movements upward and reverses to a downward movement as the club is brought down to the ball.

The corresponding acceleration curves in Figure 8-31*B* identify critical phases in the swing at which maximal accelerations are obtained. Maximum acceleration in the direction of the ball (x) occurs 40 ms prior to impact, reaching a value of 870 m/s^2 (22). Acceleration continues on through impact, even though it is small. There is also vertical acceleration, reaching maximum just prior to impact and still accelerating through the impact. These trends would look very much the same for all clubs, but there would be a reduction in the values such as club head velocity, which decreases from the driver to the nine iron because of differences in club parameters.

Linear Kinematics of Wheelchair Propulsion

CYCLE PARAMETERS

Many individuals with spinal cord injury or other serious musculoskeletal impairments use a wheelchair for locomotion. Propelling a manual wheelchair involves cyclic body actions, using sequences in which both hands are in contact with the rim or not. These sequences are defined by certain parameters. The typical wheelchair cycle includes a propulsive phase with the hand pushing on the hand rim of the wheelchair followed by a nonpropulsive phase when the hand is brought back to the start of another propulsion phase. In the nonpropulsive phase, three actions describe the phase, starting with disengagement as the hand releases the hand rim at the end of propulsion, followed by recovery as the hand is brought back up to the top of the hand rim to start the propulsion again, and finally, contact, when the hand touches the rim. The amount of time spent in contact and the range of displacement of the hand forward and backward varies with individual preferences and wheelchair configurations, such as seat position. Even in world class athletes, the cycle patterns vary. Figure 8-32 shows displacement of the hand on the rim for different propulsive styles of

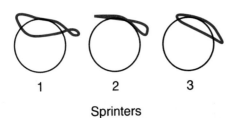

Sprinters

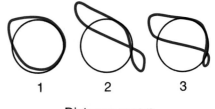

Distance racers

FIGURE 8-32 Hand displacement patterns for six Olympic wheelchair athletes illustrating differences in propulsion styles between sprinters (200 m) and distance racers (1500 m). (Higgs, C. (1984). Propulsion of racing wheelchairs. In C. Scherrell (Ed.). *Sport and Disabled Athletes*. Champaign, IL: Human Kinetics, 165–172.)

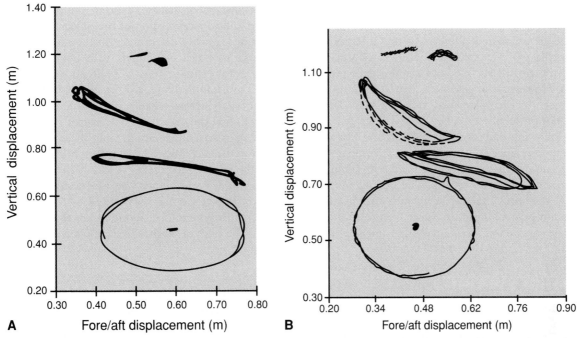

FIGURE 8-33 Vertical and fore/aft displacements of the neck, shoulder, elbow, and wrist over multiple wheelchair propulsion cycles show differences between two subjects incorporating the pumping action style **(A)** and a circular action style **(B)** (Courtesy of Joe Bolewicz, R. P. T.)

six wheelchair athletes (15). The three sprinters typically used a back-and-forth motion over the top of the hand rim, but the path of the disengagement from the rim varied as subjects' hands moved through small or large loops when they moved the hand back to make contact with the rim for propulsion. In the three distance racers, the pattern of the hand motion was more circular but still varied quite significantly between individuals.

PROPULSION STYLES

Two wheelchair propulsion styles have been identified (25). One is the pumping technique seen in the sprinters in Figure 8-33*A*, in which the hand moves back and forth horizontally with relatively large displacements away from the hand rim. The other popular technique is the circular technique (Fig. 8-33*B*), in which the hand moves in a circular path along the hand rim. The push phase in the circular pattern accounts for a larger percentage of the total propulsion cycle (43.0%) than the same phase in the pumping pattern (34.7%), suggesting that it may be more efficient.

Vertical and horizontal displacements of the wrist, elbow, shoulder, and neck during wheelchair propulsion for a moderately active individual with T3–T4 paraplegia is presented in Figure 8-33*A*. In the propulsion cycle the wrist travels forward and backward in a straight path indicating a push pattern of propulsion. The neck moved forward and backward through a range of approximately 5.9 cm and at an average of about 1 cm for every 6.735 cm of wrist movement. Peak acceleration of the hand on the rim occurred close to the end of the push phase and was in the range of 32 m/s^2.

To increase the velocity of wheelchair propulsion, the cycle time is reduced by increasing the cycle frequency. This occurs as a result of shifting the start and end angles to the front of the hand rim without changing the angular components of the push angle (28). The pattern of action in the forearm changes from a push-pull pattern in the slower velocity to more of a push pattern with support from a continuous trunk flexion.

Projectile Motion

Projectile motion refers to motion of bodies flung into the air. This type of motion occurs in many activities, such as baseball, diving, figure skating, basketball, golf, and volleyball. The motion of a projectile is a special case of linear kinematics in which, leaving aside air resistance, we know what changes in velocity and acceleration are going to occur once the object leaves the ground. For example, the horizontal velocity of a projectile remains constant while the object is airborne, resulting in zero horizontal acceleration. The vertical velocity increases by 9.81 m/s every second in flight, resulting in constant acceleration. These two characteristics of projectile kinematics allow for an easy assessment of projectile motion when the initial kinematic parameters of the projectile are known.

GRAVITY

When no other forces are acting on a body, the force of gravity on a projectile results in constant vertical acceleration. The acceleration due to gravity is approximately 9.81 m/s^2 at sea level and results from the attraction of two masses, the earth and the object. Only gravity and air resistance act on an object when the object is moving through the air unassisted. Objects in this situation are called projectiles. Gravity uniformly accelerates a projectile toward the earth's surface, and air resistance retards its progress. However, not all objects that fly through the air are projectiles. Self-propelled objects, such as airplanes, are not projectiles.

For the following discussion air resistance will be considered negligible, since it is relatively small compared to gravity. Depending on the projectile, different kinematic questions may be asked. For example, in the long jump or the shot put, the horizontal displacement is critical. In the high jump and pole vaulting, however, vertical displacement must be maximized. In biomechanics, it is important to understand the nature of projectile motion.

TRAJECTORY OF A PROJECTILE

The flight path of a projectile is called its trajectory (Fig. 8-34A). The instant at which an object becomes a projectile, such as when a pitcher releases the baseball, is known as the instant of release. Gravity continuously acts to change the vertical motion of the object once it has been released. If gravity did not act on the projectile, it would continue to travel indefinitely with the same velocity as when it was released (Fig. 8-34B). In space, beyond the earth's gravitational pull, a short firing burst of a vehicle's engine will result in a change in velocity. When the engine ceases to fire, the velocity at that instant remains constant, resulting in zero acceleration. Since there is no gravity and no air resistance, the vehicle will continue on this path until the engine fires again.

The flight path followed by a projectile in the absence of air resistance is a parabola (Fig. 8-34A). A parabola is a curve that is symmetrical about an axis through its highest point. The highest point of a parabola is its apex.

FACTORS INFLUENCING PROJECTILES

Three primary factors influence the trajectory of a projectile: the projection angle, projection velocity, and projection height (Fig. 8-35).

Projection Angle

The angle at which the object is released determines the shape of its trajectory. Projection angles generally vary from 0° (parallel to the ground) to 90° (perpendicular to the ground), although in some sporting activities, such as ski jumping, the projection angle is negative. If the projection angle is 0° (parallel to the horizontal), the trajectory is essentially the latter half of a parabola, because it has zero

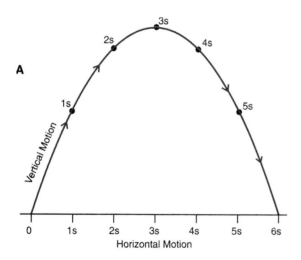

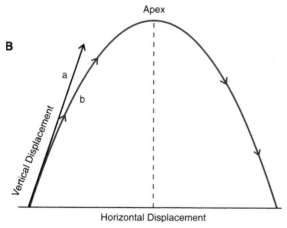

FIGURE 8-34 A. The parabolic trajectory of a projectile. **B.** Path a represents the trajectory of a projectile without the influence of gravity. Path b is a trajectory with gravity acting. Path b forms a parabola.

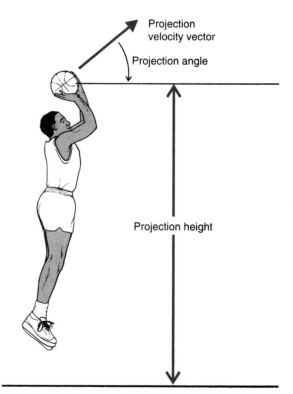

FIGURE 8-35 The factors influencing the trajectory of a projectile are **(a)** projection velocity, **(b)** projection angle, and **(c)** projection height.

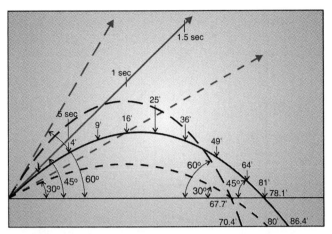

FIGURE 8-36 Theoretical trajectories of a projectile projected at different angles keeping velocity (15.2 m/s) and height (2.4 m) constant. (After Broer, M. R., Zernike, R. F. [1979]. *Efficiency of Human Movement* (4th Ed.). Philadelphia: Saunders College.)

vertical velocity and is immediately acted upon by gravity to pull it to the earth's surface. On the other hand, if the projection angle is 90°, the object is projected straight up into the air with zero horizontal velocity. In this case, the parabola is so narrow as to form a straight line.

If the projection angle is between 0° and 90°, the trajectory is truly parabolic. Figure 8-36 displays theoretical trajectories for an object projected at various angles with the same speed and height of projection.

The optimal angle of projection for a given activity is based on the purpose of the activity. Intuitively, it would appear that jumping over a relatively high object like a high jump bar would require quite a steep projection angle. This has proved to be the case, as high jumpers have a projection angle of 40 to 48° using the flop high jump technique (7). On the other hand, if one tried to jump for maximal horizontal distance such as in a long jump, the projection angle would be much smaller. This has also proved to be the case, as long jumpers have projection angles of 18 to 27° (12). Table 8-5 illustrates the projection angles reported in the research literature for several activities. Positive angles of projection indicate angles greater than zero, where the object is projected above the horizontal. Negative angles of projection refer to those less than zero, or below the horizontal. For example, in a

TABLE 8-5 **Projection Angles Used in Selected Activities**		
Activity	Angle (°)	Reference
Racing dive	5–22	14
Ski jumping	−4	19
Tennis serve	−3–15	24
Discus	−35–15	27
High jump (flop)	40–48	7

tennis serve, the serve is projected downward from the point of impact.

Projection Velocity

The velocity of the projectile at the instant of release will determine the height and distance of the trajectory as long as all other factors are held constant. The resultant velocity of projection is usually calculated and given when discussing the factors influencing the projectile. The resultant velocity of projection is the vector sum of the horizontal and vertical velocities. It is necessary, however, to focus on the components of the velocity vector, since they dictate the height of the trajectory and the distance the projectile will travel. Like other vectors, the velocity of projection has a vertical component (v_y) and a horizontal component (v_x).

The magnitude of the vertical velocity is reduced by the effect of gravity (9.81 m/s for every second of upward flight). Gravity reduces the vertical velocity of the projectile until the velocity equals zero. At that point, the projectile reaches its highest point in flight. The vertical velocity component, therefore, determines the height of the apex of the trajectory. The time it takes for gravity to reduce the vertical velocity to zero is:

$$\text{Time}_{up} = \frac{\text{vertical velocity}}{\text{gravity}}$$

If the vertical velocity is 11.2 m/s, the time to the apex is:

$$t_{up} = \frac{11.2 \text{ m/s}}{9.81 \text{ m/s}}$$

$$t_{up} = 1.14 \text{ s}$$

The vertical velocity is likewise increased by the effect of gravity on the downward flight. If the projectile lands at the same height as takeoff, t_{up} equals t_{down}. Total time in the air for this projectile would be:

$$\text{Time}_{total} = 2 * \left(\frac{\text{vertical velocity}}{\text{gravity}} \right)$$

$$t_{total} = 2 * \left(\frac{11.2 \text{ m/s}}{9.81 \text{ m/s}} \right)$$

$$t_{up} = 2.28 \text{ s}$$

The vertical velocity affects the height the projectile achieves, the time the projectile takes to reach that height, and consequently the time to fall to earth.

The horizontal component of the projection velocity is constant throughout the flight of the projectile. It is known that:

$$v_x = \frac{dx}{dt}$$

Rearranging this equation:

$$dx = v_x * dt$$

Since dx represents the change in position of the projectile during its flight, dx is determined by the product of the horizontal velocity and the flight time to that position. The magnitude of dx is the distance that the projectile travels and is called the range of the projectile. For example, if a projectile is released at a horizontal velocity of 13.7 m/s, the projectile will have traveled 13.7 m in the first second, 27.4 m after 2 s, 40.1 m after 3 s, and so on. In another example, if a shot putter releases the shot with a horizontal velocity of 10.5 m/s and it travels through the air for 2.2 s, the range of the throw would be:

$$\text{Range} = 10.5 \text{ m/s} * 2.2 \text{ s}$$
$$= 23.1 \text{ m}$$

The angle of projection will affect the relative magnitude of the horizontal and vertical velocity. If the angle of projection is 40° and the projection velocity is 13.7 m/s, the horizontal component of the projection velocity is:

$$v_x = \text{projection velocity} * \text{cosine of projection angle}$$
$$= 13.7 \text{ m/s} * \cos 40°$$
$$= 10.49 \text{ m/s}$$

The vertical component is:

$$v_y = \text{projection velocity} * \text{sine of projection angle}$$
$$= 13.7 \text{ m/s} * \sin 40°$$
$$= 8.81 \text{ m/s}$$

If the angle is altered to 35°, the horizontal component becomes:

$$v_x = 13.7 \text{ m/s} * \cos 35°$$
$$= 11.22 \text{ m/s}$$

The vertical component becomes:

$$v_y = 13.7 \text{ m/s} * \sin 35°$$
$$= 7.86 \text{ m/s}$$

To understand in general how the angle of projection affects the velocity components, consider that the cosine of 0° is 1 and decreases to zero as the angle increases. If the cosine of the angle is used to represent the horizontal velocity, the horizontal velocity decreases as the angle of projection increases from 0 to 90° (Fig. 8-37). Also, the sine of 0° is zero and increases to 1 as the angle increases. Consequently, if the sine of the angle is used to represent vertical velocity, the vertical velocity increases as the angle increases from 0 to 90° (Fig. 8-37). It can readily be seen that as the angle gets closer to 90°, the horizontal velocity becomes smaller and the vertical velocity becomes greater. As the angle gets closer to 0°, the horizontal velocity becomes greater and the vertical velocity gets smaller.

At 45°, however, the sine and cosine of the angle are equal. For any given velocity, therefore, horizontal velocity equals vertical velocity. It would appear that 45° would be the optimum angle of projection, since for any velocity the horizontal and vertical velocities are equal. This is true under certain circumstances to be discussed in relation to projection height. Generally, if the maximum range of the projectile is critical, an angle to optimize the horizontal velocity, or an angle less than 45°, would be appropriate.

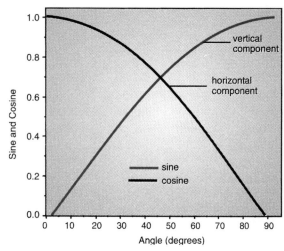

FIGURE 8-37 Graph of sine and cosine values at angles from 0 to 90°. Sin 45° = cosine 45°.

Thus, in activities such as the long jump and shot putting, the optimal angle of projection is less than 45°. If the height of the projectile is important, an angle greater than 45° should be chosen. This is the case in activities such as high jumping.

Projection Height

The height of projection of a projectile is the difference in height between the vertical takeoff position and the vertical landing position. Three situations greatly affect the shape of the trajectory. In each case, the trajectory is parabolic but the shape of the parabola may not be completely symmetrical; that is, the first half of the parabola may not have the same shape as the second half.

In the first case, the projectile is released and lands at the same height. The shape of the trajectory is symmetrical, and thus the time for the projectile to reach the apex from the point of release equals the time for the projectile to reach the ground from the apex. If a ball is kicked from the surface of a field and lands on the field's surface, the relative projection height is zero, and thus time up to the apex is equal to time down from the apex.

In the second situation, the projectile is released from a point higher than the surface on which it lands. The parabola is asymmetrical, with the initial portion to the apex less than the latter portion. In this case, time for the projectile to reach the apex is less than time to reach the ground from the apex. For example, if a shot putter releases the shot from 2.2 m above the ground and the shot lands on the ground, the height of projection is 2.2 m.

In the third situation, the projectile is released from a point below the surface on which it lands. Once again the trajectory is asymmetrical, but now the initial portion to the apex of the trajectory is greater than the latter portion. Thus, time for the projectile to reach the apex is greater than time for the projectile to reach the ground from the apex. For example, if a ball is thrown from a

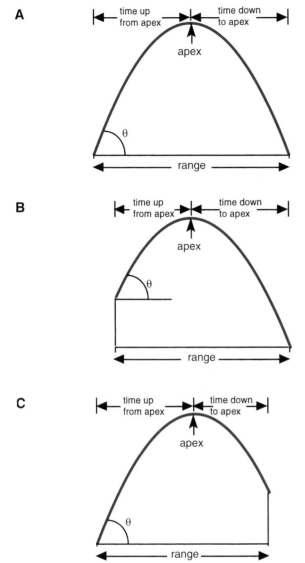

FIGURE 8-38 Influence of projection height on the shape of the trajectory of a projectile.

height of 2.2 m and lands in a tree at a height of 4 m, the height of projection is 1.8 m (Fig. 8-38).

Generally, when the projection velocity and angle of projection are held constant, the higher the point of release, the longer the flight time. If the flight time is longer, the range is greater. Also, for maximum range, when the relative height of projection is zero, the optimum angle is 45°; when the projection height is above the landing height, the optimum angle is less than 45°; and when the projection height is below the landing height, the optimum angle is greater than 45°. The effect of landings that are lower than takeoffs is shown in Figure 8-36.

OPTIMIZING PROJECTION CONDITIONS

To optimize the conditions for the release of a projectile, the purpose of the projectile must be considered. As discussed previously, the three primary factors that affect the

flight of a projectile are interrelated and will affect both the height of the trajectory and the distance traveled. It may be intuitive that since the height of the apex and the length of the trajectory of the projectile are both affected by the projection velocity, increasing the projection velocity will increase both of these parameters. However, this common perception is incorrect. The choice of an appropriate projection angle is what will dictate whether the vertical or the horizontal velocity will be increased with increasing projection velocity. In addition, the angle of projection can be affected by the height of projection.

The relative importance of these factors is illustrated in the following example. If an athlete puts the shot with a velocity of 14 m/s at an angle of 40° from a height of 2.2 m, the distance of the throw is 22 m. If each factor is increased by a given percentage (10% in this case) as the other two factors are held constant, the relative importance of each factor may be calculated. Increasing the velocity to 15.4 m/s results in a throw of 26.2 m; increasing the angle to 44° results in a throw of 22 m; and increasing the height of projection to 2.4 m results in a throw of 22.2 m. It is readily evident that increasing the velocity of projection increases the range of the throw more substantially than increasing either the angle or the height of projection. However, the three factors are interrelated, and any change in one results in a change in the others.

Equations of Constant Acceleration

THREE EQUATIONS

When a projectile is traveling through the air, only gravity and air resistance act upon it. If air resistance is ignored, only gravity is considered to act on the projectile. The acceleration due to gravity is constant, and thus the projectile undergoes constant acceleration. Using the concepts from the previous section, equations of constant acceleration, or projectile motion, can be determined based on the definitions of velocity and acceleration. There are three such expressions involving the interrelationships of the kinematic parameters time, position, velocity, and acceleration. These expressions are often referred to as the equations of constant acceleration. The first equation expresses final velocity as a function of the initial velocity, acceleration, and time.

$$v_f = v_i + at$$

The variables v_f and v_i refer to the final velocity and the initial velocity, respectively. Many of the vertical and horizontal velocity components can be described by this equation, especially in the vertical direction where acceleration is constant.

As described previously, the horizontal component of velocity, v_x, is constant throughout the flight of the projectile, so the horizontal acceleration is zero. Indeed if $a = 0$ is substituted in this equation, it can be seen that:

$$vx_f = vx_i$$

The final velocity equals the initial velocity, or the horizontal velocity of projection is constant throughout the flight period.

In the earlier discussion of the vertical velocity component, v_y, it was suggested that gravity immediately acted to decrease the magnitude of v_y after release of the projectile. If the coordinate system is oriented such that positive is up and negative is down, acceleration downward must be negative. Since gravity accelerates a projectile toward the ground, the acceleration due to gravity must be negative. Therefore, the acceleration due to gravity is -9.81 m/s^2. For the vertical component, the first equation of constant acceleration equation is:

$$vy_f = vy_i - 9.81\,t$$

This simply reaffirms that the vertical velocity at any instant is equal to the initial vertical velocity of release decreased by a value of 9.81 m/s for every second of flight until the final velocity is zero. Velocity is zero at the apex of the trajectory.

In the second equation, position is expressed as a function of initial velocity, acceleration, and time.

$$s = v_i t + \frac{1}{2}at^2$$

The variable in this expression may refer to the horizontal or vertical case and is the change in position or the distance that the object travels from one position to another. This equation is derived by integrating the first equation. If acceleration is zero, as in the horizontal velocity case, this equation becomes:

$$s = vx_i t$$

This expression reaffirms that the horizontal distance the object travels—the range—is the product of the horizontal velocity and the time of the flight.

In considering the vertical in this equation, note that the variable "a" representing acceleration due to gravity equals -9.81 m/s^2. The expression, therefore, is not as simple as for the horizontal component. If, for example, an object begins at rest and is dropped from some height, the initial vertical velocity is zero. This expression then becomes:

$$s_y = \frac{1}{2}at^2$$

$$s_y = \frac{1}{2} * 9.81 * t^2$$

The variable t is the time it takes for the projectile to reach the ground from the point at which it was dropped. This expression indicates that height may be calculated by simply knowing the length of time it took for the object to touch the ground once it was released, given that gravitational acceleration is constant.

The last equation expresses final velocity as a function of initial velocity, acceleration, and position.

$$v_f^2 = v_i^2 + 2as$$

Each of the kinematic variables in this expression appeared in one or both of the previous equations. Simplifying this expression for the horizontal case (that is $a_x = 0$) again reaffirms that horizontal velocity is constant throughout the projectile's flight. That is:

$$vx_f^2 = vx_i^2$$

For the vertical case, the example of an object dropping from some height, by beginning with a vertical velocity of zero, may be used. The expression, where $a = 9.81$ m/s^2, becomes:

$$vy_f^2 = 2as_y$$

$$vy_f^2 = 2 * 9.81 * s_y$$

The final vertical velocity is therefore a function of the acceleration due to gravity and the height, s_y, from which the object was dropped.

NUMERICAL EXAMPLE

The equations of constant acceleration all employ parameters that are basic to linear kinematics. The three equations of constant acceleration thus provide a useful method of analyzing projectile motion. If calculating the range of a projectile, for example, the following expression can be used:

$$\text{Range} = \frac{v^2 * \sin\theta * \cos\theta + v_x * \sqrt{(v_y)^2 + 2gh}}{g}$$

where v = velocity of projection, θ = angle of projection, h = height of release of projection, and g = acceleration due to gravity. This is a rather complicated expression, however. Instead, the equations of constant acceleration can be used to work through a problem of calculating the range of a projectile.

Suppose a shot putter releases the shot at an angle of 40° from a height of 2.2 m with a velocity of 13.3 m/s. Figure 8-39 illustrates what is known about the conditions of the projectile at the instant of projection and the shape of the trajectory based on our previous discussion.

Using the previous equation, the range can be calculated as follows:

Range =

$$= \frac{13.3 \text{ m/s}^2 * \sin 40 * \cos 40 + 10.19 \text{ m/s} * \sqrt{8.55 \text{ m/s}^2 + 2(9.81 \text{ m/s}^2)(2.2 \text{ m})}}{9.81 \text{ m/s}^2}$$

$$= \frac{176.89 * 0.6428 * 0.766 + 10.19 * \sqrt{73.10 + 43.16}}{9.81}$$

$$= \frac{87.09 + 10.19 * 10.78}{9.81}$$

$$= \frac{87.09 + 109.84}{9.81}$$

$$= 20.07 \text{ m}$$

The same problem can be solved in seven steps, using the equations of constant acceleration. Remember, to find

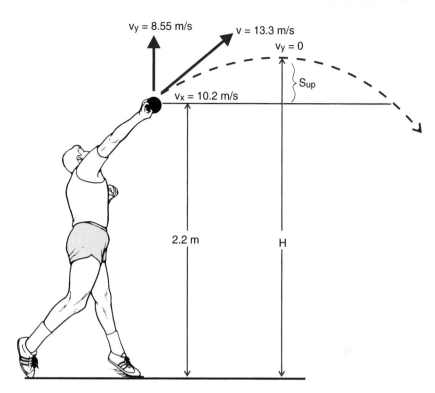

FIGURE 8-39 Conditions during the flight of the shot. Initial conditions are: v = 13.3 m/s; projection angle = 40° ; and projection height = 2.2 m.

the range of a projectile, the horizontal velocity and the length of time that the shot was in the air must be known.

Step 1. Calculate the initial vertical and horizontal velocities. (Use Appendix D for sine and cosine values).

$$v_x = v * \cos \theta$$
$$= 13.3 \text{ m/s} * \cos 40°$$
$$= 13.3 \text{ m/s} * 0.766$$
$$= 10.19 \text{ m/s}$$

$$v_y = v * \sin \theta$$
$$= 13.3 \text{ m/s} * \sin 40°$$
$$= 13.3 \text{ m/s} * 0.643$$
$$= 8.55 \text{ m/s}$$

Step 2. Use the first equation of constant acceleration to calculate the time required for the projectile to reach the apex of its trajectory. Since it is necessary to calculate the time to the apex, the equation using the vertical velocity must be used. Thus, the acceleration due to gravity, a, will act, bringing the vertical velocity to zero at the apex.

$$v_y = v_{yi} + at_{up}$$
$$0 = 8.55 \text{ m/s} - 9.81 \text{ m/s}^2 * t_{up}$$
$$t_{up} = \frac{8.55 \text{ m/s}}{9.81 \text{ m/s}^2}$$
$$t_{up} = 0.87 \text{ s}$$

Step 3. Use the third equation of constant acceleration to calculate the height of the apex of the trajectory above the release height. Remember that the height of the trajectory depends on the vertical velocity, the acceleration due to gravity is -9.81 m/s^2, and the vertical velocity at the apex is zero.

$$v_{yf}^2 = v_{yi}^2 + 2as_y$$
$$0 = (8.55 \text{ m/s})^2 - 2 * 9.81 \text{ m/s}^2 * s_{yup}$$
$$s_{yup} = \frac{8.55 \text{ m/s}^2}{2 * 9.81 \text{ m/s}^2}$$
$$s_{yup} = 3.72 \text{ m}$$

Step 4. Calculate the total height to the apex of the trajectory.

$$H = \text{projection height} + s_{yup}$$
$$= 2.2 \text{ m} + 3.72 \text{ m}$$
$$= 5.92 \text{ m}$$

Step 5. Calculate the time for the projectile to reach the ground from the apex of the trajectory. Since the projectile will land at a level lower than the release point, time for the projectile to reach the apex of the trajectory must be less than time for the projectile to reach the ground from the apex. The time down, t_{down}, can be calculated using the second equation of constant acceleration. In this equation, the displacement is negative, since it measures the distance from the apex to the ground. In addition, the initial vertical velocity of the downward flight is zero.

$$s_y = v_i t + \frac{1}{2}at^2$$
$$-5.92 \text{ m} = 0 + \frac{1}{2} * -9.81 \text{ m/s}^2 * t_{down}^2$$
$$-t_{down} = \sqrt{\frac{2 * 5.92 \text{ m}}{-9.81 \text{ m/s}^2}}$$
$$-t_{down} = \sqrt{\frac{11.84 \text{ m}}{-9.81 \text{ m/s}^2}}$$

Since time cannot be negative, each side of this equation must be multiplied by -1, resulting in the following:

$$t_{down} = 1.10 \text{ s}$$

Step 6. Calculate the total time the projectile is in the air by adding the time to reach the apex of the trajectory to the time to reach the ground from the apex.

$$\begin{aligned} T_{total} &= t_{up} + t_{down} \\ &= 0.87 \text{ s} + 1.10 \text{ s} \\ &= 1.97 \text{ s} \end{aligned}$$

Step 7. Calculate the range of the projectile.

$$\begin{aligned} \text{Range} &= v_x * T_{total} \\ &= 10.19 \text{ m/s} * 1.97 \text{ s} \\ &= 20.07 \text{ m} \end{aligned}$$

The distance that the shot traveled under these conditions is 20.1 m. In our initial discussion of projectiles and the equations of constant acceleration, air resistance was considered to be negligible. The mathematics of air resistance is well beyond the scope of this book, since it would require solving differential equations. However, it may be of interest to know that if these initial conditions were used to solve this problem taking into account air resistance, a reduction of 1.46% in the range of the throw would be found. Considering air resistance, the throw would be 0.3 m less, or a total of 19.8 m.

 Summary

Biomechanics is a quantitative discipline. One type of quantitative analysis involves linear kinematics, the study of linear motion with respect to time. Linear kinematics involves the vector quantities position, velocity, and acceleration and the scalar quantities displacement and speed. Velocity is defined as the time rate of change of position and is calculated in biomechanics, using the first central difference method as follows:

$$v = \frac{s_{i+1} - s_{i-1}}{2\Delta t}$$

Equation Review for Linear Kinematics

Purpose	Given	Formula
Vector composition, magnitude	Horizontal and vertical components	$r^2 = x^2 + y^2$
Vector composition, angle	Horizontal and vertical components	$\tan \theta = y/x$
Vector resolution, vertical	Magnitude and direction of vector	$y = r \sin \theta$
Vector resolution, horizontal	Magnitude and direction of vector	$x = r \cos \theta$
Time between video frames	Camera frame, sampling rate	Time (s) = 1/frame rate
Calculate position	Starting position relative to origin, constant velocity (zero acceleration), time	$s = s_i + v_i t$
Calculate position	Starting position at origin, constant velocity (zero acceleration), time	$s = v_i t$
Calculate position	Initial velocity, time, constant acceleration	$s = v_i t + 1/2 a t^2$
Calculate position	Initial velocity zero, time, constant acceleration	$s = 1/2 a t^2$
Calculate average velocity	Displacement and time	$v = x_2 - x_1/t_2 - t_1$
Calculate average velocity	Initial and final velocity	$v = v_i + v_f/2$
Calculate final velocity	Initial velocity, constant acceleration, and time	$v_f = v_i + at$
Calculate final velocity	Starting velocity zero, constant acceleration, time	$v = at$
Calculate final velocity	Velocity at time = zero, constant acceleration, initial position relative to origin, final position	$v = \sqrt{v_i^2 + 2a(x - x_i)}$
Calculate final velocity	Initial velocity zero, constant acceleration, initial and final position	$v_f^2 = 2as$ $v = \sqrt{2a(x - x_i)}$
Calculate acceleration	Final velocity and displacement	$a = v_f^2/2d$
Calculate average acceleration	Velocity and time	$a = v_2 - v_1/t_2 - t_1$
Calculate time	Displacement, constant acceleration	$t = \sqrt{2d/a}$
Calculate time in air for projectile beginning and landing at same height	Vertical velocity, constant acceleration	$t = 2 v_y/a$
Calculate distance of projectile	Resultant velocity, initial angle of release, constant acceleration	$s = r^2 \sin 2\theta/a$

Acceleration is defined as the time rate of change of velocity and is calculated as follows:

$$a = \frac{v_{i+1} - v_{i-1}}{2\Delta t}$$

The process of calculating velocity from position and time or acceleration from velocity and time is called differentiation. Calculating the derivative via differentiation entails finding the slope of a line tangent to the parameter–time curve. The process opposite to differentiation is called integration. Velocity may be calculated as the integral of acceleration and position as the integral of velocity. Integration implies calculating the area under the parameter–time curve. The method of calculating the area under a parameter–time curve is called the Riemann sum.

Projectile motion involves an object that undergoes constant acceleration because it is uniformly accelerated by gravity. The flight of a projectile, its height and distance, are affected by conditions at the point of release: the angle, velocity, and relative height of projection. Three equations govern constant acceleration. The first expresses final velocity, v_f, as a function of initial velocity, v_i, acceleration, a, and time, t. That is:

$$v_f = v_i + at$$

The second equation expresses position, s, as a function of initial velocity, v_i, acceleration, a, and time, t. That is:

$$s = v_i t + \frac{1}{2}at^2$$

The third equation expresses final velocity, v_f, as a function of initial velocity, v_i, acceleration, a, and position, s.

$$v_f^2 = v_i^2 + 2as$$

These equations may be used to calculate the range of a projectile.

REVIEW QUESTIONS

True or False

1. ____ Estimating the range of motion at the hip joint during stair ascent after visually observing the movement is a quantitative analysis.
2. ____ The motion of a long jumper in the air is an example of translational motion.
3. ____ The x and y axes in a two-dimensional rectangular reference system are always oriented vertically and horizontally, respectively.
4. ____ With a cartesian coordinate reference system originating at the hip joint, a sample set of coordinates for the ankle joint could be (0.5, −12).
5. ____ Both the x and y coordinates in the second quadrant of the rectangular coordinate system are negative.
6. ____ Speed is a vector quantity.
7. ____ Displacement indicates the direction and distance from the starting position.
8. ____ The slope of a secant indicates instantaneous velocity.
9. ____ Vectors are added together graphically by placing the tail of one vector at the head of the other vector.
10. ____ The slope of a displacement–time graph represents the average velocity.
11. ____ Positive acceleration indicates motion is occurring away from the origin.
12. ____ The point where the velocity is maximum in a velocity–time graph indicates the point where acceleration is maximum.
13. ____ Velocity is a measure of the area under the acceleration–time curve.
14. ____ The steepness of the slope of a velocity–time curve is an indication of the magnitude of the acceleration.
15. ____ Stride length is measured from the heel contact of one foot to the heel contact of the other foot.
16. ____ The support phase in walking accounts for a greater percentage of the total cycle than in running.
17. ____ Walking speed is increased by increasing stride length, stride rate, or both.
18. ____ Successful sprinters can usually increase their acceleration at the end of the race.
19. ____ In the golf swing, the club head should still be accelerating past contact with the ball.
20. ____ Maximum acceleration of the club head occurs at the moment of impact in the golf swing.
21. ____ Velocity of wheelchair propulsion is increased by increasing the cycle frequency.
22. ____ Horizontal motion of a projectile is a special case of constant acceleration.
23. ____ Vertical velocity of a projectile determines its time in the air.
24. ____ An airplane is a projectile.
25. ____ Releasing a projectile from a greater height extends the time in the air.

Multiple Choice

1. Convert the rectangular coordinates of (122, 10) to polar coordinates.
   a. (11.49, 4.69)
   b. (122.4, 4.69)
   c. (122.4, 85.3)
   d. (11.49, 85.3)
2. Convert the polar coordinates of (135, 182) to rectangular coordinates.
   a. (−4.71, −134.9)
   b. (134.9, 4.71)
   c. (−134.9, −4.71)
   d. (4.71, 134.9)

3. Figure 8-11 depicts the path of a runner. If the runner starts and ends at the end of each block, and if each block is a square with lengths of 200 m, what is the magnitude of the resultant displacement of the runner?
   a. 1200 m
   b. 1150 m
   c. 894 m
   d. 900 m

4. A swimmer completes six laps in a 50-m swimming pool, finishing where he started. What was the linear distance and the linear displacement?
   a. Distance = 150 m, displacement = 150 m
   b. Distance = 300 m, displacement = 300 m
   c. Distance = 300 m, displacement = 0
   d. None of the above

5. A basketball player shoots from beyond the 3-point arc. The ball leaves the hand with an initial velocity of 8 m/s angled 52° from the horizontal. What is the horizontal and vertical velocity of the basketball?
   a. v_x = 6.3 m/s v_y = 4.9 m/s
   b. v_x = 4.9 m/s v_y = 6.3 m/s
   c. v_x = 6.0 m/s v_y = 5.0 m/s
   d. v_x = 5.0 m/s v_y = 6.0 m/s

6. At takeoff, the horizontal and vertical velocities of a long jumper are 7.6 m/s and 3 m/s, respectively. What are the resultant velocity and angle of takeoff?
   a. v = 8.17 m/s θ = 11.9°
   b. v = 7.2 m/s θ = 11.9°
   c. v = 7.2 m/s θ = 21.5°
   d. v = 8.17 m/s θ = 21.5°

7. Given a right triangle with hypotenuse = 12.5 cm, side Y = 7.2 cm, find the length of side X and the size of the other two angles.
   a. Side X = 14.42 cm $θ_1$ = 31.7° $θ_2$ = 53.2°
   b. Side X = 10.2 cm $θ_1$ = 35.2° $θ_2$ = 54.8°
   c. Side X = 12.5 cm $θ_1$ = 54.8° $θ_2$ = 35.2°
   d. Side X = 14.42 cm $θ_1$ = 53.2° $θ_2$ = 31.7°

8. Suppose an individual moves from point s1 (6, 9) to point s2 (11,10) to point s3 (5, 6). What are the horizontal, vertical, and resultant displacements?
   a. Horizontal = 11 units; vertical = 5 units; resultant = 12.1 units
   b. Horizontal = 1 unit; vertical = 3 units; resultant = 3.16 units
   c. Horizontal = −1 unit; vertical = −3 units; resultant = 3.16 units
   d. Horizontal = −11 units; vertical = −5 units; resultant = 12.1 units

9. Combine the following two vectors to find the resultant vector. Vector A = 7.4 units at 30° and Vector B = 11.1 units at 120°.
   a. Resultant = 13.34 units; θ = 86.3°
   b. Resultant = 18.49 units; θ = 60.0°
   c. Resultant = 17.89 units; θ = 48.1°
   d. Resultant = 17.89 units; θ = 41.9°

10. An individual drives 50 km in 72 minutes. What was the average speed in meters per second?
    a. 1.157
    b. 11.57

c. 69.44
d. 694.44

11. A train accelerates from rest at a constant rate of 10 m/s². How fast is it going after 5 s?
    a. 500 m/s
    b. 50 m/s
    c. 5 m/s
    d. 55 m/s

12. The initial velocity of a projectile was 45 m/s at 72°. How high above the ground and how far horizontally was the object when it was 4.7 s into the flight?
    a. vertical = 92.78 m, horizontal = 65.38 m
    b. vertical = 87.54 m, horizontal = 62.34 m
    c. vertical = 94.56 m, horizontal = 70.11 m
    d. vertical = 91.56 m, horizontal = 64.87 m

13. A triple jumper needs a velocity of 9 m/s to make a good jump. If he is accelerating at 1.7 m/s², how much time does he need to reach the velocity?
    a. 4.79 s
    b. 5.33 s
    c. 5.18 s
    d. 5.29 s

14. A vaulter is trying to reach a velocity of 8 m/s at the end of a 15-m runway. How quickly must she accelerate?
    a. 2.13 m/s²
    b. 1.82 m/s²
    c. 1.90 m/s²
    d. 2.09 m/s²

15. A sprinter starts from rest and reaches a maximum velocity of 7.4 m/s in 2.5 s. What was their average acceleration from rest to maximum velocity?
    a. 3.01 m/s²
    b. 2.94 m/s²
    c. 2.87 m/s²
    d. 2.96 m/s²

16. A high jumper takes off with a vertical velocity of 4.2 m/s. How long does it take the jumper to reach the peak height of the jump?
    a. 0.86 s
    b. 0.79 s
    c. 0.43 s
    d. 0.37 s

17. Golf Ball A is driven straight out from a tee box that is 2 m above the fairway. At the instant the club contacts the ball, another golfer drops Ball B from a height of 2 m. Which ball will contact the ground first?
    a. Ball A
    b. Ball B
    c. Both balls will contact at the same time

    Questions 18 to 24: A baseball is thrown with a velocity of 31 m/s at an angle of 40° from a height of 1.8 m.

18. Calculate the vertical and horizontal velocity components.
    a. v_x = 18.65 m/s v_y = 12.58 m/s
    b. v_x = 12.58 m/s v_y = 18.65 m/s
    c. v_x = 19.93 m/s v_y = 23.75 m/s
    d. v_x = 23.75 m/s v_y = 19.93 m/s

19. Calculate the time to peak trajectory
   a. 2.03 s
   b. 2.42 s
   c. 2.32 s
   d. 1.90 s

20. Calculate the height of the trajectory from the point of release.
   a. 17.73 m
   b. 28.73 m
   c. 22.01 m
   d. 20.21 m

21. Calculate the total height of the parabola.
   a. 22.01 m
   b. 30.52 m
   c. 19.43 m
   d. 24.25 m

22. Calculate the time from the apex to the ground.
   a. 1.99 s
   b. 2.49 s
   c. 2.12 s
   d. 2.22 s

23. Calculate the total flight time.
   a. 3.89 s
   b. 4.91 s
   c. 4.15 s
   d. 4.54 s

24. Calculate the range of the throw.
   a. 98.53 m
   b. 48.94 m
   c. 63.33 m
   d. 115.8 m

25. A baseball leaving the bat at 46° at a height of 1.2 m from the ground clears a 3-m high wall 125 meters from home plate. What is the initial velocity of the ball (ignoring air resistance)?
   a. 37.3 m/s
   b. 34.9 m/s
   c. 35.02 m/s
   d. 36.9 m/s

REFERENCES

1. Bates, B. T., Haven, B. H. (1974). Effects of fatigue on the mechanical characteristics of highly skilled female runners. In R. C. Nelson, C. A. Morehouse (Eds.). *Biomechanics IV.* Baltimore: University Park Press, 119–125.

2. Bates, B. T., et al. (1979). Variations of velocity within the support phase of running. In J. Terauds and G. Dales (Eds.). *Science in Athletics.* Del Mar: Academic, 51–59.

3. Brady, R. A., et al. (2000). Foot displacement but not velocity predicts the outcome of a slip induced in young subjects while walking. *Journal of Biomechanics,* 33:803–808.

4. Brancazio, P. J. (1984). *Sport Science.* New York: Simon & Schuster.

5. Broer, M. R., Zernike, R. F. *Efficiency of Human Movement* (4th Ed.). Philadelphia: Saunders College, 1979.

6. Chow, J. W. (1987). Maximum speed of female high school runners. *International Journal of Sports Biomechanics,* 3:110–127.

7. Dapena, J. (1980). Mechanics of translation in the Fosbury flop. *Medicine and Science in Sports and Exercise,* 12:37–44.

8. Dapena, J., Chung, C. S. (1988). Vertical and radial motions of the body during the take-off phase of high jumping. *Medicine and Science in Sports and Exercise,* 20:290–302.

9. Elliott, B. C., Blanksby, B. A. (1979). A biomechanical analysis of the male jogging action. *Journal of Human Movement Studies,* 5:42–51.

10. Elliott, B., et al. (1986). A three-dimensional cinematographic analysis of the fastball and curveball pitches in baseball. *International Journal of Sport Biomechanics,* 2:20–28.

11. Fukashiro, S., Komi, P. V. (1987). Joint moment and mechanical power flow of the lower limb during vertical jump. *International Journal of Sports Medicine,* 8:15–21.

12. Hay, J. G. (1986). The biomechanics of the long jump. *Exercise and Sport Science Review,* 401–446.

13. Henry, F. M., Trafton, I. (1951). The velocity curve of sprint running. *Research Quarterly,* 23:409–422.

14. Heusner, W. W. (1959). Theoretical specifications for the racing dive: Optimum angle for take-off. *Research Quarterly,* 30:25–37.

15. Higgs, C. (1984). Propulsion of racing wheelchairs. In C. Sherrel (Ed.). *Sport and Disabled Athletes.* Champaign, IL: Human Kinetics, 165–172.

16. Holden, J. P., et al. (1997). Changes in knee joint function over a wide range of walking speeds. *Clinical Biomechanics,* 12:375–382.

17. Hoshikawa, T., et al. (1973). Analysis of running patterns in relation to speed. In *Medicine and Sport Vol. 8: Biomechanics III.* Basel: Karger, 342–348.

18. Hreljac, A. (1993). Preferred and energetically optimal gait transition speeds in human locomotion. *Medicine and Science in Sports and Exercise,* 25:1158–1162.

19. Komi, P. V., et al. (1974). *Biomechanics of ski-jumping.* Jyvaskyla: University of Jyvaskyla, 25–29.

20. Luhtanen, P., Komi, P. V. (1973). Mechanical factors influencing running speed. In E. Asmussen, K. Jorgensen (Eds.). *Biomechanics VI-B.* Baltimore: University Park Press, 23–29.

21. Mason, B. R., et al. (1996). Biomechanical golf swing analysis. In R. Bauer (ed.). *XIII International Symposium for Biomechanics in Sport: Proceedings.* Thunder Bay, Ontario: International Society for Biomechanics in Sport, 67–70.

22. Neal, R. J., Wilson, B. D. (1985). 3D Kinematics and kinetics of the golf swing. *International Journal of Sport Biomechanics,* 1:221–232.

23. Ounpuu, S. (1994). The biomechanics of walking and running. *Clinics in Sports Medicine,* 13:843–863.

24. Owens, M. S., Lee, H. Y. (1969). A determination of velocities and angles of projection for the tennis serve. *Research Quarterly,* 40:750–754.

25. Sanderson, D. J., Sommer, H. J. (1985). Kinematic features of wheelchair propulsion. *Journal of Biomechanics,* 18:423–429.

26. Sinning, W. E., Forsyth, H. L.(1970). Lower limb actions while running at different velocities. *Medicine and Science in Sports,* 2:28–34.

27. Terauds, J. (1975). Some release characteristics of international discus throwing. *Track and Field Review,* 75:54–57.

28. Vanlandewijck, Y. C., et al. (1994). Wheelchair propulsion efficiency: Movement pattern adaptations to speed changes. *Medicine and Science in Sports and Exercise*, 26:1373–1381.

29. Wagenaar, R. C., Emmerik, R. E. A. (2000). Resonant frequencies of arms and legs identify different walking patterns. *Journal of Biomechanics*, 33:853–861.

ADDITIONAL READING

Cavanagh, P. R., Kram, R. (1990). Stride length in distance running: Velocity, body dimensions, and added mass effects. In P. R. Cavanagh (Ed.). *Biomechanics of Distance Running*. Champaign, IL: Human Kinetics, 35–63.

Daish, C. B. (1972). *The Physics of Ball Games*. London: English Universities Press.

Dillman, C. J. (1974). Kinematic Analysis of Running. In *Exercise and Sports Science Review*. New York: Macmillan, 193–218.

Williams, K. R. (1985). Biomechanics of Running. In *Exercise and Sports Science Review*. New York: Macmillan, 389–441.

GLOSSARY

Apex: The highest point of a parabola and the highest point a projectile reaches in its trajectory.

Calculus: A method of calculating the derivative or integral of a function.

Cartesian Coordinate System: An x, y, z reference system with either two or three axes in which a point may be located as a distance from each of the axes.

Cosine of an Angle: In a right triangle, the ratio of the side adjacent to the angle and the hypotenuse.

Curvilinear Motion: Linear motion along a curved path.

Derivative: The result of differentiation—the slope of a line—either a secant or a tangent, on a parameter–time curve.

Differentiation: The mathematical process of calculating a derivative.

Digitization: The process of applying x, y coordinates to points on a video frame.

Dimension: A term denoting the nature of a measurable quantity.

First Central Difference Method: A method of calculating the average slope over two time intervals, as in generating velocity from position–time data or acceleration from velocity–time data.

Instantaneous Linear Acceleration: The slope of a line tangent to a velocity–time curve.

Instantaneous Linear Velocity: The slope of a line tangent to a position–time curve.

Integral: The result of the process of integration; the area under a parameter–time curve.

Integration: The mathematical process of calculating an integral.

Kinematics: The area of study that examines the spatial and temporal components of motion.

Limit: The derivative of a function when the change in time approaches zero.

Linear Acceleration: The time rate of change of linear velocity.

Linear Distance: The length of an actual path.

Linear Displacement: A vector representing the straight-line distance and direction from one position to another.

Linear Motion: See translation.

Linear Kinematics: The description of linear motion involving position, velocity, and acceleration.

Linear Velocity: The time rate of change of linear position.

Midstance: The point during locomotor support when the center of mass is directly over the foot.

Motion: The progressive change in position of an object.

Nonsupport: A phase of the gait cycle in which the leg is not supported on the ground.

Parabola: A curve that describes the trajectory of a projectile.

Projectile: An object that has been flung into the air.

Projectile Motion: The motion of a projectile.

Projection Angle: The angle at which a projectile is released.

Projection Height: The difference between the heights at which a projectile is released and at which it lands.

Projection Velocity: The velocity at which a projectile is released.

Pythagorean Theorem: A mathematical description of the relationship among the sides of a right triangle. That is, $a^2 = b^2 + c^2$, where a is the hypotenuse and b and c are the other sides of the triangle.

Qualitative Analysis: A nonnumeric description or evaluation of movement that is based on direct observation.

Quantitative Analysis: A numeric description or evaluation of movement based on data collected during execution of the movement.

Range: The distance a projectile travels.

Resultant: The sum of two vectors.

Riemann Sum: A mathematical process by which the area under a parameter–time curve can be calculated, given that the time interval, dt, is small.

Rise: The change in a parameter between two successive time intervals.

Run: The change in time between two successive locations of parameter.

Scalar: A quantity that is defined by its magnitude alone.

Secant: A line that intersects a curve at two places.

Sine of an Angle: In a right triangle, the ratio of the side opposite the angle and the hypotenuse.

Slope: The ratio of the rise to the run.

Speed: The magnitude of the velocity vector.

Stance: See support.

Step: A portion of a stride from an event occurring on one leg to the same event on the opposite leg.

Stride: A gait cycle lasting from an event by one limb to the next occurrence of that event by the same limb, as from heel strike to heel strike on the right foot.

Stride Length: The distance traveled during one stride.

Stride Rate: The number of strides per minute.

Support: The phase of the gait cycle when the foot is in contact with the ground.

Swing: See nonsupport.

Tangent: A line that touches a curve at only one place.

Trajectory: The flight path of a projectile.

Translation: Motion in a straight or curved path where different regions of the object move the same distance in the same time interval.

Vector: A quantity that is defined by both its magnitude and its direction.

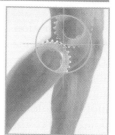

Angular Kinematics

OBJECTIVES

After reading this chapter, the student should be able to:

1. Distinguish between linear, angular, and general motion.

2. Determine relative and absolute angles.

3. Determine the direction of angular motion vectors.

4. Discuss the relationship among the kinematic quantities of angular distance and displacement, angular velocity, and angular acceleration.

5. Discuss the conventions for the calculation of lower extremity angles.

6. Discuss the relationship between angular and linear motion, particularly displacement, velocity, and acceleration.

7. Interpret angle–angle diagrams.

8. Discuss selected research studies that have used an angular kinematic approach.

9. Solve quantitative problems that employ angular kinematic principles.

Angular Motion

Angular motion occurs when all parts of a body move through the same angle but do not undergo the same linear displacement. The subset of kinematics that deals with angular motion is **angular kinematics**, which describes angular motion without regard to the causes of the motion. Consider a bicycle wheel (Fig. 9-1). Pick any point close to the center of the wheel and any point close to the edge of the wheel. The point close to the edge travels farther than the point close to the center as the wheel rotates. The motion of the wheel is angular motion.

Angular motion occurs about an axis of rotation that is a line perpendicular to the plane in which the rotation occurs. For example, the bicycle wheel spins about its axle, which is its axis of rotation. The axle is perpendicular to the plane of rotation described by the rim of the wheel (Fig. 9-1).

An understanding of angular motion is critical to comprehend how one moves. Nearly all human movement involves rotation of body segments. The segments rotate about the joint centers that form their axes of rotation. For example, the forearm segment rotates about the elbow joint during flexion and extension. When an individual moves, the segments generally undergo both rotation and translation. Sequential combinations of angular motion of multiple segments can result in linear motion of the segment end point seen in throwing and many other movements in which end point velocities are important. When the combination of rotation and translation occurs, it is described as general motion. Figure 9-2 illustrates the combination of linear and rotational motions. The gymnast undergoes translation as she moves across the ground. At the same time, she is rotating. The combination of rotation and translation is common in most human movements.

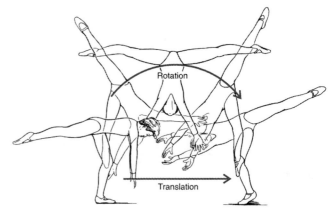

FIGURE 9-2 A gymnast completing a cartwheel as an example of general motion. The gymnast simultaneously undergoes both translation and rotation.

 Measurement of Angles

ANGLE

An **angle** is composed of two lines, two planes, or a combination that intersect at a point called the **vertex**. In a biomechanical analysis, the intersecting lines are generally body segments. If the longitudinal axis of the leg segment is one side of an angle and the longitudinal axis of the thigh segment is the other side, the vertex is the joint center of the knee. Angles can be determined from the coordinate points described in Chapter 8. Coordinate points describing the joint centers determine the sides and vertex of the angle. For example, an angle at the knee can be constructed using the thigh and leg segments. The coordinate points describing the ankle and knee joint centers define the leg segment, while the coordinate points describing the hip and knee joint centers define the thigh segment. The vertex of the angle is the knee joint center.

Definition of a segment by placing markers on the subject at the joint centers makes a technically incorrect assumption, that the joint center at the vertex of the angle does not change throughout the movement. Because of the asymmetries in the shape of the articulating surfaces in most joints, one or both bones constituting the joint may displace relative to each other. For example, while the knee is often considered a hinge joint, it is not. At the knee joint, the medial and lateral femoral condyles are asymmetrical. Therefore, as the knee flexes and extends, the tibia rotates along its long axis and about an axis through the knee from front to back. The location of the joint center, therefore, changes throughout any motion of the knee. The center of rotation of a joint at an instant in time is called the instantaneous joint center (Fig. 9-3). It is difficult to locate this moving axis of rotation without special techniques such as x-ray measurements. These measurements are not practical in most situations; thus, the assumption of a static instantaneous joint center must be made.

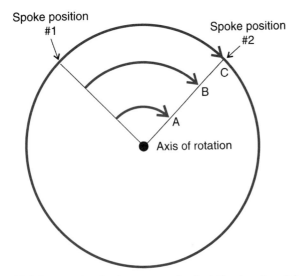

FIGURE 9-1 A bicycle wheel as an example of rotational motion. Points A, B, and C undergo the same amount of rotation but different linear displacements, with C undergoing the greatest linear displacement.

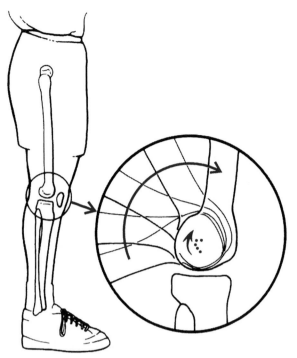

FIGURE 9-3 Instantaneous center of rotation of the knee. (After Nordin, M., Frankel, V. H. [eds.] [1979]. *Biomechanics of the Musculoskeletal System* (2nd Ed.). Philadelphia: Lea & Febiger.)

UNITS OF MEASUREMENT

In angular motion, three units are used to measure angles. It is important to use the correct units to communicate the results of this work clearly and to compare values from study to study. It is also essential to use the correct units because angle measurements may be used in further calculations. The first and most commonly used is the **degree**. A circle, which describes one complete rotation, transcribes an arc of 360° (Fig. 9-4*A*). An angle of 90° has sides that are perpendicular to each other. A straight line has a 180° angle (Fig. 9-4*B*).

The second unit of measurement describes the number of rotations or revolutions about a circle (Fig. 9-4*A*). One **revolution** is a single 360° rotation. For example, a triple jump in skating requires the skater to complete three and one-half revolutions in the air. The skater completes a rotation of 1260°. This unit of measurement is useful in qualitative descriptions of movements in figure skating, gymnastics, and diving but is not useful in quantitative analysis.

While the degree is most commonly understood and the revolution is often used, the most appropriate unit for angular measurement in biomechanics is the **radian**. A radian is defined as the measure of an angle at the center of a circle described by an arc equal to the length of the radius of the circle (Fig. 9-4*C*). That is:

$$\theta = \frac{s}{r} = 1 \text{ radian}$$

where θ = the angle equaling 1 radian, s = arc of length r, and r = radius of the circle. Since both s and r have units of length (m), the units in the numerator and denominator cancel each other out, with the result that the radian is dimensionless.

In further calculations, the radian is not considered in determining the units of the result of the calculation. Degrees have a dimension and must be included in the unit of the product of any calculation. It is necessary, therefore, to use the radian as a unit of angular measurement instead of the degree in any calculation involving linear motion because the radian is dimensionless. One radian is the equivalent of 57.3°. To convert an angle in degrees to radians, divide the angle in degrees by 57.3. For example:

$$\frac{72°}{57.3°} = 1.26 \text{ rad}$$

To convert radians to degrees, multiply the angle in radians by 57.3. For example:

$$0.67 \text{ rad} * 57.3° = 38.4°$$

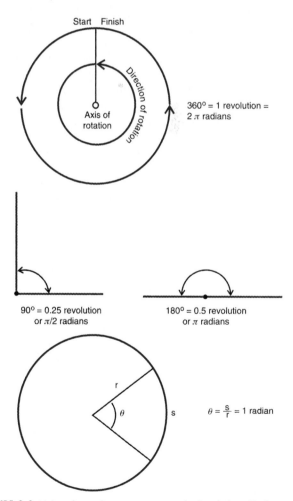

FIGURE 9-4 Units of angular measurement. **A.** Revolution. **B.** Perpendicular and straight lines. **C.** Radian.

Angular measurement in radians is often determined in multiples of pi ($\pi = 3.1416$). Since there are 2π radians in a complete circle, 180° may be represented as π radians, 90° as $\pi/2$ radians, and so on.

Although the unit of angular measurement in the Systéme International d'Unites (SI) is the radian and this unit must be used in further calculations, the angular motion concepts presented in the remainder of this chapter will use the degree for ease of understanding.

 Types of Angles

ABSOLUTE ANGLE

In biomechanics two types of angles are generally calculated. The first is the **absolute angle**, the angle of inclination of a body segment relative to some fixed reference in the environment. This type of angle describes the orientation of a segment in space. There are two primary conventions for calculating absolute angles. One involves placing a coordinate system at the proximal end point of the segment. The angle is then measured counterclockwise from the right horizontal. The most frequently used convention for calculating absolute angles, however, places a coordinate system at the distal end point of the segment (Fig. 9-5). The angle using this convention is also measured counterclockwise from the right horizontal. The absolute angles calculated using these two conventions are related and give comparable information. When calculating absolute angles, however, the convention

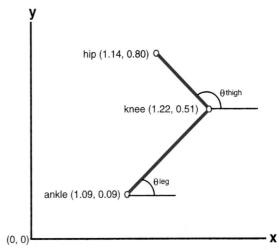

FIGURE 9-6 Absolute angles of the thigh and leg as defined in a coordinate system.

used must be stated clearly. The absolute angle of a segment relative to the right horizontal is also called the segment angle.

Absolute angles are calculated using the trigonometric relationship of the **tangent**. The tangent is defined based on the sides of a right triangle. It is the ratio of the side opposite the angle in question and the side adjacent to the angle. The angle in question is not the right angle in the triangle. If the leg and thigh segment coordinate positions are considered, the absolute angles of both the thigh and leg segments can be calculated (Fig. 9-6).

To calculate the absolute leg angle, the coordinate values of the segment end points of the leg are substituted into the formula to define the tangent of the angle:

$$\tan \theta_{leg} = \frac{y_{distal} - y_{proximal}}{x_{distal} - x_{proximal}}$$

$$= \frac{y_{knee} - y_{ankle}}{x_{knee} - x_{ankle}}$$

$$= \frac{0.51 - 0.09}{1.22 - 1.09}$$

$$= \frac{0.42}{0.13}$$

$$= 3.23$$

Next, the angle whose tangent is 3.23 is again determined using either the trigonometric tables (see Appendix D) or a calculator. This is called finding the inverse tangent and is written as follows:

$$\theta_{leg} = \tan^{-1} 3.23$$

$$= 72.8°$$

The absolute angle of the leg, therefore, is 72.8° from the right horizontal. This orientation indicates that the leg is positioned so that the knee is farther from the vertical (y) axis of the coordinate system than the ankle. That is, the knee joint is to the right of the ankle joint.

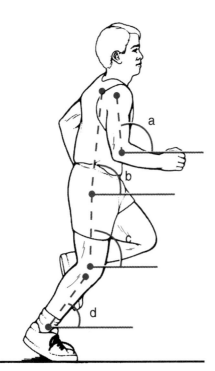

FIGURE 9-5 Absolute angles: The arm (a), the trunk (b), the thigh (c), and the leg (d) of a runner.

Similarly, to calculate the thigh angle, the coordinate values are substituted:

$$\tan \theta_{\text{thigh}} = \frac{y_{\text{hip}} - y_{\text{knee}}}{x_{\text{hip}} - x_{\text{knee}}}$$
$$= \frac{0.80 - 0.51}{1.14 - 1.22}$$
$$= \frac{0.29}{-0.08}$$
$$= -3.625$$

Once again, the angle whose tangent is -3.625 is determined as follows:

$$\theta_{\text{thigh}} = \tan^{-1} - 3.625$$
$$= -74.58°$$

This angle is clockwise from the left horizontal, since we have moved into the second quadrant with the negative x-value. To convert the angle so it is relative to the right horizontal and counterclockwise, it must be added to $180°$, resulting in an absolute angle of $105.4°$ relative to the right horizontal (Fig. 9-7). An absolute thigh angle of $105.4°$ in the second quadrant means that the thigh is oriented such that the hip joint is to the left of the vertical (y) axis running through the knee joint and above the horizontal (x) axis of the coordinate system originating at the knee joint. In this case, the thigh would be oriented with the knee to the right of the hip in this reference system. When both x and y are negative, the value is in the third quadrant, and the angle is computed counterclockwise and relative to the left horizontal, so $180°$ is still added to adjust the absolute angle so it is relative to the right horizontal. Finally, if there is only a negative y-value, the angle is in the fourth quadrant and taken clockwise and relative to the right horizontal, so $360°$ should be added to convert the absolute angle so that it is relative to the right horizontal in the counterclockwise direction.

Trunk, thigh, leg, and foot segmental end points for both the touchdown and the toe-off in walking are graphically

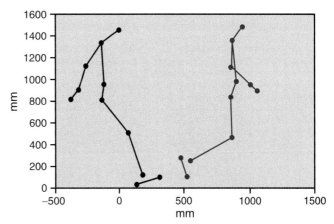

FIGURE 9-8 By plotting the segmental endpoints and creating a stick figure, the similarities or differences in position can be clearly observed. The differences in right foot touch down (black) and right foot toe off (red) phases of a walking gait are apparent. See Appendix Frame 1 and Frame 76, respectively.

illustrated in Figure 9-8. The corresponding calculations of the absolute angles shown in Table 9-1 use the conventions discussed previously to convert all angles so they are taken counterclockwise with respect to the right horizontal. For example, the leg orientation in touchdown results in a negative x-position and positive y-position, so $180°$ is added to the final angle computation to make it relative to the right horizontal. In the case of toe-off, however, both x and y are positive, so there is no adjustment. Likewise, the foot orientation in touchdown and toe-off result in both negative x and y, placing it in the third quadrant, where $180°$ is again added. These adjustments provide a consistent reference for the computation of the absolute angles.

Refer to the walking data in Appendix E: Calculate the absolute angle of the trunk (using shoulder and greater trochanter markers), the thigh, and the lower leg for frame 38, a point occurring in the midsupport phase of walking.

RELATIVE ANGLE

The other type of angle calculated in biomechanics is the **relative angle** (Fig. 9-9A). This is the angle between longitudinal axes of two segments. For example, the relative angle at the elbow describes the amount of flexion or extension at the joint. Relative angles, however, do not describe the position of the segments or the sides of the angle in space. If an individual has a relative angle of $90°$ at the elbow and that angle is maintained, the arm may be in any of a number of positions (Fig. 9-9B). The relative angle between two segments is also called the intersegmental or joint angle.

Relative angles can be calculated using the **law of cosines**. This law, simply a more general case of the Pythagorean theorem, describes the relationship between the sides of a triangle. For our purposes, the triangle is made up of the two segments B and C and a line, A, joining the distal end of one segment to the proximal end of the other (Fig. 9-10).

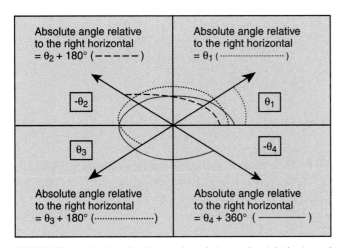

FIGURE 9-7 To calculate absolute angles relative to the right horizontal requires adjustments when the orientation is such that the differences between the proximal and distal end points indicate that the segment is not in the first quadrant.

TABLE 9-1 Absolute Angle Calculation for Touchdown and Toe-off in Walking

Frame	Trunk$_x$ = (Shoulder$_x$ to Greater Trochanter$_x$)	Trunk$_y$ = (Shoulder$_y$ to Greater Trochanter$_y$)	Absolute Angle = arctan (y/x)	Thigh$_x$ = (Greater Trochanter$_x$ to Knee$_x$)	Thigh$_y$ = (Greater Trochanter$_y$ to Knee$_y$)
1	−3.95	523.08	= −89.57° + 180° = 90.43°	−210.15	317.14
76	10.92	532.10	= 88.82°	−14.76	368.95

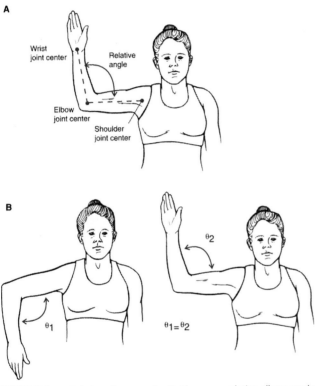

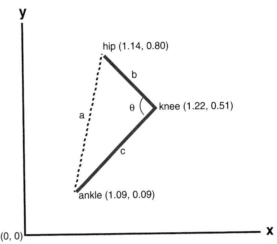

FIGURE 9-10 Coordinate points describing the hip, knee, and ankle joint center and the relative angle of the knee (θ).

FIGURE 9-9 A. Relative elbow angle. **B.** The same relative elbow angle with the arm and forearm in different positions.

In Figure 9-10, the coordinate points for two segments describing the thigh and the leg are given. To calculate the relative angle at the knee (θ), the lengths a, b, and c would be calculated using the Pythagorean relationship.

$$a = \sqrt{(x_h - x_a)^2 + (y_h - y_a)^2}$$
$$= \sqrt{(1.14 - 1.09)^2 + (0.80 - 0.09)^2}$$
$$= \sqrt{0.0025 + 0.5041}$$
$$= 0.71$$
$$b = \sqrt{(x_h - x_k)^2 + (y_h - y_k)^2}$$
$$= \sqrt{(1.14 - 1.22)^2 + (0.80 - 0.51)^2}$$
$$= \sqrt{0.0064 + 0.0841}$$
$$= 0.30$$

$$c = \sqrt{(x_k - x_a)^2 + (y_k - y_a)^2}$$
$$= \sqrt{(1.22 - 1.09)^2 + (0.51 - 0.09)^2}$$
$$= \sqrt{0.0169 + 0.1764}$$
$$= 0.44$$

The next step is to substitute these values in the law of cosines equation and solve for the cosine of the angle θ.

$$a^2 = b^2 + c^2 - 2 * b * c * \cos\theta$$
$$\cos\theta = \frac{b^2 + c^2 - a^2}{2 * b * c}$$
$$\cos\theta = \frac{0.30^2 + 0.44^2 - 0.71^2}{2 * 0.3 * 0.44}$$
$$\cos\theta = -0.833$$

To find the angle θ, the angle whose cosine is −0.833 can be determined using either trigonometric tables (see Appendix D) or a calculator with trigonometric functions. This process, known as finding the inverse cosine or arcos, is written as follows:

$$\theta = \cos^{-1} -0.833$$
$$\theta = 146.4°$$

Absolute Angle = arctan (y/x)	Leg$_x$ = (Knee$_x$ to Ankle$_x$)	Leg$_y$ = (Knee$_y$ to Ankle$_y$)	Absolute Angle = arctan (y/x)	Foot$_x$ = (Heel$_x$ to Met$_x$)	Foot$_y$ = (Heel$_y$ to Met$_y$)	Absolute Angle = arctan (y/x)
= −56.47° + 180° = 123.53°	−113.03	377.88	= −73.35° + 180° = 106.65°	−181.92	−67.95	= 20.48° + 180° = 200.48°
= −87.71° + 180° = 92.29°	313.49	218.66	= 34.90°	−51.20	169.39	= −73.18° + 180° = 106.82°

Therefore, the relative angle at the knee is 146.4°. In this case, the knee is slightly flexed (180° representing full extension).

Refer to walking data in Appendix E: Calculate the relative angle at the knee and at the hip joint for frame 38 during midsupport of the right limb. Use the law of cosines.

A relative angle can be calculated from the absolute values to obtain a result similar to computations using the law of cosines. The relative angle between two segments can be calculated by subtracting the absolute angle of the distal segment from the proximal segment. In the example using the thigh and lower leg, the following calculation is another option:

$$\theta_{relative} = \theta_{absolute\ thigh} - \theta_{absolute\ leg}$$
$$\theta_{relative} = -74.58° - 72.8°$$
$$\theta_{relative} = 147.4°$$

In clinical situations, the relative angle is most often calculated because it provides a more practical indicator of function and joint position. In quantitative biomechanical analyses, however, absolute angles are calculated more often than relative angles because they are used in a number of subsequent calculations. Regardless of the type of angle calculated, however, a consistent frame of reference must be used.

Unfortunately, many coordinate systems and systems of defining angles have been used in biomechanics, resulting in difficulty comparing values from study to study. Several organizations, such as the Canadian Society of Biomechanics and the International Society of Biomechanics, are now attempting to standardize the calculation and representation of angles to provide consistency in biomechanics research, especially in the area of joint kinematics, in which there are a number of recommendations on joint coordinate systems.

Lower Extremity Joint Angles

In discussing the angle of a joint such as the knee or ankle, it is imperative that a meaningful representation of the action of the joint be made. A special use of relative angles

to compute joint angles is very useful for clinicians and others interested in joint function. Lower extremity joint angles can be calculated using the absolute angles similar to the procedure described previously. A system of lower extremity joint angle conventions was presented by Winter (33). These lower extremity angle definitions are for use in a two-dimensional sagittal plane analysis only. In Winter's system, digitized points describing the trunk, thigh, leg, and foot are used to calculate the absolute angles of each (Fig. 9-11). In such a biomechanical analysis, it is assumed that a right side sagittal view is being analyzed. That is, the right side of the subject's body is closest to the camera and is considered to be in the x, y plane. If not, the data must be converted to represent a right side view.

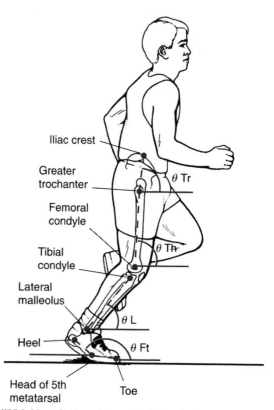

FIGURE 9-11 Definition of the sagittal view absolute angles of the trunk, thigh, leg, and foot. (After Winter, D. A. [1987]. *The Biomechanics and Motor Control of Gait*. Waterloo, Ont.: University of Waterloo Press.)

HIP ANGLE

Based on the absolute angles of the trunk and the thigh calculated, the hip angle is:

$$\theta_{hip} = \theta_{thigh\ absolute} - \theta_{trunk\ absolute}$$

In this scheme, if the hip angle is positive, the action at the hip is flexion, while if the hip angle is negative, the action is extension. If the angle is zero, the thigh and the trunk are aligned vertically in a neutral position. For, example the hip joint angle representing flexion and extension for the touchdown phase in walking (Table 9-1) would be:

$$\begin{aligned}\theta_{hip} &= \theta_{thigh} - \theta_{trunk}\\ &= 123.53° - 90.43°\\ &= 33.1°\end{aligned}$$

The joint angle of 33.1° at touchdown indicates that the thigh is flexing at the hip joint. In a human walking at a moderate pace, the hip angle oscillates ±35° about 0°, while in running, the hip angle oscillates ±45°. The relative angle between the thigh and the trunk can easily be computed by subtracting the joint angle from 180°. In this case:

$$\begin{aligned}\theta_{thigh-trunk\ relative} &= 180° - \theta_{hip}\\ &= 180° - 33.1°\\ &= 146.9°\end{aligned}$$

KNEE ANGLE

Using the absolute angle of the thigh and the leg, the knee joint angle is defined as:

$$\theta_{knee} = \theta_{thigh\ absolute} - \theta_{leg\ absolute}$$

In human locomotion, the knee angle is always positive, that is, in some degree of flexion, and it usually varies from 0 to 50° throughout a walking stride and from 0 to 80° during a running stride. Since the knee angle is positive, the knee is always in some degree of flexion. If the knee angle gets progressively greater, the knee is flexing, while if it gets progressively smaller, the knee is extending. A zero knee angle is a neutral position, while a negative angle would indicate a hyperextension of the knee. The knee angle for the touchdown phase in the walking example (Table 9-1) is:

$$\begin{aligned}\theta_{knee} &= \theta_{thigh} - \theta_{leg}\\ &= 123.53° - 106.65°\\ &= 16.88°\end{aligned}$$

This joint angle indicates knee flexion at this phase of the walking cycle. Again, the relative angle between the thigh and the leg segments:

$$\begin{aligned}\theta_{thigh-leg\ relative} &= 180° - \theta_{knee}\\ &= 180° - 16.88°\\ &= 163.12°\end{aligned}$$

ANKLE ANGLE

The ankle angle is calculated using the absolute angles of the foot and the leg:

$$\theta_{ankle\ joint\ angle} = \theta_{leg} - \theta_{foot} + 90°$$

This may seem more complicated than the other lower extremity joint angle calculations. Without adding 90° the ankle angle would oscillate about 90°, making interpretation of it difficult. Adding 90° makes the ankle angle oscillate about 0°. Thus, a positive angle represents dorsiflexion and a negative angle represents plantarflexion.

The ankle angle for the touchdown phase in the walking example (Table 9-1) is:

$$\begin{aligned}\theta_{ankle} &= \theta_{leg} - \theta_{foot} + 90°\\ &= 106.65° - 200.48° + 90°\\ &= -3.83°\end{aligned}$$

This value indicates that the ankle is in plantarflexion at touchdown. The relative angle between the leg and the foot is computed somewhat differently using this joint angle. First, the joint angle can be subtracted from 180°, as in the case of the other angles, but the 90° previously added must be subtracted. So the relative angle between the foot and leg is:

$$\begin{aligned}\theta_{leg-foot\ relative} &= 180° - \theta_{ankle} - 90°\\ &= 180° - (-3.83°) - 90°\\ &= 93.83°\end{aligned}$$

The ankle angle generally oscillates ±20° during a natural walking stride and ±35° during a running stride. Lower extremity angles calculated for a walking stride using Winter's convention are presented in Figure 9-12.

Refer to walking data in Appendix E: Calculate the joint angles at the hip and knee joints for frame 38 (mid-support in walking). Calculate the relative angle between the segments and compare with values obtained using the law of cosines.

REARFOOT ANGLE

Another lower extremity angle that is often calculated in biomechanical analyses is the rearfoot angle. The motion of the subtalar joint in a two-dimensional analysis is considered to be in the frontal plane. The rearfoot angle represents the motion of the subtalar joint. The rearfoot angle thus approximates calcaneal eversion and calcaneal inversion in the frontal plane. Calcaneal eversion and inversion are among the motions in the pronation and supination action of the subtalar joint. In the research literature, calcaneal eversion is often measured to evaluate pronation, while calcaneal inversion is measured to determine supination.

Rearfoot angle is calculated using the absolute angles of the leg and the calcaneus in the frontal plane. Two segment markers are placed on the rear of the leg to define the longitudinal axis of the leg. Two markers are also placed on the calcaneus (or the rear portion of the shoe)

A

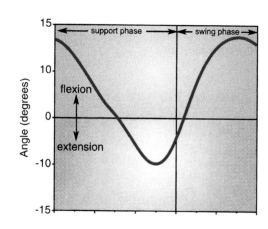

B

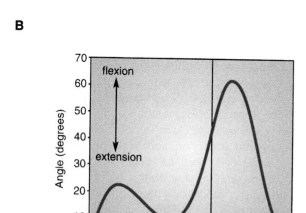

C

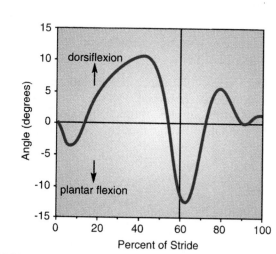

FIGURE 9-12 Graphs of the hip **(A)**, knee **(B)**, and ankle **(C)** angles during walking.

to define the longitudinal axis of the calcaneus (Fig. 9-13). These markers are used to calculate the absolute angles of the leg and heel; thus the rear foot angle is:

$$\theta_{\text{rear foot}} = \theta_{\text{leg}} - \theta_{\text{calcaneus}}$$

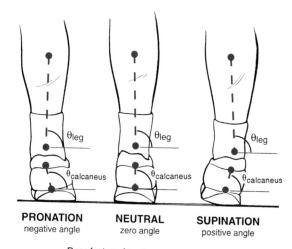

Rear foot angle = $\theta_{\text{calcaneus}} - \theta_{\text{leg}}$

FIGURE 9-13 Definition of the absolute angles of the leg and calcaneus in the frontal plane. These angles are used to constitute the rearfoot angle of the right foot.

By this calculation, a positive angle represents calcaneal inversion, a negative angle represents calcaneal eversion, and a zero angle is the neutral position.

During the support phase of the gait cycle, the rearfoot, as defined by the rearfoot angle, is in an inverted position at the initial foot contact with the ground. At this instance, the rearfoot angle is positive. From that point onward, during support until midstance, the rearfoot moves to an everted position. Thus, the rearfoot angle is negative. At midstance position, the foot becomes less everted and moves to an inverted position at toe-off. The rearfoot angle becomes less negative and eventually positive at toe-off. Figure 9-14 is a representation of a typical rearfoot angle curve during the support phase of a running stride.

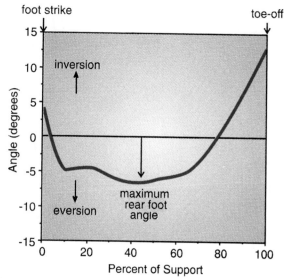

FIGURE 9-14 A typical rearfoot angle–time graph during running. Maximum rearfoot angle is indicated.

Representation of Angular Motion Vectors

It is difficult to represent angular motion vectors graphically as lines with arrows, as was done in linear kinematics. It is essential, however, to determine how the direction of rotation is determined. The direction of rotation of an angular motion vector is referred to as the **polarity** of the vector. The polarity of an angular motion vector is determined by the **right-hand rule**. The direction of an angular motion vector is determined using this rule by placing the curled fingers of the right hand in the direction of the rotation. The angular motion vector is defined by an arrow of the appropriate length that coincides with the direction of the extended thumb of the right hand (Fig. 9-15). The convention generally used is that in the sagittal plane all

segments counterclockwise from the right horizontal have positive polarity and all segments rotating in clockwise have a negative polarity.

Angular Motion Relationships

The relationships discussed in Chapter 8 on linear kinematics are comparable to those of angular kinematics. The angular case is simply an analog of the linear case.

ANGULAR POSITION AND DISPLACEMENT

The angular position of an object refers to its location relative to a defined spatial reference system. In the case of a two-dimensional system with the y-axis up and down and the x-axis running anterior to posterior, angular position is described in the x-y plane. A three-dimensional system adds a third axis, z, in the medial and lateral. Many clinicians use planes to describe angular positioning. For example, if the axes are placed with the origin at the shoulder joint, angular position of the arm in the x-y plane would be a flexion and extension position, in the y-z plane abduction and adduction, and in the x-z plane, rotation. This system works well for describing joint angles but lacks precision for describing complex movements. Absolute angles can be computed relative to a fixed reference system placed at a joint or at another fixed point in the environment. As discussed earlier, angular position can also be computed relative to another line or plane that is allowed to move. It is common to present joint angles such as those shown in Figure 9-12 to document the joint actions in a movement such as walking.

Refer to walking data in Appendix E: Calculate and graph the absolute and relative angles of lower leg for the support phase (frames 0–76).

The concepts of distance and displacement in the angular case must be discerned. Consider a simple pendulum swinging in the x-y plane through an arc of 70° (Fig. 9-16). If the pendulum swings though a single arc, the angular

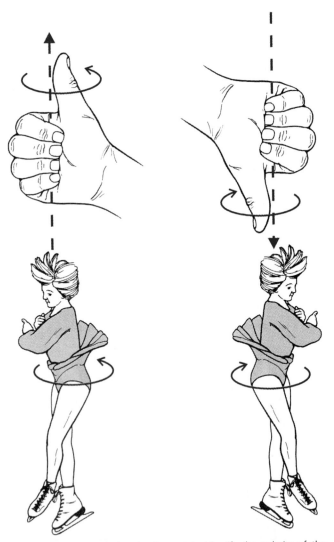

FIGURE 9-15 The right-hand rule used to identify the polarity of the angular velocity of a figure skater during a spin. The fingers of the right hand point in the direction of the rotation and the right thumb points in the direction of the angular velocity vector. The angular velocity vector is perpendicular to the plane of rotation.

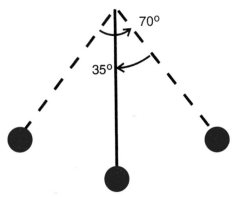

FIGURE 9-16 A swinging pendulum illustrating the angular distance over 1.5 arcs of swing.

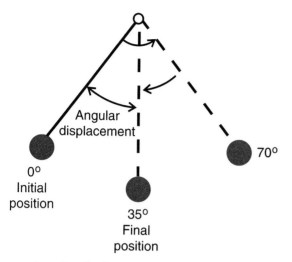

Angular displacement = 35° – 0° = 35°

FIGURE 9-17 Angular displacement is the difference between the initial position and the final position.

distance is 70°, but if it swings through 1.5 arcs, the angular distance is 105°. Angular distance is the total of all angular changes measured following its exact path. As in the linear case, however, angular distance is not the same as angular displacement.

Angular displacement is the difference between the initial and final positions of the rotating object (Fig. 9-17). In the example of the pendulum, if the pendulum swings through two complete arcs, the angular displacement is zero, since its final position is the same as the starting position. Angular displacement never exceeds 360° or 2π rad of rotation, while angular distance can be any value. In discussing angular displacement, it is necessary to designate the direction of the rotation. Counterclockwise rotation is considered to be positive (+), and clockwise rotation is negative (−). With a reference system placed at the shoulder joint, the positive y-axis would be upward, the positive x-axis would be posterior to anterior, and the positive z-axis would be medial to lateral. The corresponding positive joint movements about these axes would be internal rotation (y-axis), flexion (x-axis), and abduction (z-axis).

If the absolute angle of a segment, theta (θ), is calculated for successive positions in time, the angular displacement ($\Delta\theta$) is:

$$\Delta\theta = \theta_{final} - \theta_{initial}$$

The polarity, or sign, of the angular displacement is determined by the sign of $\Delta\theta$ as calculated and may be confirmed by the right-hand rule.

ANGULAR VELOCITY

Angular speed and **angular velocity** are analogous with linear speed and linear velocity in both definition and meaning. Angular speed is the angular distance traveled per unit of time. Angular speed is a scalar quantity and is generally not critically important in biomechanical analysis because it is not used in any further calculations.

Angular velocity, characterized by the Greek letter omega (ω), is a vector quantity that describes the time rate of change of angular position. If the measured angle is θ, then the angular velocity is:

$$\omega = \frac{\text{change in angular position}}{\text{change in time}}$$
$$= \frac{\theta_{final} - \theta_{initial}}{time_{final} - time_{initial}}$$
$$= \frac{\Delta\theta}{\Delta t}$$

If the initial angle of a segment was 34° at time 1.25 s and the segment moved to an angle of 62° at time 1.30 s, the angular velocity would be:

$$\omega = \frac{\Delta\theta}{\Delta t}$$
$$= \frac{62° - 34°}{1.30\ s - 1.25\ s}$$
$$= \frac{28°}{0.05\ s}$$
$$= 560°/s$$

Angular speed and angular velocity are generally presented in degrees per second (°/s). If, however, as noted previously, any further computation is to be done using angular velocity, the units must be radians per second (rad/s).

In the previous example, the average angular velocity was calculated over the interval from 1.25 s to 1.30 s. According to the discussion in the previous chapter, this angular velocity would represent the slope of a secant on an angular position–time graph over this interval. The instantaneous angular velocity would represent the slope of a tangent to an angular position–time graph and would be calculated as a limit.

$$\text{limit } \omega = \frac{d\theta}{dt}$$
$$dt -> 0$$

Angular velocity is thus the first derivative of angular position.

As in the linear case, the direction of the slope on an angle–time profile will determine whether the angular velocity is positive or negative, and the steepness of the slope will indicate the rate of change of angular position. If θ_{final} is greater than $\theta_{initial}$, ω is positive (i.e., the slope is positive), but if θ_{final} is less than $\theta_{initial}$, ω is negative (i.e., slope is negative). Both situations can be confirmed using the right-hand rule. If there is no change in the angle, the slope is zero and ω is zero.

The method used to calculate angular velocity over a series of frames of a kinematic analysis is the first central difference method. This method calculates the angular velocity at the same instant at which data for angular position are available. For angular velocity, this formula is:

$$\omega_i = \frac{\theta_{i+1} - \theta_{i-1}}{t_{i+1} - t_{i-1}}$$

where θ_i is the angle at time t_i. Table 9-2 represents the thigh absolute angle data collected for one support phase in walking (see Appendix E). The rate of the camera was

120 frames per second, and every third frame is presented from touchdown (frame 0) to toe-off (frame 76). The time between each frame is $1/120 = 0.0083$ s; thus the time between 3 frames is 0.0249. Using the first central difference method, the angular velocity is calculated from the absolute angular position for each frame. Once calculated, the values are typically graphed to observe the pattern of motion (Fig. 9-18). The results of the calculation

TABLE 9-2 Calculation of Angular Position, Velocity, and Acceleration for the Thigh During the Support Phase of Walking

Frame	Time (s)	Thigh Absolute Angle (°)	Thigh Angular Velocity(°/s)	Thigh Angular Acceleration (°/s/s)
Number			$\omega_i = \dfrac{\theta_{i+1} - \theta_{i-1}}{t_{i+1} - t_{i-1}}$	$\alpha_i = \dfrac{\omega_{i+1} - \omega_{i-1}}{t_{i+1} - t_{i-1}}$
0	0	123.8097		
			$\omega_3 = \dfrac{\theta_6 - \theta_0}{t_6 - t_0}$	
			$= \dfrac{122.2607 - 123.8097}{0.0498 - 0.00}$	
3	0.0249	123.094	$= -31.1032$	
				$\alpha_6 = \dfrac{\omega_9 - \omega_3}{t_9 - t_3}$
				$= \dfrac{-55.1236 - (-31.1032)}{0.0747 - 0.0249}$
6	0.0498	122.2607	-39.2284	$= -482.337$
9	0.0747	121.1404	-55.1236	-785.509
12	0.0996	119.5156	-78.3467	-956.469
15	0.1245	117.2387	-102.756	-859.349
18	0.1494	114.3983	-121.142	-588.432
21	0.1743	111.2058	-132.06	-338.676
24	0.1992	107.8218	-138.008	-178.207
27	0.2241	104.333	-140.934	-71.1306
30	0.249	100.8032	-141.551	9.8018
33	0.2739	97.28381	-140.446	79.63316
36	0.2988	93.80901	-137.585	173.4212
39	0.3237	90.43208	-131.81	313.8466
42	0.3486	87.24488	-121.955	478.1787
45	0.3735	84.35871	-107.997	620.2579
48	0.3984	81.86665	-91.0665	714.6628
51	0.4233	79.8236	-72.4064	776.5076
54	0.4482	78.26081	-52.3964	848.4548
57	0.4731	77.21426	-30.1533	982.3175
60	0.498	76.75918	-3.477	1213.751
63	0.5229	77.0411	30.29149	1517.822
66	0.5478	78.26769	72.11054	1781.703
69	0.5727	80.63221	119.0203	1846.942
72	0.5976	84.19491	164.0882	
75	0.6225	88.8038		

A

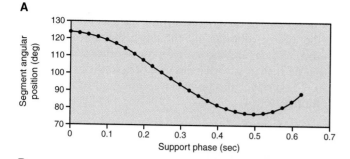

B

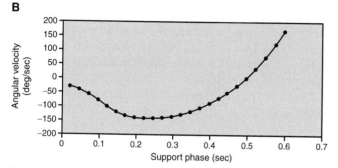

C

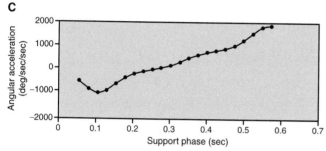

FIGURE 9-18 Graphic representations of: thigh absolute angle **(A)**, thigh angular velocity **(B)**, and thigh angular acceleration **(C)** as a function of time for the support phase of walking (data from Appendix E).

and graphing of angular kinematics of the thigh indicate that for most of the support phase the thigh is moving clockwise with respect to the knee joint. At heel strike the thigh is in extreme hip flexion that is reduced as the trunk is brought over the support limb, moving the thigh clockwise (negative angular velocity). The thigh is vertically aligned in frame 39, and the trunk continues moving over the limb, forcing the thigh to continue in its clockwise rotation about the knee joint. At the end of the support phase (frame 63), the motion of the thigh reverses and a counterclockwise movement of the thigh begins in preparation for toe-off (positive angular velocity).

Refer to the walking data in Appendix E: Using the first central difference method, calculate and graph the angular velocity of the lower leg using the absolute segment position angles.

ANGULAR ACCELERATION

Angular acceleration is the rate of change of angular velocity with respect to time and is symbolized by the Greek letter alpha (α).

$$angular\ acceleration = \frac{change\ in\ angular\ velocity}{change\ in\ time}$$

$$\alpha = \frac{\omega_{final} - \omega_{initial}}{time_{final} - time_{initial}}$$

$$\alpha = \frac{\Delta\omega}{\Delta t}$$

For ease of understanding, biomechanists generally present their results in degrees per second squared, but the most commonly used unit for angular acceleration is radians per second squared (rad/s^2).

As with the linear case and with angular velocity, angular acceleration is the derivative of angular velocity and represents the slope of a line, either a secant or a tangent. If α is the slope of a secant to an angular velocity–time profile, it represents an average acceleration over a time interval. If α is the slope of a tangent, the instantaneous angular acceleration has been calculated. This also implies that the slope may be positive (ω_{final} is greater than $\omega_{initial}$), negative (ω_{final} is less than $\omega_{initial}$), or zero (ω_{final} equals $\omega_{initial}$). The direction of the angular acceleration vector may be confirmed using the right-hand rule. The instantaneous angular acceleration is calculated by:

$$limit\ \alpha = \frac{d\omega}{dt}$$
$$dt -> 0$$

Once again, in a kinematic analysis, the usual method of calculating angular acceleration is the first central difference method. The formula for angular acceleration for this method is:

$$\alpha_i = \frac{\omega_{i+1} - \omega_{i-1}}{t_{i+1} - t_{i-1}}$$

where ω_i is the angular velocity at time t_i. Table 9-2 presents the calculated angular acceleration of the thigh for selected frames in the support phase of walking.

As in the case for linear acceleration, the sign or polarity of angular acceleration does not indicate the direction of rotation. For example, positive angular acceleration may mean increasing angular velocity in the positive direction or decreasing angular velocity in the negative direction. Also, negative angular acceleration may indicate decreasing angular velocity in the positive direction or increasing angular velocity in the negative direction. The angular position, velocity, and acceleration of the thigh is presented in Table 9-2, with a corresponding graph in Figure 9-18. The angular acceleration of the thigh is negative (increasing angular velocity in the negative direction) and then positive (decreasing angular velocity in the negative direction) during the portion of the support phase where the thigh angular velocity is negative, and the acceleration remains positive (increasing angular velocity in the positive direction) in the later stages of support, when the thigh angular velocity changes from negative to positive (direction change).

Refer to the walking data in Appendix E: Using the first central difference method, calculate and graph the angular acceleration of the lower leg.

 Relationship Between Angular and Linear Motion

In many human movements, the result of the movement is linear, while the motions of the segments constituting the movement are angular. For example, a pitcher throws a baseball that travels linearly. However, the motions of the pitcher's segments resulting in the throw are rotational. In many instances it is necessary to know the linear motion of the hand, which depends on the angular motion of the segments of the upper extremity. This example suggests a mechanical relationship between linear and angular motion.

LINEAR AND ANGULAR DISPLACEMENT

When the angular measure of an angle, the radian, was defined, it was noted:

$$\theta = \frac{s}{r}$$

where θ was the angle subtended by an arc of length s that is equal to the radius of the circle. The length of the arc can be presented as:

$$s = r\theta$$

Suppose the forearm, with length r_1, rotates about the elbow joint (Fig. 9-19). The arc described by the rotation—the distance that the wrist moves—is Δs_1, and the angle is $\Delta\theta$. The linear distance that the wrist travels is described as:

$$\Delta s_1 = r_1 \Delta\theta$$

Therefore, the linear distance that any point on the segment moves can be described if the distance of that point to the axis of rotation and the angle through which the segment rotates are known. Suppose another point on the arm is marked as s_2 with a distance of r_2 to the axis of rotation. The distance this point travels during the same angular motion is:

$$\Delta s_2 = r_2 \Delta\theta$$

Since r_1 is longer than r_2, the distance traveled by s_1 must be greater than s_2. Thus, the most distal points on a segment travel a greater distance than points closer to the axis of rotation. The value for the expression r is called the **radius of rotation** and refers to the distance of a point from the axis of rotation.

Consider that the change in the angle, $\Delta\theta$, is very small; then the length of the arc, Δs, can be approximated as a straight line. Therefore, a relationship between angular and linear displacement can be formulated. That is, when r is the radius of rotation:

linear displacement = radius of rotation * angular displacement

or

$$\Delta s = r \Delta\theta$$

or using calculus (that is, when $d\theta$ is very small)

$$ds = r \, d\theta$$

For example, if the arm segment of length 0.13 m rotates about the elbow an angular distance of 0.23 radians, the linear distance that the wrist traveled is:

$$\Delta s = r \Delta\theta$$
$$\Delta s = 0.23 \text{ rad} * 0.13 \text{ m}$$
$$\Delta s = 0.03 \text{ m}$$

Δs has a unit of length m, which is the correct unit, since it is a linear distance. Remember that radians are dimensionless, so that radians times meters results in units of meters.

LINEAR AND ANGULAR VELOCITY

The relationship between linear and angular velocity is similar to the relationship between linear and angular displacement. In the example in the last section, the arm, with length r, rotates about the elbow. The linear displacement of the wrist is the product of the distance r, the radius of rotation, and the angular displacement of the segment. Differentiating this equation with respect to time:

$$ds = r \, d\theta$$
$$\frac{ds}{dt} = r \frac{d\theta}{dt}$$
$$v = r\omega$$

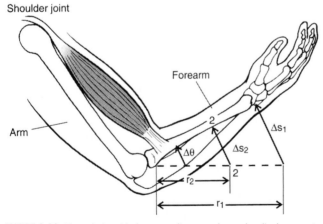

FIGURE 9-19 The relationship between linear and angular displacement.

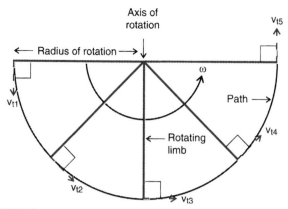

FIGURE 9-20 Tangential velocity of a rotating segment at different instants in time. The tangential velocity is perpendicular to the radius of rotation.

Thus, the linear velocity of a point on a rotating body is the product of the distance of that point from the axis of rotation and the angular velocity of the body. The linear velocity vector in this expression is instantaneously tangent to the path of the object and is referred to as the **tangential velocity**, or v_T (Fig. 9-20). That is, the linear velocity vector behaves as a tangent, touching the curved path at only one point. The vector, therefore, is perpendicular to the rotating segment.

For example, if the arm segment of length r = 0.13 m rotated with an angular velocity of 2.4 rad/s, the velocity of the wrist is:

$$v_T = r\omega$$
$$v_T = 0.13 \text{ m} * 2.4 \text{ rad /s}$$
$$v_T = 0.31 \text{ m/s}$$

Linear velocity is expressed in meters per second, which results in this instance from meters times radians per second, since radians are dimensionless.

The relationship between linear velocity and angular velocity is critical in a number of human movements, particularly those in which the performer throws or strikes an object. To increase the linear velocity of the ball, for example, the soccer player can either increase the angular velocity of the lower extremity segments or increase the length of the extremity by extending at the joints, or both, to gain the maximum range of a kick. For an individual, the major alternative is to increase the angular velocities of these segments. For example, Plagenhoef (22) reported foot velocities prior to impact of 16.33 to 24.14 m/s for several types of soccer kicks for the same individual. Since the segment lengths did not change substantially, if the foot velocity changed, the angular velocity certainly must have varied for each type of kick.

In some activities, however, the length r can change. In golf, the clubs have varying lengths and club head lofts according to the desired distance for the ball to travel (Fig. 9-21). For example, the 2-iron is longer than the 9-iron and has a different club head loft, with the 9-iron having a greater club head loft than the 2-iron. If both

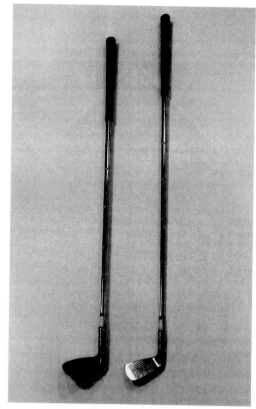

FIGURE 9-21 Comparison of the lengths of the shafts of golf clubs, a 2-iron (*left*) and a 9-iron.

clubs had the same loft, the two-iron shot would go farther than a 9-iron shot, given the same angular velocity of the golf swing, as it does for most expert golfers. Golfers often use the same club but vary the length, r, by choking up on the handle, that is, gripping the club closer to the middle of the shaft. Using this technique, the golfer may swing with the same angular velocity but vary the length, thereby varying the linear velocity of the club head.

LINEAR AND ANGULAR ACCELERATION

Remember that the linear velocity vector calculated from the product of the radius and the angular velocity is tangent to the curved path and can be referred to as the tangential velocity. As previously stated:

$$v_T = r\omega$$

If the time derivative of this expression is determined, the relationship expresses the **tangential acceleration** in terms of the radius of rotation and the angular acceleration. The expression of the derivative is:

$$a_T = \alpha r$$

where a_T is the tangential acceleration, r is the radius of rotation, and α is the angular acceleration. The tangential acceleration, like the tangential velocity vector, is a vector tangent to the curve and perpendicular to the

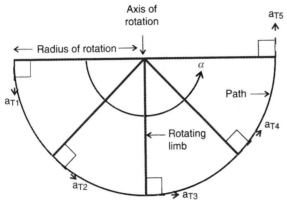

FIGURE 9-22 The tangential acceleration of a swinging segment. It is perpendicular to the swinging limb.

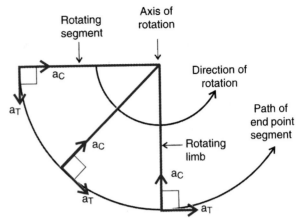

FIGURE 9-24 Tangential acceleration (a_T) and centripetal acceleration (a_C), which are perpendicular to each other. The tangential acceleration accelerates the segment end point downward, and the centripetal acceleration accelerates the end point toward the center of rotation. The result is motion along a curved path.

rotating segment (Fig. 9-22). In any activity, such as the discus, in which the performer spins to throw the implement, the purpose is to throw an implement as far as possible. An understanding of tangential velocity and tangential acceleration is therefore necessary. The time rate of change in the tangential velocity of the discus along its curved path is the tangential acceleration. The peak tangential velocity is ideally reached just prior to the release of the discus, at which time the tangential acceleration must be zero.

Consider a softball pitcher using an underhand pitch; further insight into another component of linear acceleration acting during rotational movement can be gained. As the pitcher moves the arm to the point of release of the pitch, the ball follows a curved path. Because the pitcher's arm is attached to the shoulder, the ball must follow the curved path produced by the rotation of the arm. Therefore, to continue on this path, the ball moves slightly inward and slightly downward at each instant in time until the ball is released (Fig. 9-23). That is, the ball is incrementally accelerated downward and inward toward the shoulder, or the axis of rotation.

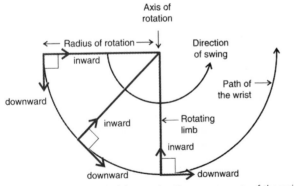

FIGURE 9-23 The directions of the acceleration components of the wrist of a softball/baseball pitcher during the downswing of the arm to the release of the ball. The wrist is accelerated in toward the shoulder and down tangential to the path of the wrist. These two vectors are perpendicular to each other.

Two components of acceleration produced by the rotation of a segment have been discussed: one tangential to the path of the segment and one along the segment toward the axis of rotation. These two accelerations are necessary for the ball in the pitcher's hand to continue on its curved path. The forward movement is the result of the tangential acceleration that has been previously discussed. Acceleration toward the axis or center of rotation, however, is called **centripetal acceleration** (Fig. 9-24). The adjective centripetal means center seeking. Centripetal acceleration is also known as **radial acceleration**. Either name is correct, although for the remainder of this discussion, the term centripetal acceleration will be used.

To derive the formula for centripetal acceleration, the resultant linear acceleration of a segment end point, such as the wrist, of a rotating segment is:

$$a = \frac{dv}{dt}$$

Since the segment is rotating, the linear velocity is:

$$v_T = \omega r$$

Substituting this into the acceleration equation, the acceleration becomes:

$$a = \frac{d(\omega r)}{dt}$$

If certain computational rules from calculus are applied, this equation becomes:

$$a = \omega * \frac{dr}{dt} + \frac{d\omega}{dt} * r$$

Since $\frac{dr}{dt}$ is the linear velocity and $\frac{d\omega}{dt}$ is the angular acceleration of the segments, this expression is:

$$a = \omega v + \alpha r$$

The linear velocity, v, is equal to ω r, so the expression for the linear acceleration of the segment end point is:

$$a = \omega\omega r + \alpha r$$

or

$$a = \omega^2 r + \alpha r$$

Remember that the resultant acceleration has two components that are perpendicular to each other. This expression illustrates these two components. This explanation requires the use of vector calculus and is much more complicated in derivation than presented. The addition (+) sign in this expression means vector addition. It was previously determined that αr was the tangential acceleration; thus $\omega^2 r$ is centripetal acceleration. The expression for centripetal acceleration is:

$$a_C = \omega^2 r$$

Centripetal acceleration may also be expressed in the following form as a function of the tangential velocity and the radius of rotation. That is, if $v = \omega r$ is substituted into the centripetal acceleration equation, the equation becomes:

$$a_C = \frac{v^2}{r}$$

From this expression, it can be seen that the centripetal acceleration will increase if the tangential velocity increases or if the radius of rotation decreases. For example, the usual difference between an indoor running track and an outdoor track is that the indoor track is smaller and thus has a smaller radius. If a runner attempted to maintain the same velocity around the indoor turn as on an outdoor track, the centripetal acceleration would have to be greater for the runner to accomplish the turn. Generally, the runner cannot accomplish the turn at the same velocity as outdoors, so race times on indoor tracks are somewhat slower than on outdoor tracks.

Since centripetal and tangential acceleration are components of linear acceleration, they must be perpendicular to each other. The acceleration vector of these components may then be constructed. The resultant acceleration (Fig. 9-25) is computed using the Pythagorean relationship:

$$a = \sqrt{a_T^2 + a_C^2}$$

In computing either the tangential or the centripetal acceleration, the units of angular velocity and angular acceleration are radians per second and radians per second squared, respectively. The units of linear acceleration (meters per second squared) can result only when a radian-based unit is used in the computation.

Angle–Angle Diagrams

In most graphical presentations of human movement, usually some parameter (e.g., position, angle, velocity) is

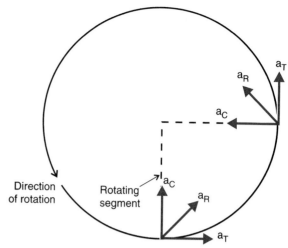

FIGURE 9-25 The resultant linear acceleration vector (a_R) composed of the centripetal and tangential acceleration components.

graphed as a function of time. In certain activities, such as locomotion, the motions of the segments are cyclic; that is, they are repetitive, with the end of one cycle at the beginning of the next. In these instances, an **angle–angle diagram** may be useful to represent the relationship between two angles during the movement. An angle–angle diagram is the plot of one angle as a function of another angle. That is, one angle is used for the x-axis and one for the y-axis. In an angle–angle diagram, one angle is usually a relative angle (angle between two segments) and the other is an absolute angle (angle relative to reference frame). For the angle–angle graph to be meaningful, a functional relationship between the angles should exist (Fig. 9-26). For example, in studying an individual running, the relationship between the sagittal view ankle and knee angles may be meaningful, whereas the relationship between the elbow angle and the ankle angle may not.

One problem with this type of diagram is that time cannot be easily represented on the graph. It can be presented, however, by placing marks on the angle–angle curve to represent each instant in time at which the data were calculated. These marks are placed at equal time intervals and give an indication of the angular distance through which each joint has moved in equal time intervals. Thus angular velocity of the movement is represented, since the further apart the marks are on the curve, the greater the velocity of the movement. Conversely, the closer together the marks, the less the velocity (Fig. 9-27).

Angle–angle diagrams have proved useful in the examination of the relationship between the rearfoot angle and the knee angle (1,31). This relationship is based on the related anatomical motions of the subtalar and knee joints. During the support phase of gait, the knee flexes at touchdown and continues to flex until midstance. At the same time, the foot lands in an inverted position and immediately begins to evert until midstance. Both knee flexion and subtalar eversion are associated with internal tibial rotation. After midstance, the knee extends and the subtalar joint

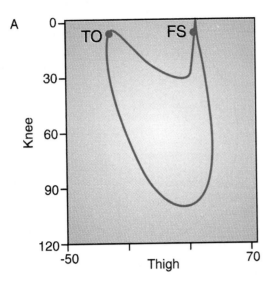

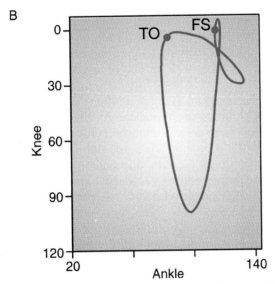

FIGURE 9-26 Angle–angle diagrams of the knee angle as a function of the thigh angle **(A)** and the knee angle plotted as a function of the ankle angle **(B)** for one complete running stride of an individual running at 3.6 m/second. TO, toe-off; FS, foot strike. (After Williams, K. R. [1985]. Biomechanics of running. *Exercise and Sports Sciences Review, 14.*)

inverts. Both of these joint actions result in external tibial rotation. These actions are presented in Figure 9-27 with the knee angle expressed as a relative angle and subtalar joint inversion and eversion expressed as an absolute angle. Figure 9-28, an angle–angle diagram presented in a paper by van Woensel and Cavanagh (31), illustrates the relationship between the knee angle and the rearfoot angle in different shoe conditions. One of the three shoes used in this study was specifically designed to force the runner to pronate during support, another to force the runner to supinate during support, and the third pair was a neutral shoe.

Angular Kinematics of Walking and Running

Many researchers have reported on how the lower extremity joint angles vary throughout the walking and running stride, particularly during the support portion of the stride. An angular kinematic analysis of walking and running will typically include a graphical presentation of joint rotations as a function of time. While some researchers have studied patterns of angular velocity and acceleration in both running and walking, the major focus of investigation has been on the characteristics of angular positions and displacements at critical events in the locomotion cycle. For both walking and running, the greatest range of motion occurs in the sagittal plane, and segment movements in this plane are often used to describe gait characteristics, even though movement in the other planes is critical to successful gait. Sagittal, frontal, and transverse plane joint angular kinematic patterns for walking, running, and sprinting are shown in Figure 9-29. Although there are obvious magnitude differences where the angular displacements increase with speed of locomotion, the patterns are similar across the speeds of locomotion with some temporal phasing differences. The one exception is at the ankle joint, where there is less and less plantarflexion at heel strike as locomotion speed increases until a

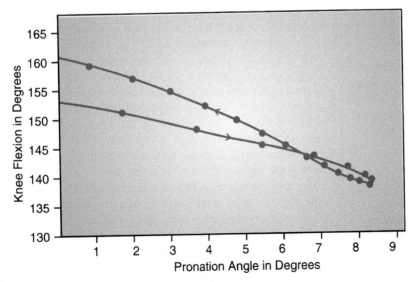

FIGURE 9-27 Angle–angle diagram of knee flexion as a function of subtalar pronation angle for an individual running at 6 minutes per mile on a treadmill. The dots on the curve indicate equal time intervals. (After Bates, B. T., et al. [1978, fall]. Foot function during the support phase of running. *Running, 24:29.*)

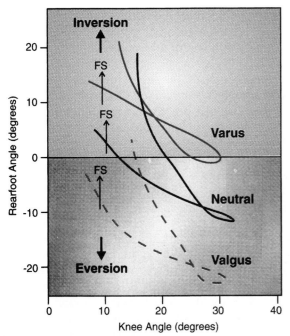

FIGURE 9-28 Knee–rearfoot angle–angle diagram of an individual in three types of running shoes. FS, foot strike. The *varus* shoe has a medial wedge, which mediates rearfoot pronation; the *valgus* shoe has a lateral wedge, which enhances rearfoot pronation; the *neutral* shoe is a normal running shoe. (After van Woensel, W., Cavanagh, P. R. [1992]. A perturbation study of lower extremity motion during running. *International Journal of Sports Biomechanics*, 8:30–47).

accompany this response are hip flexion, knee flexion, and ankle dorsiflexion. As the body continues over the foot in midstance, these movements continue until the terminal stages of stance, where there is a reversal into hip extension, knee extension, and plantarflexion.

The initial touchdown hip flexion angle for walking and running has been reported to be in the range of 35 to 40° and 45 to 50°, respectively (16,20,21). In the early phases of contact the hip adducts in the reported range of 5 to 10° and 8 to 12° for walking and running, respectively. After touchdown, the amount of hip flexion reduces over the course of the support until toe-off, at which 0 to 3° of hip extension in walking and 3 to 5° of hip extension in running is reported (16,20,21). There is also hip movement into abduction at toe-off in the range of 2 to 5° for both walking and running. When the limb is off the ground in the swing phase, hip flexion maximum values are reported in the range of 35 to 50° for walking and 55 to 65° for running. Hip abduction in the initial portion of the swing phase is similar for walking and running, reported to be in the range of 3 to 8°. Hip adduction late in the swing phase varies more between walking and running, in the range of 0 to 5° and 5 to 15°, respectively (16,20,21).

The knee angle is flexed at touchdown and has been reported in the literature to be in the range of 10 to 15° for walking (16,20,21) and 21 to 40° (1,5,8,9,16,20,21) for running. After touchdown, the knee flexes to values ranging from 20 to 25° for walking and 38 to 60° for running, with the greater flexion occurring at faster speeds (1,2). The knee flexion movement lowers the body in stance. Maximal knee flexion occurs at midstance, after which the knee extends until toe-off. Full extension is not

point in very fast running at which plantarflexion is absent (6). As contact is made with the ground in both walking and running, a loading response absorbs body weight and downward acceleration. The angular kinematics that

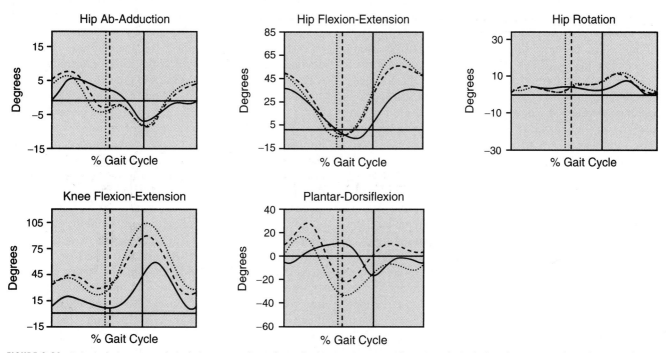

FIGURE 9-29 Gait analysis commonly includes a recording of angular kinematics across the gait cycle, including the support phase (percent of cycle up to vertical line) and the swing phase (percent of cycle past the vertical line). The angular kinematic differences and similarities between walking (solid line), running (broken line) and sprinting (dotted line) become apparent when graphed against one another (after Novacheck, T. F. [1995]. Instructional Course Lectures. Park Ridge, IL, 44:497–506.)

achieved at toe-off; values range from 10 to 40° in walking and 18 to 40° in running, depending on speed (4,8,16,20,21). Greater extension values at toe-off are generally associated with faster speeds. In the swing phase, knee flexion is important to shorten the swing leg before the hip flexion brings the limb forward. The range of knee flexion in walking and running is reported to be in the range of 50 to 65° and 100 to 125°, respectively (16,20,21).

Again, while the magnitude of the knee angles at these specific instants in time during the support phase of running vary, the profile of the curve does not. The profile of the knee joint angle appears to be relatively stable and immune to distortion from influences such as running shoe construction (9,31) or delayed-onset muscle soreness (10).

In walking, the ankle is plantar flexed in a reported range of 5 to 6° at heel strike and moves into 10 to 12° of dorsiflexion before returning to 15 to 20° of plantarflexion at toe-off. During the swing phase of walking the foot continues on through 18 to 20° of plantarflexion and then dorsiflexes in a reported range of 2 to 5° in preparation for the next heel strike. As the speed of locomotion increases, there is less plantarflexion at heel strike until dorsiflexion is the movement occurring at touchdown. Depending on the speed, the reported range of dorsiflexion at heel strike in running is 10 to 17°, increasing to 20 to 30° in midstance and then moving to plantarflexion at toe-off (range, 10 to 20°). Plantarflexion continues into the initial phases of the swing phase (range, 15 to 30°) and then moves like walking into dorsiflexion in the reported range of 10 to 15° (16,20,21).

A number of investigations have described the rearfoot angle during the support phase of walking and running. Excessive rearfoot motion during running has been hypothesized to cause a variety of lower extremity injuries, although little evidence directly relates excessive rearfoot motion and injury (5,19). In fact, a valid definition of excessive rearfoot motion has not yet been determined. From a functional standpoint, eversion of the calcaneus is necessary because it allows the foot to assume a flat position on the ground. Typically, maximum rearfoot angle values from −6 to −17° at midstance have been reported in the literature (5,11) for running and in the range of −9.2 to −12.9° for walking (13,24). This wide range in maximum values can be due to differences in the foot structure of individuals as well as the influence of footwear. It has been reported that more extreme rearfoot angles occurred at midstance in running when the subjects wore racing shoes as compared to training shoes (11). More extreme rearfoot eversion angles have also been reported for runners in a shoe with a very soft midsole than in a shoe with a firmer midsole (9). Although the rearfoot angle is related in motion to the knee angle by the action of tibial rotation, it is, unlike the knee angle, highly variable and certainly can be influenced by a number of factors.

The simultaneous actions of these two lower extremity angles has been a topic of several investigations. Since internal tibial rotation accompanies knee flexion and subtalar joint eversion and both reach a maximum at midstance, the mistiming of these joint actions has been suggested as a possible mechanism for lower extremity injury (1). Hamill et al. (9) illustrated that the rearfoot angle could be changed by a running shoe with a very soft midsole, while the knee angle could not. They reported that in a soft midsole running shoe, the maximum rearfoot angle occurred sooner in the support period than did maximum knee flexion. The subtalar joint also stayed at this maximum while the knee began to extend. Thus, it appeared that a twisting action may be applied to the tibia by the differential speeds at which the tibia rotated early in support and late in support. Since the tibia is a rigid structure and may be difficult to twist, the tibia may continue to rotate internally at the knee, even though it should externally rotate. This undesirable action at the knee may possibly cause knee pain in the runner. If these actions are repeated with each foot-to-ground contact and the runner has many foot-to-ground contacts, the runner may be subject to a knee injury that would prohibit training. This type of injury is often referred to as an **overuse injury**. It results from an accumulation of stresses, not a single high-level stress.

Alterations in the angular kinematics of the lower extremity joints during both walking and running occur in response to changes in the environment or to functional limitations in the system. For example, some individuals when running over a noncompliant surface will make a kinematic adjustment at impact by responding with more initial knee flexion at contact (7). Walking uphill brings about a number of adjustments in the lower extremity. For example, increasing the grade from 0 to 24%, the lower extremity adjustments start at heel strike with a 22% increase in dorsiflexion, 31% more knee flexion, and 23% more hip flexion (15). Over the stance phase, there are unequal adjustments at the three lower extremity joints, with the hip joint undergoing the greatest increase in the range of motion (+59%), followed by the ankle (+20%) and an actual decrease (−12%) range of motion at the knee (15). The primary adjustment to walking downhill during the stance phase occurs at the knee joint, where there is as much as 15° more knee flexion in early stance (14). Movement adjustments in the swing phase occur at the hip and ankle, with less hip flexion and less plantarflexion.

Locomotion is also influenced by a variety of medical conditions. For example, the walking gait of an individual with Parkinson's disease will usually exhibit small, quick steps and less range of motion in the lower extremity joints. A tight hip flexor (psoas) in individuals with cerebral palsy can limit the hip extension during the stance phase. This causes an increase in pelvic tilt (26). Specific adjustments in the joint kinematics of individuals with hemiplegia may show a reduction in the range of motion at the knee joint, with increases in range of motion at the ankle and excessive hip and knee motion in the swing

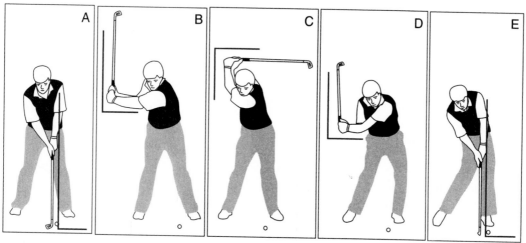

FIGURE 9-30 Critical angular positions in the address **(A)**, takeaway **(B)**, top of backswing **(C)**, downswing **(D)**, and impact **(E)** phases determine the success of the golf swing.

phase. Finally, individuals with injury to one limb will typically compensate for pain in one limb by altering range of motion in both limbs so they can increase the time spent on the limb with no pain.

 ## Angular Kinematics of Golf Swing

Chapter 8 pointed out that the linear speed and path of the club head are important determinants of a successful golf shot. These two linear kinematic components of the swing are the result of a series of angular movements; thus the angular kinematics of the golf swing is commonly the primary focus of golf instruction and evaluation. The golf swing can be accurately described using a double pendulum model, with one link being the arm rotating about the shoulder joint and the second link being the club and wrist, where the wrist acts as a hinge about which the club rotates (17). A third connected link has been suggested between the shoulder and what is referred to as the hub axis as the body rotates about a vertical axis (28). For purposes of this introduction to the golf swing, the primary focus will be on the double pendulum characteristics of the swing.

In the golf swing, the left arm sets the plane of the swing (28). The swing plane is an elliptical plane around the body that brings the club head into contact with the ball from the inside, where it ends up square to the ball. The swing is a pivot about an axis running through the base of the neck with the head stationary (27). Many beginning golfers try to create an upright swing plane with the club brought straight back and straight forward. When the club head comes down to meet the ball with this swing plane, it is never square with the ball and puts spin on the ball at contact.

The angular positions of the club at various stages of the swing are good predictors of a successful swing. A frontal view of the golf swing provides a good perspective for evaluating club position (Fig. 9-30). In the first stage of the swing, the golfer addresses the ball. This position at the beginning of the swing should be the same as the position at impact. It establishes the arm and shoulder position that will bring the club into precise alignment for impact (27). The club and the left arm should form a straight line, and the club face should be aimed down a perpendicular line from the ball forward in a straight line (Fig. 9-30A). As the club is started in the backswing, there is an initial takeaway phase where the club head is taken back away from the ball. This is initiated with a weight shift to the rear, which allows for greater range of motion at the hip and flattens the arc of the swing. A long takeaway is preferred: the club travels in a wide arc and the wrist does not allow movement of the club until the hands are chest high. This increases the distance for the club head to travel as the shoulders are rotated farther from the target. At the end of the takeaway phase, the left arm should be horizontal to the ground and the club should be vertical and perpendicular to the arm (Fig. 9-30B). Continuing to the top of the backswing, the upper body has rotated to allow the club to be positioned parallel to the ground again and parallel to the final target line for ball contact. The right elbow flexes at the end of the backswing to reduce the length and allow for more acceleration. The left arm continues to be straight and vertical. This position ensures that the club face will travel squarely to the ball at contact (Fig. 9-30C). From the top of the backswing, the downswing begins as the club shaft and the left arm drop in one piece to the position halfway down, where the left arm is again parallel to the ground and the club is vertical (Fig. 9-30D). Hip rotation and the legs initiate this movement as they drive forward, dropping the right shoulder and the shaft into place. The impact position should duplicate the initial address position, with the left arm and club forming a straight vertical line and the club face traveling in a straight line through the ball (Fig. 9-30E). If these angular positions can be obtained within the context of a fluid swing, the ball will travel far and accurately.

The interaction of the arm and club links are shown in the displacement, velocity, and acceleration curves in the downswing phase illustrated in Figure 9-31. The displacement of the arm segment in the downswing was 100 to 270°, and the displacement of the club relative to the arm was 50 to 175°. As the shoulder displacement increased in the early phases, the wrist angle remained constant until it uncocked in the later stages of the downswing (17). This uncocking increases dramatically 80 to 100 ms prior to impact as the club is brought in line with the hands (18). The interaction between the arm and the club segments enhances the velocity and acceleration of the club at impact. This is illustrated in the angular velocity graph, where the arm velocity moves through a range of 250°/s, increasing to 800°/s and reducing velocity to 500°/s at impact. The resulting effect on the club segment is a build in velocity from zero initially to a culminating 2300 to 4000°/s at impact (17,18). Angular accelerations of the club were minimal in the beginning of the downswing and increased rapidly to values approaching 10,000°/s/s at a point where the angular acceleration of the arm was reduced to zero and began the negative acceleration (17).

 ## Angular Kinematics of Wheelchair Propulsion

Angular kinematic characteristics of the trunk and joint actions at the shoulder, elbow, and wrist are the focus of many investigations of wheelchair propulsion. Both linear and angular kinematics are constrained because the hand must follow the rim (29). However, there are differences in hand position on the rim as well as different seat positions and other adjustments that can alter the angular kinematics considerably. A stick figure illustrating the sagittal angular positions of the arm, forearm, and hand segments during wheelchair propulsion is shown in Figure 9-32. The angular positions are shown for various stages in the event at a rim contact position that is −15° with respect to top dead center continuing on through +60° in 15° increments. The range of motion in the elbow and shoulder joints has been reported to be an average of 55 to 62° of elbow flexion and extension, 60 to 65° of shoulder flexion and extension, 20° of shoulder abduction and adduction, 36° of shoulder internal and external rotation, 35° of wrist flexion and extension, and 68 to 72° of wrist ulnar and radial flexion (12,23). There is also a reported approximate 37° of pronation and supination (3). The trunk contributes to wheelchair propulsion via flexion in the propulsive phase and extension in the recovery phase following hand release (30). Angular velocity and acceleration during wheelchair propulsion have not been studied extensively, but

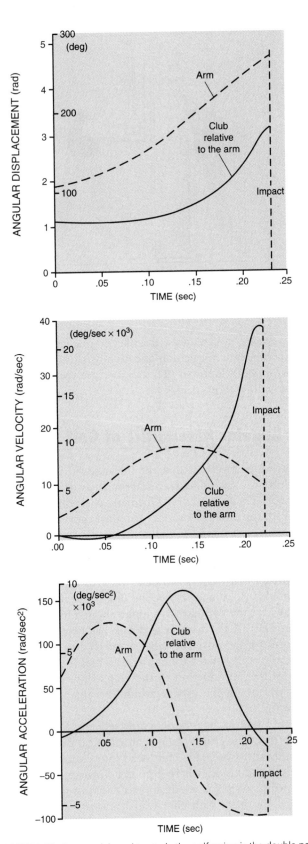

FIGURE 9-31 One model used to study the golf swing is the double pendulum. Displacement, velocity, and acceleration data for the arm (broken line) and the club motion relative to the arm (solid line) illustrate the unique motion characteristics of each segment. (After Milburn, P. D. [1982]. Summation of segmental velocities in the golf swing. *Medicine, Science in Sports and Exercise*, 14:60–64.)

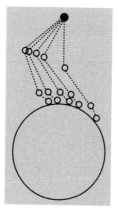

FIGURE 9-32 Angular positions of the upper extremity during wheelchair propulsion at 1.11 m/second. (After Van der Helm, F. C. T., Veeger, H. E. J. [1996]. Quasi-static analysis of muscle forces in the shoulder mechanism during wheelchair propulsion. *Journal of Biomechanics*, 29:39–52.)

reported values approach 300°/s for elbow extension even at slow speeds (1.11 m/s) (32).

If propulsion is made with a lever rather than on the hand rim, the angular kinematics change, requiring more elbow range of motion, less shoulder extension, more shoulder rotation, and more shoulder abduction (12). Likewise, speed-dependent changes are seen in angular displacement. It has been reported that with increased speed of propulsion, the trunk displacement increases and the shoulder displacement decreases (25). Propelling up a slope also influences angular kinematics, resulting in greater trunk displacement and an increase in arm displacement at the shoulder. Finally, seat adjustments influence angular kinematics depending on the direction and level of alteration (12).

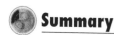 **Summary**

Nearly all purposeful human movement involves the rotation of segments about axes passing through the joint centers, and thus a knowledge of angular kinematics is necessary to understand human movement. Angles may be measured in degrees, revolutions, or radians. If the angular measurement is to be used in further calculations, the radian must be used. A radian is equal to 57.3°.

Angles may be defined as relative and absolute, and both may be used in biomechanical investigations. A relative angle measures the angle between two segments but cannot determine the orientation of the segments in space. An absolute angle measures the orientation of a segment in space relative to the right horizontal axis placed at the distal end of the segment. How segment angles are defined must be clearly stated when presenting the results of any biomechanical analysis.

The kinematic quantities of angular position, displacement, velocity, and acceleration have the same relationship

to each other as their linear analogs. Thus, angular velocity is calculated using the first order central difference method as follows:

$$\omega_i = \frac{\theta_{i+1} - \theta_{i-1}}{2\Delta t}$$

Likewise, angular acceleration is defined as:

$$\alpha_i = \frac{\omega_{i+1} - \omega_{i-1}}{2\Delta t}$$

The techniques of differentiation and integration apply to angular quantities as well as linear quantities. Thus, angular velocity is the first derivative of angular position with respect to time, and angular acceleration is the second derivative. The concept of the slope of a secant and a tangent also applies in the angular case to distinguish between average and instantaneous quantities.

It is difficult to represent angular motion vectors in the manner in which linear motion vectors were represented. The right-hand rule is used to determine the direction of the angular motion vector. Rotations that are counterclockwise are positive (+), while clockwise rotations are negative (−).

Sagittal view lower extremity angles were defined using a system suggested by Winter (36). In this convention, ankle, knee, and hip angles were defined using the absolute angles of the foot, leg, thigh, and pelvis segments. rearfoot angle measures the relative motion of the leg and the calcaneus in the frontal plane and is calculated from the absolute angles of the calcaneus and the leg.

There is a relationship between linear and angular motion. Comparable quantities of the two forms of motion may be related when the radius of rotation is considered. The linear velocity of the distal end of a rotating segment is called the tangential velocity and is calculated as:

$$v_T = \omega r$$

where ω is the angular velocity of the segment and r is the length of the segment. The derivative of the tangential velocity, the tangential acceleration is:

$$a_T = \alpha r$$

where a is the angular acceleration of the rotating segment. The other component of the linear acceleration of the end point of the rotating segment is the centripetal or radial acceleration. This is expressed as:

$$a_C = \omega^2 r$$

The tangential and centripetal acceleration components are perpendicular to each other.

A useful tool in biomechanics is the presentation angular motion in angle–angle diagrams. These diagrams generally present angles of joints that are anatomically functionally related. Time can be presented only indirectly on this type of graph, however.

Equation Review for Angular Kinematics

Purpose	Given	Formula
Relative angle between two segments using law of cosines	Length of segment a and b and distance between end of a and b (length c)	$\theta = \arccos\left(\dfrac{b^2 + c^2 - a^2}{2 * b * c}\right)$
Absolute angle	End points: horizontal and vertical components	$\theta = \arctan\left(\dfrac{y_{distal} - y_{proximal}}{x_{distal} - x_{proximal}}\right)$
Calculate position	Starting position relative to origin, constant velocity (zero acceleration), and time	$\theta = \theta_{initial} + \omega_{initial}t$
Calculate position	Starting position at origin, constant velocity (zero acceleration), and time	$\theta = \omega_{initial}\, t$
Calculate position	Initial velocity, time, constant acceleration	$\theta = \omega_i t + \dfrac{1}{2}\alpha t^2$
Calculate position	Initial velocity = zero, time, constant acceleration	$\theta = \dfrac{1}{2}\alpha t^2$
Calculate final displacement	Final angular velocity; constant angular acceleration	$\theta = \dfrac{\omega^2}{2 * \alpha}$
Calculate average velocity	Displacement and time	$\omega = \dfrac{\theta_2 - \theta_1}{t_2 - t_1}$
Calculate average velocity	Initial and final velocity	$\omega = \dfrac{\omega_{initial} + \omega_{final}}{2}$
Calculate final velocity	Initial velocity, constant acceleration, and time	$\omega_f = \omega_{initial} + \alpha t$
Calculate final velocity	Starting velocity = zero, constant acceleration, and time	$\omega = \alpha t$
Calculate final velocity	Velocity at time = zero, constant acceleration, initial position relative to origin, final position	$\omega = \sqrt{\omega_{initial}^2 + 2\alpha(\theta - \theta_{initial})}$
Calculate final velocity	Initial velocity = zero, constant acceleration, initial and final position	$\omega_f^2 = 2\alpha\theta$ $\omega = \sqrt{2\alpha(\theta - \theta_{initial})}$
Calculate acceleration	Final velocity and displacement	$\alpha = \dfrac{\omega_{final}^2}{2\theta}$
Calculate average acceleration	Velocity and time	$\alpha = \dfrac{\omega_2 - \omega_1}{t_2 - t_1}$
Calculate average acceleration	Displacement, time	$\alpha = \dfrac{2\theta}{t^2}$
Calculate time	Displacement, constant acceleration	$t = \sqrt{\dfrac{2\theta}{\alpha}}$
Calculate linear distance	Radius, angular displacement	$s = r\theta$
Calculate linear velocity (tangential)	Radius, angular velocity	$v = r\omega$
Calculate linear acceleration (tangential)	Radius, angular acceleration	$a = r\alpha$
Centripetal acceleration	Radius, angular velocity	$a_c = \omega^2 r$
Centripetal acceleration	Radius, tangential linear velocity	$a_c = \dfrac{v^2}{r}$

REVIEW QUESTIONS

True or False

1. ____ A thigh with an angular velocity of 3.2 rad/s is extending.

2. ____ Choking up on a bat in baseball is done to increase the amount of wrist action.

3. ____ With increased speed of locomotion, there is a concomitant increase in the amount of plantarflexion at heel strike.

4. ____ Angular acceleration of the golf club is maximum when the arm's angular acceleration is zero.

5. ____ All points on a thigh flexing through 75° undergo the same amount of rotation.

6. ____ Linear acceleration away from the axis of rotation in a rotating lever is termed centripetal acceleration.

7. ____ The relative angle between the trunk and the arm abducted straight out to the side is 90°.

8. ____ Trunk extension accompanies shoulder flexion and elbow extension in wheelchair propulsion.

9. ____ The absolute angle of the thigh relative to the trunk when standing straight up is 0°.

10. ____ Walking uphill results in an increase in motion at the hip, knee, and ankle joints.

11. ____ A radian is an angle formed when the length of the radius is equal to the length of the arc.

12. ____ There is minimal motion at the wrist joint during wheelchair propulsion.

13. ____ Linear displacement of a point on a lever is a function of the length of the radius and the angular displacement.

14. ____ The vertex is the angle between two segments.

15. ____ Positive angular acceleration indicates that counterclockwise movement is occurring.

16. ____ Maximum rearfoot movement occurs at heel strike in running.

17. ____ The law of cosines provides the tool for computing relative angles between two segments not at a right angle to each other.

18. ____ In human locomotion, the knee joint angle is negative at contact in the support phase.

19. ____ Angle–angle diagrams usually plot a relative angle against an absolute angle.

20. ____ Absolute angles are always computed with respect to the right horizontal.

21. ____ Most movements in running occur in the frontal plane.

22. ____ The swing plane for golf is elliptical.

23. ____ The initiation of the downswing in golf occurs with the uncocking of the wrists.

24. ____ The units for a radian are degrees.

25. ____ Angular velocity is the slope of secant to an angle–time curve.

Multiple Choice

A golf club 1.01 m long completes a downswing in 0.25 s through a range of 180°. Assume a uniform angular velocity. (Use for Questions 1–4)

1. What is the average angular velocity of the club?
   a. 12.57 rad/s
   b. 727.2°/s
   c. 11.28 rad/s
   d. 659°/s

2. What is the linear distance moved by the end of the club?
   a. 181.8 m
   b. 172.6 m
   c. 2.45 m
   d. 3.17 m

3. What is the tangential velocity of the end of the club?
   a. 12.70 m/s
   b. 13.56 m/s
   c. 11.59 m/s
   d. 3.20 m/s

4. What is the tangential acceleration of the end of the club?
   a. 101.53 m/s^2
   b. 100.52 m/s^2
   c. 50.78 m/s^2
   d. 48.34 m/s^2

5. During an elbow flexion exercise, the relative angle at the elbow was 22° at 0.3 s and 155° at 0.62 s. What was the angular velocity of the elbow?
   a. 443.9°/s
   b. −443.9°/s
   c. −415.6°/s
   d. 415.6°/s

6. If the angular velocity at 0.19 s was 3.2 rad/s and 1.2 rad/s at 0.27 s, what was the average angular acceleration over this time interval?
   a. −25 r/s^2
   b. 25 r/s^2
   c. 7.41 r/s^2
   c. −7.41 r/s^2

7. If a skater is rotating during a spin at a constant angular velocity of 2.5 rad/s for 1.1 s, what is the angular acceleration?
   a. 2.27 r/s^2
   b. −2.27 r/s^2
   c. 0 r/s^2
   d. No movement

8. An object is spinning at 4 rev/s and starts decelerating at 0.9 rev/s^2. How long will it take the object to stop?
   a. 3.6 s
   b. 3.89 s
   c. 4.44 s
   d. 4.72 s

9. The kicking phase of a soccer kick took place over 0.096 s and included hip flexion (23°) and knee extension (29°). If the thigh was 0.61 m long and the leg 0.51 m long, what is the tangential velocity of the foot resulting from these movements?
   a. 2.55 m/s
   b. 2.69 m/s
   c. 5.24 m/s
   d. 5.55 m/s

10. If a discus thrower rotates through the last 45° of a turn in 0.11 s and the distance from the axis of rotation to the center of the discus is 1.22 m, calculate the average linear velocity of the discus.
    a. 499.09 m/s
    b. 502.10 m/s
    c. 8.71 m/s
    d. 9.02 m/s

11. An object is spinning at a constant angular velocity of 13.9 rad/s. If it spins for 1.9 s, what is the angular distance traveled?
    a. 26.42 rad
    b. 7.3 rad
    c. 12.51 rad
    c. 21.22 rad

12. A hammer thrower releases the hammer after reaching an angular velocity of 14.9 rad/s. If the hammer is 1.6 m from the shoulder joint, what is the linear velocity at release?
    a. 853.77 cm/s
    b. 845.34 cm/s
    c. 23.84 m/s
    d. 21.79 m/s

13. Calculate the relative angle at the knee and the absolute angles of the leg given the following positions in degree: hip (2.128, 1.891); knee (2.122, 1.642); ankle (1.897, 1.210).
    a. Abs = 88.62°; rel = 153.9°
    b. Abs = 88.62°; rel = 62.48°
    c. Abs = 62.48°; rel = 153.9°
    d. Abs = 62.48°; rel = 26.14°

14. During the support phase of walking, the absolute angle of the thigh has the following angular velocities:

frame	time (s)	angular velocity (rad/s)
38	0.6167	1.033
39	0.6333	1.511
40	0.6500	1.882
41	0.6667	2.190

    Calculate the angular acceleration at frame 40.
    a. 25.49 rad/s²
    b. 18.44 rad/s²
    c. 21.82 rad/s²
    d. 20.33 rad/s²

15. An ice skater rotating around a vertical axis increases in angular velocity from 450°/s to 610°/s in 2.3 seconds. Find the angular acceleration.
    a. 265°/s²
    b. 1.22 rad/s²
    c. 69.57°/s²
    d. 4.63 rad/s²

16. A baseball bat is swing through 140° in 0.7 s. What is the angular acceleration?
    a. 200.0°/s²
    b. 189.1°/s²
    c. 564.3°/s²
    d. 571.4°/s²

17. Angular velocity of a rotating object changes from 650°/s to 495°/s in 1.2 seconds. What is the angular acceleration?
    a. −131.20°/s²
    b. 131.20°/s²

18. A cyclist completes 3.2 cycle revolutions in 1.4 s. What is the angular velocity in radians per second?
    a. 2.29
    b. 822.86
    c. 14.36
    d. 8.34

19. An individual's arm segment is 0.18 m long and has an angular velocity of 117°/s. What is the tangential velocity of the wrist?
    a. 21.06 m/s
    b. 2.04 m/s
    c. 0.75 m/s
    d. 0.38 m/s

20. A diver accelerates through a somersault at 950°/s. What is the angular displacement over 0.15 s?
    a. 10.69°
    b. 6333.3°
    c. 142.5°
    d. 21.38°

21. An individual is running around a turn with an 11-m radius at 3.75 m/s. What is the runner's centripetal acceleration?
    a. 32.2 m/s²
    b. 25.2 m/s²
    c. 0.34 m/s²
    d. 1.28 m/s²

22. The final angular velocity of a golf swing was 370°/s with a constant angular acceleration of 580°/s². How far did the club rotate?
    a. 210°
    b. 118°
    c. 156°
    d. 213°

23. If the linear velocity of a club head in the golf swing is 50 m/s at impact, what was the angular velocity if the club is 0.95 m long?
    a. 52.6 rad/s
    b. 47.5 rad/s
    c. 52.6°/s
    d. 47.5°/s

24. A baseball bat is rotating at 350 rpm at contact. What is the angular velocity in radians per second?
    a. 2198.9
    b. 36.7
    c. 6.1
    d. 131937.2

25. In the release phase of bowling, the bowler's arm and forearm traveled through 0.23 and 0.27 radians, respectively, in 0.03 seconds. If the length of the arm is 0.8 m and the forearm 0.5 m, what is the tangential velocity of the ball resulting from these two movements?
    a. 10.64 m/s
    b. 14.34 m/s
    c. 21.67 m/s
    d. 16.67 m/s

REFERENCES

1. Bates, B. T., et al. (1978). Foot function during the support phase of running. *Running*, 24:29.
2. Bates, B. T., et al. (1979). Functional variability of the lower extremity during the support phase of running. *Medicine and Science in Sports and Exercise*, 11(4):328–331.
3. Boniger, M. L., et al. (1997). Wrist biomechanics during two speeds of wheelchair propulsion: An analysis using a local coordinate system. *Archives Physical Medicine Rehabilitation*, 78:364–372.
4. Cavanagh, P. R., et al. (1977). A biomechanical comparison of good and elite distance runners. In P. Milvy (Ed.). *The Marathon: Physiological, Medical, Epidemiological, and Psychological Studies*. New York: New York Academy of Science, 328–345.
5. Clarke, T. E., et al. (1983). The effects of shoe design parameters of rearfoot control in running. *Medicine and Science in Sports and Exercise*, 15(5):376–381.
6. Czerniecki, J. M. (1988). Foot and ankle biomechanics in walking and running. *American Journal of Physical Medicine and Rehabilitation*, 67:246–252.
7. Dixon, S. J., et al. (2000). Surface effects on ground reaction forces and lower extremity kinematics in running. *Medicine and Science in Sports and Exercise*, 32:1919–1926.
8. Elliott, B. R., Blanksby, B. A. (1979). A biomechanical analysis of the male jogging action. *Journal of Human Movement Studies*, 5:42–51.
9. Hamill, J., et al. (1992). Timing of lower extremity joint actions during treadmill running. *Medicine and Science in Sports and Exercise*, 24:807–813.
10. Hamill, J., et al. (1990). Muscle soreness during running: Biomechanical and physiological considerations. *International Journal of Sports Biomechanics*, 7:125–137.
11. Hamill, J., et al. (1987). Effects of shoe type on cardiorespiratory responses and rearfoot control during treadmill running. *Medicine and Science in Sports and Exercise*, 20:515–521.
12. Hughes, C. J., et al. (1992). Biomechanics of wheelchair propulsion as a function of seat position and user-to-chair interface. *Archives of Physical Medicine and Rehabilitation*, 73:263–69.
13. Isacson, J., et al. (1986). Three dimensional electrogoniometric gait recording. *Journal of Biomechanics*, 19:627–35.
14. Kuster, M., et al. (1995). Kinematic and kinetic comparison of downhill and level walking. *Clinical Biomechanics*, 10:79–84.
15. Lange, G. W., et al. (1996). Electromyographic and kinematic analysis of graded treadmill walking and the implications for knee rehabilitation. *Journal of Orthopedic and Sports Physical Therapy*, 23:294–301.
16. Mann, R. A., Hagy, J. L. (1980). Biomechanics of walking, running, and sprinting. *American Journal of Sports Medicine*, 8:345–350.
17. Milburn, P. D. (1982). Summation of segmental velocities in the golf swing. *Medicine and Science in Sports and Exercise*, 14:60–64.
18. Neal, R. J., Wilson, B. D. (1985). 3D kinematics and kinetics of the golf swing. *International Journal of Sports Biomechanics*, 1:221–231.
19. Nigg, B. M., et al. (1983). Methodological aspects of sport shoe and sport surface analysis. In H. Matsui, K. Kobayashi (Eds.). *Biomechanics VIII-B*. Champaign, IL: Human Kinetics, 1041–1052.
20. Novacheck, T. F. (1995). Walking, running, and sprinting: A three dimensional analysis of kinematics and kinetics. *Instructional Course Lectures*, 44:497–506.
21. Ounpuu, S. (1994). The biomechanics of walking and running. *Clinics in Sports Medicine*, 13:843–863.
22. Plagenhoef, S. (1971). *Patterns of Human Motion*. Englewood Cliffs, NJ: Prentice-Hall.
23. Rodgers, M. M., et al. (1994). Biomechanics of wheelchair propulsion during fatigue. *Archives of Physical Medicine and Rehabilitation*, 75:85–93.
24. Ronsky, J. L., et al. (1995). Correlation between physical activity and the gait characteristics and ankle joint flexibility of the elderly. *Clinical Biomechanics*, 10:41–49.
25. Sanderson, D. J., Sommer, H. J. (1989). Kinematic features of wheelchair propulsion. *Journal of Rehabilitation Research*, 26:31–50.
26. Schwartz, M. H., et al. (2000). A tool for quantifying hip flexor function during gait. *Gait and Posture*, 12:122–127.
27. Shoup, T. E., Fabian, D. (1986). Lengths and lies: choosing golf equipment scientifically. *SOMA*, 1:16–23.
28. Turner, A. B., Hills, N. J. (1999). A three-link mathematical model of the golf swing. In M. R. Farrally, A. J. Cochran (Eds.). *Science and Golf III*. Champaign, IL: Human Kinetics, 3–12.
29. Van der Helm, F. C. T., Veeger, H. E. J. (1996). Quasi-static analysis of muscle forces in the shoulder mechanism during wheelchair propulsion. *Journal of Biomechanics*, 29:39–52.
30. Vanlandewijck, Y. C., et al. (1984). Wheelchair propulsion efficiency: movement pattern adaptations to speed changes. *Medicine and Science in Sports and Exercise*, 26:1372–1381.
31. van Woensel, W., Cavanagh, P. R. (1992). A perturbation study of lower extremity motion during running. *International Journal of Sports Biomechanics*, 8:30–47.
32. Veeger, H. E. J., et al. (1991). Load on the upper extremity in manual wheelchair propulsion. *Journal of Electromyography and Kinesiology*, 1:270–280.
33. Winter, D. A. (1987). *The Biomechanics and Motor Control of Gait*. Waterloo, Ont.: University of Waterloo.

ADDITIONAL READING

Inman, V. T., et al. (1981). *Human Walking*. Baltimore: Williams & Wilkins.

Milliron, M. J., Cavanagh, P. R. (1990). Sagittal plane kinematics of the lower extremity during distance running. In P. R. Cavanagh (Ed.). *Biomechanics of Distance Running*. Champaign, IL: Human Kinetics, 65–105.

Stacoff, A., et al. (1989). The torsion of the foot in running. *International Journal of Sports Biomechanics*, 5:375–389.

Winter, D. A. (1990). *Biomechanics and Motor Control of Human Movement* (2nd edition). New York: Wiley.

GLOSSARY

Absolute Angle: Angle of a segment as measured from the right horizontal that describes the orientation of the segment in space.

Angle: A figure formed by two lines meeting at a point, the vertex.

Angle–Angle Diagram: A graph in which the angle of one segment is plotted as a function of the angle of another segment.

Angular Acceleration: The change in angular velocity per unit time.

Angular Displacement: The difference between the final angular position and the initial angular position of a rotating body.

Angular Distance: The total of all angular changes of a rotating body.

Angular Kinematics: The description of angular motion, including angular positions, angular velocities, and angular accelerations, without regard to the causes of the motion.

Angular Motion: Motion about an axis of rotation in which different regions of the same object do not move through the same distance in the same time.

Angular Speed: The angular distance traveled divided by the time over which the angular motion occurred.

Angular Velocity: The time rate of change of angular displacement.

Axis of Rotation: The point about which a body rotates.

Centripetal Acceleration: The component of the linear acceleration directed toward the axis of rotation.

Degree: A unit of angular measurement: $1/360$ of a revolution.

General Motion: Motion that involves both translation and rotation.

Instantaneous Joint Center: The center of rotation of a joint at any instant in time.

Joint Angle: Angle between two segments that is relative and does not change with body orientation.

Law of Cosines: The general case of the Pythagorean theorem:

$$a^2 = b^2 + c^2 - 2ab \cos A$$

where a is the length of the side opposite angle A and b and c are the lengths of the other two sides in a triangle.

Overuse Injury: An injury caused by continual low-level stress on a body.

Polarity: The direction of rotation designated as positive or negative.

Radial Acceleration: See centripetal acceleration.

Radian: The measure of an angle at the center of a circle described by an arc equal to the length of the radius of the circle ($1 \text{ rad} = 57.3°$).

Radius of Rotation: The linear distance from the axis of rotation to a point on the rotating body.

Relative Angle: The angle formed by the longitudinal axes of two adjacent segments whose vertex is at the joint.

Revolution: A unit of measurement that describes one complete cycle of a rotating body.

Right-Hand Rule: The convention that designates the direction of an angular motion vector; the fingers of the right hand are curled in the direction of the rotation and the right thumb points in the direction of the vector.

Rotation: A motion that occurs when not all parts of an object undergo the same displacement.

Segment Angle: The angle of the segment with respect to the right horizontal that is absolute and that changes according to orientation of the body.

Tangent: The ratio of the side opposite an angle to the adjacent angle in a right triangle.

Tangential Acceleration: The change in linear velocity per unit time of a body moving along a curved path.

Tangential Velocity: The change in linear position per unit time of a body moving along a curved path.

Vertex: The intersection of two lines that form an angle.

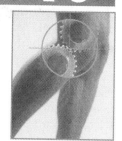

Linear Kinetics

OBJECTIVES

After reading this chapter, the student should be able to:

1. Define force and discuss the characteristics of a force.

2. Compose and resolve forces according to vector operations.

3. Discuss Newton's law of gravitation and how it affects human movement.

4. Differentiate between a contact and a noncontact force.

5. Discuss the six types of contact forces and how each affects human movement.

6. Represent the external forces acting on the human body on a free body diagram.

7. State Newton's three laws of motion and their relevance to human movement.

8. Define the impulse–momentum relationship.

9. Define the work–energy relationship.

10. Discuss the concepts of internal and external work.

11. Discuss the forces acting on an object as it moves along a curved path.

12. Discuss the relationships between force, pressure, work, energy, and power.

13. Discuss selected research studies that used an linear kinetic approach.

14. Solve quantitative problems that employ linear kinetic principles.

I. Force
  A. Characteristics of a Force
  B. Composition and Resolution of Forces

II. Types of Forces
  A. Noncontact Forces
  B. Contact Forces
    1. Ground Reaction Force
    2. Joint Reaction Force
    3. Friction
    4. Fluid Resistance
    5. Inertial Force
    6. Muscle Force
    7. Elastic Force

III. Representation of Forces Acting on a System

IV. Laws of Motion
  A. Law I: Law of Inertia
  B. Law II: Law of Acceleration

  C. Law III: Law of Action–Reaction
  D. Analysis Using Newton's Laws of Motion
    1. Effects of a Force at an Instant in Time
    2. Effects of Force Applied Over a Period of Time

V. Special Force Applications
  A. Centripetal Force
  B. Pressure
  C. Work: The Effect of a Force Applied Over a Distance
  D. Power
  E. Energy

VI. Linear Kinetics of Locomotion

VII. Linear Kinetics of the Golf Swing

VIII. Linear Kinetics of Wheelchair Propulsion

IX. Summary

Previous chapters discussed linear and angular kinematics and the description of motion. The motion described was either translatory (linear), rotational (angular), or both (general). In this chapter the concern is with the causes of motion. For example, why does a runner lean on the curve of a track? What keeps an airplane in the air? Why do golf balls slice or hook? How does a pitcher curve a baseball? How do we propel ourselves forward in running? The search for the causes of motion date to antiquity, and answers to some of these questions were suggested by such notables as Aristotle and Galileo. The culmination of these explanations was provided by the great scientist Sir Isaac Newton, who ranks among the greatest thinkers in human history for his theories on gravity and motion. In fact, the laws of motion described by Newton in his famous book *Principia Mathematica* (1687) form the cornerstone of the mechanics of human movement (13). The branch of mechanics that deals with the causes of motion is called **kinetics**. Kinetics is concerned with the forces that act on a system. If the motion is translatory, **linear kinetics** is of concern. The basis for the understanding of the kinetics of linear motion is the concept of **force**.

Force

According to Newton's principles, objects move when acted upon by a force greater than the resistance to movement provided by the object. A force involves the interaction of two objects and produces a change in the state of motion of an object by pushing or pulling it. The force may produce motion, stop motion, positively or negatively accelerate, or change the direction of the object. In each case, the acceleration of the object changes or is prevented from changing. A force, therefore, may be defined as any interaction, a push or pull, between two objects that can cause an object to accelerate either positively or negatively. For example, a push on the ground generated by a forceful knee and hip extension may be sufficient to cause the body to accelerate upward and leave the ground—that is, jump.

CHARACTERISTICS OF A FORCE

Forces are vectors and as such have the characteristics of a vector, magnitude and direction. Magnitude is the amount of force being applied. It is also necessary to state the direction of a force, because the direction of a force may influence its effect, for example, on whether the force is pushing or pulling. Vectors, as described in Chapter 8, are usually represented by arrows, with the length of the arrow indicating the magnitude of the force and the arrowhead pointing in the direction in which the force is being applied. In the International System (SI) of measurement the unit for force is the newton (N), although for

comparison value, forces are often represented in the literature as a ratio of force to body weight or force to body mass. Sample peak force values for a variety of movements, expressed as a function of body weight, are presented in Table 10-1.

Forces have two other equally important characteristics, however: the **point of application** and the **line of action**. The point of application of a force is the specific point at which the force is applied to an object. This is very important because the point of application will most

TABLE 10-1 Maximum Forces Acting on the Body

Activity	Relative Force (N/BW)
Vertical jump, peak vertical	1.4–8.3 (32)*
	2.2 (60)
Squat jump	
Countermovement	
Hopping	
Landing	1.5–5.4 (24)
On hard surface from 0.45 m	5–7 (59)
Dismount from horizontal bars	8.2–11.6 (59)
Single leg landing, double	9.3–10.6 (61)
back somersault	
Basketball rebound landing	1.3–6.0 (74)
Vertical jump, hard surface	>3 (46)
Vertical jump, soft surface	2 (46)
Triple Jump, vertical forces	
Hop	7–10 (63)
Step	8–12 (63)
Jump	7.1–12.2 (63)
Triple jump, anteroposterior forces	
Hop	2.1–3.3 (63)
Step	−1.7–3.2 (63)
Jump	−1.7–3.9 (63)
Basketball jump shot, 2-point range	
Vertical	2.6 (27)
Horizontal	−0.5 (27)
Walking (vertical)	1–1.5
Compressive forces in the ankle joint	3–5.5 (64)
Reaction forces in the ankle joint	3.9–5.2 (64)
Reaction forces in the subtalar joint	2.4–2.8 (64)
Running (vertical)	2–3.5 (68)
Bone-on-bone force in the ankle joint	13 (68)
Patellar tendon force	4.7–6.9 (68)
Patellofemoral force	7.0–11.1 (68)
Plantar fascia force	1.3–2.9 (68)
Achilles tendon force	
Walking	3.9 (32)
Running	7.7 (32)
10 (70)	
Peak forces acting at hip	
Walking	2.8–4.8 (7)
Jogging	5.5 (7)
Stumbling	7.2 (7)

*Source in parenthesis

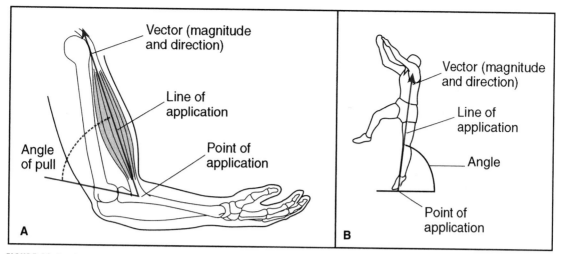

FIGURE 10-1 Characteristics of a force for an internal muscular force **(A)** and an external force generated on the ground in the high jump **(B)**.

often determine whether the resulting motion is linear or angular or both. In many instances, a force is represented by a point of application at a specific point, although there may be many points of application. For example, the point of application of a muscular force is the center of the muscle's attachment to the bone, or the insertion of the muscle. In many cases, the muscle is not attached to a single point on the bone but to many points, such as in the case of the fan-shaped deltoid muscle. In solving mechanical problems, however, it is considered to be attached to a single point. Other points of application are the contact point between the foot and the ground for activities such as jumping, walking, and running; hand contact with the ball for a baseball throw; and the contact point between the racket and the ball in tennis. The line of action of a force is a straight line of infinite length in the direction in which the force is acting. A force can be assumed to produce the same acceleration of the object if it acts anywhere along this line of action. Thus, if the force coming up from the ground in the last jump phase of a triple jumper has a line of action directed to 18° with respect to the horizontal, the jumper accelerates forward and upward in that direction. The orientation of the line of action is usually given with respect to an x, y coordinate system. The orientation of the line of action to this system is given as an angular position and is referred to as the angle of application. This angle is designated by the Greek letter theta (θ). The four characteristics of a force are illustrated in Figure 10-1A for a muscular force and in Figure 10-1B for a high-jump takeoff.

COMPOSITION AND RESOLUTION OF FORCES

Forces are vector quantities having both magnitude and direction. As presented in the discussion of kinematic vectors in Chapter 8, a single force vector may be resolved into perpendicular components, or several forces can be resolved

into one vector. That is, a single force vector can be calculated or composed to represent the net effect of all of the forces in the system. Similarly, given the resultant force, the resultant force can be resolved into its horizontal and vertical components. To do either, the trigonometric principles presented in Appendix D are applied.

However, several types of force systems must be defined to compose or resolve systems of multiple forces. Any system of forces acting in a single plane are referred to as coplanar, and if they act at a single point, they are called concurrent. Any set of concurrent **coplanar forces** may be substituted by a single force, or the resultant, producing the same effect as the multiple forces. The process of finding this single force is called **composition** of force vectors.

When force vectors act along a single line, the system is said to be collinear. In this case, vector addition is used to compose the forces. Consider the force system in Figure 10-2A. The force vectors a, b, and c all act in the same

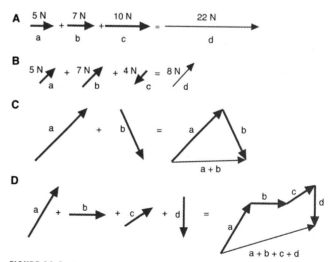

FIGURE 10-2 Force vector addition.

direction and can be replaced by a single force, d, which is the sum of a, b, and c. Thus:

$$d = a + b + c$$
$$= 5\,N + 7\,N + 10\,N$$
$$= 22\,N$$

The force vector d would have the same effect as the other three force vectors. In Figure 10-2B, however, two of the force vectors, a and b, are acting in one direction, while the vector c, is acting in the opposite direction. Thus, the force vector d is the algebraic sum of these three force vectors:

$$d = a + b - c$$
$$= 5\,N + 7\,N - 4\,N$$
$$= 8\,N$$

The force vector d still represents the net effect of these force vectors. In both of these examples, sets of **collinear force** vectors are present.

When the force vectors are not collinear but are coplanar, they may still be composed to determine the resultant force. Graphically, this can be done in exactly the same manner as described in Chapter 8 in the section on adding vectors. Consider Figure 10-2C. The force vectors a and b are not collinear, but they may be composed or added to determine their net effect. With the arrow of vector a placed at the tail of vector b, the resultant composed vector c is the distance between the tail of a and the arrow of b. This procedure is illustrated in Figure 10-2D with multiple vectors.

Multiple vectors can also be combined using trigonometric functions. First presented in Chapter 8, this involves first breaking each vector down into its components using **resolution**. Once resolved into vertical and horizontal components, the orthogonal components for each vector are added, and the resultant vector is composed. To illustrate, the four vectors shown in Figure 10-2D will be assigned values of length 10 and $\theta = 45°$ for vector A, length 6 and $\theta = 0°$ for vector B, length 5 and $\theta = 30°$ for vector C, and length 7 and $\theta = 270°$ for vector D. The first step is to resolve each vector into vertical and horizontal components.

Vector A

$$y = 10 \sin 45°$$
$$y = 10 * 0.7071$$
$$= 7.07$$
$$x = 10 \cos 45°$$
$$x = 10 * 0.7071$$
$$= 7.07$$

Vector B

$$y = 6 \sin 0°$$
$$y = 6 * 0.0$$
$$= 0$$
$$x = 6 \cos 0°$$
$$x = 6 * 1.000$$
$$= 6.00$$

Vector C

$$y = 5 \sin 30°$$
$$y = 5 * 0.500$$
$$= 2.50$$
$$x = 5 \cos 30°$$
$$x = 5 * 0.866$$
$$= 4.33$$

Vector D

$$y = 7 \sin 270°$$
$$y = 7 * -1.00$$
$$= -7.00$$
$$x = 7 \cos 270°$$
$$x = 7 * 0.00$$
$$= 0$$

To find the magnitude of the resultant vector, the horizontal and vertical components of each vector are added and resolved using the Pythagorean theorem:

	Horizontal Components	Vertical Components
Vector A	7.07	7.07
Vector B	5.00	0.00
Vector C	4.33	2.50
Vector D	0.00	−7.00
Sum (Σ)	16.40	2.57

$$C = \sqrt{x^2 + y^2}$$
$$C = \sqrt{16.40^2 + 2.57^2}$$
$$= \sqrt{268.96 + 6.61}$$
$$= \sqrt{275.57}$$
$$= 16.60$$

To find the angle of resultant vector, the trigonometric function tangent is used:

$$\tan \theta = \text{y-component/x-component}$$
$$\theta = \arctan\left(\frac{2.57}{16.40}\right)$$
$$\theta = \arctan(0.1567)$$
$$= 8.91°$$

The characteristics of the resultant vector (R = 16.60, θ = 8.91°) is clearly confirmed by examining the resultant obtained by combining vectors graphically using the head-to-tail method.

Refer to the walking ground reaction force (GRF) data in Appendix E: Using the peak anteroposterior (F_y) and vertical force (F_z) for frame 18, calculate the resultant force and the angle of force application at this point.

Types of Forces

The forces that exist in nature and affect the way humans move may be classified in a number of ways. The most common classification scheme is to describe forces as contact or **noncontact force**s (11). A contact force involves the actions, pushes or pulls, exerted by one object in direct contact with another object. These are the forces involved, for example, when a bat hits a baseball or the foot hits the floor. In contrast to contact forces are those that act at a distance. These are called noncontact forces. As implied by the name, these are forces that are exerted by objects that are not in direct contact with one another and in fact may be separated by a considerable distance.

NONCONTACT FORCES

In the investigation of human movement, the most familiar and important noncontact force is gravity. Any object released from a height will fall freely to the earth's surface, pulled by gravity. The publication of the *Principia* in 1687 by Sir Isaac Newton (1642–1727) astounded the scientific community of the day. In this book, he introduced his theories of motion and gravity and used these theories to explain a number of phenomena (13). In the law of gravitation, Newton identified gravity as the force that causes objects to fall to the earth, the moon to orbit the earth, and the planets to revolve about the sun. This law states:

> The force of gravity is inversely proportional to the square of the distance between attracting objects and proportional to the product of their masses.

In algebraic terms, the law is described by the following equation:

$$F = \frac{G m_1 m_2}{r^2}$$

where G = universal gravitational constant
m_1 = mass of one object
m_2 = mass of the other object
r = distance between the mass centers of the objects

The constant value G was estimated by Newton and determined accurately by Cavendish in 1798. The value of G is $6.67 * 10^{-11}$ Nm^2/kg^2.

The gravitational attraction of one object of a relatively small size to another object of similar size is extremely small and therefore can be neglected. In biomechanics, the objects of most concern are the earth, the human body, and projectiles. In these cases the earth's mass is considerable and gravity is a very important force. The attractive force of the earth on an object is called the **weight** of the object. This is stated as:

$$W = F_g = \frac{G m_{object} M_{earth}}{r^2}$$

The force of gravity causes an object to accelerate toward earth at a rate of 9.81 m/s². Newton determined through his theories of motion that:

$$W = ma$$

where m is the mass of the individual and a is the acceleration due to gravity. Thus:

$$W = mg$$

where g is the acceleration due to gravity. Body weight is thus the product of the individual's mass and the acceleration due to gravity. It is apparent, therefore, that an individual's mass and body weight are not the same. Body weight is a force, and the appropriate unit for body weight is the newton. To determine a person's body weight, simply multiply mass times the acceleration due to **gravity** (9.81 m/s²).

Since weight is a force, it has the attributes of a force. As a vector, it has a line of action and a point of application. An individual's total body weight is considered to have a point of application at the center of mass and a line of action from the center of mass to the center of the earth. Because the earth is so large, this line of action is straight down.

The point of origin of the weight vector is called the center of gravity. This is a point about which all particles of the body are evenly distributed. Another term used interchangeably with the center of gravity is the center of mass, a point about which the mass of the segment or body is equally distributed. They differ in that the center of gravity refers only to the vertical direction because that is the direction in which gravity acts, whereas the center of mass does not depend on a vertical orientation. The computation of both the center of mass and the center of gravity will be presented in Chapter 11.

The value for g, the acceleration due to **gravity**, depends on the square of the distance to the center of the earth. Because of the spin on its axis, the earth is not perfectly spherical. The earth is slightly flattened at the poles, resulting in shorter distances to the earth's center at the poles than at the equator. Thus, the points on the earth are not all equidistant from its center, and acceleration due to gravity, g, does not have the same value everywhere. The latitude—the position on the earth with respect to the equator—on which a long jump, for example, is performed, can have a significant effect on the distance jumped. Another factor influencing the value of g is altitude. The higher the altitude, the lower the value for g. If one were weighing oneself and a minimal weight were essential, the optimum place for the weigh-in would be on the highest mountain at the earth's equator.

CONTACT FORCES

Because **contact forces** are those resulting from an interaction of two objects, the number of such forces is considerably greater than the single noncontact force discussed.

The following contact forces are considered paramount in human movement: (*a*) ground reaction force; (*b*) joint reaction force; (*c*) friction; (*d*) fluid resistance; (*e*) inertial force; (*f*) muscle force; and (*g*) elastic force.

Ground Reaction Force (GRF)

In almost all terrestrial human movement, the individual is acted upon by the GRF at some time. This is the reaction force provided by the surface upon which one is moving. The surface may be a sandy beach, a gymnasium floor, a concrete sidewalk, or a grass lawn. If the individual is swinging from a high bar, the surface of the bar provides a reaction force. All surfaces provide a reaction force. The individual pushes against the ground with force and the ground pushes back against the individual with equal force in the opposite direction. These forces affect both parties, the ground and the individual, and do not cancel out even though they are equal in magnitude but opposite in direction. Also, the GRF changes in magnitude, direction, and point of application during the period that the individual is in contact with the surface.

Refer to the GRF data for walking in Appendix E: Calculate the resultant force using F_y (anteroposterior) and F_z (vertical) data for frames 18, 36, and 60. How does the direction of the force application change across the support phase?

As with all forces, the GRF is a vector and can be resolved into its components. For the purpose of analysis, it is commonly broken down into its components. These components are orthogonal to each other along a three-dimensional coordinate system (Fig. 10-3). The components are usually labeled: Fz, Fy, Fx.

Fz, vertical (up–down); Fy, anteroposterior (forward–backward); and Fx, mediolateral (side-to-side). However, according to the standards of the International Society of Biomechanics (ISB), in the reporting of three-

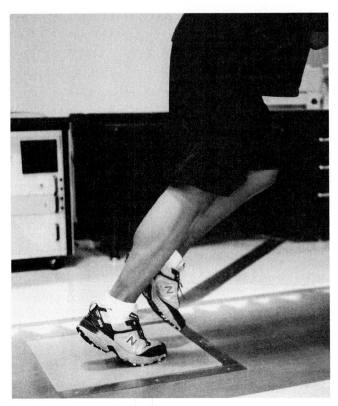

FIGURE 10-4 A typical laboratory force platform setup.

dimensional data, the components should be labeled as Fy, (vertical); Fx (anteroposterior); and Fz (mediolateral). The ISB convention conforms to the reference system for kinematics but is not the most commonly used system. The former convention will be used in this book, as it is the most often used system. In either case, the anteroposterior and mediolateral components are referred to as shear components because they act parallel to the surface of the ground.

Biomechanists measure the GRF components using a **force platform**. A force platform is a sophisticated measuring scale usually imbedded in the ground, with its surface flush with the surface on which the individual is performing. A typical force platform experimental setup for the data collected in Appendix E is shown in Figure 10-4. This device can measure the force of the collision of the sole of the foot on the performing surface or the force of an individual just standing on the platform. Force platforms have been used since the 1930s (26) but became more prominent in biomechanics research in the 1980s. While forces are measured in newtons, GRF data are generally scaled by dividing the force component by the individual's body weight, resulting in units of times body weight (BW). In other instances, GRFs may be scaled by dividing the force by body mass, resulting in a unit of newtons per kilogram of body mass.

Refer to the GRF walking data in Appendix E: Locate the maximum vertical (F_z), anteroposterior (F_y) and mediolateral (F_x) forces (N). Report peak forces scaled to body weight (BW) and to body mass (N/kg).

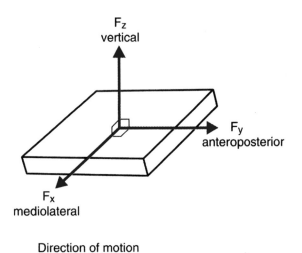

FIGURE 10-3 Ground reaction force components. The origin of the force platform coordinate system is at the center of the platform.

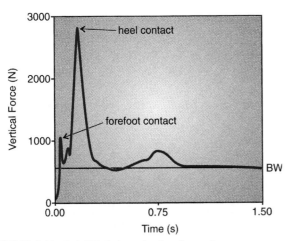

FIGURE 10-5 Vertical GRF during a landing from a jump.

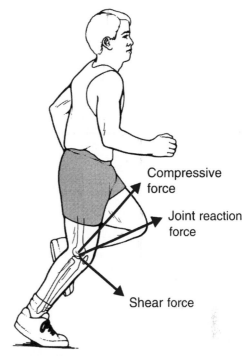

FIGURE 10-6 The joint reaction force of the knee with its shear and compressive components.

GRF data have been used in many studies to investigate a variety of activities. Most studies, however, have dealt with the load or impact on the body during landings, either from jumps or during support phase of gait. For example, GRFs have been studied during the support phase of running (16,18), walking (34), and landings from jumps (25,51).

A vertical component curve of a single foot contact of an individual landing from a jump is presented in Figure 10-5. Only the vertical component is presented, since it is of much greater magnitude than the other components and since the major interest in landings has been the effect of vertical loads or impacts on the human body. In the landing curve, the first peak represents the initial ground contact with the forefoot. The second peak is the contact of the heel on the surface. Generally, the second peak is greater than the first peak. Some individuals, however, land flat-footed and have only one **impact peak**. When the individual comes to rest on the surface, the vertical force curve settles at the individual's body weight. While the magnitude of the vertical component at impact in running is 3 to 5 times body weight, the vertical component in landing can be as much as 11 times body weight, depending on the height from which the person dropped (25,51).

Joint Reaction Force

In many instances in biomechanical analyses, individual segments are examined either singly or one at a time in a logical order. When this analysis is conducted, the segment is separated at the joints, and the forces acting across the joints must be considered. For example, if one is standing still, the thigh exerts a downward force on the leg across the knee joint. Similarly, the leg exerts an upward force of equal magnitude on the thigh (Fig. 10-6). This is the net force acting across the joint and is referred to as the **joint reaction force**. In most analyses, the magnitude of this force is unknown, but it can be calculated given the appropriate kinematic and kinetic data, in addition to anthropometric data describing the body dimensions.

There has been some confusion as to whether the joint reaction force is the force of the distal bony surface of one segment acting on the proximal bony surface of the contiguous segment. The joint reaction force does not, however, reflect this **bone-on-bone force** across a joint. The actual bone-on-bone force is the sum of the actively contracting muscle forces pulling the joint together and the joint reaction force. Since the force generated by the actively contracting muscles is not known, the bone-on-bone force is difficult to calculate, although sophisticated calculations have been done to estimate bone-on-bone forces (88).

Friction

Friction is a force acting parallel to the interface of two surfaces that are in contact during the motion or impending motion of one surface as it moves over the other. For example, the weight of a block resting on a horizontal table pulls the block downward, pressing it against the table. The table exerts an upward force on the block that is perpendicular or normal to the surface. To move the block horizontally, a horizontal force on the block of sufficient magnitude must be exerted. If this force is too small, the block will not move. In this case the table evidently exerts a horizontal force equal and opposite to the force on the block. This interaction, the frictional force, is due to the bonding of the molecules of the block and the table at the places where the surfaces are in very close contact. Figure 10-7 illustrates this example.

It appears that the area of contact influences the force of friction. However, this is not the case. The force of friction is proportional to the normal force between the surfaces, that is:

$$F_f = \mu N$$

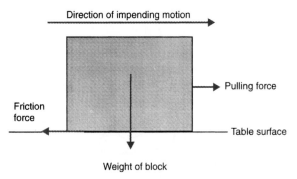

FIGURE 10-7 The forces acting on a block being pulled across a table.

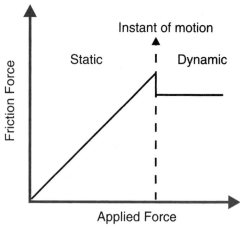

FIGURE 10-8 A theoretical representation of friction force as a function of the applied force. The applied force increases with the friction force until motion occurs.

where μ is the **coefficient of friction** and N is the normal force or the force perpendicular to the surface. The coefficient of friction is calculated by:

$$\mu = \frac{F_f}{N}$$

The coefficient of friction depends on the nature of the interfacing surfaces and is a dimensionless number. The greater the magnitude of the coefficient of friction, the greater the interaction between the molecules of the interfacing surfaces.

Continuing the block and table example, if a steadily increasing force is applied to the block, the table also applies an increasing opposite force resisting the movement. At the point where the pulling force is at a maximum and no movement results, the resisting force is called the maximum static friction force (F_{sMAX}). Prior to movement, it can be stated that:

$$F_{sMAX} \leq \mu_s N$$

where μ_s is the static coefficient of friction. At some point, however, the force is sufficiently large and the static friction force cannot prevent the movement of the block. This relationship simply means that if a block weighing 750 N is standing on a surface with μ_s of 0.5, it will take 50% of the 750 N normal force, or 375 N, of a horizontal force to cause motion between the block and the table. A μ_s of 0.1 would require a horizontal force of 75 N to cause motion and a μ_s of 0.8 would require a 600 N horizontal force. As can be seen, the smaller the coefficient of friction, the less horizontal force required to cause movement.

As the block slides along the surface of the table, molecular bonds are continually made and broken. Thus, once the two surfaces start moving relative to each other, it becomes slightly easier to maintain the motion. The result is a force of sliding friction that opposes the motion. Sliding friction and rolling friction are types of **kinetic friction**. Kinetic friction is defined as:

$$F_k = \mu_k N$$

where μ_k is the dynamic coefficient of friction or the coefficient of friction during movement. It has been found experimentally that μ_k is less than μ_s and that μ_k depends on the relative speed of the object. At speeds of one centimeter per second to several meters per second, however, μ_k is approximately constant. Figure 10-8 illustrates the friction–external force relationship.

While translational friction is important in human movement, **rotational friction** must also be considered. Rotational friction is the resistance to rotational or twisting movements. For example, the soles of the shoes of a basketball player accomplishing a pivot interact with the playing surface to resist the turning of the foot. Obviously, the player must be able to accomplish this movement during a game, and thus the rotational friction must allow this motion without influencing the other frictional characteristics of the shoe. A basketball player executing a 180° pivot in a conventional basketball shoe on a wooden floor would have a rotational friction value 4.3 times greater than in gym socks (75). The measurement of rotational friction does not yield a coefficient of friction. The values used to compare rotational friction are based on the value of the resistance to rotation, usually measured on a force platform. For example, rotational friction values for a tennis shoe on artificial turf or artificial grass have been shown to range from 15.8 to 21.2 Nm (newton-meters) and 17.1 to 21.2 Nm, respectively (57). Translational and rotational friction are not independent of each other.

Friction is a complicated but important influence on human movement. Just to walk across a room requires an appropriate coefficient of friction between the shoe outsoles and the surface of the floor. In everyday activities, one may try either to increase or to decrease the coefficient of friction, depending on the activity. For example, skaters prefer fresh ice because it has a low coefficient of friction. On the other hand, a golfer wears a glove to increase the coefficient of friction and get a better grip on the club.

Many types of athletes wear cleated shoes to increase the coefficient of friction and get better traction on the playing surface. Valiant (73) suggested that μ_s equaling 0.8 provides sufficient traction for athletic movements and

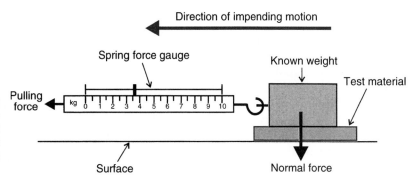

FIGURE 10-9 A towed sled device that measures applied force. The known weight constitutes the normal force, and the spring gauge measures the resistant horizontal force on the known weight. The coefficient of friction is computed by the ratio of the spring gauge force to the known weight.

any greater coefficient of friction may be unsafe. In certain situations cleated shoes may, in fact, result in too much translational and/or rotational friction. This appears to be the case with artificial turf. Many injuries, such as turf toe and anterior cruciate ligament tears, have been related to too much friction force on artificial turf.

When the coefficient of friction is too small, a slip hazard results, but when the coefficient of friction is too great, a trip hazard occurs. In the workplace, slips and falls are numerous and often cause serious injury. Cohen and Compton (19) reported that 50% of 120, 682 workers compensation cases in New York state from 1966 to 1970 were caused by slips. In England, Buck (12) cited 1982 statistics in which 14% of accidents in the manufacturing industry resulted from slips and trips. Thus, the coefficient of friction is a very important criterion in the design of any surface on which people perform, whether in the workplace or in athletics.

The static coefficient of friction of materials on different surfaces has been successfully measured using a towed sled device (2). This device, illustrated in Figure 10-9, involves an object of a known mass and a force-measuring gauge. The moving surface, usually some type of footwear, is placed beneath the mass. The gauge pulls the mass until it moves, and the force is measured by the gauge at the instant of movement. The coefficient of friction can then be calculated using the known mass and the force measured from the gauge. This type of measurement is known as a materials test measure; it does not involve human subjects.

It is difficult to measure the static or kinetic coefficient of friction accurately without sophisticated equipment. Both, however, may be measured with a force platform. The shear components F_y and F_x are, in fact, the frictional forces in the anteroposterior and mediolateral directions, respectively. If the normal force is known, the dynamic coefficient of friction may be estimated. Generally, this is done using the vertical (F_z) component as the normal force. Thus, the coefficient of friction can be determined by:

$$\mu = \frac{F_y}{F_z}$$

Several researchers have devised instruments to measure both translational and rotational friction. A device

developed in the Nike Sports Science Laboratory is one such instrument (Fig. 10-10). It has been used to measure the friction characteristics of many types of athletic shoes.

In general, the magnitude of the coefficient of friction depends on the types of materials constituting the surfaces in contact and the nature of those surfaces. For example, a rubber-soled shoe would have a higher coefficient of friction on a wood gymnasium floor than a leather-soled shoe. Jogging shoes on an artificial track register static and dynamic frictional coefficients in the range of 0.7 to 1.1 and 0.7 to 1.0, respectively (57). This is compared to football shoes on artificial turf, for which the static and dynamic coefficients of friction range from 1.1 to 1.6 and 1.0 to 1.5, respectively (57). The relative roughness or smoothness of the contacting surfaces also affects the coefficient of friction. Intuitively, a rough surface has a higher coefficient of friction than a smooth surface. The addition of lubricants, moisture, or dust to a surface will also greatly affect frictional characteristics. To determine the coefficient of friction, all of these factors must be considered.

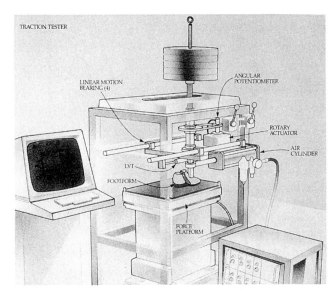

FIGURE 10-10 Device for mechanically evaluating translational and rotational friction characteristics of athletic footwear outsoles. This device was developed at the Nike Sports Research Laboratory.

Fluid Resistance

In many activities, human motion is affected by the fluid in which the activities are performed. Both air, a gas, and water, a liquid, are considered fluids. Thus, the motion of a runner is affected by the movement of air and that of a swimmer by the water or the air–water interface. Projectiles, whether humans or objects, are also affected by air. For example, anyone who has ever driven a golf ball into the wind will understand the effects of air on the golf ball.

Density and Viscosity

The two properties of a fluid that most affect objects as they pass through it are the fluid's density and viscosity. Density is defined as the mass per unit volume. Generally, the more dense the fluid, the more resistance it presents to the object. The density of air is particularly affected by humidity, temperature, and pressure. Viscosity is a measure of the fluid's resistance to flow. For example, water is more viscous than air, with the result that water resistance is greater than air resistance. Gases such as air become more viscous as the air temperature rises.

As an object passes through a fluid, it disturbs the fluid. This is true for both air and water. The degree of disturbance depends on the density and viscosity of the fluid. The greater the disturbance of the fluid, the greater the energy that is transmitted from the object to the fluid. This transfer of energy from the object to the fluid is called **fluid resistance**. The resultant fluid resistance force can be resolved into two components, lift and drag (Fig. 10-11).

Drag Force Component

Drag is a component of fluid resistance that always acts to oppose the motion. The direction of drag is always directly opposite to the direction of the velocity vector and acts to retard the motion of the object through the fluid. In most instances *drag* is synonymous with *air resistance*. The magnitude of the drag component may be determined by:

$$F_{drag} = \frac{1}{2} C_d A \rho v^2$$

where C_d is a constant, the coefficient of drag, A is the projected frontal area of the object, the Greek letter rho

(ρ) is the fluid viscosity, and v is the relative velocity of the object, that is, the velocity of the object relative to the fluid. The magnitude of the drag component is a function of the nature of the fluid, the nature and shape of the object, and the velocity of the object through the fluid.

Two types of drag must be considered. Drag as a result of friction between the object's surface and the fluid is referred to as **surface drag** or **viscous drag**. When an object moves through a fluid, the fluid interacts with the surface of the object, literally sticking to its surface. The resulting fluid layer is called the **boundary layer**. The fluid in the boundary layer is slowed down relative to the object as it passes it by. It results in the object pushing on the fluid and the fluid pushing on the object in the opposite direction. This interaction causes friction between the fluid in the boundary layer and the object's surface. This fluid friction opposes the motion of the object through the fluid. A fluid with high viscosity will generate a high drag component. In addition, the size of the object becomes more important if more surface is exposed to the fluid.

From the formula for drag force, it can be seen that drag force increases as a function of the velocity squared. The relative velocity of the fluid as it passes by the object actually determines how the object will interact with the fluid. At lower movement velocities of the object, the fluid passes the object in uniform layers of differing speed, with the slowest-moving layers closest to the surface of the object. This is called **laminar flow** (Fig. 10-12*A*). Laminar flow occurs when the object is small and smooth and the velocity is small. The drag force consists almost entirely of surface or friction drag. On every object, however, there are points, called the points of separation, at which the fluid separates from the object. That is, the fluid does not completely follow the contours of the shape of the object. As the object moves through the fluid faster, the fluid moves by the object faster. When this occurs, the points of separation move forward on the object and the fluid separates from the contours of the object closer to the front of the object. Thus, at relatively high velocities, the fluid does not maintain a laminar flow; **separated flow** occurs (Fig. 10-12*B*). Separated flow is also referred to as partially **turbulent flow**. In this instance, the fluid is unable to contour to the shape of the object, and the boundary layer separates from the surface. This produces turbulence behind the object. In power boating, for example, the turbulence behind the boat is called the wake. The wake of an object moving through a fluid is a low-pressure region. Separated flow occurs at a small relative velocity if the object is large and has a rough surface or under any conditions in which the fluid does not stick to the surface of the object.

When the fluid contacts the front of the object, an area of relatively high pressure is formed. The turbulent area behind the object is an area of pressure lower than the pressure at the front of the object. The greater the turbulence, the lower the pressure behind the object. The net pressure differential between the front and back of the

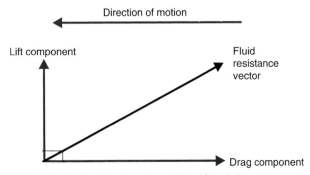

FIGURE 10-11 Fluid resistance vector with its lift and drag components.

A. Laminar Flow

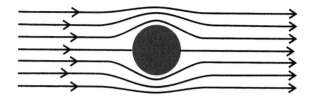

B. Separated Flow

Points of separation

Turbulent wake

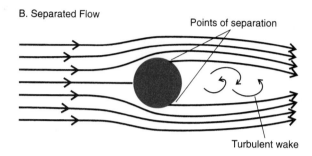

C. Turbulent Flow

Turbulent wake

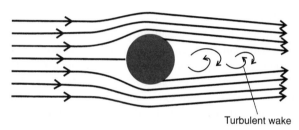

FIGURE 10-12 Flow about a sphere. **A.** Laminar flow. **B.** Separated flow. **C.** Turbulent flow.

object retards the object's movement through the fluid. With increasing flow velocity, the point at which the boundary layer separates from the surface of the object moves farther to the front of the object, resulting in an even greater pressure differential and greater resistance. Drag resulting from this pressure differential is called **form drag**. In partially turbulent flow, both form and friction drag occur. As the wake increases, form drag dominates.

As the relative velocity of the object and the fluid increases, the whole boundary layer becomes turbulent. This type of fluid flow is called turbulent flow (Fig. 10-12*C*). Interestingly, the turbulence in the boundary layer actually moves the **point of separation** toward the back of the object, reducing the ability of the boundary layer to separate from the object. The net result is a reduction in the drag force.

Moving from partially turbulent flow to fully turbulent flow, thus decreasing the drag force, can be accomplished by streamlining and smoothing the surface of the object. Contrary to what one might expect, putting dimples on a golf ball or seams on a baseball, thereby roughening the surface, actually helps in this transition.

The shift from laminar to partially turbulent flow can be forestalled, hence drag minimized, with a streamlined shape or smooth surface or both. Athletes such as sprinters, cyclists, swimmers, and skiers generally wear smooth suits during their events. A significant 10% reduction of drag occurs when a speed skater wears a smooth body suit (77). Wearing smooth clothing also prevents such things as long hair, laces, and loose-fitting clothing from increasing drag (45). Kyle (44) reported that loose clothing or thick long hair could raise the total drag 2 to 8%. He calculated that a 6% decrease in air resistance can increase the distance of a long jump by 3 to 5 cm.

Streamlining the shape of the object involves decreasing the projected frontal area. The projected frontal area of the object is the area of the surface that might come in contact with the fluid flow. Athletes in sports in which air resistance must be minimized manipulate this frontal area constantly. For example, a speed skater can assume any of a number of body positions during a race. A skater who has the arms hanging down in front presents a greater frontal area than one in an arms back racing position. The frontal areas in these speed skating positions are 42.21 m² and 38.71 m², respectively (81). Similarly, a ski racer will assume a tuck position to minimize the frontal area rather than the posture of a recreational skier. To decrease the drag component, a more streamlined position must be assumed. Streamlining helps minimize the pressure differential and thus the form drag on the object. For example, the drag coefficient for a standing human figure is 0.92, while it is 0.8 for a runner and 0.7 for a skier in a low crouch (44).

Much equipment has been designed to minimize fluid resistance. New bicycle designs; solid rear wheels on racing bicycles; clothing for skiers, swimmers, runners, and cyclists, bent poles for downhill skiers, new helmet designs, and so on have all contributed to help these athletes in their events. Research on streamlining body positions has also greatly aided athletes in many sports, such as cycling, speed skating, and sprint running (81).

Lift Force Component

Lift is the component of fluid resistance that acts perpendicular to drag. Thus, it also acts at right angles to the direction of motion. While there is always a drag force component, the lift component occurs only under special circumstances. That is, lift occurs only if the object is spinning or is not perfectly symmetrical. The **lift force** component is one of the most significant forces in aerodynamics. This is the force that helps airplanes fly. Contrary to what the name suggests, this force component does not always oppose gravity.

Lift force is produced by any break in the symmetry of the airflow about an object. This can be shown in an object having an asymmetrical shape, a flat object being tilted to the airflow, or a spinning object. The effect makes the air flowing over one side of the object follow a different path than the air flowing over the other side. The result of this differential airflow is lower air pressure on

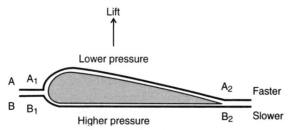

FIGURE 10-13 Bernoulli's principle in creating lift on an airfoil. Molecules of air A and B move from A_1 to A_2 and B_1 to B_2 respectively in the same amount of time, but the distance from A_1 to A_2 is greater. Thus the velocity of A is greater than the velocity of B, which causes lower pressure on top of the airfoil than underneath.

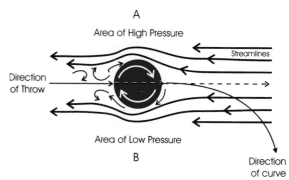

FIGURE 10-14 The Magnus effect on a spinning ball. Because of this effect, the ball will curve in the direction of B.

one side of the object and higher air pressure on the other side. This pressure differential causes the object to move toward the side that has the lower pressure. Figure 10-13 shows an airfoil (the cross-section of an airplane wing). The air flowing over the top of the airfoil moves at a higher speed than the air flowing beneath it. A principle first stated by Daniel Bernoulli in 1738 relates the speed of airflow to the pressure exerted by the fluid. **Bernoulli's principle** states that pressure is inversely proportional to the velocity of the fluid; it is expressed mathematically as:

$$P = \frac{1}{v}$$

where P is the pressure and v is the velocity of the fluid. Thus, when the velocity of a moving fluid increases, the pressure exerted by the fluid decreases and vice versa. The result is that the airfoil develops lift force in the direction of the lower pressure.

The lift force component is used on the wings of airplanes, as spoilers on cars, and in swimming. Lift can be generated by the swimmer's hands as they move through the water. The swimmer's hands resemble airfoils, and the swimmer pitches or orients the hands as they are pulled through the water. Pitching the hand puts the lift component in the desired direction of the swim (5,67). The lift component thus may also contribute to the forward motion of the swimmer.

Lift force also contributes to the curved flight of a spinning ball that is critical in baseball and most maddeningly, in golf. The spin on the ball results in the air flowing faster on one side of the ball and slower on the other side, creating a pressure differential. Consider the spinning ball in Figure 10-14. Side A of the ball is spinning against the airflow, causing the boundary layer to slow down on that side. On side B, however, because it is moving in the same direction as the airflow, the boundary layer speeds up. By Bernoulli's principle, this results in a pressure differential. This is comparable to the pressure differential about the airfoil. The ball, therefore, is deflected laterally toward the direction of the spin or the side on which there is a lower pressure area. This effect was first described by Gustav Magnus in 1852, hence is known as the **Magnus effect**. Baseball pitchers have mastered the art of putting just

enough spin on the ball to curve its path successfully. Many golfers try not to put a sideways spin on the ball to avoid slicing or hooking the ball. They do, however, try to put backspin on the golf ball. The backspin, because of the Magnus effect, creates a pressure differential between the top and the bottom of the golf ball, with the lower pressure on the top. The golf ball gains lift and thus distance.

Inertial Force

In many instances in human movement, one segment can exert a force on another segment, causing a movement in that segment that is not due to muscle action. When this occurs, an inertial force has been generated. Generally a more proximal segment exerts an inertial force on a more distal segment. For example, during the swing phase of running, the ankle is plantarflexed at takeoff and slightly dorsiflexed at touchdown. The ankle is relaxed during the swing phase, and in fact, the muscle movement about this joint is very nearly zero, indicating little muscle activity. The leg also swings through, however, and exerts an inertial force on the foot segment, causing the foot to move to the dorsiflexed position. Similarly, the thigh segment exerts an inertial force on the leg.

Muscle Force

When a force was defined, it was noted that a force constituted a push or pull that results in a change in velocity. A muscle can generate only a pulling or tensile force and therefore has only unidirectional capability. The biceps brachii, for example, pulls on its insertion on the forearm to flex the elbow. To extend the elbow, the triceps brachii must pull on its insertion on the forearm. Thus, the movements at any joint must be accomplished by opposing pairs of muscles. Gravity also assists in the motion of segments.

In most biomechanical analyses, it is assumed that a muscle force acting across a joint is a net force. That is, the force of individual muscles acting across a joint cannot be taken into consideration. Generally a number of muscles act across any joint. Each of these muscles constitutes an unknown value. Mathematically, the number of unknown values must have a comparable number of equations.

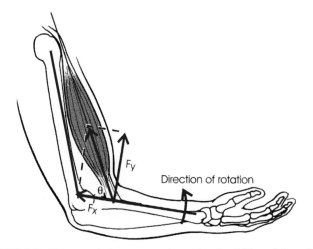

FIGURE 10-15 A muscle force vector, the angle of pull (θ), and its vertical and horizontal components.

Because there is no comparable number of equations, there cannot be a solution for each individual muscle force. If a solution were attempted, it would result mathematically in an indeterminate solution; that is, no solution.

It is also assumed that the muscle force acts at a single point. This assumption is again not completely correct, since the insertions of muscles are rarely if ever single points. Each muscle can be represented as a single force vector that is the resultant of all forces generated by the individual muscle fibers (Fig. 10-15). The force vector can be resolved into its components, one component (F_y) acting to cause a rotation at the joint and the other (F_x) acting toward the joint center. If the angle θ is considered, it can be seen that as θ gets large, such as when the joint is flexing, the rotational component increases while the component acting toward the joint center decreases. This can be assumed because:

$$F_y = F \sin \theta$$

and

$$F_x = F \cos \theta$$

At θ = 90°, the rotational component is a maximum, since the sin 90° = 1, while the component acting toward the joint center is zero, since cos θ = 0.

The actual muscle force in vivo is very difficult to measure. To do so requires either a mathematical model or the placement of a measuring device called a force transducer on the tendon of a muscle. Many researchers have developed mathematical models to approximate individual muscle forces (39,69). To do this, however, it is necessary to make a number of assumptions, including the direction of the muscle force, point of application, and whether cocontraction occurs.

For example, a simple model to determine the peak Achilles tendon force during the support phase of a running stride would use the peak vertical GRF and the point of application of that force. It must be assumed that the line of this force is a specific distance anterior to the ankle joint and the Achilles tendon is located a specific distance posterior to the ankle joint. In addition, the center of mass of the foot and its location relative to the ankle joint center must be determined. In this rather simple example, the number of anatomical assumptions that must be made is evident.

The second technique, placing a force-measuring device on the tendon of a muscle, requires a surgical procedure. Komi et al. (43) and Komi (41) have placed force transducers on the Achilles tendon of individuals. Komi (41) reported peak Achilles tendon forces corresponding to 12.5 BW while the subject ran at 6 m/s. While the technique to measure in vivo muscle forces is not well developed for long-term studies, it can be used to analyze several important parameters in muscle mechanics.

Elastic Force

When a force is applied to a material, the material undergoes a change in its length. The algebraic statement that reflects this relationship is:

$$F = k\Delta s$$

where k is a constant of proportionality and Δs is the change in length. The constant k represents stiffness, or the ability of the material to be compressed or stretched. A stiffer material requires a greater force to compress or stretch it. This relationship is often applied to biological materials and represented in stress–strain relationships. This relationship was presented in Chapter 2.

The effect of elastic force can be visualized in an example of a diver on a springboard. The diver uses body weight as the force to deflect the springboard. The deflected springboard stores an elastic force that is returned as the springboard rebounds to its original state. The result is that the diver is flung upward. A considerable amount of work has been conducted to determine the elasticity of diving springboards used in competition (9,71).

In most situations, the biological tissues—muscles, tendons, and ligaments—do not exceed their elastic limit. Within this limit, these tissues can store force when they are stretched, much as a rubber band does. When the loading force is removed, the elastic force may be returned and with the muscle force contribute to the total force of the action. For example, using a prestretch prior to a movement will increase the force output by inducing the elastic force potential of the surrounding tissues. There is, however, a time constraint on how long this elastic force can be stored. Attempts to measure the effect of stored elastic force have illustrated that using this force can affect oxygen consumption (3). Further estimates of stored elastic force in vertical jumping have been investigated by Komi and Bosco (42), who reported higher jumps using stored elastic force. It has been suggested by Alexander (1) that elastic force storage is important in the locomotion of humans and many animals, such as kangaroos and ostriches.

Representation of Forces Acting on a System

When one undertakes an analysis of any human movement, one must take into account a number of forces acting on the **system**. To simplify the problem for better understanding, a free body diagram is often used. A **free body diagram** is a stick figure drawing of the system showing the vector representations of the external forces acting on the system. External forces are those exerted outside the system rather than from inside the system. Thus, internal forces are not represented on a free body diagram. Before this discussion proceeds, however, the term *system* must be defined. In biomechanics, the system refers to the total human body or parts of the human body and any other objects that may be important in the analysis. It is critically important to define the system correctly; otherwise, extraneous variables may confound the analysis.

Once the system has been defined, the external forces acting upon the system must be identified and drawn. Figure 10-16 is a free body diagram of a total body sagittal view of a runner. The external forces acting on the runner are (*a*) the GRF; (*b*) friction; (*c*) fluid or air resistance; and (*d*) gravity as reflected in the runner's body weight. Vector representations of the external forces are drawn on the stick figure at the approximate point of application. If

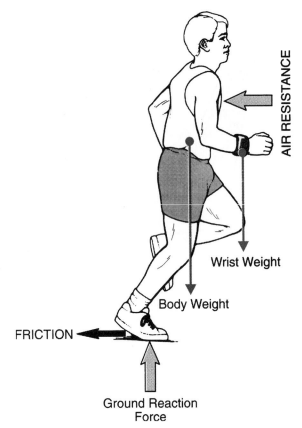

FIGURE 10-17 A free body diagram of a runner's wrist weight system.

the runner is carrying an implement, such as a wrist weight, another force vector representing the weight of this implement must be added to the free body diagram (Fig. 10-17). For the most part, however, the four external forces noted earlier are the only ones identified on a total body diagram.

When a specific segment, not the total body, is defined as the system, the interpretation of what constitutes an external force must be clarified. In drawing a free body diagram of a particular segment, the segment must be isolated from the rest of the body. The segment is drawn disconnected from the rest of the body, and all external forces acting on that segment are drawn. The muscle forces that cross the proximal or distal joints of that segment are external to the system and must be classified as external forces. As noted earlier, it is not possible to identify all of the muscles and their forces acting across a joint. An idealized net muscle force, that is, a single force vector, is used to represent the sum total of all muscle forces.

Figure 10-18 is a free body diagram of the forearm of an individual doing a biceps curl. The four external forces acting on this system that must be identified are (*a*) the net biceps muscle force, (*b*) the joint reaction force, (*c*) the force of gravity on the arm represented by the weight of the forearm, and (*d*) the force of gravity acting on the barbell or the weight of the barbell. These are drawn as they would act during this movement. In many instances the joint reaction force and the net muscle force are not

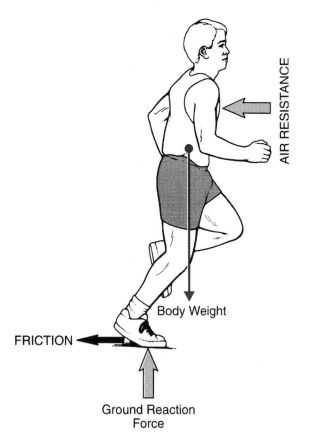

FIGURE 10-16 A free body diagram of a runner with the whole body defined as the system.

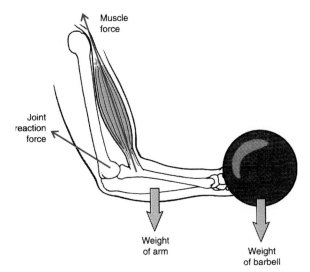

FIGURE 10-18 A free body diagram of the forearm during a biceps curl.

known but must be calculated. All other forces, such as the friction forces in the joints and the forces of the ligaments and tendons, are assumed to be negligible. Air resistance is also ignored.

Free body diagrams are extremely useful tools in biomechanics. Drawing the system and identifying the forces acting upon the system define the problem and determine how to undertake the analysis.

 ## Laws of Motion

Newton's three laws of motion have demonstrated how and when a force creates a movement and how it applies to all of the different types of forces previously identified. His work has provided the link between cause and effect that essentially forms the basis for most analyses of human movement in biomechanics. To fully understand the underlying nature of motion, it is necessary to understand the cause of the movement, not merely the description of the outcome. That is, the forces that cause motion must be fully understood. The statements of these laws are taken from a translation of Newton's *Principia* (13).

LAW I: LAW OF INERTIA

Every body continues in its state of rest, or of uniform motion in a straight line, unless it is compelled to change that state by forces impressed on it (13).

The **inertia** of an object is used to describe its resistance to motion. Inertia is directly related to the mass of the object. **Mass** is the measure of the amount of matter that constitutes an object and is expressed in kilograms. An object's mass is constant, regardless of where it is measured, so that the mass is the same whether it is calculated on earth or on the moon. The greater the mass of an object, the greater its inertia and thus the greater the difficulty in moving it or changing its current motion.

To get an object moving, the inertia of the object has to be overcome. Newton suggested that an object at rest—an object with zero velocity—would remain at rest. This point seems obvious. A chair sitting in a room has zero velocity because it is not moving. Additionally, an object moving at a constant velocity would continue to do so in a straight line. This concept is not as obvious, since the practical instances of individuals on the earth's surface rarely experience constant velocity motion. If it is noted that constant velocity results in zero acceleration just as zero velocity does, then it can be understood how this law holds for both cases. Therefore, the inertia of these objects would compel them to maintain their status at a constant velocity.

To overcome the inertia of such objects requires a net external force greater than the inertia of the object. For example, if a barbell has a mass of 70 kg, a force greater than 686.7 N, or the acceleration due to gravity (9.81 m/s^2) times 70 kg, must be exerted to lift it. If an object is subjected to an external force that can overcome the inertia, the object will be either positively or negatively accelerated. To get an object moving, the external force must positively accelerate the object. On the other hand, to stop the object from moving, the external force must negatively accelerate the object. Since body mass determines inertia, an individual with more mass will have to generate larger external forces to overcome inertia and generate acceleration.

LAW II: LAW OF ACCELERATION

The change of motion is proportional to the force impressed and is made in the direction of the straight line in which that force is impressed (13).

Newton's second law generates an equation that relates force, mass, and acceleration. This relationship is:

$$\text{Force} = \text{mass} * \text{acceleration}$$

or

$$F = ma$$

This equation can also be used to define the unit of force, the newton. By substituting the units for mass and acceleration in the right-hand side it can be seen that:

$$\text{newton} = \frac{\text{kg-m}}{\text{s}^2}$$

where kgm = kilogram-meters. In this equation, the force is the net force acting on the object in question, that is, the sum of all of the forces involved. In adding up all forces acting on an object, it is necessary to take the direction of the forces into account. If the forces exactly counteract each other, the net force is zero. If the sum of the forces is zero, the acceleration will also be zero. This case is also described by Newton's first law. If the net force produces acceleration, the accelerated object will travel in a straight line along the line of action of the net force.

Rearranging the equation described by Newton's second law allows another important concept in biomechanics to be defined. Acceleration was previously defined as dv/dt. Substituting this expression into the equation of the second law:

$$F = m\frac{dv}{dt}$$

or

$$F = \frac{mdv}{dt}$$

The product of mass and velocity in the numerator of the right-hand side of this equation is known as the momentum of an object. Momentum is the quantity of motion of an object. It is generally represented by the letter p and has units of kilogram-meters per second. For example, if a football player has a mass of 83 kg and is running at 4.5 m/s, his momentum is:

$$\begin{aligned} p &= \text{mass} * \text{velocity} \\ &= 83 \text{ kg} * 4.5 \text{ m/s} \\ &= 373.5 \text{ kgm/s} \end{aligned}$$

Newton's second law can thus be restated:

$$F = \frac{dp}{dt}$$

That is, force is equal to the time rate of change of momentum. To change the momentum of an object, an external force must be applied to the object. The momentum may increase or decrease, but in either case, an external force is required.

LAW III: LAW OF ACTION–REACTION

To every action there is always opposed an equal reaction; or, the mutual actions of two bodies upon each other are always equal and directed to contrary parts.

This law illustrates that forces never act in isolation but always in pairs. When two objects interact, the force exerted by Object A on Object B is counteracted by a force equal and opposite exerted by Object B on Object A. These forces are equal in magnitude but opposite in direction. In addition, the force—the action—and the counterforce—the reaction—act on different objects. The result is that these two forces cannot cancel each other out, since they act on and may have a different effect on the objects. For example, a person landing from a jump exerts a force on the earth, and the earth exerts an equal and opposite force on the person. Because the earth is more massive than the individual, the effect on the individual is greater than the effect on the earth. This example illustrates that while the force

and the counterforce are equal, they may not necessarily have comparable results.

In human movements, an action force is generated on the ground or implement, and the reaction force generally produces the desired movement. As shown in Figure 10-5, the jumper makes contact with the ground and generates a large downward force because of the acceleration of the body combined with forces generated by body segments at contact, and a resulting reaction force upward controls the landing. All of the contact forces previously discussed, such as reaction, friction, and fluid forces, create motion via the reaction force.

ANALYSIS USING NEWTON'S LAWS OF MOTION

There are multiple conceptual forms and variations of Newton's laws that can describe the relationship between the kinematics and the kinetics of a movement. From Newton's law of acceleration (F = ma) arise three general approaches to exploring kinematic and kinetic interactions. These approaches can be categorized as (*a*) the effect of a force at an instant in time, (*b*) the effect of a force applied over a period of time, and (*c*) the effect of a force applied over a distance (52). None of these methods can be considered better or worse than any other. The choice of which relationship to use simply depends upon which method will best answer the question. Using the appropriate analytical technique, however, makes it possible to investigate the forces causing motion more effectively.

Effects of a Force at an Instant in Time

When considering the effects of a force and the resulting acceleration at an instant in time, Newton's second law of motion is considered:

$$\Sigma F = ma$$

Two situations based upon the magnitude of the resulting acceleration can be defined. In the first situation, the resulting acceleration will have a zero value. This is the branch of mechanics known as **statics**. In the second case, the resulting acceleration is a nonzero value. This area of study is known as **dynamics**.

Static Analysis

The static case is devoted to systems at rest or moving at a constant velocity. In both of these situations, acceleration is zero. When the acceleration of a system is zero, the system is said to be in equilibrium. A system is in equilibrium when, as stated in Newton's first law, it remains at rest or it is in motion at a constant velocity.

In translational motion, when a system is in equilibrium, all forces that are acting on the system cancel each other out, and the effect is zero. That is, the sum of all

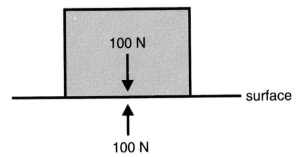

FIGURE 10-19 A free body diagram of a box on a table. The box is in equilibrium because there are no horizontal forces and the sum of the vertical forces is zero.

forces acting on the system must total zero. This is expressed algebraically as:

$$\Sigma F_{system} = 0$$

The forces in this equation can be further expressed in terms of the two-dimensional x- and y-components as:

$$\Sigma F_x = 0$$

and

$$\Sigma F_y = 0$$

Here the sum of the forces in the horizontal (x) direction must equal zero and the sum of the forces in the vertical (y) direction must equal zero.

The static case is simply a particular example of Newton's second law and can be described in terms of a cause-and-effect relationship. The left-hand side of these equations describes the cause of the motion, and the right-hand side describes the product or the result of the motion. Because all forces in the system are in balance, there is no acceleration. If the forces were not in balance, some acceleration would occur.

Figure 10-19 presents a **free body diagram** of a linear force system in which a 100-N box rests on a table. Gravity acts to pull the box downward on the table with a force of 100 N. Because the box does not move vertically, an equal and opposite force must act to support the box. In this coordinate system up is positive and down is

negative. The weight of the box, acting downward, thus has a negative sign. There are no horizontal forces acting in this example. Thus:

$$\Sigma F_y = 0$$
$$-100 \text{ N} + R_y = 0$$
$$R_y = 100 \text{ N}$$

where R_y is the reaction force to the weight of the box. Since the weight of the box acts negatively, the reaction force must act positively, or in the opposite direction to the weight of the box.

Consider a system with multiple forces acting. In Figure 10-20, a tug-of-war is presented as a linear force system. In this example, the two contestants on the right balance the three contestants on the left. The contestants on the left exert forces of 50 N, 150 N, and 300 N, respectively. These forces can be considered to act in a negative horizontal direction. Assuming a static situation, the reaction force to produce equilibrium can be calculated. Thus:

$$\Sigma F_x = 0$$
$$-50N - 150N - 300N + R_x = 0$$
$$R_x = 50N + 150N + 300N$$
$$R_x = 500 \text{ N}$$

The two contestants on the right must exert a reaction force of 500 N in the positive direction to produce a state of equilibrium.

The linear force system previously presented is a relatively simple example of the static case, but in many instances in human motion, the forces, are nonparallel. In Figure 10-21*A*, two nonparallel forces F_1 and F_2, are acting upon a rigid body in addition to the weight of the rigid body. For this system to be in equilibrium, a third force (F_3) must act through the intersection of the two nonparallel forces. The free body diagram in Figure 10-21*B* illustrates that the horizontal component of F_3, acting in a positive direction, must counterbalance the sum of the horizontal components of the nonparallel forces F_1 and F_2. Also, the vertical components F_1 and F_2 must be counterbalanced by

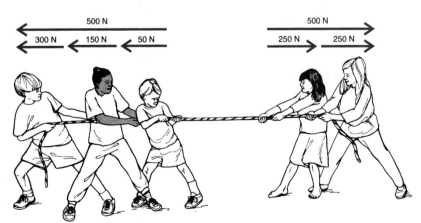

FIGURE 10-20 Tug-of-war. The system is in equilibrium because the sum of the forces in the horizontal direction is zero. No movement to the left or the right can occur.

A

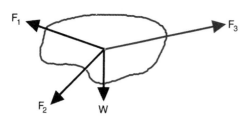

B

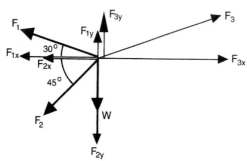

FIGURE 10-21 A. A force system in which the sum of the forces is zero. **B.** A free body diagram of the force system shows the horizontal and vertical components of all forces.

the weight of the rigid body and by the vertical component of F_3. If $F_1 = 100$ N, the components of F_1 are:

$$F_{1x} = F_1 \cos 30°$$
$$= F_1 \cos 150° \text{ (relative to right horizontal)}$$
$$= 100 \text{ N} * \cos 150°$$
$$= -86.6 \text{ N}$$

$$F_{1y} = F_1 \sin 30°$$
$$= 100 \text{ N} * \sin 150° \text{ (relative to right horizontal)}$$
$$= 100 \text{ N} * \sin 150°$$
$$= 50.0 \text{ N}$$

and if $F_2 = 212.13$ N, the components of F_2 are:

$$F_{2x} = F_2 \cos 45°$$
$$= 212.13 \text{ N} * 225° \text{ (relative to right horizontal)}$$
$$= 212.13 \text{ N} * \cos 225°$$
$$= -150 \text{ N}$$

$$F_{2y} = F_2 \sin 45°$$
$$= 212.13 \text{ N} * 225° \text{ (relative to right horizontal)}$$
$$= 212.13 \text{ N} * \sin 225°$$
$$= -150 \text{ N}$$

The weight of the rigid body, 50 N, also acts in a negative vertical direction. Thus:

$$\Sigma F_y = 0$$
$$F_{3y} + F_{1y} + F_{2y} + W = 0$$
$$F_{3y} + 50 \text{ N} - 150 \text{ N} - 50 \text{ N} = 0$$
$$F_{3y} = -50 \text{ N} + 150 \text{ N} + 50 \text{ N}$$
$$F_{3y} = 150 \text{ N}$$

F_{3y} must have a magnitude of 150 N to maintain the system in equilibrium in the vertical direction. In the horizontal direction:

$$\Sigma F_x = 0$$
$$F_{3x} + F_{1x} + F_{2x} = 0$$
$$F_{3x} - 86.6 \text{ N} - 150 \text{ N} = 0$$
$$F_{3x} = 86.6 \text{ N} + 150 \text{ N}$$
$$F_{3x} = 236.6 \text{ N}$$

To balance the two nonparallel forces in the horizontal direction, a force of 236.6 N is required. The resultant force, F_3, can be determined using the Pythagorean relationship:

$$F_3 = \sqrt{F_{3x}^2 + F_{3y}^2}$$
$$F_3 = \sqrt{236.6^2 + 150^2}$$
$$F_3 = 280 \text{ N}$$

The F_3 force orientation can be determined using trigonometric functions:

$$\theta_{F_3} = \arctan(F_y/F_x)$$
$$= \arctan(150/236.6)$$
$$= \arctan(0.6340)$$
$$= 32.37°$$

The forces F_1 and F_2 and the weight of the rigid body are counteracted by the force F_3, keeping the system in equilibrium.

A second condition that determines whether a system is in equilibrium occurs when the forces in the system are not concurrent. **Concurrent forces** do not coincide at the same point, so they cause rotation about some axis. These rotations all sum to zero, however, and as this is a static case, no rotation occurs. This will be discussed in more detail in Chapter 11.

Static models have been developed to evaluate such tasks such as material handling and lifting. A free body diagram of the joint reaction forces and forces acting at the center of mass of the segment is created. Figure 10-22 is a static lifting model (17) that shows the linear forces acting on the body at the shoulder, elbow, wrist, hip, knee, ankle joints and the ground contact. This model is not complete until the angular components are also included (see Chapter 11).

Dynamic Analysis

A static analysis may be used to evaluate the forces on the human body when acceleration is insignificant (4). When accelerations are significant, however, **dynamic analysis** must be undertaken. Dynamic analysis should be used, therefore, when accelerations are not zero. The equations for a dynamic analysis were derived from Newton's second law of motion and expanded by the famous Swiss mathematician Leonhard Euler (1707–1783). The equations of motion for a two-dimensional case are based on:

$$\Sigma F = ma$$

Linear acceleration may be broken down into horizontal (x) and vertical (y) components. As in the static two-

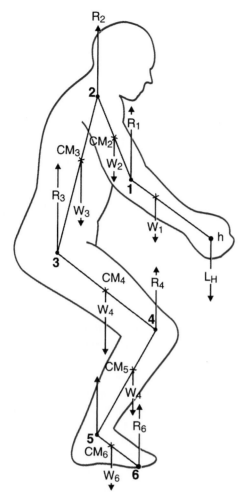

FIGURE 10-22 A free body diagram of a sagittal view static lifting model showing the linear forces at the joints and segments. (After Chaffin, D. B., Andersson, G. B. J. [1991]. *Occupational Biomechanics* (2nd Ed.). New York: Wiley.)

dimensional analysis, independent equations are used in a dynamic two-dimensional linear kinetic analysis:

$$\Sigma F_x = ma_x$$
$$\Sigma F_y = ma_y$$

where x and y represent the horizontal and vertical coordinate directions, respectively, a is the acceleration of the center of mass, and m is the body center of mass. The forces acting on a body may be any one of the previously discussed forces such as muscular, gravitational, contact, or inertial. The gravitational forces are the weights of each of the segments. The contact forces can be reactions—forces with another segment, the ground, or an external object—and the inertial forces are ma_x and ma_y. Using the equations of dynamic motion, the forces acting on a segment can be calculated.

In moving from static to dynamic analysis, the problem becomes more difficult. In the static case, no accelerations were present. In the dynamic case, linear accelerations and the inertial properties of the body segments resisting these accelerations must be considered. In addition, there is a

substantial increase in the work done to collect the data necessary to conduct a dynamic analysis. Since the forces that cause the motion are determined by evaluating the resulting motion itself, a technique called an **inverse dynamics** approach will be used. This approach calculates the forces based on the accelerations of the object instead of measuring the forces directly.

In using the inverse dynamics approach, the system under consideration must be determined. The system is usually defined as a series of segments. The analysis on a series of segments is generally conducted beginning with the most distal segment and proceeding proximally up to the next segment and so on. Several assumptions must be made when using this approach. The body is considered to be a rigid linked system with frictionless pin joints. Each link, or segment, has a fixed mass and a center of mass at a fixed point. Finally, the moment of inertia about any axis of each segment remains constant. Moment of inertia will be discussed in Chapter 11.

As was stated previously, the dynamic case is more complicated than the static case. As a result only a limited example of a single segment will be presented. In Figure 10-23 a free body diagram of the foot of an individual during the swing phase of the gait cycle is presented for the linear forces acting on the segment.

During the swing phase of gait, no external forces other than gravity act on the foot. It can be seen that the only linear forces acting on the foot are the horizontal and vertical components of the joint reaction force and the weight of the foot acting through the center of mass. The joint reaction force components can be computed with the two-dimensional linear kinetic equations defining the dynamic analysis. First, the horizontal joint reaction force may be defined:

$$\Sigma F_x = ma_x$$

Since there are no horizontal forces other than the horizontal joint reaction force, this equation becomes:

$$R_x = ma_x$$

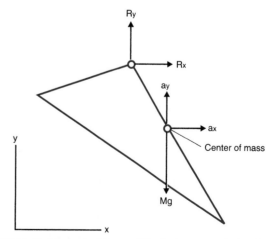

FIGURE 10-23 Free body diagram of the foot segment during the swing phase of a walking stride showing linear forces and accelerations.

If the mass of the foot is 1.16 kg and the horizontal acceleration of the center of mass of the foot is -1.35 m/s^2, the horizontal reaction force is:

$$R_x = 1.16 \text{ kg} * -1.35 \text{ m/s}^2$$
$$R_x = -1.57 \text{ N}$$

Next, the vertical joint reaction force component may be defined from:

$$\Sigma F_y = ma_y$$

There is, however, a vertical force other than the vertical joint reaction force. This force is the weight of the foot itself, and so the vertical forces are described as:

$$R_y - mg = ma_y$$

If the vertical acceleration of the center of mass of the foot is 7.65 m/s^2, then:

$$R_y = (1.16 \text{ kg} * 7.65 \text{ m/s}^2) + (1.16 \text{ kg} * 9.81 \text{ m/s}^2)$$
$$R_y = 20.3 \text{ N}$$

Refer to the walking data in Appendix E: Identify the maximum vertical peak force. Compute the vertical acceleration at that point. Repeat for the maximum anteroposterior and mediolateral forces.

Effects of Force Applied Over a Period of Time

For motion to occur, forces must be applied over time. Manipulating the equation describing Newton's second law of motion allows generation of an important physical relationship in human movement that describes the concept of forces acting over time. This relationship relates the momentum of an object to the force and the time over which the force acts.

This relationship is derived from Newton's second law:

$$F = m * a$$

Since $a = dv/dt$, this equation can be rewritten as:

$$F = m * \frac{dv}{dt}$$

and further:

$$F = d\left(\frac{m * v}{dt}\right)$$

If each side is multiplied by dt to remove the fraction on the right-hand side of the equation, the resulting equation is:

$$F * dt = d(m * v)$$

or

$$F * dt = mv_{final} - mv_{initial}$$

The left-hand side of this equation, the product of F * dt, a quantity known as an **impulse**, has units of newton-seconds (Ns). Impulse is the measure of what is required to change the motion of an object. Figure 10-24 illustrates

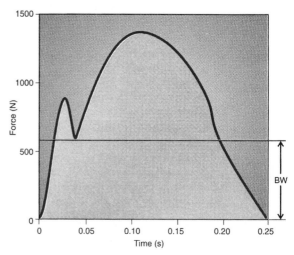

FIGURE 10-24 Vertical GRF of a subject running at 5 m/second. The vertical impulse is the shaded area under the force–time curve.

the vertical component of the GRF of a single footfall of a runner. This figure represents a force applied over time as the foot is in contact with the surface, generating a downward force and receiving an equal and opposite reaction force. Impulse may be expressed graphically as the area under a force–time curve. The right-hand side of the equation describes a change in momentum. Thus, when a force is applied to an object over time, the momentum of the object changes. The derived equation describes the **impulse–momentum relationship**.

Consider an individual with a mass of 65 kg jumping from a squat position into the air. The velocity of the person at the beginning of the jump is zero. Video analysis reveals that the velocity of the center of mass at takeoff was 3.4 m/s. The impulse can then be calculated as:

$$F * dt = mv_{final} - mv_{initial}$$
$$F * dt = (65 \text{ kg} * 3.4 \text{ m/s}) - (65 \text{ kg} * 0 \text{ m/s})$$
$$F * dt = 221 \text{ kgm/s}$$

It is assumed that the force application took place over 0.2 s. The average force applied, therefore, would be:

$$F * 0.02s = 221 \text{ kg-m/s}$$
$$F = \frac{221 \text{ kg-m/s}}{0.2 \text{ s}}$$
$$F = 1105 \text{ N}$$

The nature of the force applied and the time over which it is applied will determine how the momentum of the object is changed. To change the momentum of an object, a great force can be applied over a short period, or a small force over a long period. Of course, the tactic used depends on the situation. For example, in landing from a jump, the performer must change momentum from some initial value to zero. The initial momentum value at impact is a function of body mass times the velocity created by the force of gravity that causes the jumper to accelerate toward the ground at a rate of 9.81 m/s^2. At

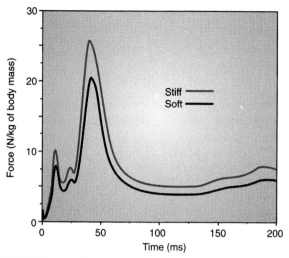

FIGURE 10-25 Vertical GRF for soft and stiff landings. Stiff landings had 23% greater linear impulse than the soft landing. (After DeVita, P., Skelly, W. A. [1992]. Effect of landing stiffness on joint kinetics and energetics in the lower extremity. *Medicine and Science in Sports and Exercise*, 24:108–115.)

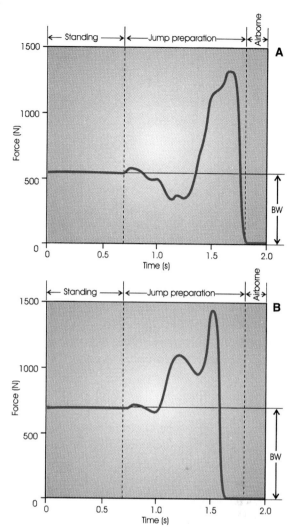

FIGURE 10-26 The vertical GRF of two types of vertical jumps: the countermovement jump **(A)** and the squat jump **(B)**.

floor impact, an impulse is generated to change the momentum and reduce it to zero as the jumper stops. If an individual lands with little knee flexion (locked knees), the impact force occurs over a very short period. If, however, the individual lands and flexes the joints of the lower extremity, the impact force is smaller and occurs over an extended time. If in both cases the jumper is landing with the same velocity and consequently the same momentum, the resulting impulses will also be the same, even though there are different force (large vs smaller force) and time (short vs extended) components. An example of soft and rigid landings is presented in Figure 10-25. This example, taken from a study by DeVita and Skelly (21), shows a large peak force in the rigid landing as compared to the smaller force in the soft landing. Because both appear to take place over about the same amount of time, there is a greater impulse in the rigid landings.

Using the data in Appendix E, graph the vertical, anteroposterior, and mediolateral ground reaction curves for the support phase of walking, and shade in the impulse for each curve.

One interesting research application for the use of the impulse–momentum relationship has been in vertical jumping. This area of research has used the force platform to determine the GRF during the vertical jump. Remember that the GRF reflects the force acting on the center of mass of the individual. Thus, researchers have used the impulse–momentum relationship on data collected from the force platform to determine the parameters necessary to investigate the height of the center of mass above its starting point during vertical jumping (42). Figure 10-26*A* shows the vertical GRF profile of an individual starting at rest on the platform and jumping into the air. This is called a countermovement jump because the

subject flexes at the knees and then swings the arms up as the knees are extended during the jump. Figure 10-26*B* illustrates a squat jump, in which the subject begins in a squat (knees flexed) and simply forcefully extends the knees to jump into the air.

In both cases, the impulse–momentum relationship can be used to calculate the peak height of the center of mass above the initial height during the jump. Consider the vertical GRF curve of a counterjump in Figure 10-27. The vertical force in the initial portion of the curve is the individual's body weight. If the body weight line is extended to the instant of takeoff, the area beneath the curve describes the body weight impulse (BW_{imp}). It may be calculated as an integral:

$$BW_{imp} = \int_{t_i}^{t_f} BW \, dt$$

where t_i to t_f represents the time interval when the subject is standing still on the force platform until the instant of takeoff. The total area under the force–time curve until

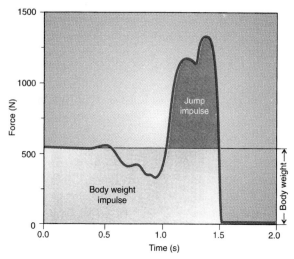

FIGURE 10-27 The vertical GRF of a countermovement jump illustrating the body weight impulse and the jump impulse.

the subject leaves the force platform may be designated as $total_{imp}$ and can be calculated as an integral:

$$total_{imp} = \int_{t_i}^{t_{jump}} F_z \, dt$$

where t_i to t_{jump} represents the time when the subject is on the platform before the jump. The impulse that propelled the subject into the air can then be determined by:

$$jump_{imp} = total_{imp} - BW_{imp}$$

The impulse–momentum relationship can then be formulated using the impulse that the subject generated to perform the jump. Thus:

$$jump_{imp} = m(v_f - v_i)$$

where v_i is the initial velocity of the center of mass and v_f is the takeoff velocity of the center of mass. Since $v_i = 0$:

$$jump_{imp} = m(v_f - 0)$$

By substituting the impulse of the jump ($jump_{imp}$) and the subject's body mass (m) in this equation, the velocity of the center of mass at takeoff for the vertical jump can be calculated. The height of the center of mass during the jump is then calculated based on the projectile equations elaborated upon in Chapter 8. Thus:

$$height_{cm} = \frac{v_m^2}{2g}$$

This calculation has proved to be in good agreement with values calculated from high-speed film data. Komi and Bosco (42) reported an error of 2% from the computation on the force platform.

Consider the force–time profile of a countermovement jump in Figure 10-27. The body weight impulse, the rectangle formed by the body weight and the time of force application, was calculated to be:

$$BW_{imp} = \int_{t0}^{t1.5} BW \, dt$$

$$BW_{imp} = 620.80 \text{ N} \cdot \text{s}$$

The total impulse, that is, the total force application from time 0 to time = 1.5 s, including the body weight, is:

$$total_{imp} = \int_{ti}^{tf} F_z \, dt$$

$$total_{imp} = 772.81 \text{ N} \cdot \text{s}$$

The jump impulse, therefore, is:

$$jump_{imp} = Total_{imp} - BW_{imp}$$
$$jump_{imp} = 772.81 \text{ N} \cdot \text{s} - 620.80 \text{ N} \cdot \text{s}$$
$$jump_{imp} = 152.01 \text{ N} \cdot \text{s}$$

Substituting this value in the impulse–momentum relationship, it is possible to solve for the velocity of the center of mass at takeoff. Thus, with the body mass of the jumper of 56.2 kg, the velocity of takeoff is:

$$jump_{imp} = m(v_f - v_i)$$
$$152.01 \text{ N} \cdot \text{s} = 56.2 \text{ kg } (v_f - 0)$$
$$v_f = \frac{152.01 \text{ N} \cdot \text{s}}{56.2 \text{ kg}}$$
$$v_f = 2.70 \text{ m/s}$$

The height of the center of mass during the jump can be calculated by:

$$Height_{cm} = \frac{v_{cm}^2}{2g}$$
$$Height_{cm} = \frac{(2.70 \text{ m/s})^2}{2 * 9.81 \text{ m/s}^2}$$
$$Height_{cm} = 0.373 \text{ m}$$

Therefore, in this particular jump, the center of mass was elevated 37.3 cm above the initial height of the center of mass.

This calculation technique was used by Dowling and Vamos (23) to identify the kinetic and temporal factors related to vertical jump performance. They found a large variation in the patterns of force application between the subjects that made it difficult to identify the characteristics of a good performance. Interestingly, they reported that a high maximum force was necessary but not sufficient for a good performance. They concluded that the pattern of force application was the most important factor in vertical jump performance.

Refer to the walking data in Appendix E: Calculate the vertical, anteroposterior, and mediolateral impulse from contact (frame 0) to the first vertical peak (frame 18). Using the impulse values, calculate the velocities generated up to that point.

Special Force Applications

CENTRIPETAL FORCE

In Chapter 9, linear and angular kinematics were related, using the situations in which an object moved along a curved path. It was demonstrated that centripetal acceleration acts toward the center of rotation when an object moves along a curved path. This is radial acceleration toward the center of the circle. The radial force occurring along a curved path that generates the acceleration is called the **centripetal force**. Using Newton's second law of motion, F = ma, a formula for the centripetal force can be generated. The force is no different from other forces and is generated by a push or pull. The force is called centripetal because of the effect: the force generates a change in the direction of the velocity. The magnitude of the centripetal or center-seeking force is calculated by:

$$F_C = m\omega^2 r$$

where F_C is the centripetal force, m is the mass of the object, ω is the angular velocity, and r is the radius of rotation. Centripetal force may also be defined as:

$$F_C = \frac{mv^2}{r}$$

where v is the tangential velocity of the segment.

Newton's third law states that for every action there is an equal and opposite reaction. For example, a runner moving along the curve of the running track applies a **shear force** to the ground, resulting in a shear GRF equal and opposite to the applied force. The shear reaction force constitutes the centripetal force. Figure 10-28 is a free body diagram of the runner moving along the curved path, showing the centripetal force, the vertical reaction force, and the resultant of these two force components. This centripetal force at the runner's foot tends to rotate the runner outward. To counteract this outward rotation, the runner leans toward the center of the curve. Hamill et al. (37) reported that this shear GRF increased as the radius of rotation decreased.

The resultant of the vertical reaction force and the centripetal force must pass through the center of mass of the runner. If the centripetal force increases, the runner leans more toward the center of rotation, and the resultant vector becomes less vertical. As mentioned in Chapter 9, banked curves on tracks reduce the shear force applied by the runner and thus reduce the centripetal force. As the centripetal force is reduced, the runner reduces the lean. The resultant force thus acts more vertically, as when the runner moves along a straight path.

PRESSURE

Up to this point in the discussion of force, the way a force causes an object to accelerate to achieve a state of motion has been considered. It is also necessary to discuss how forces, particularly impact forces, are distributed. The

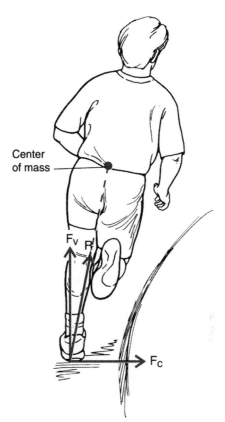

FIGURE 10-28 A free body diagram of a runner on the curve of a running track. F_C is the centripetal force, F_V is the vertical reaction force and R is the resultant of F_C and F_V.

concept of **pressure** is used to describe force distribution. Pressure is defined as the force per unit area. That is:

$$P = \frac{F}{A}$$

where F is a force and A is the area over which the force is applied. Pressure has units of N/m^2. Another unit of pressure often used is the pascal (Pa) or the kilopascal (kPa). One pascal is equal to $1\ N/m^2$. If an individual with a body weight of 650 N is supported on the soles of the feet with an approximate area of $0.018\ m^2$, the pressure on the soles of the feet would be:

$$P = \frac{650\ N}{0.018\ m^2}$$
$$P = 36.11\ kPa$$

Another individual with a smaller body weight, 500 N, and soles of the feet with an identical area would have a pressure of:

$$P = \frac{500\ N}{0.018\ m^2}$$
$$= 27.78\ kPa$$

If the heavier individual's foot soles had a larger area, 0.02 m^2 for example, the pressure would be 32.50 kPa. The pressure on the soles of the feet of the heavier individual is less than the pressure on the soles of the lighter individual, even though the body weight is different. These pressures appear quite large, but imagine if these individuals were women wearing spike-heeled shoes, which have much less surface area than ordinary shoes. A more dramatic example would be if these individuals were wearing ice skates, which have a distinctly smaller area of contact with the surface than the sole of a normal shoe or a spike-heeled shoe. On the other hand, if these individuals were using skis or snow shoes to walk in deep snow, the pressure would be quite small because of the large area of the skis or snowshoes in contact with the snow. In this way, individuals walk on snow without sinking into it.

The concept of pressure is especially important in activities in which a collision results. Generally, when a force of impact is to be minimized, it should be received over as large an area as possible. For example, when landing from a fall, most athletes attempt a roll to spread the impact force over as large an area as possible. In the martial arts, considerable time is spent in learning how to fall correctly, specifically applying the pressure as force per unit area.

A number of sporting activities in which collisions abound have special protective equipment designed to reduce pressure. Examples are shoulder pads in football and ice hockey; shin pads in ice hockey, field hockey, soccer, and baseball (for the catcher); boxing gloves; and batting helmets in baseball. In all of these examples, the point of the design of the protective padding is to spread the impact force over as large an area as possible to reduce the pressure.

With use of a force platform, it is possible to obtain a measure of the **center of pressure** (COP), a displacement measure indicating the path of the resultant GRF vector on the force platform. It is equal to the weighted average of the points of application of all of the downward-acting forces on the force platform. Since the COP is a general measurement, it may be nowhere near the maximal areas of pressure.

However, it does provide a general pattern and has been extensively used in gait analysis. Cavanagh and Lafortune (16) showed different COP patterns for rear foot and midfoot strikers. Representative COP patterns are illustrated in Figure 10-29. Cavanagh and Lafortune suggested that COP information may be useful in shoe design, but these patterns have not been related successfully to foot function during locomotion. Miller (53) noted that COP data provide only restricted information on the overall pressure distribution on the sole of the foot.

Methods of measuring the local pressure patterns under the foot or shoe have been developed in recent years. An example of the type of data available on these systems is presented in Figure 10-30. Cavanagh et al. (15) developed such a measuring system and reported distinct local areas of high pressure on the foot throughout the ground contact phase. The greatest pressures were measured at the heel, on the metatarsal heads, and on the hallux. Cavanagh et al. (15) also compared the pressure patterns during running barefoot and with vari-

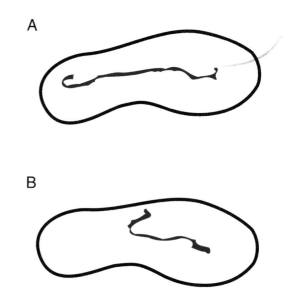

FIGURE 10-29 Center of pressure patterns for the left foot. **A.** A heel–toe footfall pattern runner. **B.** A midfoot foot strike pattern runner.

ous foam materials attached to the foot. They reported that peak pressures were reduced when wearing the foam materials, but the changes in the pressure pattern over the support period were similar. Foti et al. (30), using an in-shoe pressure measurement device, reported that softer midsole shoes distributed the foot-to-shoe pressure at heel contact during walking better than a hard midsole shoe. The implication is that softer midsole shoes provide a more cushioned feel to the wearer.

WORK: THE EFFECT OF A FORCE APPLIED OVER A DISTANCE

The term **work** is used to mean a variety of things, generally anything that demands mental or physical effort. In mechanics, however, work has a more specific and narrow meaning. Mechanical work is equal to the product of the magnitude of a force applied against an object and the distance the object moves in the direction of the force

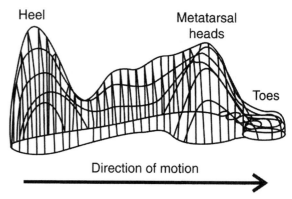

FIGURE 10-30 Pressure distribution pattern of a normal foot during walking. (After Cavanagh, P. R. [1989]. The biomechanics of running and running shoe problems. In B. Segesser, W. Pforringer (Eds.). *The Shoe in Sport.* London: Wolfe, 3–15.)

while the force is applied to the object. For example, in moving an object along the ground, an individual pushes the object with a force parallel to the ground. If the force necessary to move the object is 100 N and the object was moved 1 m, the work done would be 100 Nm. The case cited, however, is a very specific one. More generally, work is:

$$W = F * \cos \theta * s$$

where F is the force applied, s is the displacement, and θ is the angle between the force vector and the line of displacement. The unit of mechanical work is derived from the product of force in newtons and displacement in meters. The most commonly used units are the newton-meter and the joule (J). These are equivalent units:

$$1 \text{ Nm} = 1 \text{ J}$$

In Figure 10-31*A*, the force is applied to a block parallel to the line of displacement, that is, at an angle of 0° to the displacement. Since cos 0° = 1, the work done is simply the product of the force and the distance the block is displaced. Thus if the force applied is 50 N and the block is displaced 0.1 m, the mechanical work done is:

$$W = 50 \text{ N} * \cos 0° * 0.1 \text{ m}$$
$$= 50 \text{ N} * 1 * 0.1 \text{ m}$$
$$= 5 \text{ Nm}$$

If the same force is applied at an angle of 30° over the same distance, d, (Fig. 10-31*B*), the work done is:

$$W = 50 \text{ N} * \cos 30° * 0.1 \text{ m}$$
$$W = 50 \text{ N} * 0.866 * 0.1 \text{ m}$$
$$W = 4.33 \text{ Nm}$$

Therefore, more work is done if the force is applied parallel to the direction of motion than if the force is applied at an angle.

As this discussion of work implies, work is done only when the object is moving and its motion is influenced by the applied force. If a force acts on an object and does not cause the object to move, no mechanical work is done because the distance moved is zero. During an isometric contraction, for example, no work is done, since there is no movement. A weightlifter who holds an 892-N (200 lb) barbell overhead is doing no mechanical work. In lifting the barbell overhead, however, mechanical work was done. If the barbell is lifted 1.85 m, the work done is:

$$W = 892 \text{ N} * 1.85 \text{ m}$$
$$= 1650.2 \text{ J}$$

assuming that the bar was lifted straight up.

POWER

In evaluating the amount of work done by a force, the time over which the force is applied is not taken into

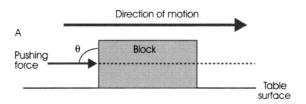

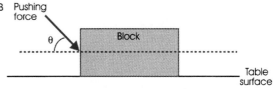

FIGURE 10-31 The mechanical work done on a block. **A.** A force is applied parallel to the surface ($\theta = 0°$; thus cos $\theta = 1$). **B.** A force is applied at an angle to the direction of motion ($\theta = 30°$; thus cos $\theta = 0.866$).

account. When the work done by the weightlifter to raise the barbell overhead was calculated, the time it took to raise the barbell was not taken into consideration. Regardless of how long it took to raise the barbell, the amount of work done was 647.5 J. The concept of **power** takes into consideration the work done per unit of time. Power is defined as the rate at which a force does work:

$$P = \frac{dW}{dt}$$

where W is the work done and dt is the time period in which the work was done. Power has units of watts (W). The change in work is expressed in joules and the change in time in seconds. Thus:

$$1 \text{ W} = 1 \text{ J/s}$$

If power is plotted on a graph as a function of time, the area under the curve equals the work done.

If the weightlifter raises the bar in 0.5 s, the power developed is:

$$P = 647.5 \text{ J}/0.5 \text{ s}$$
$$= 1295 \text{ J/s}$$
$$= 1295 \text{ W}$$

Decreasing the time over which the bar is lifted to 0.35 s increases the power developed by the weightlifter to 1850 W. While the work done remains constant, greater power must be developed to do the mechanical work more quickly.

Another definition for power can be developed by rearranging the formula. If the product of the force (F) and the distance over which it was applied (s) is substituted for the mechanical work done, the equation becomes:

$$P = \frac{d(F * s)}{dt}$$

And rearranging this equation:

$$P = F * \frac{ds}{dt}$$

Since ds/dt was defined in a previous chapter as the velocity in the s-direction, it can be readily seen that:

$$P = F * v$$

where F is the applied force and v is the velocity of the force application.

Power is often confused with force, work, energy, or strength. Power, however, is a combination of force and velocity. In many athletic endeavors, power, or the ability to use the combination of force and velocity, is paramount. One such activity, weightlifting, has already been discussed, but there are many others, such as shot putting, batting in baseball, and boxing. Jumping also requires power. To generate a takeoff velocity of 2.61 m/s in a vertical jump, Harman et al. (38) reported a peak power generation of 3896 watts. In comparisons of jump techniques, researchers have noted differences in peak power output between countermovement jumps (males = 4708 W; females = 3069 W) and squat jumps (males = 4620 W; females = 2993 W) (66).

ENERGY

As with work, the mechanical term **energy** is often misused. Simply stated, energy is the capacity to do work. There are many types of energy, some of which are light, heat, nuclear, electrical, and mechanical. In biomechanics the main concern is with mechanical energy. The unit of mechanical energy in the metric system is the joule. Mechanical energy has two forms, kinetic and potential.

Kinetic energy (KE) refers to the energy resulting from motion. An object possesses kinetic energy when it is in motion, that is, when it has some velocity. Linear kinetic energy is expressed algebraically as:

$$KE = \frac{1}{2} mv^2$$

where m is the mass of the object and v is the velocity. Since this expression includes the square of the velocity, any change in velocity greatly increases the amount of energy in the object. If the velocity is zero, the object has no kinetic energy. An approximate value for the kinetic energy of a 625-N runner would be 3600 J, while a swimmer of comparable body weight would have a value of 125 J. A moving body must have some energy, because a force must be exerted to stop it. To start an object moving, a force must be applied over a distance. Kinetic energy, therefore, is the ability of a moving object to do work resulting from its motion. The generation of a sufficient level of kinetic energy is especially important when projecting an object or body, such as in long jumping, throwing, and batting. For example, kinetic energy is developed in a baseball over the collision phase with the bat and will project the ball at velocities more than 100 mph. The kinetic energy before the collision has been demonstrated to be in the range of 320 J and 115 J for the bat and ball, respectively. After the contact, the kinetic energy of the bat is reported to be reduced to 156 J and the ball's kinetic energy increased to 157 J (28). With bat speeds in the range of 55 to 80 mph and incoming ball speeds of 85 to 100 mph, there is considerable interchange of kinetic energy.

Potential energy (PE) is the capacity to do work because of position or form. An object may contain stored energy, for example, simply because of its height or its deformation. In the first case, if a 30-kg barbell is lifted overhead to a height of 2.2 m, 647.5 J of work is done to lift the barbell. That is:

$$\begin{aligned} W &= F * s \\ &= (30 \text{ kg} * 9.81 \text{ m/s}^2) * 2.2 \text{ m} \\ &= 647.5 \text{ J} \end{aligned}$$

As the barbell is held overhead, it has the potential energy of 647.5 J. The work done to lift it overhead is also the potential energy. Potential energy gradually increases as the bar is lifted. If the bar is lowered, the potential energy decreases. Potential energy is defined algebraically as:

$$PE = mgh$$

where m is the mass of the object, g is the acceleration due to gravity, and h is the height. The more work done to overcome gravity, therefore, the greater the potential energy.

An object that is deformed may also store potential energy. This type of potential energy has to do with elastic forces. When an object is deformed, the resistance to the deformation increases as the object is stretched. Thus, the force that deforms the object is stored and may be released as elastic energy. This type of energy, **strain energy** (SE), is defined as:

$$SE = \frac{1}{2}k * \Delta x$$

where k is a proportionality constant and Δx is the distance over which the object was deformed. The proportionality constant depends on the material deformed and is often called the stiffness constant because it represents the object's ability to store energy. It has already been discussed how certain tissues, such as muscles and tendons, and certain devices, such as springboards for diving, may store this strain energy and release it to aid in human movement. In athletics numerous pieces of equipment achieve such an end. Examples are trampolines, bows in archery, and poles in pole vaulting. Perhaps the most sophisticated use of elastic energy storage is the design of the tuned running track at Harvard University. McMahon and Greene (50) analyzed the mechanics of running and the energy interactions between the runner and the track to develop an optimum design for the track surface. In the first season on this new track, an average speed advantage of nearly 3% was observed. Further, it was determined that there was a 93% probability that any given individual will run faster on this new track (49).

Many instances in human motion can be understood in terms of the interchanges between kinetic and potential energy. The mathematical relationship between the different forms of energy was formulated by the German scientist von Helmholtz (1821–1894). In 1847 he defined what has come to be known as the **law of conservation of energy**. The main point of this law is that energy cannot be created or destroyed. No machine, including the human machine, can generate more energy than it takes in. It follows, therefore, that the total energy of a closed system is constant, since energy does not enter or leave a closed system. A closed system is one that is physically isolated from its surroundings. This point can be phrased mathematically by stating:

$$TE = KE + PE$$

where TE is a constant representing the total energy of the system. In human movement, this occurs only when the object is a projectile, whereby the only external force acting upon it is gravity, since fluid resistance is neglected.

Consider the example of a projectile traveling up. At the point of release, the projectile has zero potential energy and large kinetic energy. As the projectile ascends, the potential energy increases while the kinetic energy decreases, because gravity is slowing the flight. At the peak of the trajectory, the velocity of the projectile is zero and the kinetic energy is zero, but the potential energy is a maximum. The total energy of the system did not change, since increases in potential energy resulted in equal decreases in kinetic energy. On the downward flight, the reverse change in the forms of energy occurs. These changes in energy are illustrated in Figure 10-32.

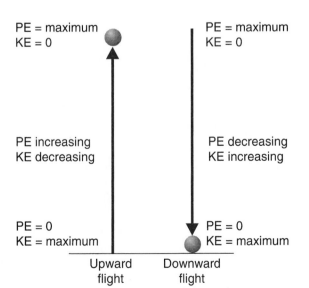

FIGURE 10-32 Changes in potential energy (PE) and kinetic energy (KE) as a ball is projected straight up and as it falls back to earth.

When an object is moved, mechanical work is said to have been done on the object. Thus, if no movement occurs, no mechanical work is done. Intuitively, there should be some **work–energy relationship**, the capacity to do work. This very useful relationship is called the **work–energy theorem**. This theorem states that the work done is equal to the change in energy:

$$W = \Delta E$$

where W is the work done and ΔE is the change in energy. That is, for mechanical work to be done, a change in the energy level must occur. The change in energy refers to all types of energy in the system, kinetic, potential, chemical, heat, light, and so on. For example, if a trampolinist weighs 780 N and is at a peak height of 2 m above a trampoline bed, the potential energy based on the height above the trampoline bed is:

$$PE = 780 \text{ N} * 2 \text{ m}$$
$$PE = 1560 \text{ J}$$

Assuming no horizontal movement, at impact the kinetic energy is 1560 J, while the potential energy is zero. The kinetic energy has this initial value, and as the bed deforms, the potential strain energy increases while the kinetic energy goes to zero. The work done on the trampoline bed is:

$$W = \Delta KE$$
$$W = 1560 \text{ J} - 0 \text{ J}$$
$$W = 1560 \text{ J}$$

This value, 1560 J, is also the value of the potential strain energy of the trampoline bed. As the bed reforms, the potential strain energy changes from this value to zero and constitutes the work done by the trampoline bed on the trampolinist.

To evaluate the work done, the energy level of a system must be evaluated at different instants in time. This change in energy represents the work done on the system. For example, a system has an energy level of 26.3 J at position 2 and 13.1 J at position 1. The work done is:

$$W = \Delta E$$
$$W = 26.3 \text{ J} - 13.1 \text{ J}$$
$$W = 13.2 \text{ J}$$

Because this work has a positive value, it is considered positive work, and work is said to be done by the system in the form of concentric muscle actions. On the other hand, if the energy level is 22.4 J at position 1 and 14.5 J at position 2, then:

$$W = \Delta E$$
$$W = 14.5 \text{ J} - 22.4 \text{ J}$$
$$W = -7.9 \text{ J}$$

Now the work done is negative and work is said to have been done on the system. That is, the muscles are undergoing eccentric contractions.

The work–energy relationship is useful in biomechanics to analyze human motion. Researchers have used this analytical method to determine the work done during a number of movements; however, the greatest use of this technique has been in the area of locomotion. The calculation of the total work done resulting from the motion of all of the body's segments is called **internal work**. This calculation has been used by many researchers, particularly those studying locomotion (58,62,82,84,87).

For a single segment, the linear work done on the segment is:

$$W_s = \Delta KE + \Delta PE$$

$$W_s = \Delta\left(\frac{1}{2}mv^2\right) + \Delta(mgh)$$

where W_s is the work done on the segment, ΔKE is the change in linear kinetic energy of the center of mass of the segment, and ΔPE is the change in potential energy of the segment center of mass. The work done on the total body is the sum of the work done on all segments and is calculated as:

$$W_b = \sum_{i-1}^{n} W_{si}$$

where W_b is the total body work and W_{si} is the work done on the ith segment. One major limitation of this calculation is that it does not account for all of the energy of a segment and so does not account for the energy of the total body. For example, the strain energy due to the deformation of tissue and the angular kinetic energy are not considered. Angular work will be discussed in Chapter 11.

External work, on the other hand, may be defined as the work done by a body on an object. For example, the work done by the body to elevate the total body center of mass while walking up an incline is considered to be external work. External work is often calculated during an inclined treadmill walk or run as:

External work = BW * treadmill speed *
percent grade * duration

where BW is the body weight of the subject, percent grade is the incline of the treadmill, and duration is the length of time of the walk or run. The product of the treadmill speed, percent grade, and the duration is the total vertical distance traveled. If the percent grade is zero, that is, the walking surface is level, the vertical distance traveled is zero. Thus, walking on a level surface results in no external work being done.

Internal work of the total body for a particular movement is derived by summing the changes in the segment energies over time. That is, the change in energy at each instant in time is summed for the length of time that the

movement lasts. Usually, this period in locomotion studies is the time for one stride. The analysis of the mechanical work done is extremely valuable as a global parameter of the body's behavior without a detailed knowledge of the motion. A variety of algorithms may be used to calculate work (14,58,62,82,84,87). These models have incorporated factors to quantify such parameters as positive and negative work, the effect of muscle elastic energy, and the amount of negative work attributable to muscular sources. The major difference among these algorithms is the way energy is transferred within a segment and between segments. Energy transfer within a segment refers to changes from one form of energy to another, as in the change from potential to kinetic. Energy transfer between segments refers to the exchange of the total energy of a segment from one segment to another. Presently, there is no consensus as to which model is most appropriate. Thus, values of mechanical work for a single running stride may range from 532 W to 1775 W (83).

If it is considered that all energy is transferred between segments, the point in the stride at which the transfer occurs can be illustrated. Figure 10-33 graphically illustrates the magnitude of between-segment energy transfer during the running stride. The magnitude of energy transfer decreases during support and increases from midstance to a maximum after toe-off (83).

When work is calculated over time, such as a locomotor stride, the result is often presented as power with units of watts. These power values have generally been scaled to body mass, resulting in units of watts per kilogram of body mass. Hintermeister and Hamill (40) investigated the relationship between mechanical power and energy expenditure. They reported that mechanical power significantly influenced energy expenditure independent of the running speed. Using several algorithms representing different methods of energy transfer, however,

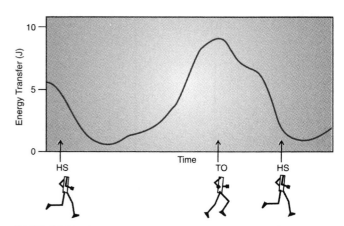

FIGURE 10-33 The magnitude of between-segment transfer during a single running stride. (After Williams, K. R. [1980]. A biomechanical and physiological evaluation of running efficiency. Unpublished doctoral dissertation, The Pennsylvania State University.)

mechanical power explained at best only 56% of the variance in energy expenditure.

The law of conservation of energy can explain this rather weak relationship between mechanical work and energy expenditure. This law states that energy is neither created nor destroyed but may be changed from one form to another. That is, potential energy may be changed to kinetic energy or heat energy. However, not all of the energy can be or is used to perform mechanical work. In fact, most of the available energy of the muscle will go to maintain the metabolism of the muscle; only about 25% of the energy is used for mechanical work. Thus, the work–energy theorem, when used to determine the mechanical work of the body, does not account for all of the energy in the system.

Linear Kinetics of Locomotion

The GRFs in locomotion represent the algebraic sum of the all of the segmental accelerations. GRF profiles continually change with time and are generally presented as a function of time. The magnitude of the GRF components for running are much greater than for walking. The magnitude of the GRFs will also vary as a function of locomotor speed (36,54), increasing with running speed. The vertical GRF component is much greater in magnitude than the other components and has received the most attention from biomechanists (Fig. 10-34). In walking, the vertical component has a maximum value of 1 to 1.2 BW, and in running, the maximum value can be 3 to 5 BW. The vertical force component in walking has a characteristic bimodal shape; that is, it has two maximum values. The first modal peak occurs during the first half of support and characterizes the portion of support when the total body is lowered after foot contact. The force rises above body weight as full weight bearing takes place and the body mass is accelerated upward. The force then lowers as the knee flexes, partially unloading. The second peak represents the active push against the ground to move into the next step. Figure 10-35 presents a comparison of walking and running vertical GRF component profiles.

In running, the shape of the vertical GRF component depends on the footfall pattern of the runner (Fig. 10-36). The heel strike runner's curve has two discernible peaks. The first peak occurs very rapidly after the initial contact and is often referred to as the **passive peak**. The term passive peak refers to the fact that this phase is not under muscular control (56) and is influenced by impact velocity, contact area between the surface and the foot, the joint angles at impact, surface stiffness, and the motion of the segments (22). This peak is also referred to as the **impact peak**. The second peak occurs during midsupport and generally has greater magnitude than the impact peak. Nigg (56) refers to the second peak as the **active peak**,

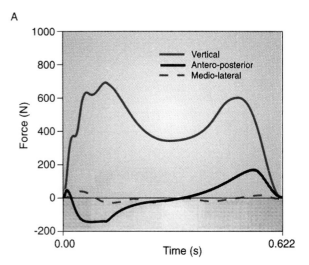

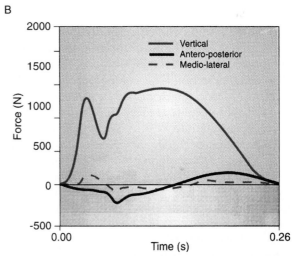

FIGURE 10-34 Ground reaction force for walking **(A)** and running **(B)**. Note the difference in magnitude between the vertical component and the shear components.

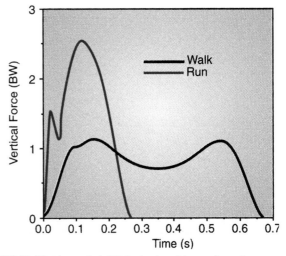

FIGURE 10-35 The vertical GRF for both walking and running.

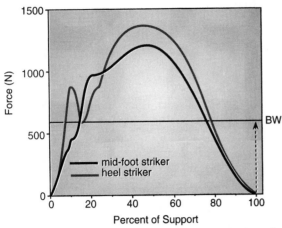

FIGURE 10-36 Vertical GRF profiles of a runner using a heel–toe footfall pattern and a runner who initially strikes the ground with the midfoot.

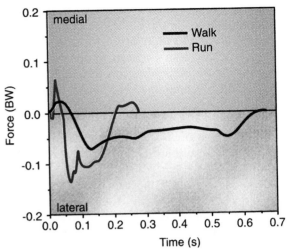

FIGURE 10-38 Mediolateral (side to side) GRF for both walking and running.

indicating the role the muscles play in the force development to accelerate the body off the ground. The midfoot strike runner has little or no impact peak.

The anteroposterior GRF component also exhibits a characteristic shape similar in both walking and running but of different magnitude (Fig. 10-37). The Fy component reaches magnitudes of 0.15 BW in walking and up to 0.5 BW in running. During locomotion, this component shows a negative phase during the first half of support as a result of a backward horizontal friction force between the shoe and the surface. This moves to positive near midstance, as force is generated by the muscles pushing back against the ground.

The mediolateral GRF component is extremely variable and has no consistent pattern from individual to individual. It is very difficult to interpret this force component without a video or film record of the foot contact. Figure 10-38 illustrates walking and running profiles for the same individual. The great variety in foot placement

regarding toeing in (forefoot adduction) and toeing out (forefoot abduction) may be a reason for this lack of consistency in the mediolateral component. The range of foot placement was shown in one study to be from 12° of toeing in to 29° of toeing out, and toeing out at heel strike has been shown to generate greater medial lateral forces and impulses (70). The magnitude of the mediolateral component ranges from 0.01 BW in walking to 0.1 BW in running.

Biomechanists have investigated GRFs to attempt to relate these forces to the kinematics of the lower extremity, particularly to foot function. Efforts have been made to relate these forces to the rear foot supination and pronation profiles of runners to identify possible injuries or aid in the design of athletic footwear (33,35). The use of GRF data for these purposes is probably extrapolating beyond the information provided by the GRFs.

To illustrate this point, a method of calculating the vertical GRF component proposed by Bobbert et al. (8) will be presented. In this method, Bobbert and associates used the kinematically derived values of the accelerations of the centers of mass of each of the body's segments. The vertical GRF component reflects the accelerations of the individual body segments resulting from the motion of the segments. The sum of the vertical forces of all body segments, including the effect of gravity is the vertical GRF component. That is:

$$F_z = \sum_{i-1}^{n} m_i(a_{zi} - g)$$

where F_z is the vertical force component (forces directed upward are defined as positive), m_i is the mass of the ith segment, n is the number of segments, a_{zi} is the vertical acceleration of the ith segment (upward accelerations are defined as positive), and g is the acceleration due to gravity. The anteroposterior GRF component reflects the horizontal (i.e., in the direction of motion) accelerations of

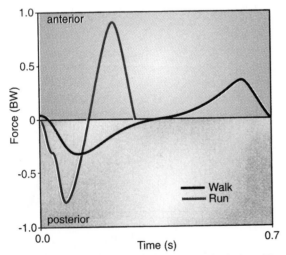

FIGURE 10-37 Anteroposterior (front to back) GRF for both walking and running.

the individual body segments. Using similar methods, this force component can be computed as:

$$F_y = \sum_{i-1}^{n} (m_i \, a_{yi})$$

where a_{yi} is the horizontal acceleration of the ith segment. Similarly, the mediolateral GRF component reflects the side-to-side accelerations of the individual body segments:

$$F_x = \sum_{i-1}^{n} (m_i \, a_{xi})$$

where a_{xi} is the side-to-side acceleration of the ith segment. If the center of mass is a single point that represents the mass center of all the body's segments, the vertical component is:

$$F_z = m(a_z - g)$$

where m is the total body mass, a_z is the vertical acceleration of the center of mass, and g is the acceleration due to gravity. Similarly, the other components may be represented as the total body mass times the acceleration of the center of mass. That is:

$$F_y = ma_y$$
$$F_x = ma_x$$

Therefore, the GRF represents the force necessary to accelerate the total body center of gravity (53) and cannot be directly associated with lower extremity function. Caution, then, should be exercised in describing lower extremity function using GRF data.

Since the GRF relates to the motion of the total body center of mass, the anteroposterior force profile can be related to the acceleration profile of the center of mass during support. Chapter 8 discusses a study by Bates et al. (6), illustrating the horizontal velocity pattern of the center of mass during the support phase of the running stride (Fig. 10-39A). When this curve was differentiated, an acceleration curve was generated (Fig. 10-39B). This curve has the characteristic shape of the anteroposterior force component in that it has negative acceleration followed by positive acceleration. According to Newton's second law of motion, if each point along this curve was multiplied by the runner's body mass (m), the anteroposterior GRF component would be generated as follows:

$$F_y = ma_y$$

Conversely, the acceleration curve could be calculated by dividing the F_y force component by the runner's body mass.

$$a_y = \frac{F_y}{m}$$

Either generating the curves using the kinematic procedure or collecting the anteroposterior GRF component leads to the same conclusion. The negative portion of the force component indicates a force against the runner

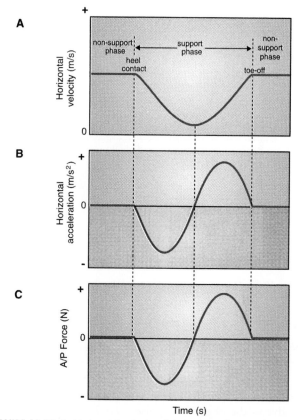

FIGURE 10-39 A. Horizontal velocity of the center of mass of a runner. **B.** If the velocity curve in **A** is differentiated, a horizontal acceleration curve of the center of mass is generated. **C.** Multiplying each point along this curve by the runner's body mass, the anteroposterior GRF is generated.

serving to brake the runner, that is, to decrease velocity. The positive portion of the component indicates a force in the direction of motion serving to accelerate the runner, so to increase velocity. If the running speed is constant, the negative and positive phases will be symmetrical, indicating no loss in velocity. If the negative portion of the curve is greater than the positive portion, the runner will slow down more than speed up. Conversely, if the positive portion is greater than the negative, the runner is speeding up.

Applying the impulse–momentum relationship, again confirms that the runner does indeed slow down during the first portion of support and speed up in the latter portion (Fig. 10-40). The area under the negative portion of the force component or the negative impulse serves to slow the runner down, that is, to change incoming velocity to some lesser velocity value. The positive area or the positive impulse of the component serves to accelerate the runner, that is, to change velocity from some lesser value to some outgoing velocity. If the positive change in velocity equals the negative change in velocity, the individual is running at a constant speed. Figure 10-41 illustrates the changes in the braking and propelling impulses across a range of running speeds (36). In many instances in the laboratory during collection of GRF data, the ratio of the

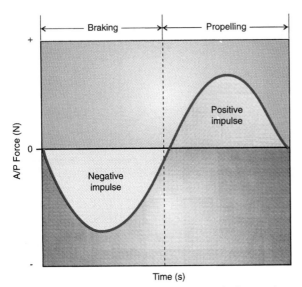

FIGURE 10-40 Anteroposterior GRF illustrating the braking and propulsion impulses.

negative impulse to the positive impulse is checked to determine if the runner is at a constant velocity, speeding up, or slowing down. However, even if the individual is maintaining a constant running speed, the ratio of the positive to the negative impulse is rarely 1.0 for any given support period of a stride. The average ratio over a number of footfalls approaches the ratio of 1.0, however.

There is an exchange of mechanical energy during both running and walking, although there are differences in the energy fluctuations. External work in walking has two components, one due to inertial forces as a result of speed changes in the forward direction and the other due to the cyclic upward displacement of the center of gravity. The work done to accelerate in the lateral direction is only a small fraction of the total work, as is evidenced by the small forces and small displacements (72). The

motion of the center of gravity in walking has been modeled as an inverted pendulum. In each step, the center of gravity is either behind or in front of the contact point between the foot and the ground (20). When the center of gravity is behind the point of contact, as during the heel strike phase of support, the GRFs cause a negative acceleration and there is a decrease in kinetic energy due to loss of forward speed. A concomitant occurrence with the loss of kinetic energy is a rise in the center of gravity as the body vaults over the support limb. This increases the gravitational potential energy, which reaches a maximum level in the middle of stance. As the center of gravity moves forward of the point of the contact, the kinetic energy increases because gravitational potential energy decreases with the reduction in the height of the center of gravity. This pendulumlike exchange between potential and kinetic energy allows savings as much as 65% of muscular work (72). This conservation of energy is not perfect, so the total energy of the center of gravity fluctuates (20). The net change in the overall mechanical energy in walking is actually small.

In running, the mechanical energy fluctuates more. Kinetic energy in running is similar to walking, reaching minimum levels at midstance due to deceleration caused by the horizontal GRF and increasing in the latter half of the support phase. The potential energy is different than in walking since it is minimum at midstance because of compliance and flexion in the support limb (29). The overall vertical excursion of the center of mass is also less as the speed of running increases (29). There is not the pendulum-like exchange between potential and kinetic energy seen in walking because they are in phase with each other, compared to walking where they are 180° out of phase (29). The exchange of energy conserves less than 5% of the mechanical work required to lift and accelerate the center of mass (29). However, substantial mechanical energy is conserved through the storage and return of elastic energy in the tissues.

Linear Kinetics of the Golf Swing

In the golf swing, substantial linear forces are generated on the ground in response to segmental accelerations. Other important force application sites are between the hand and the club and—most important—between the club head and the ball at contact. The GRFs vary between right and left limbs. High vertical GRFs are generated between the right foot and the ground in the backswing (right-handed golfer) and there is a rapid transfer of force to the left foot prior to impact, resulting in a peak force that is more than 1 BW (85). In the mediolateral direction, a lateral GRF develops in the right foot up through the backswing and from the top of the backswing to just before impact and a medial force propels the body toward the direction of the ball. At impact, this reverses to slow

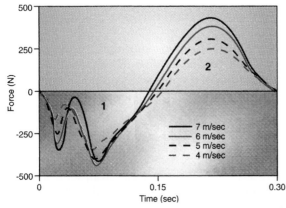

FIGURE 10-41 Changes in the anteroposterior GRF as a function of running speed. Area 1 is the braking impulse, and area 2 is the propulsion impulse. (After Hamill, J., et al. [1983]. Variations in GRF parameters at different running speeds. *Human Movement Science*, 2:47–56.)

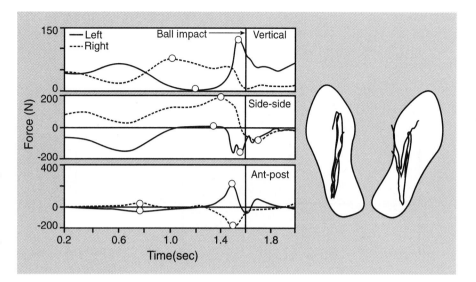

FIGURE 10-42 Ground reaction forces and center of pressure for the front (*left*) and back (*right*) foot during the golf swing. (After Williams, K. R., Sih, B. L. [1999]. Ground reaction forces in regular-spike and alternative-spike golf shoes. In M. R. Farrally, A. J. Cochran (Eds.). *Science and Golf III: Proceedings of the 1998 World Scientific Congress of Golf.* Champaign, IL: Human Kinetics, 568–575.).

the movement of the body from right to left (85). In the anteroposterior direction, a force is generated as the body rotates around a vertical axis, resulting in a backward force on the left foot and a forward force on the right foot in the backswing. This reverses in the downswing as the body rotates to impact (85). The patterns of GRF generation using the different clubs is essentially the same, with changes in force magnitudes only. A sample of the GRFs and the center of pressure patterns for both feet are illustrated in Figure 10-42. Maximum vertical GRF values for a representative subject wearing regular spikes were 1096 N at the front foot and 729 N at the rear foot (86). The maximum anteroposterior force in the anterior was 166 N generated in the front foot and was −143 N in the posterior direction, generated in the back foot. The maximum lateral force was generated in the front foot and was in the range of 161 N (86).

The forces acting on the body as a result of the swing have been shown to range between 40 and 50% of body weight (47). These forces must be controlled by the golfer to produce a good swing. A good golfer will start the downswing slowly, and the forces acting on the golfer consequently produce a smooth acceleration. An inexperienced golfer will initiate the downswing with greater acceleration. The centripetal force produced by this rapid acceleration rotates the club, reduces the acceleration, and can actually cause negative acceleration later. Forces acting on the body as a result of the swing reach values around 40% of body weight in the final third of the downswing (Fig. 10-43). These forces are directed backward and must be resisted by knee flexion and a wide base of support. The force produced by the swing is maximum at contact and is vertically directed and easily resisted by the body (47).

As a result of forces acting on the body, significant forces are generated at the knee joint. Compressive forces in the front and back knees reach values approximating

100% and 72% of body weight for the front and back knee joints, respectively (31). Shear forces are also developed. An anterior shear force is developed in the back knee (10% body weight) and posterior shear forces are present in both the front and back knee joints, approximating 39% and 20% of body weight in the front and back knee joints, respectively (31).

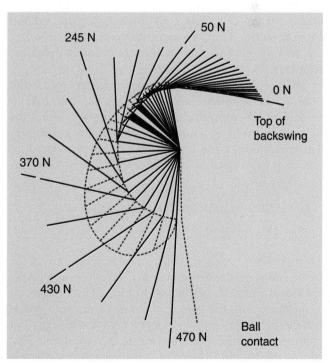

FIGURE 10-43 Forces generated as a result of the swing are shown for the golfer Bobby Jones. (After Mather, J. S. B. [2000]. Innovative golf clubs designed for the amateur. In A. J. Subic, S. J. Haake (Eds.). *The Engineering of Sport: Research, Development and Innovation.* Malden: Blackwell Science, 61–68.)

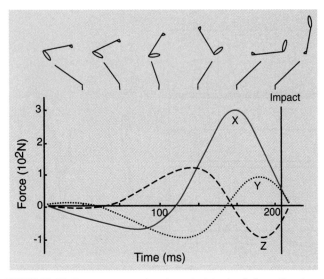

FIGURE 10-44 Forces generated at the wrist joint in all three directions. (After Neal, R. J., Wilson, B. D. [1985]. 3D kinematics and kinetics of the golf swing. *International Journal of Sports Biomechanics*, 1:221–232.)

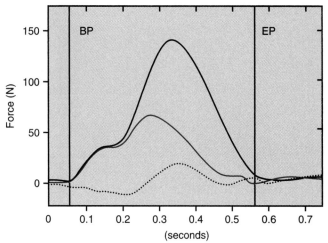

FIGURE 10-45 Vertical forces (black), anteroposterior forces (red), and mediolateral forces (dotted) applied to the rim of the wheelchair by the hand. (After Veeger, H. E., et al. [1989]. Wheelchair propulsion technique at different speeds. *Scandinavian Journal of Rehabilitation Medicine*, 21:197–203.)

Linear forces have also been measured at the wrist and shoulder. Resultant forces acting at the wrist and shoulder are shown in Figure 10-44. It is important to measure these forces because they determine the eventual acceleration of the club. Peak forces in the direction of the ball are greater for the arm segment (650 N) than the club segment (approximately 300 N), and the shoulder peak force occurred 85 ms from impact, as compared to 60 ms from impact for the club (55). Peak forces in the vertical and anteroposterior directions also occurred earlier in the arm segment, suggesting some timing interaction between the segments.

The golf ball travels upward as a reaction to the club head action downward with the face of the club held in place. The contact with the ball is not upward, and if the swing is up, the likely result is a topped ball that goes down. The magnitude of the impact force has been reported in one study to be up to 15 kN applied for about 500 ms (48).

 ## Linear Kinetics of Wheelchair Propulsion

To propel a wheelchair, the hand grasps the rim of the wheel and generates a pushing force. After the push phase, the hands return to the initial position before contact is again made with the rim. In this passive recovery phase, the inertial forces from the upper body movements can continue to influence the motion of the wheelchair (78) so that the backward swing of the trunk causes a reaction force that can propel the wheelchair forward.

The hand pushes on the rim at an angle, but only the force component tangential to the rim contributes to the propulsion (65). The propulsion force vector tangential to the rim is directed upward at the hand position of −15° to

top dead center and directed downward at +60° from top dead center (76). This force has been shown to be only 67% of the total force applied to the hand rim. A representative sample of the hand rim forces produced at a velocity of 1.39 m/s and a power output of 0.5 W/kg is illustrated in Figure 10-45 (79). In this example, the downward forces applied to the hand rim were nearly twice the horizontal forward directed forces. The outward force was the lowest of the three forces and increased only in the last third of the push phase. The actual propelling force can be calculated by dividing the torque at the hand rim by the radius from the wheel axle to the hand rim (80).

One of the main factors that determines the force application direction is the cost associated with each particular force application. If a force is applied perpendicular to a line from the hand to the elbow or from the hand to the shoulder, the cost increases at each joint (65). The posture of each individual influences the cost and effect as a result of each individual sitting in the wheelchair and holding the rim at a certain point. Large joint reaction forces generated in the shoulder joint change with hand position. For example, the shoulder joint mean forces at top dead center and at 15° relative to top dead center were computed to be 1900 and 1750 N, respectively, and were approximately 10 times the mean net forces at the joint (76).

The propulsion technique also influences the output. A circular propulsion technique has been shown to generate less mean power (37.1 watts) than the pumping technique (44.4 watts) (81). Individual differences in shoulder and elbow positions can also influence propulsion effectiveness. For example, if an individual lowers the shoulder during the push phase, a more vertical and less effective propulsive force might result.

The construction of the wheelchair can also influence propulsion. The axle position relative to the shoulder changes the push rim biomechanics significantly. If the vertical distance between the axle and the shoulder is increased, the push angle is decreased and the force available for propulsion is diminished (10). Improvements in wheelchair propulsion have been shown to be associated with a wheelchair having a more forward axle position (10). Also, cambered rear wheels whose top distance between the wheels is smaller than the bottom orient the hand rim to more closely resemble the force application. This facilitates a more effective use of elbow extension (80).

Summary

Linear kinetics is the branch of mechanics that deals with the causes of linear motion, or forces. All forces have magnitude, direction, point of application, and line of action. Forces may be categorized as noncontact or contact. The most important noncontact force acting during human movement is gravity. The contact forces include the GRF, joint reaction force, friction, fluid resistance, inertial force, muscle force, and elastic force. The GRF, a direct application of Newton's third law, has three components: a vertical component and two shear components acting parallel to the surface of the ground. The joint reaction force, the net force acting across a joint, has compressive and shear components. Friction results from interaction between two surfaces and is a force acting parallel to the interface of the two surfaces and in a direction opposite to the motion. The coefficient of friction is the quantification of the interaction of the two surfaces. Fluid resistance refers to the transfer of energy from an object to the fluid through which the object is moving. The fluid resistance vector has two components, lift and drag. Drag acts in a direction opposite to the direction of motion and lift is perpendicular to the drag component. Inertia results from the force applied by one segment on another that is not due to muscle actions. A muscle force is the pull of the muscle on its insertion, resulting in motion at a joint. Muscle forces are generally calculated as net forces, not individual muscle forces, although intricate mathematical procedures can evaluate individual muscle forces. An elastic force results from the rebound of a material to its original length once it has been deformed.

A free body diagram is a schematic illustration of a system with all external forces represented by vector arrows at their points of application. Internal forces are not presented on free body diagrams. Muscle forces are generally not represented on these diagrams unless the system involves a single segment.

These mechanical laws governing the motion of objects were developed by Sir Isaac Newton and form the basis for the mechanical analysis of human motion:

1. Law of inertia: Every body continues in its state of rest or uniform motion in a straight line unless acted upon by an external force.

2. Law of acceleration: The rate change of change of momentum of a body is proportional to the force causing it, and the change takes place in the direction of the force.

3. Law of action–reaction: For every action there is an equal and opposite reaction.

Analyses using Newton's law are usually conducted using one of three calculations: (*a*) the effect of a force at an instant in time (F = ma); (*b*) the effect of a force applied over time (impulse–momentum relationship); and (*c*) the effect of a force applied over a distance (work–energy theorem).

In the first technique, the analysis may be a static case (when a = 0) or a dynamic case (when a = 0). The static two-dimensional linear case is determined using the following equations:

$$\Sigma F_x = 0 \text{ for the horizontal component}$$
$$\Sigma F_y = 0 \text{ for the vertical component}$$

The 2-dimensional dynamic case uses the following equations:

$$\Sigma F_x = ma_x \text{ for the horizontal component}$$
$$\Sigma F_y = ma_y \text{ for the vertical component}$$

The impulse–momentum relationship relates the force applied over time to the change in momentum:

$$F * dt = mv_{final} - mv_{initial}$$

The left-hand side of the equation (F * dt) is the impulse, while the right-hand side ($mv_{final} - mv_{initial}$) describes the change in momentum. Impulse is defined as the area under the force–time curve and thus is equal to the change in momentum. This type of analysis has been used in research to evaluate the jump height of the center of mass in vertical jumping in association with the equations of constant acceleration.

Special force applications include definitions for centripetal force, pressure, mechanical work, energy, and power. Pressure is the force per unit area. Work is the product of the force applied and the distance over which the force is applied. Energy, the capacity to do work, has two forms, kinetic and potential. The relationship between work and energy is defined in the work–energy theorem, which states that the amount of work done is equal to the change in energy. Mechanical work is calculated via the change in mechanical energy. That is:

$$W = \Sigma KE + \Sigma PE$$

where KE is the translational kinetic energy and PE is the potential energy. Work can be calculated for either a single segment or for the total body. When this is done segment by segment, internal work or the work done on the segments by the muscles to move the segments is calculated. When the amount of work done is related to the time over which the work was done, the power developed is being evaluated.

Equation Review for Linear Kinetics

Calculation	Given	Formula
Vector composition: magnitude of resultant force	Horizontal, vertical forces	$R^2 = F_x^2 + F_y^2$
Angle of force application	Horizontal, vertical forces	$\tan \theta = \dfrac{F_y}{F_x}$
Vertical force	Resultant force, angle of application	$F_y = R \sin \theta$
Horizontal force	Resultant force, angle of application	$F_x = R \cos \theta$
Acceleration (a)	Force (F), mass (m)	$a = \dfrac{F}{m}$
Vertical acceleration (a)	Vertical force (F_y), mass (m)	$a_y = \dfrac{(F_y - mg)}{m}$
Force	Acceleration, mass	$F = ma$
Weight (W)	Mass	$W = ma = mg$
Momentum (p)	Mass, velocity	$p = mv$
Impulse	Momentum (m * v)	$\text{Impulse} = mv_{final} - mv_{initial}$
Velocity	Force, time, mass	$V = \dfrac{F * t}{m}$
Force	Momentum, time of force application	$F = \dfrac{mv}{t}$
Friction force (F_f)	Normal force (N), coefficient of friction μ	$F_f = \mu N$
Coefficient of friction	Frictional force and normal force	$\mu = \dfrac{F_f}{N}$
Coefficient of friction	Ground reaction force data	$\mu = \dfrac{F_y}{F_z}$
Fluid resistance drag force	Coefficient of drag (C_d), frontal area of object (A), fluid viscosity (ρ), velocity of object relative to the fluid (v)	$F_{drag} = \dfrac{1}{2} C_d\, A\, \rho\, v^2$
Centripetal force	Mass of object (m), tangential velocity (v), radius of rotation (r)	$F_c = \dfrac{m\, v^2}{r}$
Centripetal force	Mass of object (m), angular velocity (ω), radius of rotation (r)	$F_c = m\, \omega^2\, r$
Pressure	Force, area	$P = \dfrac{F}{A}$
Work	Force, displacement (s)	$W = Fs$
Work	Changes in kinetic energy (KE)	$W = \dfrac{1}{2}mv_2^2 - \dfrac{1}{2}mv_1^2$
Horizontal work	Force, angle of force application, displacement	$W = F \cos \theta\, s$
Potential energy (PE)	Mass, vertical height (h)	$PE = mgh$
Kinetic energy (KE)	Mass, velocity	$KE = \dfrac{1}{2}mv^2$
Strain energy (SE)	Proportionality constant (k), distance object deformed (Δx)	$SE = \dfrac{1}{2}k\, \Delta x$
Power	Work (W), time (t)	$P = \dfrac{W}{t}$
Power	Force, velocity	$P = Fv$

REVIEW QUESTIONS

True or False

1. ____ Weight is a good measure of inertia.

2. ____ Muscle forces are always applied via a pull rather than a push.

3. ____ When a force vector is resolved into horizontal and vertical components, the orthogonal components are always less than the magnitude of the resultant vector.

4. ____ The force of gravity is the same no matter where in the world a person is.

5. ____ The force applied to a javelin by air resistance can both assist and retard its flight.

6. ____ The anteroposterior GRF in walking is much greater than the vertical GRF.

7. ____ An object cannot move unless a force is applied to it.

8. ____ The rate at which work is performed is termed potential energy.

9. ____ Force is a scalar quantity.

10. ____ Concurrent forces acting in the same plane can be combined using composition.

11. ____ A spinning ball will curve in the direction of the spin because of the Magnus effect.

12. ____ An efficient force application to the rim in wheelchair propulsion is not always directed tangentially along the rim.

13. ____ Impulse can be measured directly by calculating the area under a force–time curve.

14. ____ All segmental movements in the body occur as a result of a contact force generated by muscles.

15. ____ An object with a mass of 100 kg cannot be lifted unless the force applied is greater than 981 N.

16. ____ Two individuals are being measured on the force platform as they perform vertical jumps. The lighter of the two will always generate a lower vertical impulse value.

17. ____ The anteroposterior GRF for a runner moving at a constant pace is constant.

18. ____ A heavier person will have an easier time walking across an icy pond because of higher friction.

19. ____ Laminar flow usually occurs only at high velocities.

20. ____ The larger the area, the greater the pressure.

21. ____ Center of pressure is a displacement measure.

22. ____ A long jumper in flight has only kinetic energy and no strain or potential energy.

23. ____ Successful golfers maximize the acceleration of the club in the initial stages of the downswing.

24. ____ In static analysis, the sum of all of the forces acting on the body always equals zero.

25. ____ Mechanical work can be computed by measuring the change in energy.

Multiple Choice

1. What are the horizontal and vertical components of a force with a magnitude of 72 N acting at 16° to the horizontal?
   a. $F_y = 15.22$ N $F_x = 4.94$ N
   b. $F_x = 19.85$ N $F_y = 69.21$ N
   c. $F_y = 19.85$ N $F_x = 69.21$ N
   d. $F_x = 15.22$ N $F_y = 4.94$ N

2. The horizontal and vertical components of a force are 32.52 N and 12.23 N, respectively. What is the magnitude of the resultant vector?
   a. 1207.12 N
   b. 30.13 N
   c. 907.98 N
   d. 34.74 N

3. How much force must be exerted to accelerate a 240-N weight to 5.7 m/s²?
   a. 136.45 N
   b. 1368 N
   c. 42.1 N
   d. 413.1 N

4. What is the coefficient of friction if the friction force is 77.4 N the normal force is 120 N?
   a. 1.37
   b. 1.55
   c. 0.65
   d. 0.74

5. If an individual's thigh exerts a force of 9.1 N at a velocity of 1.4 m/s, what is the power generated by the thigh?
   a. 1.30 W
   b. 7.70 W
   c. 6.50 W
   d. 12.74 W

6. If the static coefficient of friction of a basketball shoe on a particular playing surface is 0.51 and the normal force is 820 N, what horizontal force is necessary to cause the shoe to slide?
   a. 1607.8 N
   b. 42.6 N
   c. 418.2 N
   d. 163.89

7. An individual lifts a 95-kg weight to a height of 2.13 m. When the weight is held overhead, what is the potential energy? What is the kinetic energy?
   a. PE = 202.4 Nm, KE = 202.4 Nm
   b. PE = 202.4 Nm, KE = 0.0 Nm
   c. PE = 1985.1 Nm, KE = 0.0 Nm
   d. PE = 1985.1 Nm, KE = 1985.1 Nm

8. Calculate the impulse in the following graph.

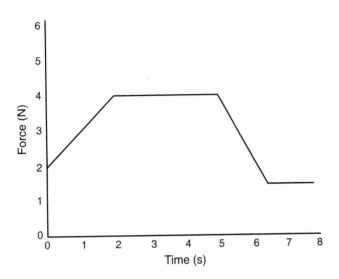

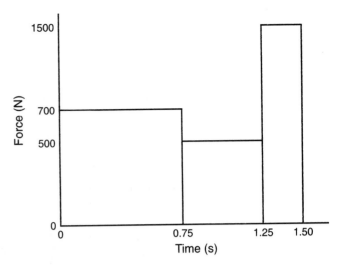

a. 32.0 Ns
b. 25.5 Ns
c. 29.0 Ns
d. 28.5 Ns

9. Consider the following free body diagram. Using static analysis, solve for the horizontal and vertical forces of C that will maintain this system in equilibrium if A = 110 N, B = 85 N, and W = 45 N.

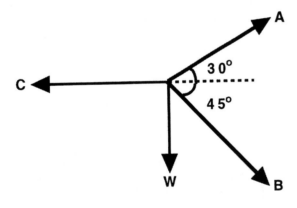

a. $F_y = 50.1$ N, $F_x = 155.4$ N
b. $F_y = 160.1$ N, $F_x = 155.4$ N
c. $F_y = 50.1$ N, $F_x = 35.2$ N
d. $F_y = 160.1$ N, $F_x = 35.2$ N

10. Calculate the height of the center of mass above its starting height during a squat jump based on the following information: body weight = 670 N; total vertical force = 788 N; time of force application = 0.9 s.
a. 0.78 m
b. 5.50 m
c. 0.12 m
d. 1.45 m

11. Calculate the height of the center of mass above its starting height during a jump based on the following hypothetical graph (jumper's weight = 700 N).

a. 0.31 m
b. 0.22 m
c. 1.03 m
d. 0.10 m

12. An object accelerates at 4.7 m/s^2 after a force of 810 N is applied. What is the mass of the object?
a. 78.33 kg
b. 82.56 kg
c. 165.14 kg
d. 172.34 kg

13. An object weighing 1100 N accelerates upward at a rate of 4.1 m/s^2. How much force was applied?
a. 1559.73 N
b. 459.73 N
c. 4510 N
d. 268.29 N

14. A 7000-kg truck starts to roll down a road with a 30° incline. People rush to stop it. How much force must they apply to stop it? How much force is required to prevent a 5000-kg truck from rolling down a 40° incline?
a. 68670 N
b. 3500 N
c. 34335 N
d. 59468 N

15. A 115-kg football player is running toward you at 12 m/s. What impulse will you have to generate to stop him?
a. 9.6 N
b. 94 N
c. 13538 N
d. 1380 N

16. A basketball player massing 105 kg applied a vertical force of 2980 N against the ground for 0.11 s. How high did his center of mass rise during his rebound?
a. 0.46 m
b. 0.21 m
c. 0.50 m
d. 0.34 m

17. What is the momentum of a 70-kg runner sprinting at 6.3 m/s?
a. 44.1 kgm/s
b. 441 kgm/s

c. 4326.21 Nm/s

d. 432.6 Nm/s

18. A woman massing 60 kg dives from a 10-m platform. What is her potential and kinetic energy 3 m into the dive?

a. KE = 420 J, PE = 420 J

b. KE = 0 J, PE = 420 J

c. KE = 0, PE = 4120.2 J

d. KE = 4120.2 J, PE = 4120.2 J

19. A 75-kg high jumper raises his center of mass 2.5 m. What is his potential energy and kinetic energy 0.1 s after he clears the bar?

a. $PE_{0.1 s}$ = 1839.38 J , $KE_{0.1 s}$ = 36.1 J

b. $PE_{0.1 s}$ = 1803.28 J, $KE_{0.1 s}$ = 36.1 J

c. $PE_{0.1 s}$ = 1839.38 J, $KE_{0.1 s}$ = 0 J

d. $PE_{0.1 s}$ = 1803.28 J, $KE_{0.1 s}$ = 0 J

20. A constant force of 160 N acts on a body in the horizontal direction. The force moves the object forward 75 m in 2.3 s. What is the mass of the body?

a. 231.27 kg

b. 11.28 kg

c. 5.64 kg

d. 60 kg

21. A 15, 000-kg truck is traveling at 25 m/s. What would be the velocity of a 6500-kg truck with the same momentum?

a. 32.69 kgm/s

b. 56.59 kgm/s

c. 57.69 kgm/s

d. 35.67 kgm/s

22. A running back is tackled with a force of 3800 N by a linebacker weighing 1000 N. What was the acceleration of the linebacker?

a. 37.3 m/s^2

b. 3.8 m/s^2

c. 26.2 m/s^2

d. 4.1 m/s^2

23. What is the pressure on the bottom of the foot for a 75-kg person on the balls of one foot making contact over an area of approximately 100 cm^2?

a. 7500 N/cm^2

b. 0.75 N/cm^2

c. 7.36 N/cm^2

d. 73.6 N/cm^2

24. The work calculated at Time 1 and Time 2 was 178 Nm and 345 Nm, respectively. Calculate the power if the time interval was 0.049 s.

a. 8.183 W

b. 167 W

c. 10673.5 W

d. 3408.2 W

25. How much power is generated in the horizontal direction by a force of 850 N applied to an object at an angle of 25°, causing the object to move horizontally 4 m in 1.6 s?

a. 2125.0 W

b. 1925.9 W

c. 898.1 W

d. 3081.5 W

REFERENCES

1. Alexander, R. M. (1984). Elastic energy stores in running vertebrates. *American Zoologist*, 24:85–94.

2. Andres, R. O., Chaffin, D. B. (1985). Ergonomic analysis of slip-resistance measurement devices. *Ergonomics*, 28:1065–1079.

3. Asmussen, E., Bonde-Peterson, F. (1974). Apparent efficiency and storage of elastic energy in human muscles during exercise. *Acta Physiologica Scandinavica*, 92:537–545.

4. Ayoub, M. M., Mital, A. (1989). *Manual Materials Handling*. London: Taylor & Francis.

5. Barthels, K. M., Adrian, M. J. (1975). Three-dimensional spatial hand patterns of skilled butterfly swimmers. In L. Lewillie, J . P. Clarys (Eds.). *Swimming II*. Baltimore: University Park, 154–160.

6. Bates, B. T., et al. (1979). Variations of velocity within the support phase of running. In J. Terauds, G. Dales (Eds.). *Science in Athletics*. Del Mar: Academic, 51–59.

7. Bergmann, G., et al. (1995). Is staircase walking a risk for the fixation of hip implants? *Journal of Biomechanics*, 28:535–553.

8. Bobbert, M. F., et al. (1991). Calculation of vertical ground reaction force estimates during running from positional data. *Journal of Biomechanics*, 24:1095–1105.

9. Boda, W. L., Hamill, J. (1990). A mechanical model of the Maxiflex "B" springboard. *Proceedings of the VI biannual meeting of the Canadian Society of Biomechanics*. Quebec City: 109–110.

10. Boniger, M. L., et al. (1997). Wrist biomechanics during two speeds of wheelchair propulsion: An analysis using a local coordinate system. *Archives Physical Medicine Rehabilitation*, 78:364–371.

11. Brancazio, P. J. (1984). *Sports Science*. New York: Simon & Schuster.

12. Buck, P. C. (1985). Slipping, tripping and falling accidents at work: a national picture. *Ergonomics*, 28:949–958.

13. Cajori, F. (1934). Sir Isaac Newton's Mathematical Principles (translated by Andrew Motte in 1729). Berkeley, CA: University of California.

14. Cavagna, G. A., et al. (1976). The sources of external work in level walking and running. *Journal of Physiology*, 262:639–657.

15. Cavanagh, P. R. (1989). The biomechanics of running and running shoe problems. In B. Segesser, W. Pforringer (Eds.). *The Shoe in Sport*. London: Wolfe, 3–15.

16. Cavanagh, P. R., Lafortune, M. A. (1980). Ground reaction forces in distance running. *Journal of Biomechanics*, 15:397–406.

17. Chaffin, D. B., Andersson, G. B. J. (1991). *Occupational Biomechanics* (2nd Ed.). New York: Wiley.

18. Clarke, T. E., et al. (1983). The effects of shoe cushioning upon ground reaction forces in running. *International Journal of Sports Medicine*, 4:376–381.

19. Cohen, H. H., Compton, D. M. J. (1982, June). Fall accident patterns. *Professional Safety*, 16–22.

20. Detrembleur, C., et al. (2000). Motion of the body center of gravity as a summary indicator of the mechanics of human pathological gait. *Gait and Posture*, 12:243–250.

21. DeVita, P., Skelly, WA. (1992). Effect of landing stiffness on joint kinetics and energetics in the lower extremity. *Medicine and Science in Sports and Exercise*, 24:108–115.

22. Dixon, S. J., et al. (2000). Surface effects on ground reaction forces and lower extremity kinematics in running. *Medicine and Science in Sports and Exercise,* 32:1919–1926.

23. Dowling, J. J., Vamos, L. (1993). Identification of kinetic and temporal factors related to vertical jump performance. *Journal of Applied Biomechanics,* 9:95–110.

24. Dufek, J. S., Bates, B. T. (1990). The evaluation and prediction of impact forces during landings. *Medicine and Science in Sports and Exercise,* 22:370–377.

25. Dufek, J. S., Bates, B. T. (1991). Dynamic performance assessment of selected sport shoes on impact forces. *Medicine and Science in Sports and Exercise,* 23:1062–1067.

26. Elftman, H. (1939). Forces and energy changes in the leg during walking. *American Journal of Physiology,* 125:339–356.

27. Elliott, B. C., White, E. (1989). A kinematic and kinetic analysis of the female two point and three point jump shots in basketball. *Australian Journal of Science and Medicine in Sport,* 21:7–11.

28. Fallon, L. P., et al. (2000). Determining baseball bat performance using a conservation equations model with field test validation. In A. J. Subic, S. J. Haake (Eds.). *The Engineering of Sport: Research, Development, and Innovation.* Oxford: Blackwell Science, 201–211.

29. Farley, C. T., Ferris, D. P. (1998). Biomechanics of walking and running: Center of mass movements to muscle action. In J. Holloszy (Ed.). *Exercise and Sport Science Reviews,* 253–281.

30. Foti, T., et al. (1992). Influence of footwear on weight-acceptance plantar pressure distribution during walking. In R. Rodano (Ed.). *Biomechanics in Sports X.* Milan: Edi-Ermes, 243–246.

31. Gatt, C. J., et al. (1999). A kinetic analysis of the knees during a golf swing. In M. R. Farrally, A. J. Cochran (Eds). Science and Golf III: Proceedings of the 1998 World Scientific Congress of Golf. Champaign, IL: Human Kinetics, 20–28.

32. Giddings, V. L., et al. (2000). Calcaneal loading during walking and running. *Medicine Science in Sports and Exercise,* 32:627–634.

33. Hamill, J., Bates, B. T. (1988). A kinetic evaluation of the effects of in vivo loading on running shoes. *Journal of Orthopaedic and Sports Physical Therapy,* 10:47–53.

34. Hamill, J., et al. (1984). Ground reaction force symmetry during walking and running. *Research Quarterly for Exercise and Sport,* 55:289–293.

35. Hamill, J., et al. (1989). Relationship between selected static and dynamic lower extremity measures. *Clinical Biomechanics,* 4:217–225.

36. Hamill, J., et al. (1983). Variations in ground reaction force parameters at different running speeds. *Human Movement Science,* 2:47–56.

37. Hamill, J., et al. (1987). The effect of track turns on lower extremity function. *International Journal of Sports Biomechanics,* 3:276–286.

38. Harman, E. A., et al. (1990). The effects of arms and countermovement on vertical jumping. *Medicine and Science in Sports and Exercise,* 22:825–833.

39. Hawkins, D., Hull, M. L. (1993). Muscle force as affected by fatigue: Mathematical model and experimental verification. *Journal of Biomechanics,* 26:1117–1128.

40. Hintermeister, R. A., Hamill, J. (1992, August). Mechanical power and energy in level treadmill running. *Proceedings of the North American Congress Of Biomechanics II.* Chicago, 213–214.

41. Komi, P. V. (1990). Relevance of in vivo force measurements to human biomechanics. *Journal of Biomechanics,* 23:23–34.

42. Komi, P. V., Bosco, C. (1978). Utilization of stored elastic energy in leg extensor muscles by men and women. *Medicine and Science in Sports,* 10:261–265.

43. Komi, P. V., et al. (1987). In vivo registration of Achilles tendon forces in man. I. Methodological development. *International Journal of Sports Medicine,* 8:3–8, Supplement.

44. Kyle, C. R. (1989). The wind resistance of the human figure in sports. *Proceedings of the First IOC World Congress on Sports Sciences.* Colorado Springs, 287–288.

45. Kyle, C. R., Caizzo, V. L. (1986). The effect of athletic clothing aerodynamics upon running speed. *Medicine and Science in Sports and Exercise,* 18:509–513.

46. Lees, A. (1981). Methods of impact absorption when landing from a jump. *Engineering Medicine,* 10:207–211.

47. Mather, J. S. B. (2000). Innovative golf clubs designed for the amateur. In A. J. Subic, S. J. Haake (Eds.). *The Engineering of Sport: Research, Development and Innovation.* Malden: Blackwell Science, 61–68.

48. Mather, J. S. B., Jowett, S. (2000). Three-dimensional shape of the golf club during the swing. In A. J. Subic, S. J. Haake (Eds.). *The Engineering of Sport: Research, Development and Innovation.* Malden: Blackwell Science, 77–85.

49. McMahon, T. A., Greene, P. R. (1978). Fast running tracks. *Scientific American,* 239(6):148–163.

50. McMahon, T. A., Greene, P. R. (1979). The influence of track compliance on running. *Journal of Biomechanics,* 12:893–904.

51. McNitt-Gray, J. L. (1991). Kinematics and impulse characteristics of drop landings from three heights. *International Journal of Sports Biomechanics,* 7:201–224.

52. Miller, D. I., Nelson, R. C. (1973). *Biomechanics of Sport.* Philadelphia: Lea & Febiger.

53. Miller, D. I. (1990). Ground reaction forces in distance running. In P. R. Cavanagh (Ed.). *Biomechanics of Distance Running.* Champaign, IL: Human Kinetics, 203–224.

54. Munro, C. F., et al. (1987). Ground reaction forces in running: a re-examination. *Journal of Biomechanics,* 20:147–155.

55. Neal, R. J., Wilson, B. D. (1985). 3D kinematics and kinetics of the golf swing. *International Journal of Sports Biomechanics,* 1:221–232.

56. Nigg, B. M. (1983). External force measurements with sports shoes and playing surfaces. In B. M. Nigg, B. Kerr (Eds.). *Biomechanical Aspects of Sports Shoes and Playing Surfaces.* Calgary: University of Calgary, 11–23.

57. Nigg, B. M., et al. (2000). *Biomechanics and Biology of Movement.* Champaign, IL: Human Kinetics.

58. Norman, R. W., et al. (1976). Re-examination of the mechanical efficiency of horizontal treadmill running. In P. V. Komi (Ed.). *Biomechanics V-B.* Baltimore: University Park, 87–93.

59. Ozguven, H. N., Berme, N. (1988). An experimental and analytical study of impact forces during human jumping. *Journal of Biomechanics,* 21:1061–1066.

60. Pandy, M. G., Zajac, F. E. (1991). Optimal muscular coordination strategies for jumping. *Journal of Biomechanics,* 24:1–10.

61. Panzer, V. P, et al. (1988). Lower extremity loads in landings of elite gymnasts. In G. deGroot et al. (Eds.). *Biomechanics XI*. Amsterdam: Free University Press, 727–735.

62. Pierrynowski, M. R., et al. (1980). Mechanical energy transfer in treadmill walking. *Ergonomics*, 24: 1–14.

63. Ramey, M. R., Williams, K. R. (1985). Ground reaction forces in the triple jump. *International Journal of Sport Biomechanics*, 1: 233–239.

64. Rogers, M. M. (1988). Dynamic biomechanics of the normal foot and ankle during walking and running. *Physical Therapy*, 68:1822–1830.

65. Rozendaal, L. A., Veeger, H. E. J. (2000). Force direction in manual wheel chair propulsion: balance between effect and cost. *Clinical Biomechanics*, 15:S39–S41.

66. Sayers, S. P., et al. (1999). Cross-validation of three jump power equations. *Medicine and Science in Sports and Exercise*, 31:572–577.

67. Schleihauf, R. E. (1979). A hydrodynamic analysis of swimming propulsion. In J. Terauds, E. W. Bedington (Eds.). *Swimming III*. Baltimore: University Park Press, 70–109.

68. Scott, S. H., Winter, D. A. (1990). Internal forces at chronic running injury sites. *Medicine and Science in Sports and Exercise*, 22:357–369.

69. Scott, S. H., Winter, D. A. (1991). Talocrural and talocalcaneal joint kinematics and kinetics during the stance phase of walking. *Journal of Biomechanics*, 24:743–752.

70. Simpson, K. J., Jiang, P. (1999). Foot landing position during gait influences ground reaction forces. *Clinical Biomechanics*, 14:396–402.

71. Sprigings, E., et al. (1989). Development of a model to represent an aluminum springboard in diving. *International Journal of Sport Biomechanics*, 5:297–307.

72. Tesio, L., et al. (1998). The 3-D motion of the center of gravity of the human body during level walking. I. Normal subjects at low and intermediate walking speeds. *Clinical Biomechanics*, 13:77–82.

73. Valiant, G. A. (1987). Ground reaction forces developed on artificial turf. In H. Reilly and A. Lees (Eds.). *Proceedings of the First World Congress of Science and Medicine in Football*. London: E&FN, 143–158.

74. Valiant, G. A., Cavanagh, P. R. (1985). A study of landing from a jump: Implications for the design of a basketball shoe. In D. A. Winter et al. (Eds.) *Biomechanics IX-B*. Champaign, IL: Human Kinetics, 117–122.

75. Valiant, G. A., et al. (1986). Measurements of the rotational friction of court shoes on an oak hardwood playing surface. *Proceedings of the North American Congress on Biomechanics*. 295–296.

76. Van der Helm, F. C. T., Veeger, H. E. J. (1996). Quasi-static analysis of muscle forces in the shoulder mechanism during wheelchair propulsion. *Journal of Biomechanics*, 29:39–52.

77. van Ingen Schenau, G. J. (1982). The influence of air friction in speed skating. *Journal of Biomechanics*, 16:449–453.

78. Vanlandewijck, Y. C., et al. (1994). Wheelchair propulsion efficiency: Movement pattern adaptations to speed changes. *Medicine and Science in Sports and Exercise*, 26:1373–1381.

79. Veeger, H. E., et al. (1989). Wheelchair propulsion technique at different speeds. *Scandinavian Journal of Rehabilitation Medicine*, 21:197–203.

80. Veeger, H. E. J., et al. (1991). Load on the upper extremity in manual wheelchair propulsion. *Journal of Electromyography and Kinesiology*, 1:270–280.

81. Walpert, R. A., Kyle, C. J. (1989). Aerodynamics of the human body in sports. *XII International Congress of Biomechanics Proceedings*. 346–347.

82. White, S. C., Winter, D. A. (1985). Mechanical power analysis of the lower limb musculature in race walking. *International Journal of Sports Biomechanics*, 1:15–24.

83. Williams, K. R. (1980). A biomechanical and physiological evaluation of running efficiency. Unpublished doctoral dissertation, The Pennsylvania State University.

84. Williams, K. R., Cavanagh P. R. (1983). A model for the calculation of mechanical power during distance running. *Journal of Biomechanics*, 16: 115–128.

85. Williams, K. R., Cavanagh, P. R. (1983). The mechanics of foot action during the golf swing and implications for shoe design. *Medicine and Science in Sports and Exercise*, 15:247–255.

86. Williams, K. R., Sih, B. L. (1999). Ground reaction forces in regular-spike and alternative-spike golf shoes. In M. R. Farrally, A. J. Cochran (Eds.). *Science and Golf III: Proceedings of the 1998 World Scientific Congress of Golf*. Champaign, IL: Human Kinetics, 568–575.

87. Winter, D. A. (1979). A new definition of mechanical work done in human movement. *Journal of Applied Physiology*, 46: 79–83.

88. Winter, D. A. (1990). *Biomechanics and Motor Control of Human Movement* (2nd Ed.). New York: Wiley.

ADDITIONAL READING

Alexander, R. M. (1988). *Elastic Mechanisms in Animal Movement*. Cambridge: Cambridge University Press.

Bobbert, M. F., van Ingen Schenau, G. J. (1988). Coordination in vertical jumping. *Journal of Biomechanics*, 21:249–262.

Frohlich, C. (1981). Aerodynamic effects on discus flight. *American Journal of Physics*, 49:1125–1132.

Greene, P. R. (1980). Sprinting with banked turns. *Journal of Biomechanics*, 20:667–680.

Pugh, L. (1971). The influence of wind resistance in running and walking and the mechanical efficiency of work against horizontal and vertical forces. *Journal of Physiology*, 213:255–276.

Nigg, B. M., Herzog, W. (1995). *Biomechanics of the Musculoskeletal System*. New York: Wiley.

Putnam, C. A., Kozey, J. W. (1985). Substantive issues in running. In C. L. Vaughn (Ed.). *Biomechanics of Sport*. Boca Raton, FL: CRC, 1–33.

Schirer, E. W., Allman, W. F. (1984). *Newton at the Bat: The Science in Sports*. New York: Scribner.

van Ingen Schenau, G. J., Cavanagh, P. R. (1990). Power equations in endurance sports. *Journal of Biomechanics*, 23:865–881.

Whiting, W. C., Zernicke, R. F. (1998). *Biomechanics of Musculoskeletal Injury*. Champaign, IL: Human Kinetics.

Winter, D. A. (1987). Mechanical power in human movement: Generation, absorption, and transfer. In B. van Gheluwe and J. Atha (Eds.). *Current Research in Sports Biomechanics*. New York: Karger, 34–45.

GLOSSARY

Active Peak: The second of the two peaks in a vertical ground reaction force curve during running.

Angle of Application: The angle at which a force vector acts.

Bernoulli's Principle: The relationship between pressure and velocity that states that pressure is inversely proportional to velocity.

Bone-on-Bone Force: The force at a joint that includes the joint reaction force and the forces due to muscles and ligaments.

Boundary Layer: The thin layer of a fluid adjacent to the surface of an object moving through the fluid.

Center of Pressure: The point of application of a force.

Centripetal Force: The force acting toward the center of rotation resulting when an object moves along a curved path.

Coefficient of Friction: The ratio of the friction force to the normal force pressing two surfaces together.

Collinear Forces: Forces whose lines of action are the same.

Composition: The process by which the resultant of two vectors is determined.

Concurrent Forces: Forces whose lines of action operate at the same point.

Contact Force: The pushes or pulls exerted by one object in direct contact with another object.

Coplanar Forces: Forces whose lines of action all act in the same plane.

Density: Mass per unit volume.

Dynamic Analysis: A calculation of the forces and moments when there are significant linear and/or angular accelerations.

Dynamics: The branch of mechanics that studies accelerating systems.

Energy: The capacity to do work.

External Work: The work done by a body on another body.

Fluid Resistance: The transfer of energy from an object to the fluid through which the object is moving.

Force: Interaction between two objects in the form of a push or pull that may or may not cause motion.

Force Platform: A device that measures ground reaction force.

Form Drag: Net resistance force caused by a pressure differential between the leading and trailing edges of an object moving through a fluid.

Free Body Diagram: A diagram in which all force vectors are drawn.

Friction: The force that resists the motion of one surface upon another.

Impact Peak: The initial peak on a vertical ground reaction force.

Impulse: The product of the magnitude of a force and its time of application; the area under a force–time curve.

Impulse–Momentum Relationship: The relationship stating that the impulse is equal to the change in momentum.

Inertia: The resistance of a body to a change in its state of motion.

Internal Work: The total work done resulting from the motion of all of the body's segments.

Inverse Dynamics: An analytical approach calculating the forces and moments based on the accelerations of the object.

Joint Reaction Force: The force acting across a joint.

Kinetic Energy: The ability of a body to do work by virtue of its motion.

Kinetics: The branch of mechanics that deals with forces acting on a system.

Kinetic Friction: Friction between two surfaces as they slide on each other.

Laminar Flow: At slow flow velocities, the flow of a fluid smoothly over the surface of an object.

Law of Conservation of Energy: The law that states that energy can neither be created nor destroyed but can only change form.

Linear Kinetics: The branch of kinetics that deals with translational motion.

Line of Action: The line along which a force acts.

Lift Force: A component of fluid resistance force that acts perpendicular to the direction of motion.

Loading Peak: See active peak.

Magnus Effect: The curve in the path of a spinning ball caused by a pressure differential on either side of the ball.

Mass: The measure of a body's inertia.

Maximum Static Friction Force: The maximum friction force measured just prior to the impending motion of an object.

Noncontact Force: A force that acts at a distance from an object.

Passive Peak: See impact peak.

Point of Application: The point at which a force acts.

Point of Separation: The point at which the boundary layer separates from an object.

Potential Energy: The ability of a body to do work by virtue of its position.

Power: The quantity of work done per unit time.

Pressure: Force per unit area.

Resolution: The breakdown of a vector into its horizontal and vertical components.

Rotational Friction: The resistance in rotation of one surface upon another.

Separated Flow: The type of fluid flow in which the boundary layer separates from the object, creating turbulence and thus resisting the motion of the object.

Shear Force: A force that acts parallel to the surface.

Statics: The branch of mechanics in which the system being studied undergoes no acceleration.

Strain Energy: The capacity to do work by virtue of the deformation of an object.

Surface Drag: The fluid drag force acting on a body resulting from the friction between the surface of the object and the fluid.

System: A defined set of forces.

Turbulent Flow: The type of fluid flow in which the boundary layer becomes so turbulent that the point of separation moves farther back on the object, thus reducing drag.

Viscous Drag: See surface drag.

Viscosity: The measure of a fluid's resistance to flow.

Weight: The force of the earth's gravitational attraction to a body's mass.

Work: The product of the force applied to a body and the distance through which the force is applied.

Work–Energy Theorem: The relationship between work and energy stating that the work done is equal to the change in energy.

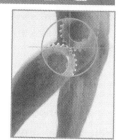

Angular Kinetics

OBJECTIVES

After reading this chapter, the student should be able to:

1. Define torque and discuss the characteristics of a torque.

2. Define the concept of center of mass.

3. Discuss the different methods of determining body segment parameters for the calculation of center of mass.

4. Calculate the segment center of mass and the total body center of mass.

5. Discuss the concept of moment of inertia.

6. Differentiate between the three classes of levers.

7. State the angular analogs of Newton's three laws of motion and their impact on human movement.

8. Understand the impact of angular momentum on human motion.

9. Discuss the relationships between torque, angular work, rotational kinetic energy, and angular power.

10. Define and conduct a static analysis on a single joint motion.

11. Define stability and discuss its effect on human movement.

12. Define and conduct a dynamic analysis on a single joint motion.

13. Define the impulse–momentum relationship.

14. Discuss selected research studies that have used an angular kinetic approach.

15. Solve quantitative problems that employ angular kinetic principles.

Chapter 10 discussed the notion that movement does not occur unless an external force is applied. Also discussed were the characteristics of a force, two of which were the line of action and the point of application. If the line of action and the point of application of a force are critical, it would appear that the type of motion produced may depend on these characteristics. For example, a nurse pushing a wheelchair exerts two equal forces, one on each handle. The result is that the lines of action and points of application of the two forces cause the wheelchair to move in a straight line. What happens, though, when the nurse pushes the chair with only one arm, applying a force to only one of the handles? A force is still applied, but the motion is totally different. In fact, the wheelchair will translate and rotate (Fig. 11-1). The situation that has just been described actually represents most of the types of motion that occur when humans move. It is rare that a force or a system of forces cause pure translation. In fact, the majority of force applications in human movement cause simultaneous translation and rotation.

The branch of mechanics that deals with the causes of motion is called kinetics. The branch of mechanics that deals with the causes of angular motion is called **angular kinetics**.

Torque or Moment of Force

When a force causes a rotation, the rotation occurs about a pivot point, and the line of action of the force must act at a distance from the pivot point. When a force is applied so that it causes a rotation, the product of that force and the perpendicular distance to its line of action is referred to as a **torque** or a **moment of force**. These terms are synonymous and are used interchangeably in the literature. A torque is not a force but merely the effect of a force in causing a rotation. A torque is defined, therefore, as the tendency of a force to cause a rotation about a specific axis.

CHARACTERISTICS OF A TORQUE

There are two important components of a torque: magnitude of the force and the shortest or perpendicular distance from the pivot point to the line of action of the force. Also, any discussion of a torque must be with reference to a specific axis serving as the pivot point. Mathematically, torque is:

$$T = F * r$$

where T is the torque, F is the applied force in newtons, and r is the perpendicular distance in meters from the line of action of the force to the pivot point. Since torque is

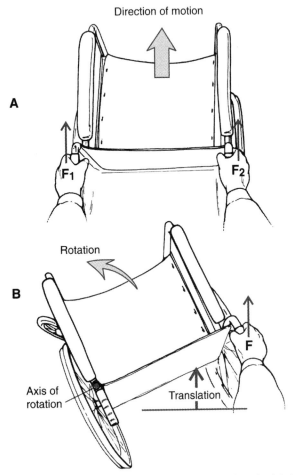

FIGURE 11-1 An overhead view of a wheelchair. **A.** The wheelchair is translated forward by forces F_1 and F_2. **B.** The wheelchair will rotate and translate if only one force, F_1, is applied.

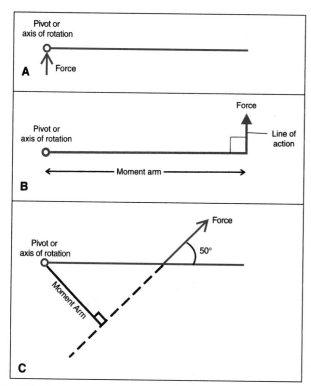

FIGURE 11-2 When a force is applied, it will cause no rotation if it is applied through the pivot point **(A)**, or it will generate a torque if the force is applied a distance from the axis **(B and C)**. The moment arm (MA) is the perpendicular distance from the line of action of the force to the axis of rotation.

the product of a force, with units of newtons, and a distance, with units of meters, torque has units of newton-meters (Nm). The distance, r, is referred to as the **moment arm** of the force. This concept is illustrated in Figure 11-2. If the force acts directly through the pivot point or the axis of rotation, the torque is zero, because the moment arm would be zero regardless of how great the force (Fig. 11-2*A*). In Figure 11-2*B*, a force of 20 N is applied perpendicular to a lever at a point 1.1 m from the axis. Because the force is applied perpendicular to the lever, the shortest distance to the axis is the distance from the point of contact of the force to the axis. The torque generated by this force can be computed as:

$$T = F * r$$
$$T = 20\,N * 1.1\,m$$
$$T = 22\,Nm$$

The torque generated by a nonperpendicular force applied to a lever can be calculated using trigonometric functions. An example of a 20-N force applied 1.1 m from the axis or rotation at an angle of 50° to the lever is shown in Figure 11-2*C*. The torque can be computed one of two ways. One way is to compute the vertical component of the force and multiply that value by the distance from the point of attachment to the axis. The computation would be:

$$T = F \sin \theta * r$$
$$T = 20 \sin 50° * 1.1\,m$$
$$T = 15.32\,M * 1.1\,m$$
$$T = 16.85\,Nm$$

The second computation of torque is the actual length of the moment arm multiplied by the resultant original force value. Identifying the adjacent angle and computing the side adjacent to that angle determine the length of the moment arm. The computation:

$$T = F * r \cos \theta$$
$$T = 20\,N * 1.1\,m \cos 40°$$
$$T = 20\,N * 1.1\,m * 0.766$$
$$T = 16.85\,Nm$$

When the force is not applied through the pivot point, as in Figure 11-2, *B* and *C*, a torque is said to result from an **eccentric force**, literally an off-center force. While an eccentric force primarily causes rotation, it also causes translation.

Examples of torque applications are illustrated in Figure 11-3. Force can be generated by muscles pulling a distance away from the joint (Fig. 11-3*A*), by the weight of a body segment acting downward away from a joint (Fig. 11-3*B*), or by a force coming up from the ground acting a distance away from the center of gravity (Fig. 11-3*C*).

Torque is a vector quantity and thus has magnitude and direction. The magnitude is represented by the quantity of

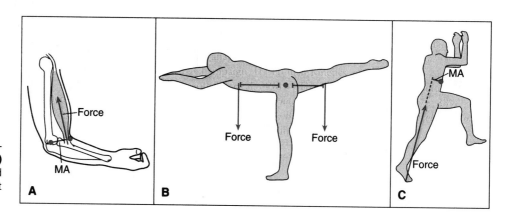

FIGURE 11-3 How torques are commonly generated by muscle force **(A)** gravitational force **(B)**, and a ground reaction force **(C)**. MA, movement arm.

the magnitude of the force times the magnitude of the moment arm. The direction is determined by the convention of the right-hand rule. As noted with angular measurement, a counterclockwise direction is considered positive (23) and a clockwise direction is negative. Thus, a counterclockwise torque is positive, while a clockwise torque is negative. Torques in a system may be evaluated through vector operations as has been described for forces. That is, torques may be composed into a resultant torque.

The concept of torque is prevalent in everyday life, for example, in the use of a wrench to loosen the nut on a bolt. Applying a force to the wrench produces rotation, causing the nut to loosen. Intuitively, the wrench is grasped at the end as in Figure 11-4A. Grasping it in this way maximizes the moment arm and hence the torque. If the wrench were grasped at its midpoint, the torque would be halved, even though the same force is applied (Fig. 11-4B). To achieve the same torque as in the first case, the force must be doubled. Thus, increasing the force, increasing the moment arm, or both, can increase a torque.

The concept of torque is often used in rehabilitation evaluation. For example, if an individual has an injured elbow, the therapist may use a manual resistance technique to evaluate the joint. The therapist would resist the individual's elbow flexion by exerting a force at the midforearm position. This creates torque, which the patient must overcome. As the individual progresses, the therapist may exert approximately the same force level at the wrist instead of the mid forearm. By increasing the moment arm while keeping the force constant, the therapist has increased the torque that the patient must overcome. This rather simple technique can be helpful to the therapist in developing a program for the individual's rehabilitation.

FORCE COUPLE

A gymnast who wishes to execute a twist about a longitudinal axis applies not one but two parallel forces in opposite directions. By applying a backward force with one foot and a forward force with the other, the gymnast creates two torques that produce rotation about the longitudinal axis (Fig. 11-5). Such a pair of forces is called a **force couple**. A force couple is two parallel forces that are equal in magnitude and that act in opposite directions. These two forces act at a distance from an axis and produce rotation about the axis. A force couple can be thought of as two moments of force, each creating a rotation about the longitudinal axis of the gymnast. Torques, however, also cause a translation, but because the translation caused by each torque is in the opposite direction, the translation of the body is canceled out. Thus, a force couple causes a pure rotation about an axis with no translation. By placing the feet slightly farther apart, the gymnast in Figure 11-5 can increase the moment arm and thus cause a great deal more rotation.

A force couple is calculated by:

$$\text{force couple} = Fd$$

where F is one of the equal and opposite forces and d is the distance between the lines of actions of the two forces. While no true force couples exist in human anatomy, the human body often uses force couples. For example, a force couple is created when one uses the thumb and forefinger to screw open the top on a jar.

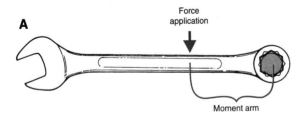

A

Force application

Moment arm

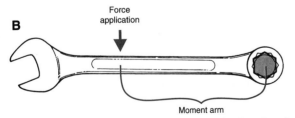

B

Force application

Moment arm

FIGURE 11-4 A wrench with two points of force application. Grasping the wrench at the end **(A)** generates more torque than a grasp near the point of rotation **(B)** because the moment arm is greater at **A** than at **B**.

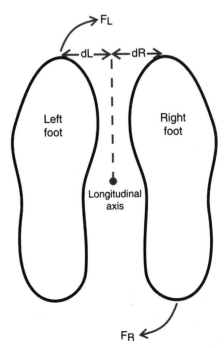

FIGURE 11-5 A torque $F_R * d_R$ is created by the right foot while another torque, $F_L * d_L$, is created by the left foot. Since these two torques are equal and in the same angular direction, the force couple will result in a rotation about the longitudinal axis through the center of mass.

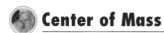 **Center of Mass**

An individual's body weight is a product of the mass and the acceleration due to gravity. The body weight vector originates at a point referred to as the **center of gravity**, or the point about which all particles of the body are evenly distributed. The point about which the body's mass is evenly distributed is referred to as the **center of mass**. The terms center of mass and center of gravity are often used synonymously. The center of gravity refers only to the vertical direction because that is the direction in which gravity acts. The more general term is the center of mass.

If the **center of mass** is the point about which the mass is evenly distributed, it must also be the balancing point of the body. Thus, the center of mass can be further defined as the point about which the sum of the torques equal zero. That is:

$$\Sigma T_{cm} = 0$$

Figure 11-6 shows an object consisting of two point masses. Point A results in a counterclockwise torque about Point C, while Point B results in a clockwise torque, also about Point C. If these two torques are equal, the object is balanced and Point C may be considered the center of mass. This does not imply that the mass of these two point masses is the same but that the torques created by the masses are equal (Fig. 11-6).

The center of mass is a theoretical point whose location may change from instant to instant during a movement. The change in position of the center of mass results from the rapidly changing positions of the body segments during movement. In fact, the center of mass does not necessarily have to be inside the limits of the object. For example, the center of mass of a doughnut is within the inner hole but outside the physical mass of the doughnut. In the case of a human performer, the positions of the segments can also place the center of mass outside the body. In activities such as high jumping and pole vaulting, in which the body must curl around the bar, the center of mass is certainly outside the limits of the body (23).

CENTER OF MASS CALCULATION: SEGMENTAL METHOD

Segment Center of Mass Calculation

There are number of ways to compute the center of mass of an object using balancing techniques, such as hanging or balancing on a reaction board. The most common method is to compute the center of mass of individual segments, which are then combined to provide the location of the center of mass of the total system. This approach, called the **segmental method**, involves knowledge of the masses and the location of the centers of mass of each of the body's segments. Two-dimensional coordinates from digitized data (x, y) and the previously mentioned properties of the segments are used to analyze one segment at a time and then calculate the total body center of mass. The estimation of the total body center of mass position is obtained by applying a model that assumes that the body is a set of rigid segments. The center of mass of the total body is calculated using the inertial parameters of each segment and its position. Before presenting the computations for this method, the source of the information concerning the body segments must be approached. At least three methods for deriving this information have been utilized. They are (*a*) measures based on cadaver studies, (*b*) mathematical geometric modeling, and (*c*) mass scanning.

Several researchers have presented formulae that estimate the mass and the location of the center of mass of the various segments based on cadaver studies (8–10,36). These researchers have generated regression or prediction equations that make it possible to estimate the mass and the location of the center of mass. Table 11-1 presents the prediction equations from Chandler et al. (8). These predicted parameters are based on known parameters, such as the total body weight or the length or circumference of the segment. An example of a regression equation based

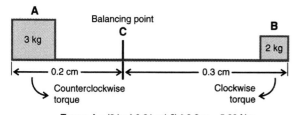

Torque A = (3 kg * 9.81 m/s²) * 0.2 m = 5.89 Nm

Torque B = (2 kg * 9.81 m/s²) * 0.3 m = 5.89 Nm

FIGURE 11-6 A two-point force system balanced at the center of mass.

TABLE 11-1 **Segment Weight Prediction Equations and Location of Center of Mass**

Segment	Weight (N)	Center of Mass[a]
Head	0.032 BW + 18.70	66.3
Trunk	0.532 BW − 6.93	52.2
Upper arm	0.022 BW + 4.76	50.7
Arm	0.013 BW + 2.41	41.7
Hand	0.005 BW + 0.75	51.5
Thigh	0.127 BW − 14.82	39.8
Leg	0.044 BW − 1.75	41.3
Foot	0.009 BW + 2.48	40.0

[a]Location from proximal end as a percentage.
From Chandler, R. F. et al. (1975). Investigation of inertial properties of the human body. AMRL Technical Report. Wright-Patterson Air Force Base, 74–137.

on Clauser et al. (9) for estimating the segment mass of the leg is as follows:

leg mass = 0.111 calf circumference
          + 0.047 tibial height
          + 0.074 ankle circumference − 4.208

where all dimensions of length are measured in centimeters. The location of the center of mass of the segment is usually presented as a percentage of the segment length from either the proximal or distal end of the segment.

Other researchers have used mathematical geometric models to predict the segment masses and locations of the center of mass. This has been done by representing the individual body segments as regular geometric solids (1,20–22). Using this method, the body segments are represented as truncated cones (e.g., upper arm, forearm, thigh, leg, and foot), cylinders (e.g., trunk), or elliptical spheres (e.g., head and hand). One such model, the Hanavan model, is presented in Figure 11-7. Regression equations based on the geometry of these solids requires the input of several measurements for each segment. For example, the thigh segment requires measurement of the circumference of the upper and lower thigh, the length of the thigh, and the total body mass to estimate the desired parameters for the segment.

The third method of determining the necessary segment characteristics is the gamma-scanning technique suggested by Zatsiorsky and Seluyanov (65). A measure of a gamma-radiation beam is made before and after it has passed through a segment. This allows calculation of the

mass per unit surface area and thus generates prediction equations to determine the segment characteristics. The following example equation is based on these data and predicts the mass of the leg segment:

$$y = -1.592 + 0.0362 * \text{body mass} \\ + 0.0121 * \text{body height}$$

where y is the leg mass in kilograms. The following equation will predict the location of the center of mass along the longitudinal axis for the same segment:

$$y = -6.05 - 0.039 * \text{body mass} \\ + 0.142 * \text{body height}$$

where y is the location of the center of mass as a percentage of the segment length.

All of these methods have been used in the literature to determine the segment characteristics of the center of mass, and all give reasonable estimates of these parameters. In a typical biomechanical analysis, researchers will collect height and weight measurements, collect position data on the segmental end points, and calculate the location of the center of mass and the proportionate weight of the segment using information provided by past cadaver or immersion studies. Tables 11-2 and 11-3 present estimates of the center of mass location and proportionate weights generated from four studies (8–10,41). The thigh segment at toe-off (frame 76) from Appendix E will be used as an example to calculate these parameters. The subject in Appendix E is a female weighing 50 kg. Using Plagenhoef's data shown in Table 11-2 (41), the mass of the thigh of a female is 0.1175 times her total body mass. Thus, for the female subject in Appendix E, the mass of the thigh would be:

$$m_{\text{thigh}} = 0.1175 * 50 \text{ kg} \\ m_{\text{thigh}} = 5.88 \text{ kg}$$

According to Plagenhoef's segmental data, the center of mass is at 42.8% of the length of the thigh measured from the proximal end along the long axis of the segment. Consider the segment end point coordinates at toe-off in Figure 11-8. The location of the center of mass would be:

$$x_{\text{cm}} = x_p - (\text{length of the segment in x-direction} \\ * 0.428) \\ = x_p + [(x_p - x_d) * 0.428] \\ = 846.6 + [(846.6 - 861.4) * 0.428] \\ = 852.9 \text{ mm}$$

where x_{cm} is the location of the center of mass, x_p is the location of the hip joint, and x_d is the location of the knee joint, all in the horizontal direction. Similarly:

$$y_{\text{cm}} = y_p - (\text{length of the segment in y-direction} \\ * 0.428) \\ = y_p + [(y_p - y_d) * 0.428] \\ = 833.2 - [(833.2 - 464.3) * 0.428] \\ = 675.3 \text{ mm}$$

where y_{cm} is the location of the center of mass, y_p is the location of the hip joint, and y_d is the location of the knee

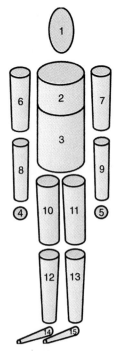

FIGURE 11-7 A representation of the human body using geometric solids. (After Miller, D. I., Morrison, W. E. [1975]. Prediction of segmental parameters using the Hanavan human body model. *Medicine and Science in Sports*, 7(3):207–212.)

TABLE 11-2 COM Location: Percent of Segment Length From Proximal End

	Plagenhoef et al., 1983 (7 males, 9 females)	Clauser, 1969 (13 male cadavers)	Dempster, 1955 (8 male cadavers)	Chandler et al., 1975 (6 male cadavers)
Head, neck	M = 55.0 F = 55.0	M = 46.4	M = 50.0	M = 66.3
Trunk	M = 44.5 F = 39.0	M = 43.8	M = 45.0	M = 52.2
Whole trunk	M = 63.0 F = 56.9		M = 60.4	
Upper arm	M = 43.6 F = 45.8	M = 51.3	M = 43.6	M = 50.7
Forearm	M = 43.0 F = 43.4	M = 39.0	M = 43.0	M = 41.7
Hand	M = 46.8 F = 46.8	M = 48.0	M = 49.4	M = 51.5
Thigh	M = 43.3 F = 42.8	M = 437.2	M = 43.3	M = 39.8
Lower Leg	M = 43.4 F = 41.9	M = 37.1	M = 43.3	M = 41.3
Foot	M = 50.0 F = 50.0	M = 44.9	M = 42.9	M = 40.0

joint, all in the vertical direction. The center of mass of the segment is (852.9, 675.3) in the reference frame. The center of mass must be between the values for the proximal and distal ends of the segments. This procedure must be carried out for each segment, using the coordinates of the joint centers to define the segments.

Refer to the walking data in Appendix E. Compute the location of the center of gravity of the lower leg from touchdown (frame 0) to toe-off (frame 79), alternating every fourth frame. Plot the path of the center of gravity of the lower leg.

TABLE 11-3 Segment Weight: Percent of Total Body Weight

	Plagenhoef et al., 1983 (37 males, 100 females)	Clauser, 1969 (13 male cadavers)	Dempster, 1955 (8 male cadavers)	Chandler et al., 1975 (6 male cadavers)
Head, neck	M = 8.26 F = 8.2	M = 7.30	M = 7.9	M = 7.35
Trunk	M = 46.8 F = 45.22	M = 50.7	M = 51.1	M = 51.66
Whole trunk	M = 55.1 F = 53.2			
Upper arm	M = 3.25 F = 2.90	M = 2.60	M = 2.70	M = 3.26
Forearm	M = 1.87 F = 1.57	M = 1.60	M = 1.60	M = 1.84
Hand	M = 0.65 F = 0.50	M = 0.70	M = 0.60	M = 0.67
Thigh	M = 10.50 F = 11.75	M = 10.3	M = 9.70	M = 9.4
Lower Leg	M = 4.75 F = 5.35	M = 4.30	M = 4.50	M = 4.01
Foot	M = 1.43 F = 1.33	M = 1.50	M = 1.40	M = 1.45

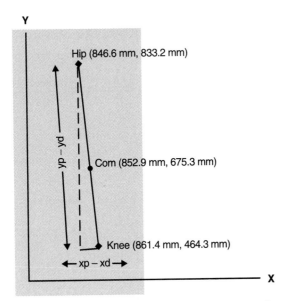

FIGURE 11-8 The thigh segment and the segment end point coordinates at an instant during toe-off in walking (See Appendix E). COM, center of mass.

Total Body Center of Mass Calculation

Once the segment center of mass locations have been determined, the total body center of mass can be calculated. Consider the illustration of a hypothetical three-segment model in Figure 11-9. The mass and the location of the center of mass of each segment has been previously determined. To determine the horizontal location of the center of mass, the torque about the y-axis is calculated, using the concept that the sum of the torques about the total system center of mass is zero. There are four torques to consider, three created by the segment centers of mass and one by the total system center of mass. Thus:

$$m_1gx_1 + m_2gx_2 + m_3gx_3 = Mgx_{cm}$$

where m is the mass of the respective segments, M is the total system mass, g is the acceleration due to gravity, x is

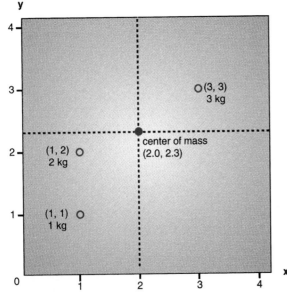

FIGURE 11-9 Location of the center of mass in a three-point mass system.

the location of the segment centers of mass, and x_{cm} is the location of the system center of mass. Since the term g appears in every term in the equation, it can be removed from the equation, resulting in:

$$m_1x_1 + m_2x_2 + m_3x_3 = Mx_{cm}$$

After substitution of the values from Figure 11-8 in this equation, there is only one unknown quantity, x_{cm}. Thus:

$$1(1) + 2(1) + 3(3) = 6x_{cm}$$

$$x_{cm} = \frac{12}{6}$$

$$x_{cm} = 2$$

Therefore, the center of mass is 2 units from the y-axis.

Using the same procedure, the vertical location of the system center of mass can be located by determining the torques about the x-axis. Thus, the vertical location of the system center of mass can be calculated by:

$$m_1y_1 + m_2y_2 + m_3y_3 = My_{cm}$$

$$1(1) + 2(1) + 3(3) = 6y_{cm}$$

$$y_{cm} = \frac{14}{6}$$

$$y_{cm} = 2.3$$

The center of mass is 2.3 units from the x-axis. Thus, the center of mass of this total system is (2, 2.3). In the x-direction, the mass is evenly distributed between the left and right sides and thus the location of the center of mass is basically in the center. This is not the case in the y-direction. The total mass is not proportioned evenly between the top and bottom because most of the mass is nearer the top of the system. As such, y_{cm} is closer to most of the mass of the system. The location of the system center of mass is represented on Figure 11-9 by the intersection of the broken lines.

The previous example can be used to generalize the procedure for calculating the total body center of mass. In the previous example, for either the horizontal or vertical position, the products of the coordinate of the segment center of mass and the segment mass for each segment were added and then divided by the total body mass. In algebraic terms:

$$X_{cm} = \frac{\sum\limits_{i=1}^{n} m_i x_i}{M}$$

where x_{cm} is the horizontal location of the total body center of mass, n is the total number of segments, m_i is the mass of the ith segment, M is the total body mass, and x_i is the horizontal location of the ith segment center of mass. Similarly, for the vertical direction:

$$y_{cm} = \frac{\sum\limits_{i=1}^{n} m_i y_i}{M}$$

where y_{cm} is the vertical location of the total body center of mass, n is the total number of segments, m_i is the mass of the ith segment, M is the total body mass, and y_i is the vertical location of the ith segment center of mass.

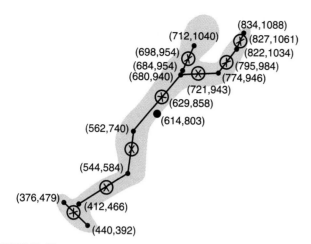

(834,1088)
(827,1061)
(712,1040)
(822,1034)
(698,954)
(795,984)
(684,954)
(774,946)
(680,940)
(721,943)
(629,858)
(614,803)
(562,740)
(544,584)
(376,479)
(412,466)
(440,392)

FIGURE 11-10 Segmental end points, segment centers of mass, and the total body center of mass for a jumper. The total body center of mass is designated by an asterisk.

This technique for calculating the total body center of mass is used in many studies in biomechanics. The computation is based on the segment characteristics and the coordinates determined from a kinematic analysis. For most situations, the body is thought of as a 14-segment model (head, trunk, and two each of upper arms, lower arms, hands, thighs, legs, and feet). In certain situations in which the actions of the limbs are symmetrical, an eight-segment model (head, trunk, upper arm, lower arm, hand, thigh, leg, and foot) will suffice, although the mass of the segments not digitized must be included. As an example of this technique, consider the illustration of the jumper in Figure 11-10, which shows the coordinates of the segmental end points of the jumper. Using an eight-segment model (head and neck, trunk, upper arm, forearm, hand, thigh, lower leg, foot), the coordinates of the location of each segment's center of mass is computed using one of the sets of available anthropometric data. For example, if it is assumed that the jumper is a male (body mass = 70 kg), segmental center of gravity locations can be calculated using Dempster's cadaver data (10). The location of the segmental center of mass measured from the proximal end is calculated in for each segment using estimated locations of the center of mass (Table 11-4).

$$COM_x = x_{proximal} + [\text{estimated COM location as \%}$$
$$\text{of segment length}) * (x_{distal} - x_{proximal})]$$
$$COM_y = y_{proximal} + [(\text{estimated COM location as\%}$$
$$\text{of segment length}) * (y_{distal} - y_{proximal})]$$

In this example, the center of mass of each segment is calculated as a distance from the proximal end point. The x and y coordinate locations of the center of mass are next used to calculate each segmental torque by multiplying the center of mass location times the segment mass proportions. That is:

$$Segment\text{-}torque_x = segment\text{-}cm_x$$
$$\text{*estimated segment mass proportion}$$
$$Segment\text{-}torque_y = segment\text{-}cm_y$$
$$\text{*estimated segment mass proportion}$$

The x_{cm} can then be calculated by summing the segmental products, and the y_{cm} is similarly calculated. The total body center of mass coordinates in digitizing units, therefore, are (614,803) and are indicated on Figure 11-10 by the bigger solid circle.

Refer to the data in Appendix E. Using Plagenhoef's data for a female, calculate the location of the center of mass of a three-link system, including the thigh, lower leg, and foot, for frame 15).

Rotation and Leverage

DEFINITIONS

The outcome of a torque is to produce a rotation or pivoting about an axis. If rotations about a fixed point are considered, the effects of the lever can be discussed. A **lever** is a rigid rod that is rotated about a fixed point or axis called the **fulcrum**. A lever consists of a **resistance force**, an **effort force**, a barlike structure, and a fulcrum. In addition, there are two moment or lever arms designated as the **effort arm** and the **resistance arm**. The effort arm is the perpendicular distance from the line of action of the effort force to the fulcrum. The resistance arm is the perpendicular distance from the line of action of the resistance force to the fulcrum. Since both the effort and resistance forces act at a distance from the fulcrum, they create torques about the fulcrum. An anatomical example, such as the forearm segment, can be used to illustrate a lever (Fig. 11-11). The long bone of the forearm segment is the rigid barlike structure, and the elbow joint is the fulcrum. The resistance force may be the weight of the segment and possibly an added load carried in the hand or at the wrist. The effort force is produced by the tension developed in the muscles to flex the elbow. Figure 11-12 illustrates several examples of simple machines that are in effect different types of levers.

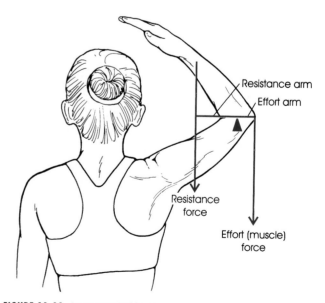

Resistance arm
Effort arm

Resistance force

Effort (muscle) force

FIGURE 11-11 An anatomical lever.

TABLE 11-4 Calculation of Total Body Center of Mass

Segment	Segment COM location equation	Segment Mass * Segment COM − x	Segment Mass * Segment COM − y
Head, neck $x, y_{top\ of\ head} = (712, 1040)$ $x, y_{midshoulder} = (684, 954)$	$x = x_{top\ of\ head} + 0.50\ (x_{mid\ shoulder} - x_{top\ of\ head}) = 712 + 0.5\ (684 - 712) = 698$ $y = y_{top\ of\ head} + 0.50\ (y_{mid\ shoulder} - y_{top\ of\ head}) = 1040 + 0.5\ (954 - 040) = 997$ $COM_{head\ and\ neck} = (698, 997)$	Weight ratio$_{head\ and\ neck}$ * COM − X = 0.079 * 698 = 55.14	Weight ratio$_{head\ and\ neck}$ * * COM − Y = 0.079 * 997 = 78.76
Trunk $x, y_{mid\ shoulder} = (684, 954)$ $x, y_{mid\ hips} = (562, 740)$	$x = x_{mid\ shoulder} + 0.45\ (x_{mid\ hip} - x_{mid\ shoulder}) = 684 + 0.45(562 - 684) = 629.1$ $y = y_{mid\ shoulder} + 0.45\ (y_{mid\ hip} - y_{mid\ shoulder}) = 954 + 0.45(740 - 954) = 857.7$ $COM_{trunk} = (629.1, 857.7)$	Weight ratio$_{trunk}$ * COM − X = 0.511 * 629.1 = 321.47	Weight ratio$_{trunk}$ * COM − Y = 0.511 * 857.7 = 438.29
R&L Upper arm $x, y_{elbow} = (774, 946)$ x, $y_{shoulder} = (680, 940)$	$x = x_{shoulder} + 0.436(x_{elbow} - x_{shoulder}) = 680 + 0.436(774 - 680) = 721$ $y = y_{shoulder} + 0.436(y_{elbow} - y_{shoulder}) = 940 + 0.436(946 - 940) = 942.6$ $COM_{upper\ arm} = (721, 942.6)$	Weight ratio$_{arm}$ * COM − X = 0.027 * 721 = 19.47	Weight ratio$_{arm}$ * COM − Y = 0.027 * 942.6 = 25.45
R&L forearm $x, y_{wrist} = (822, 1034)$ $x, y_{elbow} = (774, 946)$	$x = x_{elbow} + 0.43\ (x_{wrist} - x_{elbow}) = 774 + 0.43(822 - 774) = 794.6$ $y = y_{elbow} + 0.43\ (y_{wrist} - y_{elbow}) = 946 + 0.43(1034 - 946) = 983.8$ $COM_{forearm} = (794.6, 983.8)$	Weight ratio$_{forearm}$ * COM − X = 0.016 * 794.6 = 12.71	Weight ratio$_{forearm}$ * COM − Y = 0.016 * 983.8 = 15.74
R&L hand $x, y_{tip\ of\ finger} = (834, 1088)$ $x, y_{wrist} = (822, 1034)$	$x = x_{wrist} + 0.494\ (x_{tip\ of\ finger} - x_{wrist}) = 822 + 0.494(834 - 822) = 827.9$ $y = y_{wrist} + 0.494(y_{tip\ of\ finger} - y_{wrist}) = 1034 + 0.494(1088 - 1034) = 1060.7$ $COM_{hand} = (827.9, 1060.7)$	Weight ratio$_{hand}$ * COM − X = 0.006 * 827.9 = 4.97	Weight ratio$_{hand}$ * COM − Y = 0.006 * 1060.7 = 6.36
R&L thigh $x, y_{hip} = (562, 740)$ $x, y_{knee} = (544, 584)$	$x = x_{hip} + 0.433(x_{knee} - x_{hip}) = 562 + 0.433(544 - 562) = 554.2$ $y = y_{hip} + 0.433(y_{knee} - y_{hip}) = 740 + 0.433(584 - 740) = 672.5$ $COM_{thigh} = (554.2, 672.5)$	Weight ratio$_{thigh}$ * COM − X = 0.097 * 554.2 = 53.76	Weight ratio$_{thigh}$ * COM − Y = 0.097 * 672.5 = 65.23
R&L lower leg $x, y_{knee} = (544, 584)$ $x, y_{ankle} = (412, 466)$	$x = x_{knee} + 0.433(x_{ankle} - x_{knee}) = 544 + 0.433(412 - 544) = 486.8$ $y = y_{knee} + 0.433(y_{ankle} - y_{knee}) = 584 + 0.433(466 - 584) = 532.9$ $COM_{lower\ leg} = (486.8, 532.9)$	Weight ratio$_{lower\ leg}$ * COM − X = 0.045 * 486.8 = 21.91	Weight ratio$_{lower\ leg}$ * COM − Y = 0.045 * 532.9 = 23.98
R&L foot $x, y_{heel} = (376, 474)$ $x, y_{tip\ of\ toe} = (440, 392)$	$x = x_{heel} + 0.429(x_{tip\ of\ toe} - x_{heel}) = 376 + 0.429(440 - 376) = 403.5$ $y = y_{heel} + 0.429(y_{tip\ of\ toe} - y_{heel}) = 474 + 0.429(392 - 474) = 438.8$ $COM_{foot} = (403.5, 438.8)$	Weight ratio$_{foot}$ * COM − X = 0.014 * 403.5 = 5.65	Weight ratio$_{foot}$ * COM − Y = 0.014 * 438.8 = 6.14
	TOTAL BODY COM (x, y)	$COM_x = \Sigma Segmental$ $COM_x = 55.14 + 321.47 + 19.47 + 19.47 + 12.71 + 12.71 + 4.97 + 4.97 + 53.76 + 53.76 + 21.91 + 21.91 + 5.65 + 5.65 = 613.55$	$COM_y = \Sigma Segmental$ $COM_y = 78.76 + 438.29 + 25.45 + 25.45 + 15.74 + 15.74 + 6.36 + 6.36 + 65.23 + 65.23 + 23.98 + 23.98 + 6.14 + 6.14 = 802.76$

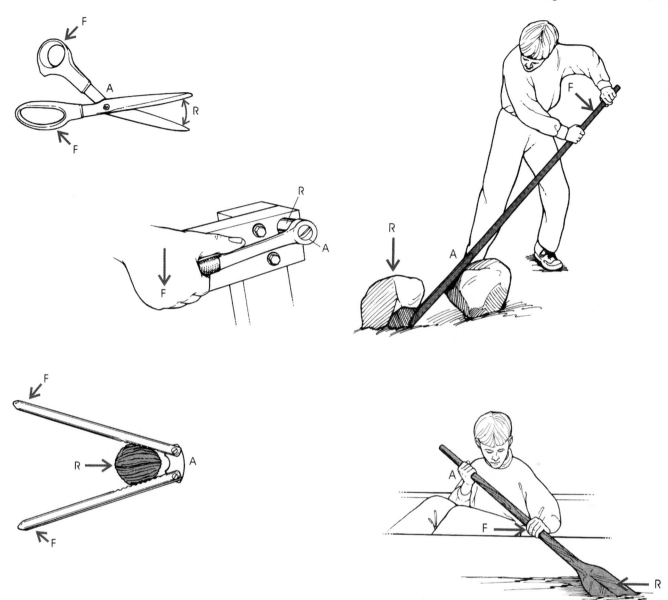

FIGURE 11-12 Levers.

A lever may be evaluated for its mechanical effectiveness by computing its mechanical advantage. **Mechanical advantage** is defined as the ratio of the effort arm to the resistance arm. That is:

$$MA = \frac{\text{effort arm}}{\text{resistance arm}}$$

In the construction of a lever, any of three situations may define the function of the lever. The simplest case is when MA = 1, when the effort arm equals the resistance arm. In this case, the function of the lever is to alter the direction of motion or balance the lever but not to magnify either the effort or resistance force. The second case is when the MA is greater than 1, when the effort arm is greater than the resistance arm. In this case, the greater effort arm magnifies the torque created by the effort force. Thus, when MA is greater than 1, the lever is said

to magnify the effort force. In the third situation, MA is less than 1, the effort arm is less than the resistance arm. In this case, a much greater effort force is required to overcome the resistance force. The effort force acts over a small distance, however, with the result that the resistance force is moved over a much greater distance in the same amount of time (Fig. 11-13). When MA is less than 1, therefore, velocity or speed of movement is said to be magnified.

CLASSES OF LEVERS

There are three classes of levers. In a **first-class lever**, the effort force and the resistance force are on opposite sides of the fulcrum. Everyday examples of this lever configuration are the seesaw, the balance scale, and the crowbar. A first-class lever may be configured many ways and may

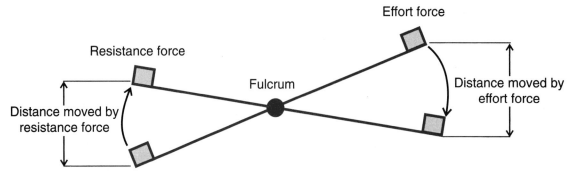

FIGURE 11-13 A first-class lever in which the moment arm is less than 1, that is, the effort arm is less than the resistance arm. The linear distance moved by the effort force, however, is less than that moved by the resistance force in the same time.

have a mechanical advantage of 1, more than 1, or less than 1. First-class levers exist in the musculoskeletal system of the human body. The agonist and antagonist muscles simultaneously acting on opposite sides of a joint create a first-class lever. In most instances, however, the first-class lever in the human body acts with a mechanical advantage of 1. That is, the lever acts to balance or change the direction of the effort force. An example of the former is the action of the splenius muscles acting to balance the head on the atlanto-occipital joint (Fig. 11-14). The latter situation, in which the lever changes the direction of the effort force, is seen in the action of many bony prominences called processes. This type of first-class lever is a pulley. One such example is

action of the patella in knee extension. Here the angle of pull of the quadriceps muscles is altered by the riding action of the patella on the condylar groove of the femur.

SECOND-CLASS LEVER

In a **second-class lever**, the effort force and the resistance force act on the same side of the fulcrum. In this class of lever, the resistance force acts between the fulcrum and the effort force. That is, the resistance force arm is less than the effort arm and thus the mechanical advantage is greater than 1. One example of a second-class lever in everyday situations is the wheelbarrow (Fig. 11-15). Using the wheelbarrow, effort forces can be applied to act against

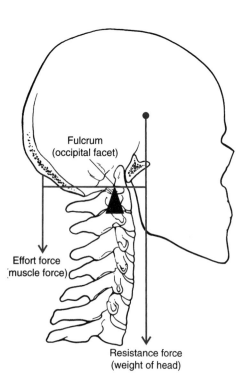

FIGURE 11-14 An anatomical first-class lever in which the weight of the head is the resistance force, the splenius muscles provide the effort force, and the fulcrum is the atlanto-occipital joint.

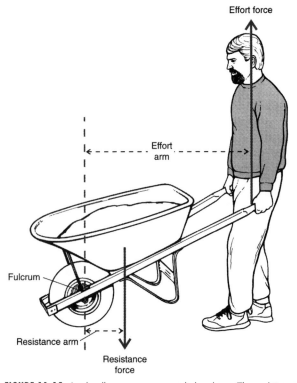

FIGURE 11-15 A wheelbarrow as a second-class lever. The resistance force is between the fulcrum and the effort force. Since the effort arm is greater than the resistance arm, MA > 1 and the effort force is magnified.

very significant resistance forces provided by the load carried in the wheelbarrow. There are very few examples of second-class levers in the human body, although the act of rising onto the toes is often proclaimed and also disputed as one. This action is used in weight training and is known as a calf raise. Since there are so few examples of second-class levers in the human body, it is safe to say that humans are not designed to apply great forces via lever systems.

THIRD-CLASS LEVER

The effort force and the resistance force are also on the same side of the fulcrum in a **third-class lever**. In this arrangement, however, the effort force acts between the fulcrum and the line of action of the resistance force. As a result, the effort force arm is less than the resistance force arm and thus the mechanical advantage is less than 1. An example of this type of lever is the shovel when the hand nearest the spade end applies the effort force (Fig. 11-16). Therefore, it would appear that a large effort force must be applied to overcome a moderate resistance force. In a third-class lever, a large effort force is applied to gain the advantage of increased speed of motion. This is the most prominent type of lever arrangement in the human body, with nearly all joints of the extremities acting as third-class levers. It is probably safe to conclude that from a design standpoint, greater speed of movement exemplified by third-class levers appears to be emphasized in the musculoskeletal system to the exclusion of greater effort force application ability of the second-class lever. Figure 11-17 illustrates a third-class lever arrangement in the human body.

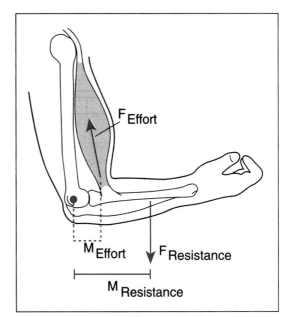

FIGURE 11-17 The arm held in flexion at the elbow is an anatomical third-class lever: the resistance force is the weight of the arm, the fulcrum is the elbow joint, and the effort force is provided by the elbow flexor muscles.

Types of Torque

A torque acting on a body is created by a force acting a distance away from the axis of rotation. Thus any of the different types of forces discussed in Chapter 10 can produce a torque if applied in a direction that does not go through the axis or pivot point. Gravity, a noncontact force, generates a torque anytime the line of gravity is not passing through the pivot point. As illustrated in Figure

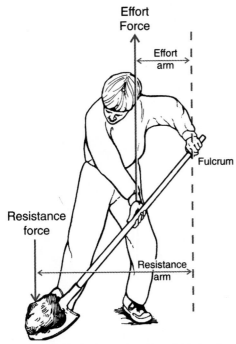

FIGURE 11-16 An individual using a shovel is a third-class lever.

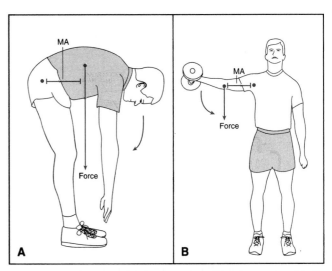

FIGURE 11-18 The gravitational torques created by the weight of body segments acting at a distance from the joint in movements such as trunk flexion **(A)** and an arm lateral raise **(B)** must be countered by muscular torques acting in the opposite direction.

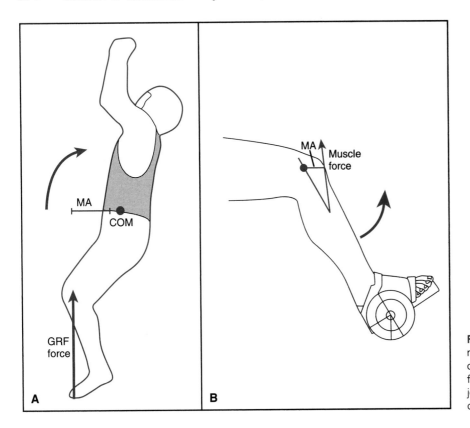

FIGURE 11-19 Contact forces such as ground reaction forces **(A)** and muscular forces **(B)** create torques because the line of action of the force does not go through the center of mass or joint axis, respectively. MA, moment arm; COM, center of mass; GRF, ground reaction force.

11-18, gravity acting on the trunk segment produces a clockwise torque about the lumbar vertebrae (Fig. 11-18A), and the weight of the arm and dumbbell produces a clockwise torque about the shoulder joint (Fig. 11-18B). A muscular torque in the clockwise direction to hold the positions statically must counteract both of these gravitational torques.

Contact forces also produce torques if applied correctly. For example, torques are generated about the center of gravity in events such as diving and gymnastics by using the vertical ground reaction force in conjunction with body configurations that move the center of mass in front of or behind the force application. Consider Figure 11-19A, in which the ground reaction force generated in a backward somersault is applied a distance from the center of mass, causing a clockwise rotation about the center of mass. Another important contact force, muscle force, also generates torques about joint axes, as shown in Figure 11-19B.

 Representation of Torques Acting on a System

A free body diagram illustrating torques acting on a system is usually combined with linear forces to identify and analyze the causes of motion. Many biomechanical analyses start with a free body diagram for each body segment.

Known as the linked segment model, it can generate either a static or dynamic model. Consider the model of the dead lift shown in Figure 11-20 showing the lift (Fig. 11-20A) and the free body diagram for the lower leg, thigh, trunk, arm, and forearm segments (Fig. 11-20B). If a link segment model is developed, forces acting at the joints (F_x, F_y) and the center of mass (W) can be indicated along with moments (M) acting at the joints.

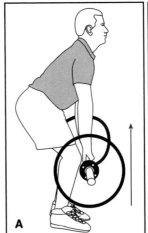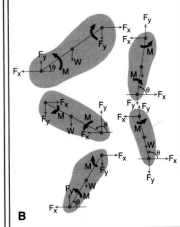

FIGURE 11-20 A squat **(A)** as free body diagram **(B)** using a linked segment model illustrating forces acting at the joints and the centers of mass, along with the moments acting at the joints.

Newton's Laws of Motion: Angular Analogs

The linear case of Newton's laws of motion was presented in Chapter 10. These laws can be restated to represent the angular analogs. Each linear quantity has a corresponding angular analog. For example, the angular analog of force is torque, of mass is moment of inertia, and of acceleration is angular acceleration. These analogs can be directly substituted into the linear laws to create the angular analogs.

FIRST LAW: LAW OF INERTIA

A rotating body will continue in a state of uniform angular motion unless acted on by an external torque.

According to Newton's first law of motion, inertia is an object's tendency to resist a change in velocity. The measure of an object's inertia is its mass. The angular counterpart to mass is the **moment of inertia**. It is a quantity that indicates the resistance of an object to a change in angular motion. Unlike its linear counterpart, mass, the moment of inertia of a body is dependent not only on the mass of the object but also on the distribution of mass with respect to the axis of rotation. The moment of inertia will also have different values because there are many axes about which an object may rotate. That is, the moment of inertia is not fixed but changeable. If a gymnast rotating in the air in a layout body position is used as an example, the way in which the moment of inertia changes can be illustrated. Suppose the gymnast twists about a longitudinal axis passing through the center of mass. The mass of the gymnast is distributed along and relatively close to this axis (Fig. 11-21A). If the gymnast rotates about a transverse axis through the center of mass, the same mass is distributed much farther from the axis of rotation (Fig. 11-21B). Since

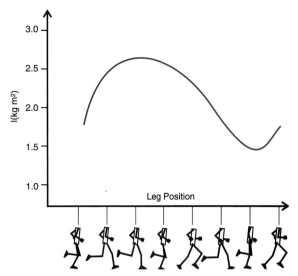

FIGURE 11-22 The changes in the leg's moment of inertia during the stride.

there is a greater mass distribution rotating about the transverse axis than about the longitudinal axis, the moment of inertia is greater in the latter case. That is, there is a **greater resistance to rotation about the transverse axis than about the longitudinal axis.** The gymnast may also alter mass distribution about an axis by changing body position, as with assuming a tuck position, bringing more body mass closer to the transverse axis, thus decreasing the moment of inertia. In multiple aerial somersaults, gymnasts will assume an extreme tuck position by almost placing the head between the knees in an attempt to reduce the moment of inertia. They do this to provide less resistance to angular acceleration and thus complete the multiple somersaults.

The concept of reducing the moment of inertia to enhance angular motion is also seen in running (Fig. 11-22). During the swing phase, the foot is brought forward from behind the body to the point on the ground where the next contact will be made. Once the foot leaves the ground, however, the leg flexes considerably at the knee and the foot is raised up close to the buttocks. The effect of this action is to decrease the moment of inertia of the lower extremity relative to a transverse axis through the hip joint. This enables the limb to rotate forward more quickly than would be the case if the lower limb were not flexed. This action is a distinguishing feature of the lower extremity action of sprinters. Figure 11-22 illustrates the change in the moment of inertia of the lower extremity during the recovery action in running.

If all objects are considered to be made up of a number of small particles, each with its own mass and its own distance from the axis of rotation, the moment of inertia can be represented in mathematical terms:

$$I = \sum_{i-1}^{n} m_i r_i^2$$

where I is the moment of inertia, n represents the number of particle masses, m_i represents the mass of the ith particle, and r_i is the distance of the ith particle from the

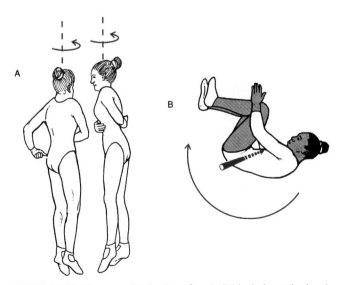

FIGURE 11-21 The mass distribution of an individual about the longitudinal axis through the total body center of mass **(A)** and about a transverse axis through the total body center of mass **(B)**.

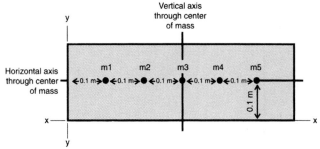

FIGURE 11-23 A hypothetical five-point mass system.

axis of rotation. That is, the moment of inertia equals the sum of the products of the mass and the distance from the axis of rotation squared of all mass particles comprising the object. A dimensional analysis results in units of kilogram-meters squared (kgm^2) for moment of inertia.

Consider the illustration in Figure 11-23. This hypothetical object is composed of five-point masses, each with a mass of 0.5 kg. The distances r_1 to r_5 represent the distance from the axis of rotation. The point masses are each 0.1 m apart, with the first mass being 0.1 m from the y-y axis. Each point mass is 0.1 m from the x-x axis. The moment of inertia about the y-y axis is:

$$I_{y-y} = \sum_{i-1}^{n} m_i - r_i^2$$
$$= m_1r_1^2 + m_2r_2^2 + m_3r_3^2 + m_4r_4^2 + m_5r_5$$
$$= 0.5 \text{ kg} * (0.1 \text{ m})^2 + 0.5 \text{ kg} * (0.2 \text{ m})^2 + 0.5 \text{ kg} * (0.3 \text{ m})^2 + 0.5 \text{ kg} * (0.4 \text{ m})^2 + 0.5 \text{ kg} * (0.5 \text{ m})^2$$
$$= 0.005 \text{ kgm}^2 + 0.02 \text{ kgm}^2 + 0.045 \text{ kgm}^2 + 0.08 \text{ kgm}^2 + 0.125 \text{ kgm}^2$$
$$= 0.275 \text{ kgm}^2$$

If the axis of rotation is changed to the x-x axis, the moment of inertia of the object about this axis would be:

$$I_{x-x} = \sum_{i-1}^{n} m_i r_i^2$$
$$= m_1r_1^2 + m_2r_2^2 + m_3r_3^2 + m_4r_4^2 + m_5r_5^2$$
$$= 0.5 \text{ kg} * (0.1 \text{ m})^2 + 0.5 \text{ kg} * (0.1 \text{ m})^2 + 0.5 \text{ kg} * (0.1 \text{ m})^2 + 0.5 \text{ kg} * (0.1 \text{ m})^2 + 0.5 \text{ kg} * (0.1 \text{ m})^2$$
$$= 0.005 \text{ kgm}^2 + 0.005 \text{ kgm}^2 + 0.005 \text{ kgm}^2 + 0.005 \text{ kgm}^2 + 0.005 \text{ kgm}^2$$
$$= 0.025 \text{ kgm}^2$$

The change in the axis of rotation from the y-y axis to the x-x axis thus dramatically reduces the moment of inertia, resulting in less resistance to angular motion about the x-x axis than about the y-y axis. If an axis that passes through the geometric center of mass is used, the mass of Point 3 would not influence the moment of inertia because the axis passes directly through this point. Thus:

$$I_{cm} = \sum_{i-=1}^{n} m_i r_i^2$$
$$= m_1r_1^2 + m_2r_2^2 + m_4r_4^2 + m_5r_5^2$$
$$= 0.5 \text{ kg} * (0.2 \text{ m})^2 + 0.5 \text{ kg} * (0.1 \text{ m})^2 + 0.5 \text{ kg} * (0.1 \text{ m})^2 + 0.5 \text{ kg} * (0.2 \text{ m})^2$$

$$= 0.02 \text{ kgm}^2 + 0.005 \text{ kgm}^2 + 0.005 \text{ kgm}^2 + 0.02 \text{ kgm}^2$$
$$= 0.05 \text{ kgm}^2$$

From these examples, it should now be clear that the moment of inertia changes according to the axis of rotation.

In the human body, the segments are not as simply constructed as in the example. Each segment is made up of different tissue types, such as bone, muscle, and skin, that are not uniformly distributed. The body segments are also irregularly shaped. This means that a segment is not of uniform density, and thus it would be impractical to determine the moment of inertia of human body segments using the particle–mass method. Values for the moment of inertia of each body segment have been determined using a number of methods. Experimentally, moment of inertia values have been obtained in much the same way as the parameters for the center of mass. The values were generated from cadaver studies (10), mathematical modeling (20,21) and from gamma-scanning techniques (65). Jensen (27) has developed prediction equations specifically for children based on the body mass and height of the child.

It is necessary for a high degree of accuracy to calculate a moment of inertia that is unique for a given individual. Most of the techniques that provide values for segment moments of inertia provide information on the segment radius of gyration, and from this the moment of inertia may be calculated. The **radius of gyration** denotes the segment's mass distribution about the axis of rotation and is the distance from the axis of rotation to a point at which the mass can be assumed to be concentrated without changing the inertial characteristics of the segment. Thus, a segment's moment of inertia may be calculated by:

$$I = m(\rho l)^2$$

where I is the moment of inertia, m is the mass of the segment, l is the segment length, and the Greek letter rho, ρ, is the radius of gyration of the segment as a proportion of the segment length. For example, consider the leg of an individual with a mass and length of 3.6 kg and 0.4 m, respectively. The proportion of the radius of gyration to segment length is 0.302 based on the data of Dempster (10). This information is sufficient to calculate the moment of inertia of the leg about an axis through the center of mass. Thus:

$$I_{cm} = m(\rho_{cm})^2$$
$$= 3.6 \text{ kg} * (0.302 * 0.4 \text{ m})^2$$
$$= 0.0525 \text{ kgm}^2$$

The moment of inertia about an axis through the center of mass is 0.0525 kgm^2. Table 11-5 illustrates the radius of gyration as a proportion of the segment length values from Dempster (10).

Using the radius of gyration technique, the moment of inertia about a transverse axis through the proximal and distal ends of the segment may also be calculated. The radius of gyration as a proportion of segment length about the proximal end of the leg in the previous example is

TABLE 11-5 Radii of Gyration as a Proportion of Segment Length About a Transverse Axis			
Segment	Center of Mass	Proximal	Distal
Head, neck, trunk	0.503	0.830	0.607
Upper arm	0.322	0.542	0.645
Arm	0.303	0.526	0.647
Hand	0.297	0.587	0.577
Thigh	0.323	0.540	0.653
Leg	0.302	0.528	0.643
Foot	0.475	0.690	0.690

From Dempster, W. T. (1955). Space requirements of the seated operator. *WADC Technical Report*. Wright-Patterson Air Force Base, 55–159.

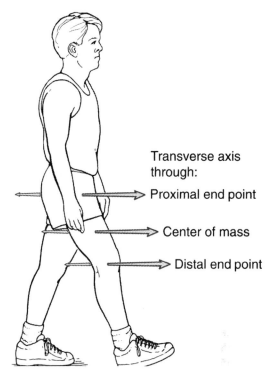

Transverse axis through:

→ Proximal end point

→ Center of mass

→ Distal end point

FIGURE 11-24 Parallel transverse axes through the proximal, distal, and center of mass points of the thigh.

0.528. Therefore, the moment of inertia about the proximal end of the segment is calculated as:

$$I_{cm} = m(\rho_{prox}l)^2$$
$$= 3.6 \text{ kg} * (0.528 * 0.4 \text{ m})^2$$
$$= 0.161 \text{ kgm}^2$$

At the distal end point of the leg segment, the moment of inertia is:

$$I_{cm} = m(\rho_{dist}l)^2$$
$$= 3.6 \text{ kg} * (0.643 * 0.4 \text{ m})^2$$
$$= 0.238 \text{ kgm}^2$$

Refer to the walking data in Appendix E. Calculate the radius of gyration and the moment of inertia from both the proximal and distal end point of the thigh segment for frame 2.

The moment of inertia value for any segment is usually given for an axis through the center of mass of the segment. This moment of inertia value is the smallest possible value of any parallel axis through the segment. For example, in Figure 11-24, three parallel transverse axes are drawn through the leg segment. These axes are through the proximal end point, through the center of mass, and through the distal end point. Since the mass of the segment is distributed evenly about the center of mass, the moment of inertia about the center of mass axis is small, and the moments of inertia about the other axes are greater but not equal. This was illustrated in the moment of inertia calculations. Since the mass of most segments is distributed closer to the proximal end of the segment, the moment of inertia about the proximal axis is less than about a parallel axis through the distal end point.

The moment of inertia can be calculated about any parallel axis, given the moment of inertia about one axis, the mass of the segment, and the perpendicular distance between the parallel axes. This calculation is known as the **parallel axis theorem**. Assume that the moment of inertia about a transverse axis through the center of mass of a segment is known and it is necessary to calculate the moment of inertia about a parallel transverse axis through the proximal end point. This theorem would state that:

$$I_{prox} = I_{cm} + mr^2$$

where I_{prox} is the moment of inertia about the proximal axis, I_{cm} is the moment of inertia about the center of mass axis, m is the mass of the segment, and r is the perpendicular distance between the two parallel axes. From the calculation in the example of the leg, it was determined that the moment of inertia about an axis through the center of mass was 0.0525 kgm². If the center of mass is 43.3% of the length of the segment from the proximal end, the moment of inertia about a parallel axis through the proximal end point of the segment can be calculated. If the length of the segment is 0.4 m, the distance between the proximal end of the segment and the center of mass is:

$$d = 0.433 * 0.4 \text{ m}$$
$$= 0.173 \text{ m}$$

The moment of inertia about the proximal end point, then, is:

$$I_{prox} = I_{cm} + mr^2$$
$$= 0.0525 \text{ kgm}^2 + 3.6 \text{ kg} * (0.173 \text{ m})^2$$
$$= 0.161 \text{ kgm}^2$$

This value is the same as was calculated using the radius of gyration and segment length proportion from

Dempster's data (10). It can be seen that the moment of inertia about an axis through the center of mass is less than the moment of inertia about any other parallel axis through any other point on the segment.

SECOND LAW: LAW OF ANGULAR ACCELERATION

An external torque will produce an angular acceleration of a body that is proportional to and in the direction of the torque and inversely proportional to the moment of inertia of the body.

This law may be stated algebraically as:

$$T = I\alpha$$

where T is the external torque, I is the moment of inertia of the object, and α is the angular acceleration of the object. For example, if an individual abducts the arm from the body to a horizontal position, the torque at the shoulder results in an angular acceleration of the arm. The greater the moment of inertia of the arm about an axis through the shoulder, the less the angular acceleration of the segment.

By rearranging the equation, one can substitute angular acceleration by $d\omega/dt$:

$$T = I\frac{d\omega}{dt}$$

or

$$T = I\frac{d\omega}{dt}$$

The product of moment of inertia and angular velocity in the numerator of the right-hand side of the equation is known as **angular momentum**. Thus:

$$H = I\omega$$

where H is the angular momentum, I is the moment of inertia, and ω is the angular velocity. **Angular momentum** is the quantity of angular motion of an object. Angular momentum has the units of $kgm^2 * s^{-1}$. These units for angular momentum can be determined by a unit analysis. That is:

$$H = I\omega$$

$$H = kgm^2 * \frac{rad}{s}$$

$$H = \frac{kg\text{-}m^2}{s}$$

Radians are dimensionless and disappear from the final unit of angular momentum. Angular momentum is a vector, and the right-hand rule determines the direction of the vector. Once again, counterclockwise rotations are positive, while clockwise rotations are negative.

The expression of the relationship in Newton's second law is once again analogous to the linear case. That is, the sum of the external torques is equal to the time rate of change in angular momentum. That is:

$$T = I\alpha$$

$$T = I\frac{\Delta\omega}{\Delta t}$$

$$T = I\frac{\Delta\omega}{\Delta t}$$

where $I\Delta\omega$ is the angular momentum. Newton's second law can thus be restated:

$$T = \frac{dH}{dt}$$

That is, torque is equal to the time rate change of angular momentum. To change the angular momentum of an object, external torque must be applied to the object. The angular momentum may increase or decrease, but in either case, external torque is required.

When gravity is the only external force acting on an object, as in projectile motion, the angular momentum generated at takeoff remains constant for the duration of the flight. This principle is known as the **conservation of angular momentum** and is derived from Newton's first law, that the angular momentum of a system will remain constant unless an external torque is applied to the system. Angular momentum is conserved during flight because the body weight vector, acting through the total body center of gravity, creates no torque, since the moment arm is zero. No internal movements or torques generated at the segments can influence the angular momentum generated at takeoff. This principle enables divers and gymnasts to accomplish aerial maneuvers by manipulating their moments of inertia and angular velocities because their angular momentum is constant.

Consider the angular momentum of a gymnast performing an aerial somersault about a transverse axis through the total body center of mass (Fig. 11-25). The torque applied over time at the point of takeoff determines the quantity of angular momentum. During the flight phase, angular momentum does not change. However, the gymnast may manipulate the moment of inertia to spin faster or slower about the transverse axis. At takeoff, the gymnast is in a layout position with a relatively large moment of inertia and a relatively small angular velocity or rate of spin. As the gymnast assumes a tuck position, the moment of inertia decreases and the angular velocity increases accordingly because the quantity of angular momentum is constant. Having completed the necessary rotation and in preparation to land, the gymnast opens up, assuming a layout position, increasing the moment of inertia and slowing the rate of spin. If these actions are done successfully, the gymnast will land on the feet.

To this point only angular momentum about a single axis has been discussed. Angular momentum about one axis may be transferred to another axis. This occurs in many activities in which the body is a projectile. While the

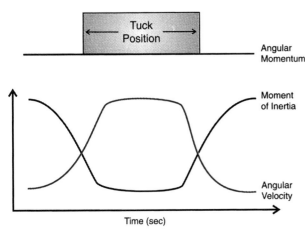

FIGURE 11-25 The angular momentum, moment of inertia, and angular velocity of a diver completing an aerial somersault. Throughout the aerial portion of the dive, the total body angular momentum of the diver is constant. When the diver is in a layout position, the moment of inertia decreases and the angular velocity increases in proportion. During the tuck portion of the dive, the angular velocity increases and the moment of inertia decreases in proportion.

total angular momentum is constant, it may be transferred, for example, from a transverse axis through the center of mass to a longitudinal axis through the center of mass. For example, a diver may twist about the longitudinal and initiate actions that produce a somersault about the transverse axis. This dive is known as a full twisting one-and-a-half somersault. Researchers have investigated arm and hip movements to accomplish this change in angular momentum (15,55,58,59). Other activities that use the principles of transferring angular momentum are freestyle skiing and gymnastics.

Rotations may be initiated in midair even when the total body angular momentum is zero. These are called zero momentum rotations. A prime example of this is the action of a cat when dropped from an upside-down position. The cat initiates a zero momentum rotation and lands on its feet. As the cat begins to fall, it arches its back, or pikes, to create two body sections, a front and a hind section, and two distinct axes of rotation (Fig. 11-26A). The cat's front legs are brought close to its head, decreasing the moment of inertia of the front section, and the upper trunk is rotated 180° (Fig. 11-26B). The cat extends its hind limbs and rotates the hind section in the opposite direction to counteract the rotation of the front segment. Since the moment of inertia of the hind section is greater than that of the front section, the angular distance that the hind section moves is relatively small. To complete the rotation, the cat brings the hind legs and tail into line with its trunk and rotates the back section about an axis through the hind section (Fig. 11-26C). The reaction of the front portion of the cat to the hind section rotation is small because the cat creates a large moment of inertia by extending its front legs. Finally, the cat has rotated sufficiently to land upright on its four paws (Fig. 11-26D). The use of such actions in sports

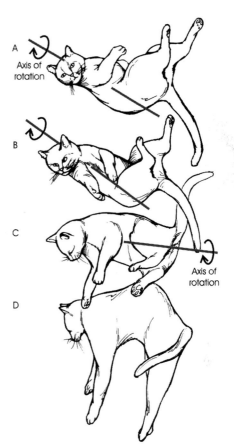

FIGURE 11-26 A cat initiating a rotation in the air in the absence of external torque.

such as diving and track and field has received considerable attention (12,15).

During human movement, multiple segments rotate. When this happens, each individual segment has angular momentum about the segment's center of mass and also about the total body center of mass. The angular momentum of a segment about its own center of mass is referred to as the **local angular momentum** of the segment. The angular momentum of a segment about the total body center of mass is referred to as the **remote angular momentum** of the segment. A segment's total angular momentum is made up of both local and remote aspects (Fig. 11-27). Expressed algebraically:

$$H_{total} = H_{local} + H_{remote}$$

If the total angular momentum of an individual is calculated, the local aspects of each segment and the remote aspects of each segment must be included. Therefore:

$$H_{total} = \sum_{i-1}^{n} H_{local} + \sum_{i-1}^{n} H_{remote}$$

where i represents each segment and n is the total number of segments.

Local angular momentum is expressed as:

$$H_{local} = I_{cm}\omega$$

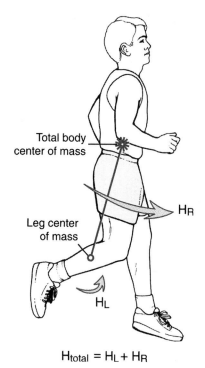

FIGURE 11-27 An illustration of the local (H_L) and remote (H_R) angular momenta of the leg segment.

$$H_{total} = H_L + H_R$$

where H_{local} is the local angular momentum of the segment, I_{cm} is the moment of inertia about an axis through the segment center of mass, and ω is the angular velocity of the segment about an axis through the segment center of mass. The remote aspect of angular momentum is calculated as:

$$H_{remote} = md\omega'^2$$

where H_{remote} is the remote angular momentum, m is the mass of the segment, d is the distance from the segment center of mass to the total body center of mass, and ω' is the angular velocity of the segment about an axis through the total body center of mass (24). Figure 11-28 illustrates the proportion of local and remote angular momentum of the total angular momentum in a forward two-and-a-half

rotation dive. In this instance, the remote angular momentum makes up a greater proportion of the total angular momentum than does the local angular momentum.

This technique for calculating total body angular momentum has been used in a number of biomechanical studies. Diving, for example, has been an area of study concerning the angular momentum requirements of many types of dives. Hamill et al. (19) found that the angular momentum of tower divers increased as the number of rotations required in the dive increased (Fig. 11-29). Values as great as 70 kgm^2/s have been reported for springboard dives (37). The inclusion of a twisting movement with a multiple rotation dive further increases the angular momentum requirements (49).

Hinrichs (25) analyzed the motion of the upper extremities during running by considering angular momentum. He used a three-dimensional analysis to determine angular momentum about the three cardinal axes through the total body center of mass. Hinrichs reported that the arms made a meaningful contribution only about the vertical longitudinal axis. The arms generated alternating positive and negative angular momenta and tended to cancel out the opposite angular momentum pattern of the legs. These findings are illustrated in Figure 11-30. The upper portion of the trunk was found to rotate in conjunction with the arms, while the lower portion of the trunk rotated in conjunction with the legs.

THIRD LAW: LAW OF ACTION–REACTION

For every torque exerted by one body on another body, there is an equal and opposite torque exerted by the latter body on the former.

Generally, the torque generated by one body part to rotate that part results in a countertorque by another body part. This concept applies in activities such as long jumping. For example, the long jumper swings the legs forward and upward in preparation for landing. To counteract this lower body torque, the remainder of the body moves forward and downward, producing a torque equal

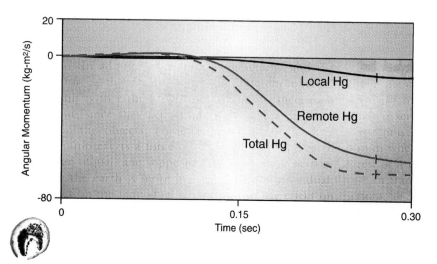

FIGURE 11-28 The relationship of total body angular momentum, total local angular momentum, and total remote angular momentum of a diver during a forward two-and-a-half rotation dive. The hash mark denotes the instant of takeoff. (After Hamill, J., et al. [1986]. Angular momentum in multiple rotation nontwisting dives. *International Journal of Sports Biomechanics*, 2:78–87.)

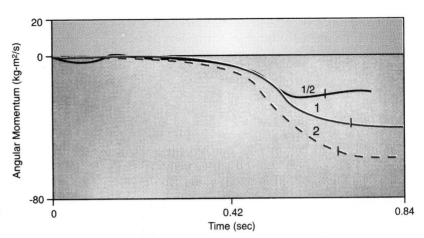

FIGURE 11-29 Profiles of back dives with half a rotation, one rotation, and two rotations depicting the buildup of angular momentum on the platform. The hash marks denote the instants of takeoff. (After Hamill, J., et al. [1986]. Angular momentum in multiple rotation non-twisting dives. *International Journal of Sports Biomechanics*, 2:78–87.)

and opposite to the lower body torque. While the torque and countertorques are equal and opposite, the angular velocity of these two body portions is different because the moments of inertia are different.

When equal torques are applied to different bodies, however, the resulting angular acceleration may not be the same because of the difference in the moments of inertia of the respective bodies. That is, the effect of one body on another may be greater than the latter body on the former. For example, when executing a pivot during a double play, the second baseman jumps into the air and throws the ball

to first base. In throwing the ball, the muscles in the second baseman's throwing arm create a torque as the arm follows through. The rest of the body must counter this torque. These torques are equal and opposite but have a much different effect on the respective segments. While the arm undergoes a large angular acceleration, the body angularly accelerates much less because the moment of inertia of the body is greater than that of the arm.

Analysis Using Newton's Laws of Motion

Chapter 10 presents three variations of Newton's laws that describe the relationship between the kinematics and the kinetics of a movement. An angular analog can be generated for each of the three approaches. In most biomechanical analyses, both the linear and angular relationships are determined to describe the cause-and-effect relationship in the movement. The linear analyses previously discussed presented three approaches categorized as (*a*) the effect of a force at an instant in time, (*b*) the effect of a force over a period of time, and (*c*) the effect of a force applied over a distance. A thorough analysis will also include the angular counterpart and examine (*a*) the effect of a torque at an instant in time, (*b*) the effect of a torque over time, and (*c*) the effect of a torque applied over a distance. Each approach provides different information and is useful in relation to the specific question asked about torque and angular motion.

EFFECTS OF A TORQUE AT AN INSTANT IN TIME

Newton's second law of motion is considered with the effects of a torque and the resulting angular acceleration. Thus:

$$\Sigma T = I\alpha$$

When the angular acceleration is zero, a static case is evaluated. A **dynamic analysis** results when the acceleration is not zero.

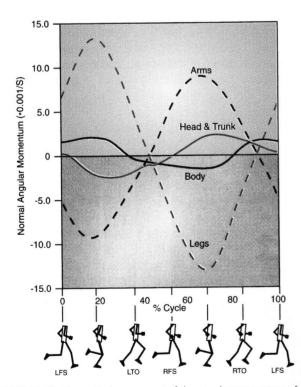

FIGURE 11-30 The vertical component of the angular momentum of the arms, head and trunk, legs, and total body of a runner at a medium running speed. (After Hinrichs, R. N. [1987]. Upper extremity function in running. II: Angular momentum considerations. *International Journal of Sports Biomechanics*, 3:242–263.)

The application of Newton's second law for both angular and linear cause and effect relationships would consider both linear and angular equations.

$$\Sigma F = ma$$
$$\Sigma T = I\alpha$$

In linear motion, the effects of a force and the resulting accelerations at an instant in time are determined. For angular motion, the effects of a torque and the resulting angular accelerations are determined.

Static Analysis

The static case involves systems at rest of moving at a constant velocity. A state of **equilibrium** exists when the acceleration of the system is zero. As illustrated in Chapter 10, linear equilibrium exists when the sum of the forces acting on the system equal zero. Equilibrium also depends on the balancing of torques acting on the system when forces are not concurrent. Concurrent forces do not coincide at the same point and thus cause rotation about some axis. These rotations all sum to zero, and the resulting system remains at rest or moves at a constant angular velocity. That is, the sum of the moments of force in the system must sum to zero. Stated algebraically, therefore:

$$\Sigma M_{system} = 0$$

Previously, a convention was suggested in which moments causing a counterclockwise rotation were considered to be positive, while clockwise torques were considered negative. To satisfy this condition of equilibrium, therefore, the sum of the counterclockwise moments must equal the sum of the clockwise moments, and no angular acceleration can occur.

Consider the free body diagram in Figure 11-31, in which a first-class lever system is described. On the left side of the fulcrum, A weighs 670 N and is 2.3 m from the axis of rotation. This individual would cause a counterclockwise or positive moment. B on the right side weighs 541 N, is 2.85 m from the fulcrum, and would cause a clockwise or negative moment. For this system to be in equilibrium, the clockwise moment must equal the counterclockwise moment. Thus:

$$M_A = 670 \text{ N} * 2.3$$
$$M_A = 1541 \text{ Nm}$$

and

$$M_B = 541 \text{ N} * 2.85 \text{ m}$$
$$M_B = 1541 \text{ Nm}$$

For this system to be in equilibrium:

$$\Sigma M = 0$$
$$M_A - M_B = 0$$
$$M_A = M_B$$

Since M_A is positive and M_B is negative and their magnitudes are equal, these moments cancel each other, and no rotation occurs. When the individual on the left pushes up with no further external forces, this system will come to rest in a balanced position.

Typically, multiple torques act on a system involving human movement. In Figure 11-32A shows the forearm of an individual holding a barbell. To determine the action at the elbow joint, it would be helpful to know the moment caused by the muscles about the elbow joint. If the elbow joint is considered to be the axis of rotation, there are two negative moments in this system. One negative moment is a result of the weight of the forearm and hand acting through the center of mass of the forearm–hand system, and the other is the result of the weight of the barbell. The counterclockwise or positive moment is a result of the muscle force acting across the elbow joint. The net moment of the muscles must be equal to the two negative moments for the system to be in equilibrium. Thus:

$$\Sigma M = 0$$
$$M_{Fm} - M_{arm\ hand} - M_{barbell} = 0$$

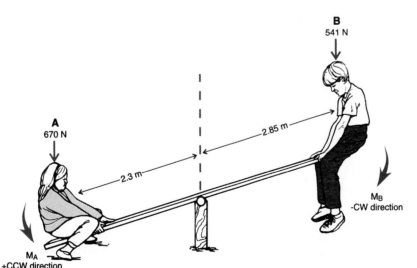

FIGURE 11-31 A first-class lever, a seesaw.

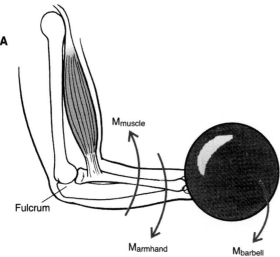

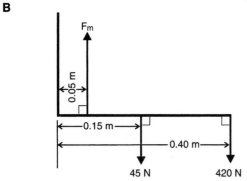

FIGURE 11-32 The forearm during an instant of a biceps curl **(A)** and a free body diagram of the system **(B)**.

Consider the free body diagram of this system illustrated in Figure 11-32B. The muscle moment that is necessary to keep the system in equilibrium can be calculated from the information in the free body diagram. The forearm–hand complex weighs 45 N, and the center of mass is 0.15 m from the elbow joint. The weight of the barbell is 420 N, and the center of mass of the barbell is 0.4 m from the elbow joint. The moment due to the weight of the arm and hand is:

$$M_{arm-hand} = (45\ N * 0.15\ m) = 6.75\ Nm$$

and the moment due to the barbell is:

$$M_{barbell} = (420\ N * 0.4\ m) = 168\ Nm$$

The moment due to the muscle force can then be calculated:

$$M_{Fm} - M_{arm-hand} + M_{barbell} = 0$$
$$M_{Fm} - (45\ N * 0.15\ m) - (420\ N * 0.4\ m) = 0$$
$$M_{Fm} = (45\ N * 0.15\ m) + (420\ N * 0.4\ m)$$
$$M_{Fm} = 6.75\ Nm + 168\ Nm$$
$$M_{Fm} = 174.75\ Nm$$

The muscle must create a torque of 174.75 Nm to counteract the weight of the forearm, hand, and barbell. This muscle moment cannot be directly attributed to any

one muscle that crosses the joint. The muscle moment calculated is the net sum of all muscle actions involved. In this case, since the arm is being held in flexion, the net muscle moment is due to the action of the elbow flexors, but it cannot be said exactly which elbow flexors are most involved. In fact, it might be surmised that since this is a static posture, there may be considerable cocontraction.

To determine the muscle action, the net torque about the joint must be considered. The net torque is the sum of all torques acting at the joint, in this case the elbow. Thus:

$$M_{elbow} = M_{Fm} - M_{arm-hand} - M_{barbell}$$
$$M_{elbow} = 174.75 - 6.75 - 168$$
$$M_{elbow} = 0$$

The net moment about the elbow joint is zero, indicating that the muscle action must be isometric.

If the moment arm of the elbow flexors was estimated to be 0.05 m from the elbow joint, the muscle force would be:

$$F_m = \frac{M_{Fm}}{0.05\ m}$$
$$F_m = \frac{174.75\ Nm}{0.05\ m}$$
$$F_m = 3495\ N$$

It can be seen that the muscle force must be considerably greater than the other two forces, because the moment arm for the muscle is very small compared to the moment arms for the forearm-hand or the barbell.

Consider Figure 11-33. In this free body diagram, the arm is placed in a posture similar to that in Figure 11-32, but this barbell weighs 100 N, and the measured muscle

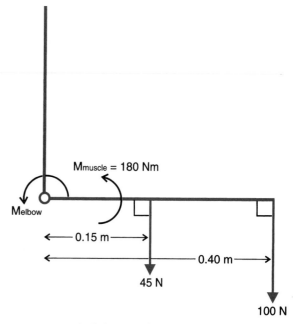

FIGURE 11-33 Free body diagram of a biceps curl at an instant when the forearm is horizontal.

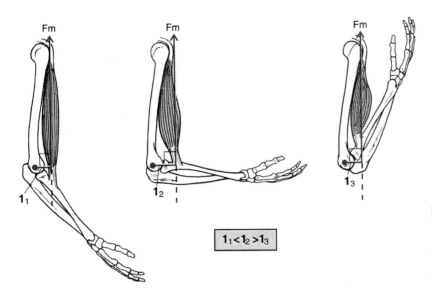

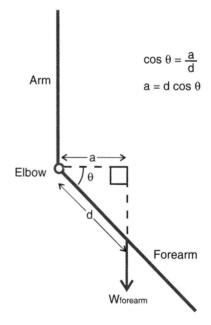

FIGURE 11-34 The change in moment of the moment arm of the biceps muscle throughout the range of motion. As the elbow flexes from an extended position, the moment arm becomes longer. As the arm continues to flex from the horizontal forearm position, the moment arm becomes shorter.

torque at the elbow is 180 Nm. All other measures in this situation are the same as in the previous example. Thus, evaluating the net moment at the elbow:

$$M_{elbow} = M_{Fm} + M_{arm-hand} + M_{barbell}$$
$$M_{elbow} = 180 \text{ Nm} - (45 \text{ N} * 0.15 \text{ m}) + (100 \text{ N} * 0.4 \text{ m})$$
$$M_{elbow} = 180 \text{ Nm} - 6.75 \text{ Nm} - 40 \text{ Nm}$$
$$M_{elbow} = 133.25 \text{ Nm}$$

Since the net moment at the elbow is positive, the rotation is counterclockwise, and the muscle action therefore is a flexor action.

In the previously described situations, the arm was parallel to the ground, and the moment arms from the axis of rotation were simply the distances measured along the segment to the lines of action of the forces. As the arm flexes or extends at the elbow joint, however, the moment arms change. In Figure 11-34, the moment arms for the muscle force are illustrated with the arm in three positions. With the elbow extended, the moment arm is rather small. As flexion occurs at the elbow, the moment arm increases until the arm is parallel to the ground. When flexion continues past this point, the moment arm becomes smaller once again. The magnitude of the moment arm of the muscle force, therefore, depends on how much flexion or extension occurs at a joint. The change in moment arm during flexion and extension of the limb is also true for the moment arms for both the weight of the forearm and hand and for anything held in the hand.

In Figure 11-35, the arm is held at some angle θ below the horizontal. The value d describes the distance from the axis of rotation to the center of mass of the arm. The moment arm for the arm weight, however, is the distance a. The lines a and d form the sides of a right triangle with the line of action of the force. Therefore, with the angle θ, the cosine function can be used to calculate the length a. Thus:

$$\text{Cos } \theta = \frac{a}{d}$$
$$a = d * \cos \theta$$

Consider that the arm has a 0° angle when it is parallel to the ground. As the arm extends, the angle increases until it is 90° at full extension. The cosine of 0° is 1, and as the angle becomes greater, the cosine gets smaller, until at 90° the cosine is 0. If the angle θ becomes greater as the arm is extended, the moment arm should become correspondingly smaller because the distance d does not change. When the angle θ is 90°, the arm is fully extended and the moment arm is zero because the line of action of the force due to the weight of the arm passes through the axis of rotation.

Consider an individual performing a biceps curl with a weight. The arm is positioned 25° below the horizontal, so that the elbow is slightly extended (Fig. 11-36A). The corresponding free body diagram is presented in Figure

FIGURE 11-35 The cosine of the angle of inclination of the forearm is used to calculate the moment arm when the forearm is not parallel to the horizontal.

weight of the arm and the weight of the barbell negative, then:

$$M_{Fm} - M_a - M_b = 0$$

Substituting all known values into this equation and rearranging it results in:

$$(F_m * 0.05 \text{ m}) = (45 \text{ N} * 0.14 \text{ m}) + (420 \text{ N} * 0.36 \text{ m})$$

This equation can be solved to determine the muscle force necessary to maintain this position in a static posture. Thus:

$$F_m = \frac{6.3 \text{ Nm} + 151.2 \text{ Nm}}{0.05 \text{ m}}$$

$$F_m = 3150 \text{ N}$$

The muscle must exert a force much greater than the weight of the arm and the barbell, because the moment arm for the muscle is relatively small. It would appear that our body is at a great disadvantage when it comes to producing large moments of force about a joint. Most of our joints are arranged as third-class levers, however, indicating that range of motion is magnified. Muscles can, therefore, exert large forces, but only over very short periods of time.

Static Equilibrium: Stability and Balance

The concept of stability is closely related to that of equilibrium. **Stability** may be defined in much the same way as equilibrium; that is, as the resistance to both linear and angular acceleration. The ability of an individual to assume and maintain a stable position is referred to as **balance**. Even in a stable or balanced position, an individual may be subject to external forces.

If a body is in a state of static equilibrium and is slightly displaced by a force, the object may return to its original position, continue to move away from its original position, or stop and assume a new position. If the object is displaced as a result of work done by a force and returns to its original position, it is said to be in a state of **stable equilibrium**. If the object is displaced and tends to increase its displacement, it is in a state of **unstable equilibrium**. A state of **neutral equilibrium** exists if the object is displaced by a force and returns to the position from which it was displaced.

Figure 11-37 illustrates these states of equilibrium. In Figure 11-37A, a ball on a concave surface exemplifies stable equilibrium. When it is displaced along one side of the surface by some force, it will return to its original position. In Figure 11-37B, an example of unstable equilibrium is presented: a force displaces a ball on a convex surface. The ball will come to rest in a new position, not its original position. Figure 11-37C illustrates neutral equilibrium. In this case, when a ball is placed on a flat surface and a force is applied, the ball will move to a new position.

The human body with its multiple segments is much more complex than a ball, but it can assume the different

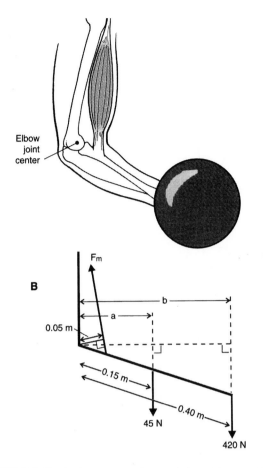

FIGURE 11-36 The forearm at an instant during a biceps curl **(A)** and the free body diagram of this position **(B)**. The arm is inclined below the horizontal.

11-36B. The moment arm for the weight of the arm can be calculated from the distance from the axis of rotation to the center of mass and the angle at which the arm is positioned:

$$a = 0.15 \text{ m} * \cos 25°$$
$$a = 0.15 \text{ m} * 0.9063$$
$$a = 0.14 \text{ m}$$

Similarly, the moment arm for the weight of the barbell held in the hand can be calculated:

$$b = 0.4 \text{ m} * \cos 25°$$
$$b = 0.4 \text{ m} * 0.9063$$
$$b = 0.36 \text{ m}$$

The moment arms are smaller than they would be if the arm were held parallel to the ground.

This problem may be solved for the muscle force using the same principles of a static analysis that were discussed previously. That is:

$$\Sigma M = 0$$

If, by convention, the moment due to the muscle is considered to be positive and the moments due to the

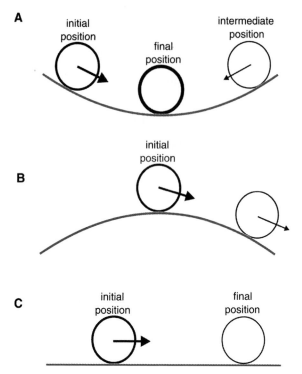

FIGURE 11-37 Examples of a ball. **A.** Stable equilibrium. **B.** Unstable equilibrium. **C.** Neutral equilibrium.

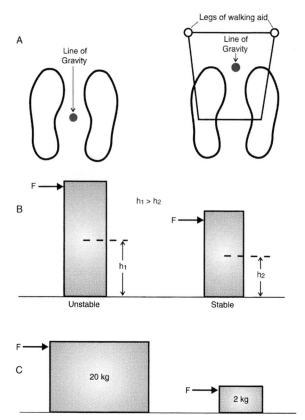

FIGURE 11-38 Factors that influence the stability of an object. **A.** Increasing the base of support. **B.** Lowering the center of mass. **C.** Increasing the mass of the system.

states of equilibrium. An individual doing a headstand, for example, is in a position of unstable equilibrium, and a child sitting on a swing is in a state of stable equilibrium.

Several factors determine the stability of an object. The first factor is where the line of gravity falls with respect to the base of support. An object will be most stable if the line of gravity is in the geometric center of the base of support. Increasing the area of the base of support generally increases the stability. However, a body may be stable in one direction and not in another. For example, spreading one's feet apart increases the area of the base of support and makes the individual stable if pushed in the transverse plane. It does not, however, help stability in the anteroposterior plane. Increasing the base of support to allow the line of gravity to fall within the base of support may be illustrated by the example of an individual using a walker. Figure 11-38A illustrates this case. The base of support is produced by the positions of the individual's legs and the legs of the walker. The walker increases the base of support, and the individual is positioned so that the line of action of the center of mass is in the geometric center of this base.

The stability of an object is also inversely proportional to the height of the center of mass. That is, an object with a low center of mass will tend to be more stable than an object with a high center of mass (Fig. 11-38B). If the two objects in Figure 11-38B undergo the same angular displacement as a result of the forces indicated, the line of gravity of the center of mass of the object on the left will move outside the limit of the base of support sooner than that of the object on the right. Therefore, the work done to dislodge the object on the left would be less than for

the object on the right. In football, for example, defensive linemen crouch in a three-point stance to keep their center of mass low. This enhances their stability so that they are less likely to be moved by the offensive linemen.

The final factor influencing stability is the mass of the object. According to the equations of motion, the greater the mass of an object, the greater its stability (Fig. 11-38C). Newton's second law states that the force applied to an object is proportional to the mass of the object and its acceleration. Thus, it takes more force to move an object with a greater mass. Moving a piano, for example, is extremely difficult because of its mass. Many sports such as wrestling and judo, in which stability is critical, take body mass into consideration by dividing the contestants into weight divisions because of the disproportionate stability of heavier individuals.

Applications of Statics

It would appear that static analyses are limited in their usefulness, since they describe situations in which no motion or motion at a constant velocity occurs. However, the **static analysis** of muscle forces and moments has been used extensively in ergonomics, even though the task may involve some movement. The evaluation of workplace tasks, such as lifting and manual materials handling, has been examined in considerable detail with static analyses. Use of static analysis to determine an individual's static or isometric

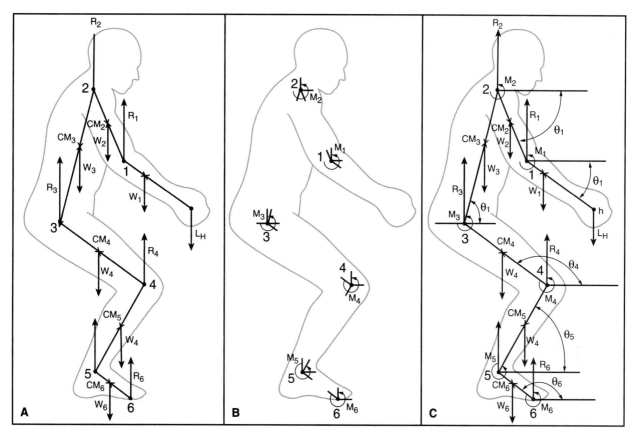

FIGURE 11-39 A free body diagram of a sagittal view static lifting model showing the linear reactive forces **(A)** and moments of forces **(B)** at the joints. These are combined to generate the total lifting model **(C)**. (After Chaffin, D. B., Andersson, G. B. J. [1991]. Occupational Biomechanics (2nd Ed.). New York: Wiley.)

strength is widely accepted in determining the ability of the person's lifting ability. Many researchers have suggested that this static evaluation should be used as a preemployment screening evaluation for applicants for manual materials handling tasks (7,29,42). Lind et al. (32) reported that the static endurance in a manual materials handling task is influenced by the posture of the individual performing the task. A model to evaluate static strength evaluations of jobs has been developed by Garg and Chaffin (17). A free body diagram of one such lifting model is presented in Figure 11-39 (6). This model was presented in Chapter 10 to illustrate a free body diagram for the linear forces acting on the system (Fig. 11-39A). Adding the moments of forces at each joint (Fig. 11-39B) allows the total lifting model to be evaluated (Fig. 11-39C).

Static analysis techniques have also been used in clinical rehabilitation. Quite often no movement of a body or a body segment is desirable, and thus a static evaluation may be undertaken. For example, placing a patient in traction demands that a static force system be implemented. Many bracing systems for skeletal problems, such as scoliosis and genu valgum (knock-knee), use a static force system to counteract the forces causing the problem (Fig. 11-40). Static analyses have been used in the calculation of muscle forces and have been performed by multiple researchers on many joints (18,39,44).

Dynamic Analysis

As pointed out in Chapter 10, a dynamic analysis should be used when the accelerations are not zero. Newton's second law establishes the basis for the dynamic analysis by examining the force–acceleration relationship. In the linear case, the equations of motion for a two-dimensional case are:

$$\Sigma F_x = ma_x$$
$$\Sigma F_y = ma_y$$

where the linear acceleration is broken down into its horizontal (x) and vertical (y) components. The angular equivalent looking at the torque–angular acceleration relationship is:

$$\Sigma T = I\alpha$$

in which I is the moment of inertia and α is the angular acceleration. In a two-dimensional system, angular acceleration occurs about the z-axis. If $\alpha = 0$, the motion is purely linear. If $a_x = 0$ and $a_y = 0$, the motion is purely rotational. If $\alpha = a_x = a_y = 0$, a static case exists.

The torques acting on a body are created by a contact or gravitational force acting a distance from the axis or rotation. $I\alpha$ is the inertial torque similar to ma_x and ma_y.

Angular accelerations and the inertial properties of the body segments resisting these accelerations must be considered in the dynamic case. As discussed in Chapter 10, in

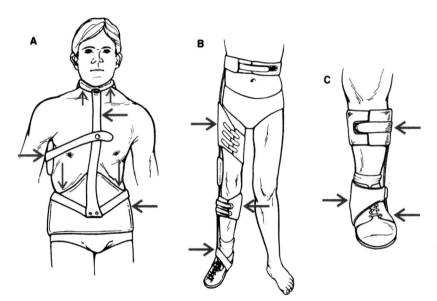

FIGURE 11-40 Bracing systems that illustrate static force systems. **A.** A neck brace. **B.** A three-point pressure brace to correct genu valgum. **C.** A brace to correct a foot deformity.

an **inverse dynamics** approach, each segment is evaluated from the most distal segment and works systematically up the segment links. Consider Figure 11-41, which illustrates a free body diagram of the foot during the swing phase of the gait cycle. In Chapter 10, a dynamic analysis of the linear forces was conducted by applying the two-dimensional linear kinetic equations. Joint reaction forces at the ankle were determined to be −1.57 N for R_x and 20.3 N for R_y.

To determine the net moment acting at the ankle joint, all moments acting on the system must be evaluated. If the center of mass of the foot is considered as the axis of rotation, three moments are acting on this system, two as a result of the joint reaction forces and the net ankle moment itself. Because the joint reaction forces and their

moment arms, the moment of inertia of the foot about an axis through the center of mass, and the angular acceleration of the foot are known, the net ankle moment can be calculated. Thus:

$$\Sigma M_{cm} = I_{cm}\alpha$$

$$M_{ankle} - M_{Rx} - M_{Ry} = I_{cm}\alpha$$

where M_{ankle} is the net muscle moment at the ankle, M_{Rx} is the moment resulting from the horizontal reaction force at the ankle, M_{Ry} is the moment resulting from the vertical reaction force at the ankle, and $I_{cm}\alpha$ is the product of the moment of inertia of the foot and the angular acceleration of the foot. In the general equation of moments acting on the foot, the moments M_{Rx} and M_{Ry} will cause clockwise rotation of the foot about the center of mass of the foot. By convention, clockwise rotations are negative and thus these moments are negative. Substituting the appropriate values from Figure 11-41 and those calculated in the previous equations and rearranging the equation:

$$M_{ankle} = I\alpha + M_{Rx} + M_{Ry}$$

$$M_{ankle} = (0.0096 \text{ kgm}^2 * -14.66 \text{ rad/s}^2) + (.07 \text{ m} * -1.57 \text{ N}) + (.07 \text{ m} * 20.3 \text{ N})$$

$$M_{ankle} = -0.141 \text{ Nm} - 0.110 \text{ Nm} + 1.421 \text{ Nm}$$

$$M_{ankle} = 1.17 \text{ Nm}$$

The net moment at this instant in time is positive, resulting in a counterclockwise rotation. A counterclockwise rotation of the foot indicates dorsiflexion activity. As with the static case, the exact muscles acting cannot be determined from this type of analysis. Thus, it cannot be stated whether the muscle activity is dorsiflexor concentric or dorsiflexor eccentric.

It was stated that a **dynamic analysis** usually proceeds from the more distal joints to the more proximal joints. The data from this calculation of the foot segment analysis

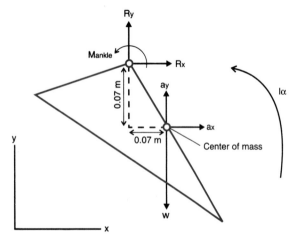

mass of foot = 1.16 kg, I = 0.0096 kg-m²
α = −14.66 rad/s²
a_x = −1.35 m/s², a_y = 7.65 m/s²
R_x = 1.57 N R_y = 20.3 N
(See Chapter 10)

FIGURE 11-41 Free body diagram of the foot during the swing phase of a walking stride. Convention dictates that moments and forces at the proximal joint are positive, as indicated on the free body diagram.

is used to calculate the net muscle moment at the knee. The calculation continues to the thigh to calculate the hip moment. The analysis is conducted for each joint at each instant in time of the movement under consideration to create a profile of the net muscle moments for the complete movement.

Applications of Dynamics

Dynamic analyses have been used in many biomechanical studies on a number of activities to determine the net moments at various joints. These activities include cycling (43), asymmetrical load carrying (11), weightlifting (31), jumping (56) and throwing (14). Figure 11-42 illustrates the net torques for the hip, knee, and ankle joints in a comparison study of one-legged and two-legged countermovement jumps by 10 volleyball players (56). The joint torques across the push-off phase demonstrated that the one-legged jump generated higher peak joint torques in all three joints and greater mean torques in the hip and ankle joints.

EFFECTS OF TORQUE APPLIED OVER A PERIOD OF TIME

For angular motion to occur, torques must be applied over a period of time. The application of a torque over time is known as angular **impulse**, derived from Newton's second law of motion:

$$T = I\alpha$$

$$T = I * \frac{d\omega}{dt}$$

$$T = \frac{d(I * \omega)}{dt}$$

$$T * dt = d(I * \omega)$$

or

$$T * dt = I\omega_{final} - I\omega_{initial}$$

The left side of the equation is angular impulse, and the right side of the equation describes a change in angular momentum. Known as the **impulse–momentum relationship**, the equation demonstrates that when a torque is applied over a period of time, a change in the angular momentum occurs. Consider the handspring vault in Figure 11-43. The gymnast is coming into contact with the horse after generating a large linear horizontal velocity during the approach, which is converted to some vertical velocity and angular momentum. On contact with the horse, the blocking action generates two torques. Since the gymnast is coming in to the horse at an angle, the contact with the horse generates both a vertical force (F_y) and a horizontal force (F_x). The vertical force on the horse increases the vertical velocity off the vault but creates a clockwise torque about the center of mass, which is the product of F_y and d_x. This angular impulse (T * t) changes the angular momentum and decreases the counterclockwise turning created by

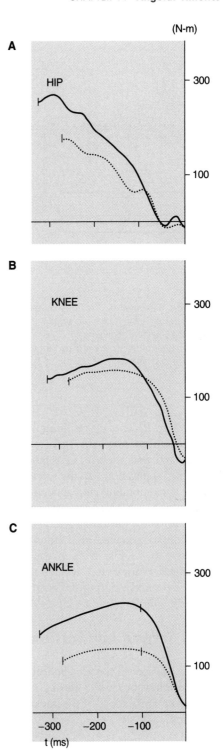

(N-m)

FIGURE 11-42 Hip **(A)**, knee **(B)**, and ankle **(C)** joint torques produced in the push-off phase of one-legged (*solid*) and two legged (*dotted*) countermovement jumps. (Modified from Van Soest, A. J., et al. [1985]. A comparison of one-legged and two-legged countermovement jumps. *Medicine and Science in Sports and Exercise*, 17:635–639.)

the angular momentum generated at takeoff from the board. The horizontal force on the horse acts in an opposite manner by decreasing horizontal velocity and increasing angular momentum generated on the board. A counterclockwise torque about the center of mass is generated via the

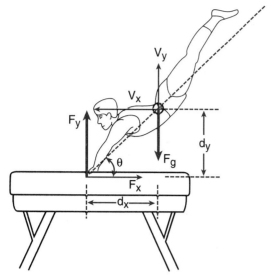

FIGURE 11-43 Torques generated on the horse by the vertical ($F_y * d_x$) and anteroposterior force ($F_x * d_y$) generate angular impulses about the center of mass of the vaulter. (Modified from Takei, Y. [1992]. Blocking and post flight techniques of male gymnasts performing the compulsory vault at the 1988 Olympics. *International Journal of Sport Biomechanics*, 8:87–110.)

impulse generated by F_x times d_y, resulting in an increase in the angular momentum from that generated at takeoff. Takei (53) indicated that the loss in angular momentum generated by the application of the vertical force was greater than the corresponding gain generated by the horizontal force, resulting in a loss of angular momentum while on the horse. In elite Olympic gymnasts the angular momentum at contact averaged 95.3 kgm²/s in the highest scored vaults and 92.4 kgm²/s in the lowest scored vaults, and the angular momentum was reduced by −33 and −27.4 kgm²/s, respectively, during the horse contact phase as a result of these angular impulses (52).

 Special Torque Applications

Angular motion has special torque applications comparable to the force applications in the linear case. Many of the angular applications are analogs of the linear case and have similar definitions.

ANGULAR WORK: EFFECTS OF TORQUE APPLIED OVER A DISTANCE

Mechanical **angular work** is defined as the product of the magnitude of the torque applied against an object and the angular distance that the object rotates in the direction of the torque while the torque is being applied. Expressed algebraically:

$$\text{Angular work} = T * \Delta\theta$$

where T is the torque applied and $\Delta\theta$ is the angular distance. Since torque has units of Nm and angular distance

has units of radians, the units for angular work are newton-meters (Nm) or joules (J), the same units as in the linear case. For example, if a 40.5 Nm torque is applied over a rotation of 0.79 radians, the work done in rotation is:

$$\begin{aligned} \text{Work} &= T * \Delta\theta \\ &= 40.5 \text{ Nm} * 0.79 \text{ rad} \\ &= 32.0 \text{ Nm} \end{aligned}$$

Thus 32 Nm of work is said to be done by the torque, T.

When a muscle contracts and produces tension to move a segment, a torque is produced at the joint and the segment is moved through some angular displacement. The muscles that rotated the segment do mechanical angular work. To differentiate between the kinds of muscle actions angular work done by muscles is characterized as either positive or negative work. **Positive work** is associated with concentric muscle actions or actions in which the muscle is shortening as it creates tension. For example, if a weight lifter performs a biceps curl on a barbell, the phase in which the elbows flex to bring the barbell up is the concentric phase (Fig. 11-44*A*). During this

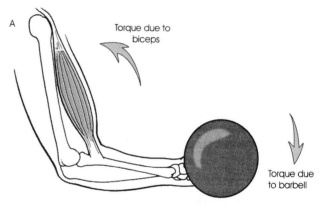

Torque due to biceps > torque due to barbell

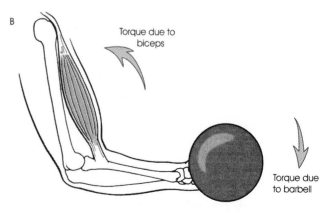

Torque due to biceps < torque to barbell

FIGURE 11-44 Positive muscular work **(A)** and negative muscular work **(B)** during a biceps curl of a barbell.

motion, the flexor muscles of the weightlifter do work on the barbell. **Negative work**, on the other hand, is associated with eccentric muscle actions, or actions in which the muscle is lengthening as it creates tension. In a biceps curl, when the weight lifter is lowering the barbell, resisting the pull of gravity, the flexor muscles are doing negative work (Fig. 11-44*B*). In this instance, the barbell is doing work on the muscles. While it has been found that positive work requires a greater metabolic expenditure than negative work, no direct relationship has been reported between mechanical work of muscles and physiological work.

ANGULAR POWER

In Chapter 10, power was defined in the linear case as the work done per unit time or the product of force and velocity. **Angular power** may be similarly defined as:

$$\text{Power} = \frac{dW}{dt}$$

where dW is the angular work done and dt is the time in which the work was done. Angular power may also be defined as in the linear case, using the angular analogs of force and velocity, torque, and angular velocity. **Angular power** is the angular work done per unit time and is calculated as the product of torque and angular velocity:

$$\text{angular power} = T * \omega$$

where T is the torque applied in newton-meters and ω is the angular velocity in radians per second. Angular power thus has units of newton-meters per second, or watts. The concept of angular power is often used to describe mechanical muscle power.

Muscle power is determined by calculating the net torque of the muscle acting across the joint and the angular velocity of the joint. The net muscle moment describes the net muscle activity across a joint and does not represent any one particular muscle that crosses the joint. It also does not take into account the situation in which biarticulate muscles may be acting. This net muscle activity at a joint is simply described as flexor or extensor actions, but whether the muscle activity is concentric or eccentric cannot be ascertained. The net muscle moment can, however, be used in conjunction with the angular velocity of the joint to determine the concentric or eccentric nature of the muscular action. As discussed previously, concentric actions of muscles are related to the positive work of muscles and eccentric actions as the negative work of muscles. Because the work done by muscles is rarely constant with time, the concept of muscle power should be used. Muscle power is the time rate of change of work and is defined as the product of the net muscle moment and the joint angular velocity. It is expressed algebraically as:

$$P_m = M_j * \omega_j$$

where P_m is the muscle power in units of watts (W), M_j is the net muscle moment in newton-meters, and ω_j is the joint angular velocity in radians per second.

Muscle power may be either positive or negative. Since power is the time rate of change of work, the area under the power–time curve is the work done. Thus, positive muscle power represents positive work or a net concentric action, while negative muscle power represents negative work or a net eccentric action. For example, if M_j and ω_j are either both positive or both negative, muscle power will be positive. If they have opposite polarity, muscle power will be negative. Figure 11-45 illustrates the positive and negative work possibilities of the elbow joint. In Figure 11-45*A*, M_j and ω_j are positive, indicating a flexor moment with the arm moving in a flexor direction. The resulting muscle power is positive, indicating a concentric action of the elbow flexors. In Figure 11-45*B*, both M_j and ω_j are negative, resulting in a positive muscle power or a concentric action. The arm is extending, indicating the muscle action is a concentric action of the elbow extensors. In Figure 11-45*C*, M_j is positive or a flexor moment, but the arm has a negative ω_j indicating extension. In this case, an external force is causing the arm to extend while the elbow flexors resist. This results in an eccentric action

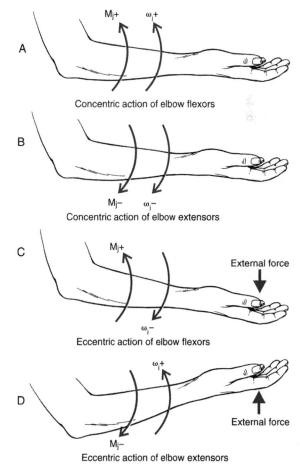

FIGURE 11-45 The definition of positive and negative power at the elbow joint: **A** and **B** result in positive power; **C** and **D** result in negative power.

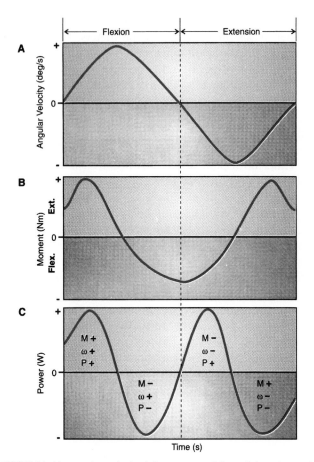

FIGURE 11-46 Angular velocity **(A)**, moment of force **(B)**, and muscle power **(C)** profiles during an elbow flexion–extension motion.

of the elbow flexors and is verified by the negative muscle power. Figure 11-45*D* illustrates the case in which an eccentric action of the elbow extensors result.

Figure 11-46 illustrates the angular velocity–time, net muscle moment–time, and the muscle power–time profiles during an elbow flexion followed by elbow extension. In the flexion phase of the movement, the net muscle moment initially is positive, but it becomes negative as the arm becomes more flexed. The initial portion, therefore, results in a positive power or a concentric contraction of the flexor muscles. In the latter portion of the flexor phase, the power is negative, indicating an eccentric muscle contraction. The eccentric contraction of the elbow extensor muscles occurs to decelerate the limb. Because the power is negative at this point, however, it does not mean that there is no flexor muscle activity. It simply means that the predominant activity is extensor. In the extension portion of the movement, the situation is reversed. In the initial portion of extension, the muscle activity is concentric extensor activity. In the latter portion, the muscle power profile indicates flexor concentric activity once again to decelerate the limb.

The analysis of net muscle moments of force and muscle power have been widely used in research in biomechanics. Winter and Robertson (64) and Robertson and

Winter (46) have investigated the power requirements in walking. Robertson (45) described the power functions of the leg muscles during running to identify any common characteristics among a group of runners. Gage (16) reported on the use of the moment of force and the muscle power profiles as a preoperative and postoperative comparison. The analysis of muscle power in the lower extremity during locomotion, therefore, appears to be a powerful research and diagnostic tool.

ENERGY

In Chapter 10, translational kinetic energy was defined in terms of mass and velocity. **Rotational kinetic energy** may also be defined similarly, using the angular analogs of mass and velocity, moment of inertia and angular velocity. Thus, rotational kinetic energy is defined algebraically as:

$$RKE = \frac{1}{2} I\omega^2$$

where RKE is the rotational kinetic energy, I is the moment of inertia, and ω is the angular velocity. Thus, when the total energy of a system is defined, the rotational kinetic energy must be added to the translational kinetic energy and the potential energy. Total mechanical energy is therefore defined as:

total energy = translational kinetic energy +
potential kinetic energy + rotational kinetic energy

or

$$TE = TKE + PE + RKE$$

In the discussion of angular kinematics, it was noted that single segments undergo large angular velocities during running. Thus, if a single segment was considered, it might be intuitively expected that the rotational kinetic energy might influence the total energy of the segment more significantly than the translational kinetic energy. Winter et al. (63), for example, hypothesized that angular contributions of the leg would be important to the changes in total segment energy in running. Williams (60) offered the following example to illustrate that this is not the case.

Consider a theoretical model of a lower extremity segment undergoing both translational and rotational movements (Fig. 11-47). If the leg segment is considered, the linear velocity of the center of mass of the leg is:

$$v_{LEGcm} = \omega r$$

where ω is the angular velocity of the leg and r is the distance from the knee to the center of mass of the leg. If the body segment values of the leg are moment of inertia = 0.0393 kgm^2, mass = 3.53 kg, and r = 0.146 m, the magnitude of the rotational kinetic energy is:

$$\begin{aligned}
RKE &= \frac{1}{2} I\omega^2 \\
&= 0.05 * 0.0393 * \omega^2 \\
&= 0.0192\omega^2
\end{aligned}$$

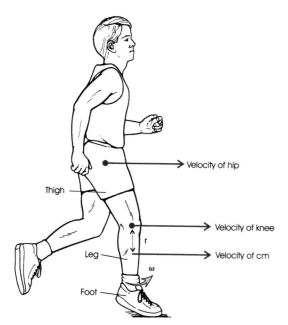

FIGURE 11-47 Theoretical representation of the translational and rotational velocities of the thigh and leg during running. (After Williams, K. R. [1980]. *A Biomechanical and Physiological Evaluation of Running Efficiency.* Unpublished doctoral dissertation, The Pennsylvania State University.)

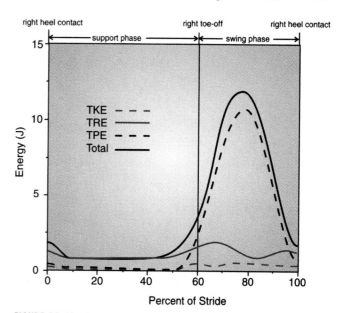

FIGURE 11-48 The relationship between total energy (*Total*), rotational kinetic energy (*RKE*), translational kinetic energy (*TKE*), and potential energy (*PE*) of the foot during a walking stride.

The translational kinetic energy of the leg under the same circumstances is:

$$TKE = \frac{1}{2}\, mv^2$$

where m and v are the mass and the linear velocity of the leg. Substituting the expression ωr into this equation for the linear velocity, v, the equation becomes:

$$
\begin{aligned}
TKE &= \frac{1}{2}\, m(\omega r)^2 \\
&= 0.5 * 3.53\,(0.146\omega)^2 \\
&= 0.0376\omega^2
\end{aligned}
$$

Since ω^2 is the same in both answers, the two types of energy can be evaluated, based on the values of 0.0192 times ω^2 for the rotational energy and 0.0376 times ω^2 for the translational energy. Thus, the translational kinetic energy is almost double that of the rotational kinetic energy. In fact, Williams stated that the rotational kinetic energy of most segments will be much less than the translational kinetic energy. Figure 11-48 illustrates the relationship between the energy components of the foot during a walking stride. In this figure, the magnitude of the total energy is almost completely made up of the translational kinetic energy.

Work-Energy Relationship

Mechanical angular work has been defined as the product of a torque applied to an object and the distance that the object moved during the torque application. Angular work is said to have been done on an object when movement occurs through some angular distance. Rotational energy also has been defined as the capacity to do angular work. Therefore the **work–energy theorem**, W = ΔE, also applies. That is, for mechanical work to be done, a change in the energy level must occur. The angular work done on an object is:

$$
\begin{aligned}
W_{angular} &= \Delta RE \\
W_{angular} &= \Delta\left(\frac{1}{2}\, I\omega^2\right)
\end{aligned}
$$

where $W_{angular}$ is the angular work done on the object and ΔRE is the change in rotational kinetic energy about the center of mass. To calculate the total work done on the object, the other forms of energy, such as potential and kinetic energy, must also be considered. With the inclusion of these two additional forms of energy, the work done on the object becomes:

$$
\begin{aligned}
W_{object} &= \Delta KE + \Delta PE + \Delta RE \\
W_{object} &= \Delta(\tfrac{1}{2}\, mv^2) + \Delta(mgh) + \Delta(\tfrac{1}{2}\, I\omega^2)
\end{aligned}
$$

where W_{object} is the work done on the object, ΔKE Is the change in the linear kinetic energy of the center of mass of the object [$\Delta(1/2\ mv^2)$], ΔPE is the change in potential energy of the object center of mass [$\Delta(mgh)$], and ΔRE is the change in rotational energy about the center of mass of the object [$\Delta(1/2\ I\omega^2)$]. For example, in baseball batting, the goal is to generate maximum energy at contact so maximum work can be generated in the ball. Both the linear and rotational kinetic energy of the bat are important. Potential energy is also a factor, as the bat stores potential energy in the handle that is later transferred as local kinetic energy at impact (13).

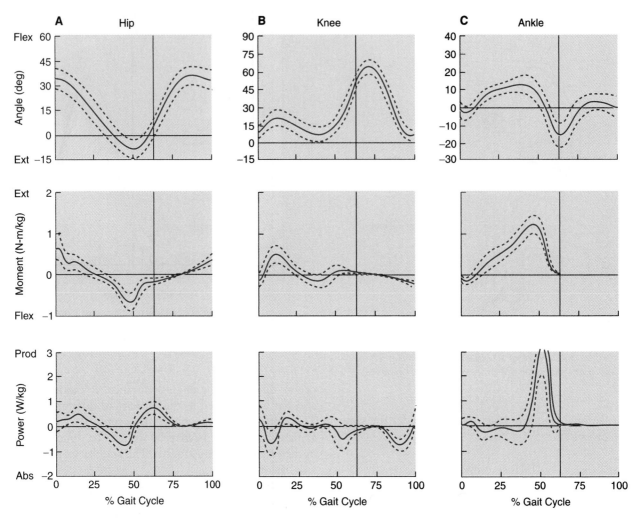

FIGURE 11-49 Angular displacement, moments of force, and power during a single walking stride. **A.** Hip, **B.** Knee. **C.** Ankle. The transition from support to swing is indicated at the solid line. (After Ounpuu, S. [1994]. The biomechanics of walking and running. *Foot and Ankle Injuries*, 13:843–863.)

Angular Kinetics of Locomotion

The angular kinetics of locomotion, specifically the joint moments of force of the lower extremity, have been widely researched (3,61,62). Winter (61) stated that the resultant moment of force provided powerful diagnostic information when comparing injured gait to uninjured gait. Another common area of investigation for gait is muscle mechanical power. Muscle power is the product of the net muscle moments and the angular velocity. Positive power results when the net joint moments are producing movement concentrically, such as flexor moments accompanying segment movement in the flexion direction. Negative power is associated with eccentric muscle action, when the net muscle moments of force are occurring in the opposite direction to the segment movement. For example, negative power would result when a net knee extension moment is generated as the knee is moving into flexion. It is not uncommon to see power fluctuate between negative and positive multiple times across the cycle in both walking and running.

Figure 11-49 illustrates the joint kinematics, the net muscle moments of force, and the corresponding powers of the net moments at the hip, knee, and ankle during a walking stride. At the hip joint, there is a net hip extensor moment during the initial loading phase of support continuing through midsupport into late stance. In late stance there is a new power absorption as hip extension is decelerated via hip flexors (40). In preparation for toe-off, the hip flexors shorten to produce power for the initiation of the swing phase. Hip flexion continues into swing via power production via flexor moments until it is terminated in late swing by a hip extensor moment.

At the knee joint, the loading response involves knee flexion controlled by the knee extensors moving into midsupport where there is a net knee extensor moment under control by the knee extensors. In late stance, there is again a knee flexor moment that moves to a small knee extensor moment controlled by the knee extensors. During swing, there is minimal power production until the terminal phase of swing, when there is a net knee

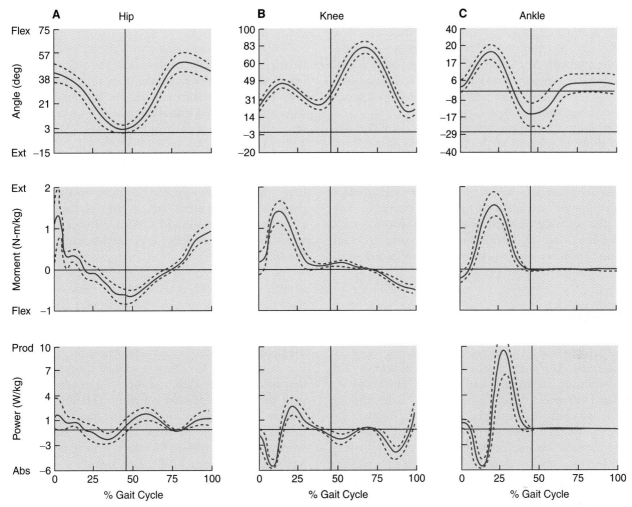

FIGURE 11-50 Angular displacement, moments of force, and power during a single running stride. **A.** Hip, **B.** Knee. **C.** Ankle. The transition from support to swing is indicated at the solid line. (After Ounpuu, S. [1994]. The biomechanics of walking and running. *Foot and Ankle Injuries*, 13:843–863.)

flexor moment controlled eccentrically to slow knee extension for contact.

The ankle joint exhibits a net dorsiflexor moment during the loading phase of stance as the foot is lowered to the ground. A transition to a net ankle plantarflexion moment first occurs through eccentric plantarflexion actions to control the body's movement over the foot. This is followed by a continuation of a net plantarflexion moment as the plantar flexors concentrically advance the limb into the swing phase. At the actual initiation of the swing phase, plantarflexion continues under the control of eccentric dorsiflexion activity. Once in the swing phase, minimal power is produced at the ankle.

The joint moment and power patterns can change with the speed of walking. For example, there are three basic moment patterns at the knee joint: a biphasic pattern, a flexor moment resisting an external extensor moment, and an extensor moment after heel strike (26). At slower speeds there is more use of a flexor moment, with little knee flexion and small knee moments through midstance resulting in negative joint power (26). In a faster walk,

there are more knee flexion and extension moments and more energy generation early in the stance phase followed by energy absorption during early stance.

Figure 11-50 illustrates the joint kinematics, the net muscle moments of force, and the corresponding powers of the net moments at the hip, knee, and ankle during a running stride (40). The moments of force and powers in running are greater in magnitude than those in walking. The lower extremity moments of force increase in magnitude with increases in locomotor speed. Cavanagh et al. (4) and Mann and Sprague (34) reported considerable variability in the magnitudes of the moments of force between subjects running at the same speed. For slow running this variability is generally smallest at the ankle and greatest at the hip.

Similar to walking, the hip joint extends during both loading and propulsive stages of stance initially via concentric hip extension and later during support via eccentric hip flexion. Concentric hip flexion continues in the swing phase as the thigh is brought forward. This continues into late swing, when the hip extensors terminate the hip flexion movement and initiate a hip extension (40).

At the knee joint, the loading response is similar to that of walking, involving flexion controlled by the knee extensors moving into midsupport, where there is a net knee extensor moment. At the start of the swing phase, a small net knee extensor moment controls knee flexion. Later in the swing phase, a net knee flexor moment slows the rapidly extending knee.

Ankle joint net joint moments and powers are also similar to those of walking, depending on the style of running. For runners with a typical heel strike pattern, the ankle joint exhibits a small net dorsiflexor moment during the loading phase followed by a net ankle plantarflexion moment for the remainder of the stance phase. In midstance the net ankle plantarflexion moment controls rapid dorsiflexion, and in later stance, the plantarflexion moment produces rapid plantarflexion. Minimal ankle power is generated in the swing phase.

Angular Kinetics of the Golf Swing

The actual physical dimensions and characteristics of the club influence the angular kinetics of a golf swing. The composition of the materials of both the shaft and the club head influences swing characteristics. Shafts made of graphite or composite materials are usually lighter and stronger. A golfer can swing a lighter club faster while producing the same amount of angular work. Adding mass to a club increases the joint torque at the shoulder and the trunk in the last half of the swing (30). Stiffer shafts hit straighter; flexible shafts hit farther but are difficult to control, which influences accuracy (51). The reason the stiffer staff offers better control is because it has less bend and twist and it compresses the ball more, creating a flight that is more representative of the actual angle of the club (35). A steel club with good direction control may be better for a novice golfer than a graphite club that can achieve more distance but is harder to control. The most desirable physical characteristics of the club are a high moment of inertia and a low center of gravity (50).

The physical characteristics of the club head can also influence the performance. An increase in the mass of the club head increases the joint torque at both the shoulder and the trunk for the latter half of the swing (30). Also, if the weight in the club head can be distributed to the periphery of the face, the sweet spot is increased, offering greater tolerance to off-center hits (50). If the center of gravity of the club head can be lowered, it can produce a higher flight path, and if the center of gravity can be moved toward the heel of the club, a right-to-left spin is promoted (50).

Club lengths influence the amount of torque generated in the shoulder, and the longer club produces an increase in the torque. This opens up the shoulder earlier and increases the linear acceleration of the wrist (30). Drivers are 5% longer than they were 10 years ago, and even if they can produce better results, they are more difficult to swing and control (35).

The angle the shaft makes with the ground is called the lie angle, and this determines how the face of the club is oriented. Lie angles range from approximately 55° for a one-wood to approximately 63° for the nine-iron. The lie angle can be altered if the club length does not match the physical dimensions of the golfer. Sample club lengths are 110 cm for a one-wood to 90 cm for a nine-iron (51). If a club is too short for a golfer, the drive is usually shorter because of lower velocities. Likewise, if the club is too long, the golfer is required to stand up more and may choke up on the shaft, which reduces the control and changes the lie angle (51). With a lower lie angle the sweet spot of the club face is raised, leading to topping of the ball.

Altering the length of the club affects the angular acceleration. For example, at the top of the backswing, the club lever is shortened by right elbow flexion. In the downswing, the club lever is lengthened (33). When the club is reversed at the top of the upswing, the torque applied to the shaft actually causes it to bend where the head trails the line of the shaft (35). Torque applied through the shoulders accelerates the club, and there is a rigid body rotation with the wrist angle held constant. This brings the shaft perpendicular to the swing. Next, the hands allow the club to accelerate about the wrist, and in the last part of the swing, the shaft is rotated 90° at the wrist to bring the shaft face square into impact (35). The distance a golf ball travels is related to the speed of the club head at contact. This speed is determined by the torque the golfer applies to the arm–club system and the management of the torque on the club by the wrists (28). If the wrists can be uncocked later in the downswing, greater club head speed is generated for a given torque. In the follow-through phase, the angular momentum of the swing takes the right arm over the left and stimulates rotation of both the trunk and the head (33).

The torque generated at the wrist about the vertical (y), anteroposterior (z), and mediolateral (x) axes in the swing of a professional golfer is shown in Figure 11-51. In the backswing, a positive torque is generated about the anteroposterior axis (z) as the angle between the club and the arm is maintained. At the initiation of the downswing, a negative torque is generated about the same axis to keep the club back and maintain the same angle between the club and the arm. At the bottom of the downswing a large positive torque is developed as the wrist uncocks and accelerates the club to impact (38). Rotations about the mediolateral axis are maximum as the club is taken back behind the head. Torques about the vertical and the anteroposterior axes are zero at this point, since the club is parallel to the vertical–anteroposterior plane. Torque about the vertical axis is maximum at the initiation of the downswing as the body rotates around the support.

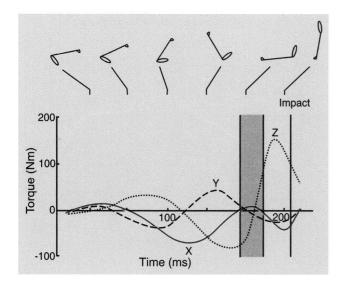

FIGURE 11-51 Joint torques acting at the wrist joint about the vertical (*Y*), anteroposterior (*Z*), and mediolateral (*X*) axes. The solid line indicates impact. (After Neal, R. J., Wilson, B. D. [1985]. 3D kinematics and kinetics of the golf swing. *International Journal of Sports Biomechanics,* 1:221–232.)

Angular Kinetics of Wheelchair Propulsion

Hand rim wheelchair locomotion is strenuous and involves a significant amount of mechanical work production by the upper extremity muscles. The size of the joint moments at the shoulder and elbow joints are influenced by the direction of application of the linear force. A large elbow moment is present when the force application to the rim is perpendicular to a line from the hand to the elbow and is minimized when the force is applied along the line from the hand to the elbow (48). Likewise, propelling forces, which are perpendicular to the line between the hand and the shoulder, result in large shoulder moments.

The shoulder joint torques account for the majority of the external power in wheelchair propulsion (54). The peak torques in the shoulder joint are greater than those generated in the elbow joint (57). Very small torques are generated in the wrist joint, where a braking effect is generated (57). The torques generated at the elbow and wrist joints are one-third and one-fifth of the torques at the shoulder joint (5). Joint torques ranges for the joints approximate 5 to 9 Nm at the wrist joint, 9 to 25 Nm at the elbow joint, and 25 to 50 Nm at the shoulder joint (47,54).

At low speeds and resistances, wheelchair propulsion is generated primarily by upper extremity sagittal plane movement, and half of the shoulder joint work is lost as negative work at the wrist and elbow (5). As the workload and speed increase, there is a concomitant increase in the direction and magnitudes of the joint torques. More extension and abduction at the shoulder coupled with more torque at the elbow joint contribute to the

increased output (5). The increase in shoulder abduction is speculated to be a forced abduction because of rotation of the arm in a closed chain system (54). A sample of the shoulder flexion and extension, shoulder adduction, elbow flexion, and wrist flexion and extension torque patterns for wheelchair propulsion are shown in Figure 11-52. The highest torques were generated via shoulder flexion and shoulder adduction. The shoulder flexion torque peaked just prior to the peak in elbow extension torque. Shoulder adduction torque controlled the shoulder abduction created as a result of arm movement in a closed chain. There is a net flexor torque at the elbow at the beginning of the propulsion phase that shifts to an extensor torque continuing on through the rest of propulsion. Wrist torques are primarily extension throughout the majority of the propulsion phase. There is also a pronation and a larger radial deviation moment acting at the wrist over the majority of the propulsive phase (2).

Summary

Torque, or the moment of force, results when the line of action does not pass through the center of mass of an object. Torques cause rotational motion of an object about an axis. Torques are vectors and thus must be considered in terms of magnitude and direction. The right-hand rule defines whether the torque is positive (counterclockwise rotation) or negative (clockwise rotation).

The concept of torque can be used to define the center of mass of an object. The sum of the torques about the center of mass of an object equals zero. That is:

$$\Sigma T = 0$$

This relationship defines the center of mass as the balancing point of the object.

The center of mass is commonly computed using the segmental method, which requires the computation of body segment parameters, such as the location of the center of mass and the segment proportion of the total body mass. The location of a segment center of mass requires the coordinates of both the proximal and distal ends of the segment. It is defined as:

$$s_{cm} = s_{prox} - (ds * \%\text{length from segment's proximal end})$$
$$= s_{prox} - [(s_{prox} - s_{distal}) * \%L]$$

where s_{cm} is the location of the segment center of mass, s_{prox} is the coordinate point of the proximal end of the segment, s_{distal} is the coordinate point of the distal end of the segment, ds is the length of the segment, and $\%L$ is the location of the segment center of mass as a proportion of the segment length from the proximal end of the segment. Locating the total body center of mass with the segmental method also uses the concept that the sum of the

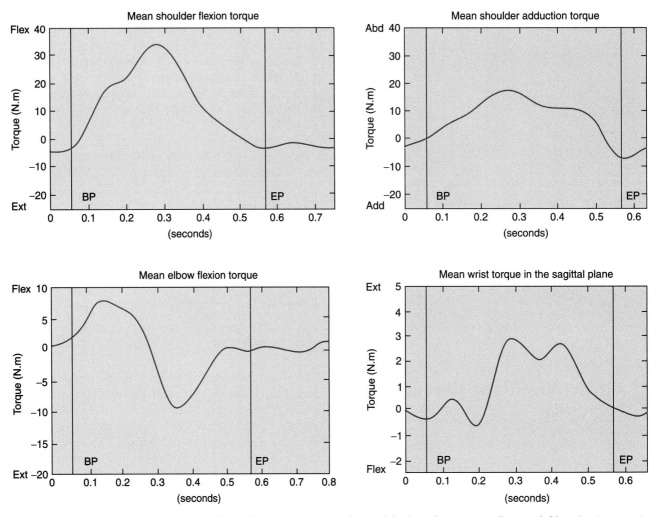

FIGURE 11-52 Shoulder flexion torque **(top left)**, shoulder adduction torque **(top right)**, elbow flexion torque **(bottom left)**, and wrist torque in the sagittal plane **(bottom right)** for the propulsive stage of wheelchair propulsion. BP, beginning propulsion; EP, end propulsion. (After Veeger, H. E. J., et al. [1991]. Load on the upper extremity in manual wheelchair propulsion. *Journal of Electromyography and Kinesiology*, 1:270–280.)

torques about the center of mass is zero. This computation uses the formula:

$$s_{cm} = \sum_{i=1}^{n} \frac{m_i s_i}{M}$$

where s_{cm} is the location of the total body center of mass, n is the number of segments, m_i is the mass of the ith segment, s_i is the location of the segment center of mass, and M is the total body center of mass.

A lever is a simple machine with a balancing point called the fulcrum and two forces, an effort force and a resistance force. The mechanical advantage (MA) of a lever is defined as the ratio of the effort arm to the resistance arm. Levers can magnify force (MA > 1), magnify speed of rotation (MA < 1), or change the direction of pull (MA = 1). The three classes of levers are based on the relationship of the effort and resistance forces to the fulcrum. In the human body, however, the third-class lever magnifying the speed of movement predominates. Most of the levers in the extremities are third-class levers.

Moment of inertia is the angular analog of mass. The moment of inertia of an object, or the resistance to angular motion, depends on the axis about which the object is rotating. The calculation of the segment moment of inertia can be calculated using the radius of gyration as:

$$I_{cm} = m(\rho_{cm} L)^2$$

where I_{cm} is the moment of inertia about a transverse axis through the center of mass, m is the mass of the segment, ρ_{cm} is a proportion describing the ratio of the radius of gyration about the center of mass to the segment length, and L is the segment length.

Angular momentum is the angular analog of linear momentum and refers to the quantity of rotation of an object. The angular momentum of a multisegment body must be understood in terms of local and remote angular momentum. Local angular momentum is the angular momentum of a segment about its own center of mass. Remote angular momentum is the angular momentum of a segment about the total body center of mass. The total segment angular momentum is the sum of the segment's local and remote aspects. The total body angular momentum is the sum of the local and remote aspects of all segments. The angular analog of Newton's first law of motion is a statement of the law of conservation of angular momentum.

Newton's laws of motion can be restated from the linear case to their angular analogs. The angular analogs of these laws:

1. A rotating body will continue in a state of uniform angular motion unless acted on by an external torque.
2. An external torque will produce an angular acceleration of a body that is proportional to and in the direction of the torque and inversely proportional to the moment of inertia of the body.
3. For every torque exerted by one body on another body, an equal and opposite torque is exerted by the latter body on the former.

Special torque applications include angular work, rotational kinetic energy, and angular power. These concepts may be developed by substituting the appropriate angular equivalent in the linear case. Angular work is defined as:

$$\text{angular work} = T * d\theta$$

where T is the torque applied and $d\theta$ is the angular distance over which the torque was applied. Angular work can be used to define the action of muscles as concentric (positive angular work) or eccentric (negative angular work). Rotational kinetic energy of a segment is defined as:

$$\text{RKE} = \frac{1}{2} I\omega^2$$

where I is the moment of inertia of the segment about its center of mass and ω is the angular velocity of the segment. Angular power is defined as either the rate of doing angular work:

$$\text{angular power} = \frac{dW}{dt}$$

Equation Review for Angular Kinetics

Calculation	Given	Formula
Torque	Force (F), moment arm (r)	$T = Fr$
Torque	Moment of inertia (I), angular acceleration (α)	$T = I\alpha$
Angular acceleration(α)	Torque (T), moment of inertia (I)	$\alpha = \frac{T}{I}$
Center of mass of system (x_{cm}, y_{cm})	Mass (m), location (x, y)	$x_{cm} = \frac{m_1x_1 + m_2x_2 + \cdots m_nx_n}{\text{total mass}}$ $y_{cm} = \frac{m_1y_1 + m_2y_2 + \cdots m_ny_n}{\text{total mass}}$
Mechanical advantage (MA)	Length of effort arm (EA), resistance arm (RA)	$MA = \frac{EA}{RA}$
Moment of inertia (I)	Mass (m), distance from axis (r)	$I = mr^2$
Moment of inertia (I)	Angular acceleration (α), torque (T)	$I = \frac{T}{\alpha}$
Moment of inertia (I)	Mass (m), length (l), radius of gyration (ρ)	$I = m (\rho * l)^2$
Angular momentum (p)	Moment of inertia (I), angular velocity (ω)	$H = I\omega$
Angular impulse	Angular momentum (I * ω)	$\text{Angular impulse} = I\omega_{final} - I\omega_{initial}$
Angular velocity	Torque, time, moment of inertia	$\omega = \frac{T * t}{I}$
Angular work	Torque and displacement (θ)	$W = T\theta$
Angular work	Changes in rotational kinetic energy (RKE)	$W = \frac{1}{2} I \omega_2^2 - \frac{1}{2} I \omega_1^2$
Horizontal work	Force, angle of force application, displacement	$W = F \cos \theta \, s$
Potential energy (PE)	Mass and vertical height (h)	$PE = mgh$
Rotational kinetic energy (RE)	Moment of inertia, angular velocity	$RE = \frac{1}{2} I \omega^2$
Angular power	Angular work (W), time (t)	$P = \frac{W}{t}$
Angular power	Torque, velocity	$P = T\omega$

where W is the mechanical work done and dt is the time period over which the work is done or the product of torque and angular velocity:

$$\text{angular power} = T * \omega$$

where T is the torque and ω is the angular velocity.

Angular motion analysis can be conducted using one of three techniques: (*a*) the effect of a torque at an instant in time ($T = I\alpha$), (*b*) the effect of a torque applied over time (impulse–momentum relationship), and (*c*) the effect of a torque applied over a distance (work-energy theorem).

In the first technique, the static two-dimensional case is determined using the following equations:

$$\Sigma F_x = 0 \text{ for the horizontal component}$$
$$\Sigma F_y = 0 \text{ for the vertical component}$$
$$\Sigma T_z = 0 \text{ for rotation}$$

while the dynamic two-dimensional case uses the following equations:

$$\Sigma F_x = ma_x \text{ for the horizontal component}$$
$$\Sigma F_y = ma_y \text{ for the vertical component}$$
$$\Sigma T_z = I\alpha \text{ for rotation}$$

The purpose in both cases is to determine the net muscle moment about a joint.

The impulse–momentum relationship relates the torque applied over time to the change in momentum:

$$T * dt = I\omega_{final} - I\omega_{initial}$$

The left-hand side of the equation ($T * dt$) is the angular impulse, while the right-hand side ($I\omega_{final} - I\omega_{initial}$) describes the change in angular momentum. In the third type of analysis, mechanical angular work is calculated via the change in mechanical energy. That is:

$$W = \Delta RE$$

where RE is the rotational kinetic energy.

REVIEW QUESTIONS

True or False

1. ____ A force that causes rotation acts through the pivot point.

2. ____ Counter-clockwise torques are considered to be positive.

3. ____ A third-class lever is not favorable for force production.

4. ____ A first-class lever always favors range of motion.

5. ____ Reducing the moment of inertia about the shoulder joint requires more muscle force to move the limb.

6. ____ Angular momentum can be reduced in the air by extending arms and legs.

7. ____ The moment arm for muscle force changes throughout the range of motion.

8. ____ A ground reaction force applied in front of the center of mass will create a clockwise turning effect.

9. ____ A negative net muscle moment can indicate an eccentric muscle action.

10. ____ The sum of torques about the center of mass of an object always equals zero.

11. ____ The mechanical advantage of the second-class lever is always less than one.

12. ____ Remote angular momentum is the angular momentum of a segment about its own center of mass.

13. ____ The only torque acting on an arm held out to the side is the torque generated by the muscle force.

14. ____ Angular power is the product of net muscle moment and the joint angular velocity.

15. ____ The moment arm is always measured from the point of application of the force to the axis of rotation.

16. ____ A higher center of gravity in the golf club results in desirable flight paths.

17. ____ A force couple produces rotation and translation.

18. ____ Total body angular momentum can be increased during a dive by forcefully swinging arms downward.

19. ____ The moment of inertia about an axis through the center of mass is less than the moment of inertia about any other parallel axis running through any other point on the segment.

20. ____ The final acceleration in the golf club during the downswing is attributed to the wrists uncocking.

21. ____ Using action-reaction in the air, the legs can be brought up by swing the arms up.

22. ____ The angular acceleration of a rotating body is not influenced by the moment of inertia.

23. ____ During the stance phase of running, positive power is produced at the hip, knee and ankle joints.

24. ____ The shoulder joint torques contribute more power in wheelchair propulsion than the elbow joint torques.

25. ____ The moment of inertia about the center of mass for the longitudinal and the transverse axes are equal.

Multiple Choice

1. A force of 213 N is exerted 0.25 m from the axis of rotation. What is the resulting moment of force?
   a. 53.25 Nm
   b. 532.50 Nm
   c. 852.00 Nm
   d. 85.20 Nm

2. An object has a moment of inertia of 150 kgm². A torque of 72 Nm is applied to the object. What is the angular acceleration?
   a. 2.08 r/s²
   b. 10,800 r/s²
   c. 0.48 r/s²
   d. 983 r/s²

3. A 70-kg gymnast applies a vertical ground reaction force of 1300 N at 0.2 m behind the center of mass. What is the torque generated about the center of mass?
a. 122.7 Nm
b. −122.7 Nm
c. 260 Nm
d. −260 Nm

4. If a force of 120 N acting 0.29 m from the axis of rotation is balanced by another force of 92 N, what is the moment arm of the second force?
a. 2.64 m
b. 0.51 m
c. 8.12 m
d. 0.15 m

5. What is the torque generated at the elbow by a 90-N force pulling on the forearm at an angle of 110° from the horizon at a point 18 cm from the elbow's axis of rotation. The forearm was positioned horizontal to the ground.
a. 16.2 Nm
b. 15.22 Nm
c. 5.54 Nm
d. 19.8 Nm

6. How much torque must be generated by the deltoid muscle to hold a 60-N dumbbell straight out at a 90° arm position? The dumbbell is 0.6 m from the shoulder joint. The center of mass of the arm, weighing 30 N, is 0.25 m from the shoulder joint. The moment arm for the deltoid muscle is 0.05 m.
a. 870 Nm
b. −870 Nm
c. 43.5 Nm
d. −43.5 Nm

7. Calculate the rotational energy of a segment, given mass of the segment = 4.59 kg; moment of inertia = 0.057 kgm^2; σ = 1.90 rad/s.
a. 0.10 J
b. 0.47 J
c. 0.21 J
d. 0.05 J

8. A force of 200 N is applied at a point 1.3 m from the axis of rotation, causing a revolving door to accelerate at 6.2 rad/s^2. What is the moment of inertia of the door from its axis of rotation?
a. 953 kgm^2
b. 1612 kgm^2
c. 24.81 kgm^2
d. 41.94 kgm^2

9. If the net moment at a joint is 25.15 Nm and the angular velocity at the same instant in time is 1.64 rad/s, what is the angular power at that joint?
a. 4.13 W
b. 41.25 W
c. 1.53 W
d. 15.34 W

10. The center of mass of the following three-point system with masses of 8, 5.4, and 9 kg at the coordinates (4, 7), (9.2, 5.6), and (7, 4), respectively, is ____.
a. 4.74, 4.82
b. 6.46, 5.46

c. 4.9, 7.47
d. 5.10, 5.98

11. What is the angular momentum if the force = 54 N, the lever arm = 5.4 m, and the time = 2.7 s?
a. 27.0 kgm^2/s
b. 108 kgm^2/s
c. 787.32 kgm^2/s
d. 145.8 kgm^2/s

12. What are the coordinates of the center of mass of a segment with the proximal end (5.7, 3.2) and the distal end (7.9, 4.1) if the center of mass is 48.6% from the proximal end of the segment?
a. 4.63, 2.77
b. 2.77, 4.63
c. 6.77, 3.64
d. 3.64, 6.77

13. Calculate the moment of inertia of a baseball bat about its proximal end if its mass is 2 kg and has a radius of gyration of 0.55 and a length of 0.864 m.
a. 0.452 kgm^2
b. 0.950 kgm^2
c. 0.903 kgm^2
d. 0.542 kgm^2

14. A torque of 68 Nm results in a rotation through 0.57 rad in 0.3 s. How much angular work was done?
a. 38.8 J
b. 129.2 J
c. 11.63 J
d. 119. 30 J

15. How much power was developed in the example presented in Question 11?
a 38.8 J
b. 129.2 J
c. 11.6 J
d. 119.3 J

16. Consider the following free body diagram. Using static analysis, solve for the muscle torque that will place this system in equilibrium, given mass of the leg and foot = 5.3 kg; distance from the knee joint to the center of mass of the leg–foot system = 0.152 m; weight of the barbell = 150 N; distance from the knee joint to the center of mass of the barbell = 0.521 m.
a. 78.96 Nm
b. 8.77 Nm
c. 15.86 Nm
d. 86.05 Nm

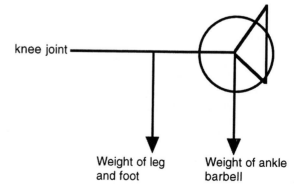

knee joint

Weight of leg and foot

Weight of ankle barbell

17. If the leg is at an angle of 15° below the horizontal, calculate the moment arm of the torque caused by the weight of the leg, given that the distance to the center of mass of the leg = 0.17 m.
   a. 0.17 m
   b. 0.16 m
   c. 0.15 m
   d. 0.14 m

18. Consider the following free body diagram. Using static analysis, solve for Achilles tendon force that will place this system in equilibrium if d1 = 0.045 m, d2 = 0.045 m, and d3 = 0.13 m.
   a. 5500.10 N
   b. 5477. 70 N
   c. 11.10 N
   d. 11.14 N

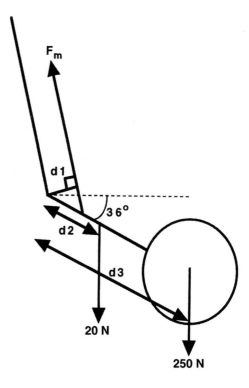

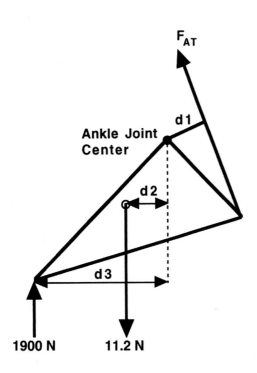

19. An object has a moment of inertia of 164 kgm². A torque of 89.3 Nm is applied to the object in 5 s. What is the angular acceleration?
   a. 2.72 rad/s²
   b. 0.272 rad/s²
   c. 5.55 rad/s²
   d. 0.55 rad/s²

20. Consider the following free body diagram. Using static analysis, solve for the moment at the elbow if d1 = 0.04 m; d2 = 0.14 m; and d3 = 0.46 m. What is the net muscle force?
   a. 2945.0 N
   b. 2872.4 N
   c. 2367.5 N
   d. 2250.5 N

21. Consider the following diagram of the biceps brachii acting on the radius in two joint positions. The angle of pull of the biceps brachii force changes from 15 to 30°. If the muscle force is 900 N and the attachment site of the muscle is 0.04 m from the joint axis, what is the change in joint torque applied by the biceps brachii from 15 to 30°?
   a. 3.59 Nm
   b. 7.19 Nm
   c. 9.0 Nm
   d. 18.0 Nm

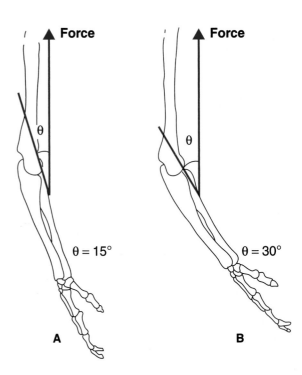

22. What is total energy of the segment, given that mass = 4.2 kg; g = 9.81 m/s2; vx = − 0.18 m/s; vy = 3.45 m/s; moment of inertia = 0.07234 kgm^2; angular velocity = 6.3 rad/s^2; height of center of mass = 0.39 m.
    a. 42.57 J
    b. 26. 43 J
    c. 42.43 J
    d. 27.01 J

23. What is the work done on the segment given the following information?

	TKE	RKE	PE
Frame 2	18.7	0.98	18.0
Frame 100	9.2	0.2	7.5
a.	2.078 J		
b.	20.78 J		
c.	10.28 J		
d.	1.028 J		

24. During a knee extension exercise, the knee extensor muscle group is applying a torque of 230 Nm in an isometric contraction against the machine pad. If the knee joint angle is being held at an angle of 40° below the horizontal and the machine pad is 0.35 m from the knee joint, how much force is being applied at the pad?
    a. 61.67 N
    b. 657.14 N
    c. 80.50 N
    d. 858.21 N

25. While exercising, an athlete holds a position with 90° of flexion at the hip joint and 90° of flexion at the knee joint. Considering only the iliopsoas muscle group, determine the amount of force necessary to maintain this position, given moment arm of iliopsoas = 10.5 cm from hip joint; mass of lower extremity = 11 kg; moment arm of CM of lower extremity = 38 cm from hip joint.
    a. 3.981 N
    b. 39.81 N
    c. 390.53 N
    d. 3905.30 N

26. During walking, the knee joint generated 50 Nm of extensor force during the same interval of the stance phase when the knee joint moved from 0.14 rad of flexion to 0.2 rad of flexion in 0.02 s. Determine the power of the knee joint muscles.
    a. 50 W
    b. −50 W
    c. 150 W
    d. −150 W

REFERENCES

1. Amar, J. (1920). *The Human Motor*. London: G. Routledge & Sons.

2. Boniger, M. L., et al. (1997). Wrist biomechanics during two speeds of wheelchair propulsion: An analysis using a local coordinate system. *Archives Physical Medicine Rehabilitation*, 78:364–371.

3. Cavanagh, P. R., Gregor, R. J. (1976). Knee joint torque during the swing phase of normal treadmill walking. *Journal of Biomechanics*, 8:337–344.

4. Cavanagh, P. R., et al. (1977). A biomechanical comparison of elite and good distance runners. *Annals of New York Academy of Sciences*, 301–328.

5. Cerquiglini, S., et al. (1981). Biomechanics of wheelchair propulsion. In A. Moretti, et al. (Eds.). *Biomechanics VII-A*. Baltimore: Park Press, 411–419.

6. Chaffin, D. B., Andersson, G. B. J. (1991). Occupational Biomechanics (2nd Ed.). New York: Wiley.

7. Chaffin, D. B., et al. (1977). Pre-employment strength testing in selecting workers for materials handling jobs. Cincinnati: National Institute for Occupational Safety and Health. Pub. No. CDC-99–74–62.

8. Chandler, R. F., et al. (1975). Investigation of inertial properties of the human body. *AMRL Technical Report*. Wright-Patterson Air Force Base, 74–137.

9. Clauser, C. E. (1969). Weight, volume, and center of mass of segments of the human body. *AMRL Technical Report*. Wright-Patterson Air Force Base, 69–70.

10. Dempster, W. T. (1955). Space requirements of the seated operator. *WADC Technical Report*. Wright-Patterson Air Force Base, 55–159.

11. Devita, P., et al. (1991). Effects of asymmetric load carrying on the biomechanics of walking. *Journal of Biomechanics*, 24:119–1129.

12. Dyson, G. (1973). *The Mechanics of Athletics*. London: University of London.

13. Fallon, L. P., et al. (2000). Determining baseball bat performance using a conservation equations model with field test validation. In A. J. Subic, S. J. Haake (Eds.). *The Engineering of Sport: Research, Development, and Innovation*. Oxford: Blackwell Science, 201–211.

14. Feltner, M. E., Dapena, J. (1986). Dynamics of the shoulder and elbow joints of the throwing arm during the baseball pitch. *International Journal of Sports Biomechanics*, 2: 235–259.

15. Frolich, C. (1979). Do springboard divers violate angular momentum conservation? *American Journal of Physics*, 47:583–592.

16. Gage, J. R. (1992). Millions of bits of data: How can we use it to treat cerebral palsy? *Proceedings of the Second North American Congress on Biomechanics*, 291–294.

17. Garg, A., Chaffin, D. B. (1975). A biomechanical computerized simulation of human strength. *Transactions of the American Institute of Industrial Engineers*, 7:1–15.

18. Ghista, D. N., Roaf, R. (1981). *Orthopaedic Mechanics: Procedures and Devices*, Vol. 2. New York: Academic Press.

19. Hamill, J., et al. (1986). Angular momentum in multiple rotation non-twisting platform dives. *International Journal of Sports Biomechanics*, 2:78–87.

20. Hanavan, E. P. (1964). A mathematical model of the human body. *AMRL Technical Report*. Wright-Patterson Air Force Base, 64–102.

21. Hatze, H. (1980). A mathematical model for the computational determination of parameter values of anthropomorphic segments. *Journal of Biomechanics*, 13:833–843.

22. Hatze, H. (1981). Estimation of myodynamic parameter values from observations on isometrically contracting muscle groups. *European Journal of Applied Physiology*, 46:325–338.

23. Hay, J. G. (1975). Straddle or flop. *Athletic Journal*, 55:83–85.

24. Hay, J. G., et al. (1977). A computational technique to determine the angular momentum of a human body. *Journal of Biomechanics*, 10:269–277.

25. Hinrichs, R. N. (1987). Upper extremity function in running. II: Angular momentum considerations. *International Journal of Sports Biomechanics*, 3:242–263.

26. Holden, J. P., et al. (1997). Changes in knee joint function over a wide range of walking speeds. *Clinical Biomechanics*, 12:375–382.

27. Jensen, R. K. (1987). The growth of children's moment of inertia. *Medicine and Science in Sports and Exercise*, 18:440–445.

28. Jorgensen, T. (1970). On the dynamics of the swing of a golf club. *American Journal of Physics*, 38:644–651.

29. Kamon, E., et al. (1982). Dynamic and static lifting capacity and muscular strength of steelmill workers. *American Industrial Hygiene Association Journal*, 43:853–857.

30. Kaneko, Y., Sato, F. (2000). The adaptation of golf swing to inertia property of golf club. In A. J. Subic, S. J. Haake (Eds.). *The Engineering of Sport: Research, Development and Innovation*. Malden, MA: Blackwell Science, 469–476.

31. Lander, J. E. (1984). Effects of center of mass manipulation on the performance of the squat exercise. Unpublished doctoral dissertation, University of Oregon.

32. Lind, A. R., et al. (1978). Influence of posture on isometric fatigue. *Journal of Applied Physiology*, 45:270–274.

33. Maddalozzo, G. F. (1987). An Anatomical and Biomechanical Analysis of the full Golf Swing. *National Strength and Conditioning Association*, 9:6–8;77–79.

34. Mann, R., Sprague, P. (1982). Kinetics of sprinting. In J. Terauds (Ed.). *Biomechanics of Sports*. Del Mar, CA: Academic.

35. Mather, J. S. B., Jowett, S. (2000). Three-dimensional shape of the golf club during the swing. In A. J. Subic, S. J. Haake (Eds.). *The Engineering of Sport: Research, Development and Innovation*. Malden: Blackwell Science, 77–85.

36. Miller, D. I., Morrison, W. E. (1975). Prediction of segmental parameters using the Hanavan human body model. *Medicine and Science in Sports*, 7:207–212.

37. Miller, D. I., Munro, C. F. (1984). Body segment contributions to height achieved during the flight of a springboard dive. *Medicine and Science in Sports and Exercise*, 16:234–242.

38. Neal, R. J., Wilson, B. D. (1985). 3D kinematics and kinetics of the golf swing. *International Journal of Sports Biomechanics*, 1:221–232.

39. Olsen, V. L., et al. (1972). The maximum torque generated by the eccentric, isometric and concentric contractions of the hip abductor muscles. *Physical Therapy*, 52:149–158.

40. Ounpuu, S. (1994). The biomechanics of walking and running. *Foot and Ankle Injuries*, 13:843–863.

41. Plagenhoef, S., et al. (1983). Anatomical data for analyzing human motion. *Research Quarterly for Exercise and Sport*, 54:169–178.

42. Pytel, J. L., Kamon, E. (1981). Dynamic strength test as a predictor for maximal and acceptable lifting. *Ergonomics*, 24:663–672.

43. Redfield, R., Hull, M. L. (1986). On the relation between joint moments and pedalling rates at constant power in cycling. *Journal of Biomechanics*, 19:317–324.

44. Reilly, D. T., Martens, M. (1972). Experimental analysis of the quadriceps muscle force and the patello-femoral joint reaction force for various activities. *Acta Orthopaedica Scandinavica*, 43:126–137.

45. Robertson, D. G. E. (1987). Functions of the leg muscles during the stance phase of running. In B. Jonsson (Ed.). *Biomechanics X-B*. Champaign, IL: Human Kinetics, 1021–1027.

46. Robertson, D. G. E., Winter, D. A. (1980). Mechanical energy generation, absorption, and transfer amongst segments during walking. *Journal of Biomechanics*, 13:845–854.

47. Rogers, M. M. (1988). Dynamic biomechanics of the normal foot and ankle during walking and running. *Physical Therapy*, 68:1822–1830.

48. Rozendaal, L. A., Veeger, H. E. J. (2000). Force direction in manual wheel chair propulsion: balance between effect and cost. *Clinical Biomechanics*, 15:S39-S41.

49. Sanders, R. H., Wilson, B. D. (1990). Angular momentum requirements of the twisting and non-twisting forward 1 $1/2$ somersault dive. *International Journal of Sports Biomechanics*, 3:47–53.

50. Shira, C. (2000). Advanced materials in golf clubs. In A. J. Subic, S. J. Haake (Eds.). *The Engineering of Sport: Research, Development and Innovation*. Malden, MA: Blackwell Science, 51–59.

51. Shoup, T. E., (1986). The anthropometric basis for fitting of golf clubs. In E. D. Rekow (Ed). *Medical Devices and Sporting Equipment*. New York: American Society of Mechanical Engineers, 13–16.

52. Takei, Y. (1991). A comparison of techniques used in performing the men's compulsory gymnastic vault at the 1988 Olympics. *International Journal of Sport Biomechanics*, 7:54–75.

53. Takei, Y. (1992). Blocking and postflight techniques of male gymnasts performing the compulsory vault at the 1988 Olympics. *International Journal of Sport Biomechanics*, 8:87–110.

54. Van der Helm, F. C. T., Veeger, H. E. J. (1996). Quasi-static analysis of muscle forces in the shoulder mechanism during wheelchair propulsion. *Journal of Biomechanics*, 29:39–52.

55. van Gheluwe, B. (1981). A biomechanical simulation model for airborne twists in backward somersaults. *Human Movement Studies*, 7:1–22.

56. Van Soest, A. J., et al. (1985). A comparison of one-legged and two-legged countermovement jumps. *Medicine and Science in Sports and Exercise*, 17:635–639.

57. Veeger, H. E. J., et al. (1991). Load on the upper extremity in manual wheelchair propulsion. *Journal of Electromyography and Kinesiology*, 1:270–280.

58. Yeadon, M. R., Atha, J. (1985). The production of a sustained aerial twist during a somersault without the use of asymmetrical arm action. In D. A. Winter et al. (Eds.). *Biomechanics IX-B*. Champaign, IL: Human Kinetics, 395–400.

59. Yeadon, M. R. (1989). Twisting techniques used in springboard diving. *Proceedings of the First IOC World Congress on Sport Sciences*, 307–308.

60. Williams, K. R. (1980). *A Biomechanical and Physiological Evaluation of Running Efficiency*. Unpublished doctoral dissertation, The Pennsylvania State University.

61. Winter, D. A. (1983). Moments of force and mechanical power in jogging. *Journal of Biomechanics*, 16:91–97.

62. Winter, D. A. (1984). Kinematic and kinetic patterns in human gait: variability and compensating effects. *Human Movement Science*, 3:51–76.

63. Winter, D. A., et al. (1976). Analysis of instantaneous energy of normal gait. *Journal of Biomechanics*, 9:253–257.

CHAPTER 11 **Angular Kinetics**   **425**

64. Winter, D. A., Robertson, D. G. E. (1978). Joint torque and energy patterns in normal gait. *Biological Cybernetics*, 142:137–142.

65. Zatsiorsky, V., Seluyanov, V. (1983). The mass and inertia characteristics of the main segments of the human body. In H. Matsui and K. Kobayashi (Eds.). *Biomechanics VIII-B.* Champaign, IL: Human Kinetics, 1152–1159.

ADDITIONAL READING

Frolich, C. (1980). The physics of somersaulting and twisting. *Scientific American*, 242:154–164.

Townend, M. S. (1984). *Mathematics in Sport*. London: Ellis Horwood.

Tricker, R. A. R.. Tricker, B. J. K. (1967). *The Science of Movement*. New York: American Elsevier.

van Ingen Schenau, G. J., Cavanagh, P. R. (1990). Power equations in endurance sports. *Journal of Biomechanics,* 23:865–881.

Winter, D. A. (1987). Mechanical power in human movement: Generation, absorption, and transfer. In B. van Gheluwe, J. Atha (Eds.). *Current Research in Sports Biomechanics*. New York: Karger, 34–45.

Yeadon, M. R. (1987). Theoretical models and their application to aerial movement. In B. van Gheluwe, J. Atha (Eds.). *Current Research In Sports Biomechanics*. New York: Karger, 86–106.

GLOSSARY

Angular Kinetics: The branch of mechanics that deals with the causes of rotations.

Angular Momentum: The quantity of angular motion determined by the product of the object's angular velocity and its moment of inertia.

Angular Power: The time rate of change of angular work determined by the product of the torque and the angular velocity.

Angular Work: The product of torque applied to an object and the angular distance over which the torque is applied.

Balance: The ability of an individual to assume and maintain a stable position.

Center of Gravity: The point at which all of the body's mass seems to be concentrated; the balance point of the body; the point about which the sum of the torques equals zero.

Center of Mass: A balance point of a body; the point about which all of the mass particles of the body are evenly distributed.

Conservation of Angular Momentum: The concept that angular momentum is constant unless the object is acted on by an external force.

Dynamic Analysis: A calculation of the forces and moments when there are significant linear and/or angular accelerations.

Dynamics: The branch of mechanics in which the system being studied undergoes acceleration.

Eccentric Force: A force that is not applied through the center of mass of an object.

Effort Arm: See moment arm.

Effort Force: A force applied to a lever, causing movement of the lever.

Equilibrium: The state of a system whose acceleration is unchanged.

External Work: The work done by a body on another body.

First-Class Lever: A lever in which the fulcrum is between the effort force and the resistance force.

Force Couple: Two forces that are equal in magnitude, act in opposite directions at a distance from an axis of rotation, and produce rotation with no translation.

Fulcrum: The axis of rotation of a lever.

Impulse: The product of the magnitude of a torque and its time of application.

Impulse–Momentum Relationship: The relationship stating that the impulse is equal to the change in momentum.

Internal Work: The total work done resulting from the motion of all of the body's segments.

Inverse Dynamics: An analytical approach calculating forces and moments based on the accelerations of the object.

Lever: A mechanism for doing work that consists of a fulcrum and two eccentric forces.

Local Angular Momentum: The angular momentum of a body segment about its own center of mass.

Mechanical Advantage: The ratio of the effort arm to the resistance arm of a lever.

Moment: See torque.

Moment Arm: The perpendicular distance of the line of action of a force to the axis of rotation.

Moment of Force: See torque.

Moment of Inertia: The resistance of a body to angular acceleration.

Muscle Power: The product of the net muscle moment and the angular velocity of the joint.

Negative Work: The work done on a system when the loading torque is greater than the torque exerted by the muscle.

Neutral Equilibrium: The state of a body in which the body will remain in a location if displaced from another location.

Parallel Axis Theorem: A theorem stating the relationship between the moment of inertia about an axis through the body's center of mass (I_{cm}) and any other parallel axis (I_{axis}) such that:

$$I_{axis} = I_{cm} + mr^2$$

where m is the mass of the body and r is the perpendicular distance between the axes.

Positive Work: The work done by a system when the torque exerted by a muscle is greater than the torque of the external load.

Radius of Gyration: A measure of the distribution of a body's mass about an axis of rotation.

Remote Angular Momentum: The angular momentum of a segment about the total body center of mass.

Resistance Arm: See moment arm.

Resistance Force: A force that resists the effort force in a lever.

Rotational Kinetic Energy: The capacity to do angular work; the product of half the moment of inertia and the angular velocity squared.

Second-Class Lever: A lever in which the resistance force acts between the fulcrum and the effort force.

Segmental Method: A method of calculating the total body center of mass of a multisegment body by summing the product of the locations of the centers of mass of the segments and the mass of the respective segment and dividing by the total body mass.

Stability: Resistance to a disturbance in the body's equilibrium.

Stable Equilibrium: The state of a body in which the body will return to its original location if it is displaced.

Statics: The branch of mechanics in which the system being studied undergoes no acceleration.

Third-Class Lever: A lever in which the effort force acts between the fulcrum and the line of action of the resistance force.

Torque: The product of the magnitude of a force and the perpendicular distance from the line of action of the force to the axis of rotation.

Unstable Equilibrium: The state of a body in which the body continues to increase its displacement if it is displaced.

Work–Energy Theorem: The relationship between work and energy stating that the work done is equal to the change in energy.

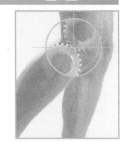

Ligaments

TABLE A-1 **Ligaments Supporting the Shoulder Complex**

Ligament	Insertion	Action
Acromioclavicular	Acromion process TO clavicle	Prevents separation of clavicle and scapula
Coracoacromial	Coracoid process TO acromion process	Forms arch over shoulder
Coracoclavicular: trapezoid, conoid	Coracoid process TO clavicle	Maintains relationship between scapula and clavicle; prevents anterior, posterior scapula movements; prevents upward and downward movements of clavicle on scapula
Coracohumeral	Coracoid process TO greater and lesser tuberosity on humerus	Checks upward displacement of humeral head; checks external rotation; supports weight of arm
Costoclavicular	Clavicle TO first rib	Checks clavicle elevation and anterior, posterior, lateral movement; supports weight of upper extremity
Glenohumeral: inferior, middle, superior	Upper anterior edge of glenoid TO over, in front of, below humeral head	Taut with external rotation, abduction; prevents anterior dislocation of humerus
Interclavicular	Clavicle TO clavicle	Checks motion of clavicle; supports weight of upper extremity
Sternoclavicular: anterior, posterior	Clavicle TO sternum	Prevents anterior and posterior dislocation; supports weight of upper extremity
Transverse	Across bicipital groove	Keeps biceps tendon in groove

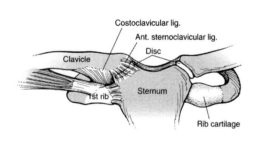

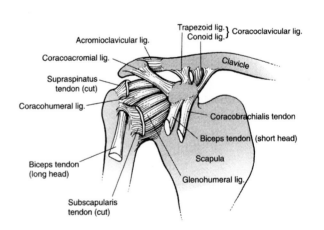

TABLE A-2 **Ligaments Supporting the Elbow and Radioulnar**

Ligament	Insertion	Action
Annular	Anterior margin of radial notch TO posterior margin of radial notch	Surrounds, supports head of radius; maintains radius in joint
Radial collateral	Lateral epicondyle TO annular ligament	Supports lateral joint
Ulnar collateral: posterior, transverse, anterior	Medial epicondyle; olecranon process TO coronoid process	Supports medial joint, resists valgus forces

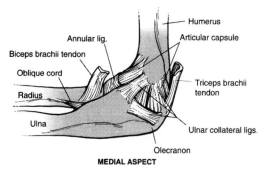

MEDIAL ASPECT

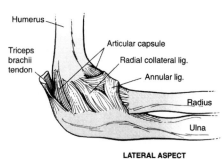

LATERAL ASPECT

 TABLE A-3 **Ligaments Supporting the Wrist and Fingers**

Ligament	Insertion	Action
Collateral	Phalanx TO phalanx; sides of MP, PIP, and DIP joints	Supports sides of fingers; prevents varus, valgus forces
Dorsal intercarpal	First row of carpals TO second row of carpals	Keeps carpals together
Deep transverse	MP of finger TO MP of adjacent finger	Taut in finger flexing, disallowing abduction
Dorsal radiocarpal	Lower end of radius TO scaphoid; lunate; triquetrum	Connects radius to carpals; supports posterior side of wrist
Palmar intercarpal	Scaphoid TO lunate; lunate TO triquetrum	Keeps carpals together
Palmer plates	Across the anterior joint of MP, PIP, DIP	Supports anterior MP, PIP, and DIP joints
Palmar radiocarpal	Lower radius TO scaphoid; lunate; triquetrum	Connects radius to carpals; supports anterior side of wrist
Radial collateral	Radius TO scaphoid; trapezium	Supports lateral side of wrist; resists valgus forces
Ulnar collateral	Ulna TO pisiform; triquetrum	Supports medial side of wrist; resists varus forces

MP, metaphalangeal; PIP, proximal interphalangeal; DIP, distal interphalangeal.

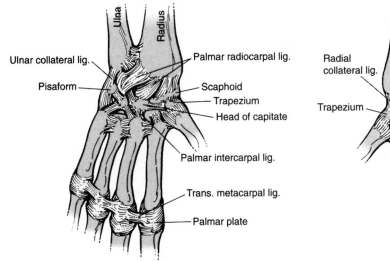

PALMAR ASPECT

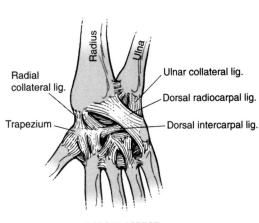

DORSAL ASPECT

TABLE A-4 Ligaments Stabilizing the Pelvis and Hip

Ligament	Insertion	Action
Dorsal sacroiliac	Posterior, inferior spine of ilium TO pelvic surface of sacrum	Maintain relationship between sacrum and ilium
Iliofemoral	Anterior, inferior iliac spine TO intertrochanteric line of femur	Supports anterior hip; resists in movements of extension, internal rotation, external rotation
Interosseous (SI)	Tuberosity of ilium TO tuberosity of sacrum	Prevents downward displacement of sacrum due to body weight
Ischiofemoral	Posterior acetabulum TO iliofemoral ligament	Resists adduction and internal rotation
Ligament of head	Acetabular notch and transverse ligament TO pit on head of femur	Transmits vessels to head of femur; no mechanical function
Pubic	Transverse fiber from body of pubis TO body of pubis	Maintains relationship between right and left pubic bones
Pubofemoral	Pubic part of acetabulum; superior rami TO intertrochanteric line	Resists abduction and external rotation
Ventral sacroiliac	Thin; pelvic surface of sacrum TO pelvic surface of ilium	Maintains relationship between sacrum and ilium

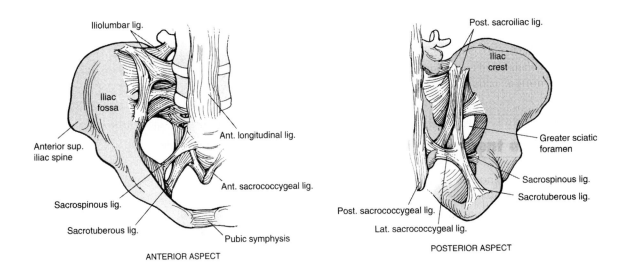

ANTERIOR ASPECT

POSTERIOR ASPECT

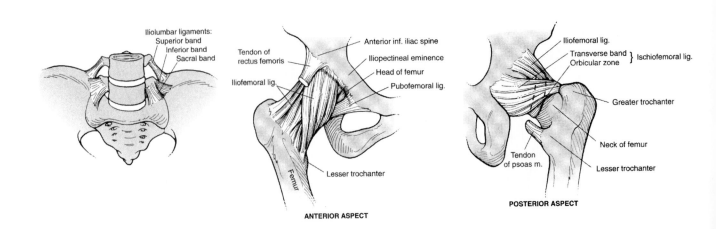

ANTERIOR ASPECT

POSTERIOR ASPECT

TABLE A-5 Ligaments Stabilizing the Knee Joint

Ligament	Insertion	Action
Anterior cruciate	Anterior intercondylar area of tibia TO medial surface of lateral condyle	Prevents anterior tibial displacement; resists extension, internal rotation, flexion
Arcuate	Lateral condyle of femur TO head of fibula	Reinforces back of capsule
Coronary	Meniscus TO tibia	Holds menisci to tibia
Medial collateral	Medial epicondyle of femur TO medial condyle of tibia and medial meniscus	Resists valgus forces; taut in extension; resists internal, external rotation
Lateral collateral	Lateral epicondyle of femur TO head of fibula	Resists varus forces; taut in extension
Patellar	Inferior patella TO tibial tuberosity	Transfers force from quadriceps to tibia
Posterior cruciate	Posterior spine of tibia TO inner condyle of femur	Resists posterior tibial movement; resists flexion and rotation
Posterior oblique	Expansion of semimembranosus muscle	Supports posterior, medial capsule
Transverse	Medial meniscus TO lateral meniscus in front	Connects menisci to each other

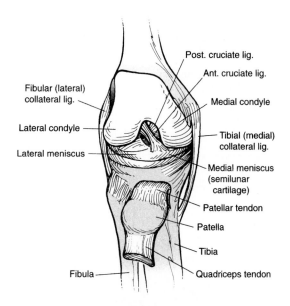

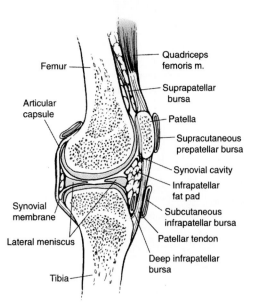

TABLE A-6 Ligaments Supporting the Foot and Ankle

Ligament	Insertion	Action
Anterior talofibular	Lateral malleolus TO neck of talus	Limits anterior displacement of foot or talar tilt; limits plantarflexion and inversion
Anterior talotibial	Anterior margin of tibia TO front margin on talus	Limits plantarflexion and abduction of foot
Calcaneocuboid	Calcaneus TO cuboid on dorsal surface	Limits inversion of foot
Calcaneofibular	Lateral malleolus TO tubercle on outer calcaneus	Resists backward displacement of foot; resists inversion
Deltoid	Medial malleolus TO talus, navicular, calcaneus	Resists valgus forces to ankle; limits plantarflexion, dorsiflexion, eversion, abduction of foot
Dorsal (tarsometatarsal)	Tarsals TO metatarsals	Supports arch; maintains relationship between tarsals and metatarsals
Dorsal calcaneocuboid	Calcaneus TO cuboid on dorsal side	Limits inversion
Dorsal talonavicular	Neck of talus TO superior surface of navicular	Supports talonavicular joint; limits inversion
Interosseous (intertarsal)	Connects adjacent tarsals	Supports arch of foot, intertarsal joints
Interosseous (talocalcaneal)	Undersurface of talus TO upper surface of calcaneus	Limits pronation, supination, abduction, adduction, dorsiflexion, plantarflexion
Plantar calcaneocuboid	Undersurface of calcaneus TO undersurface of cuboid	Supports arch
Plantar calcaneonavicular	Anterior margin of calcaneus TO undersurface of navicular	Supports arch; limits abduction
Posterior talofibular	Inner, back lateral malleolus TO posterior surface of talus	Limits plantarflexion, dorsiflexion, inversion; supports lateral ankle
Posterior talotibial	Tibia TO talus behind articulating facet	Limits plantarflexion; supports medial ankle
Talocalcaneal	Connecting ant./posterior, medial, lateral talus TO calcaneus	Supports subtalar joint

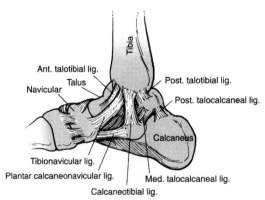

MEDIAL ASPECT

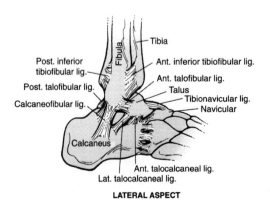

LATERAL ASPECT

TABLE A-7 **Ligaments Supporting the Vertebral Column**

Ligament	Insertion	Action
Alar	Apex of dens TO medial occipital	Limits lateral flexion, rotation of head; holds dens in atlas
Apical	Apex of dens TO front foramen magnum	Holds dens in atlas and skull
Anterior longitudinal	Sacrum; anterior vertebral body and disc TO above anterior body and disc; atlas	Limits hyperextension of spine; limits forward sliding of vertebrae
Costotransverse	Tubercles of ribs TO transverse process of vertebrae	Supports rib attachment to thoracic vertebrae
Cruciform	Odontoid bone TO arch of atlas	Stabilizes odontoid, atlas; prevents posterior movement of dens in atlas
Iliolumbar	Transverse process of L5 TO iliac crest	Limits lumbar motion in flexion, rotation
Interspinous	Spinous process TO spinous process	Limits flexion of trunk; limits shear forces acting on vertebrae
Intertransverse	Transverse process TO transverse process	Limits lateral flexion of trunk
Ligamentum flavum	Laminae TO laminae	Limits flexion of trunk; assists extension of trunk; maintains constant tension on disc
Ligamentum nuchae	Laminae TO laminae in cervical region; connects with supraspinous ligament	Limits cervical flexion; assists extension; maintains constant disc load
Posterior longitudinal	Posterior vertebral body and disc TO posterior body and disc of next vertebra	Limits flexion of trunk
Radiate	Head of rib TO body of vertebra	Maintains rib to thoracic vertebra
Supraspinous	Spinous process TO spinous process of next vertebra	Limits flexion of trunk; resists forward shear force on spine

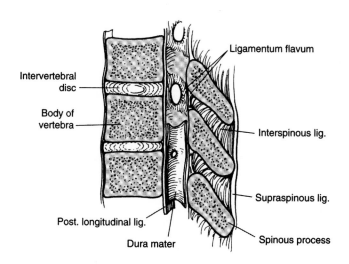

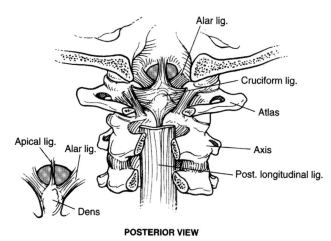

POSTERIOR VIEW

Muscles

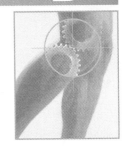

TABLE B-1 Muscles Acting on the Shoulder Complex

Muscle	Insertion	Action	Nerve Supply
Biceps brachii	Supraglenoid tubercle; corocoid process TO radial tuberosity	Arm abduction	Musculocutaneous nerve; C5, C6
Coracobrachialis	Coracoid process of scapula TO medial surface adjacent to deltoid tuberosity	Arm horizontal flexion	Musculocutaneous nerve; C6, C7
Deltoid	Lateral third of clavicle; acromion process; spine of scapula TO deltoid tubercle on humerus	Arm abduction, flexion, horizontal flexion, horizontal extension, internal rotation	Axillary nerve; C5, C6
Infraspinatus	Infraspinous fossa TO greater tubercle on humerus	Arm external rotation, horizontal extension	Subscapular nerve; C5, C6
Latissimus dorsi	Spinous process of thoracic vertebrae 6–12, L1–L5; lower 3–4 ribs; iliac crest; inferior angle of scapula TO intertubercular groove on humerus	Arm internal rotation, adduction, extension	Thoracodorsal nerve; C6–C8
Levator scapula	Transverse process of C1–C4 TO superior angle of scapula	Shoulder girdle elevation	Cervical plexus via C3, C4; dorsal scapular nerve; C5
Pectoralis major	Clavicle; sternum; ribs 1–6 TO greater tubercle of humerus, intertubercular groove	Arm internal rotation, horizontal flexion, flexion, extension	Musculocutaneous nerve; C6, C7
Pectoralis minor	Ribs 3–5 TO corocoid process	Shoulder girdle depression, downward rotation, protraction	Medial anterior thoracic nerve; C8, T1
Rhomboid	Spinous process of C7, T1–T5 TO medial border of scapula	Shoulder girdle retraction, elevation	Dorsal scapular nerve; C5
Serratus anterior	Ribs 1–8 TO underside of scapula along medial border	Shoulder girdle protraction, elevation, upward rotation	Long thoracic nerve; C5–C7
Subclavius	Costal cartilage of rib 1 TO underside of clavicle	Shoulder girdle depression	Brachial plexus; C5, C6
Subscapularis	Whole underside of scapula TO lesser tubercle on humerus	Arm internal rotation	Subscapular nerve; C5–C7
Supraspinatus	Supraspinous fossa of scapula TO lesser tubercle of humerus	Arm abduction, flexion	Subscapular nerve; C5
Teres major	Posterior surface of scapula at inferior angle TO lesser tubercle of humerus	Arm internal rotation, extension, adduction	Subscapular nerve; C5, C6
Teres minor	Lateral border of posterior scapula TO greater tubercle on humerus	Arm internal rotation, adduction, extension	Axillary nerve; C5
Trapezius	Occipital bone; ligamentum nuchae; spinous process of C7, T1–T12 TO acromion process; spine of scapula; lateral clavicle	Shoulder girdle upward rotation, elevation, retraction; arm abduction	Accessory nerve–spinal portion of 11th cranial nerve; C3, C4

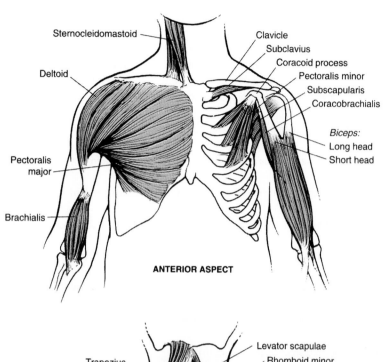

Sternocleidomastoid

Deltoid

Pectoralis
major

Brachialis

Clavicle
Subclavius
Coracoid process
Pectoralis minor
Subscapularis
Coracobrachialis

Biceps:
Long head
Short head

ANTERIOR ASPECT

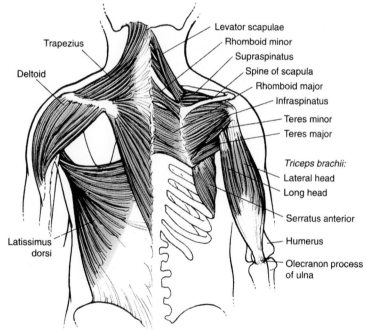

Trapezius

Deltoid

Latissimus
dorsi

Levator scapulae
Rhomboid minor
Supraspinatus
Spine of scapula
Rhomboid major
Infraspinatus
Teres minor
Teres major

Triceps brachii:
Lateral head
Long head

Serratus anterior

Humerus

Olecranon process
of ulna

POSTERIOR ASPECT

TABLE B-2 Muscles Acting on the Forearm

Muscle	Insertion	Action	Nerve Supply
Anconeus	Lateral epicondyle of humerus TO olecarnon process on ulna	Forearm extension	Radial nerve; C7, C8
Biceps brachii	Supraglenoid tubercle; corocoid process TO radial tuberosity	Forearm flexion, supination	Musculocutaneous nerve; C5, C6
Brachialis	Anterior surface of lower humerus TO coronoid process on ulna	Forearm flexion	Musculocutaneous nerve; C5, C6
Brachioradialis	Lateral supracondylar ridge of humerus TO styloid process of radius	Forearm flexion	Radial nerve; C5, C6
Extensor carpi radialis brevis	Lateral epicondyle of humerus TO base of 3rd metacarpal	Forearm flexion	Radial nerve; C6, C7
Extensor carpi radialis longus	Lateral supracondylar ridge of humerus TO base of 2nd metacarpal	Forearm flexion	Radial nerve; C6, C7
Extensor carpi ulnaris	Lateral epicondyle TO base of 5th metacarpal	Forearm extension	Posterior interosseous branch of radial nerve; C6–C8
Pronator quadratus	Distal anterior surface of ulna TO distal anterior surface of radius	Forearm pronation	Anterior interosseous nerve from median nerve; C8, T1
Pronator teres	Medial epicondyle of humerus, coronoid process on ulna TO mid lateral surface of radius	Forearm pronation, flexion	Median nerve; C5, C6
Supinator	Lateral epicondyle of humerus TO upper lateral side of radius	Forearm supination	Posterior interosseous nerve; C6
Triceps brachii	Infraglenoid tubercle on scapula; mid posterior shaft of humerus; lower shaft of humerus TO olecranon process	Forearm extension	Radial nerve; C7, C8

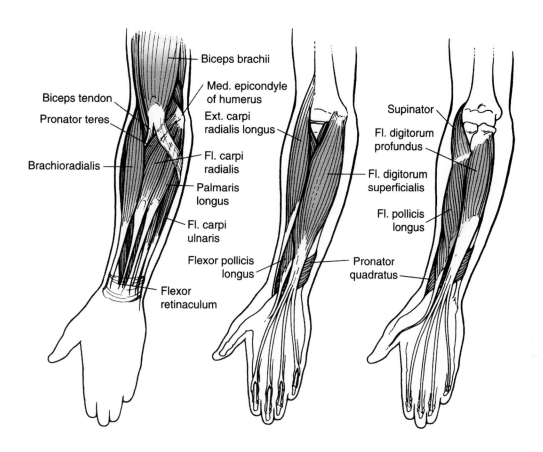

Biceps brachii

Med. epicondyle of humerus

Biceps tendon

Pronator teres

Ext. carpi radialis longus

Fl. carpi radialis

Brachioradialis

Palmaris longus

Fl. carpi ulnaris

Flexor pollicis longus

Flexor retinaculum

Supinator

Fl. digitorum profundus

Fl. digitorum superficialis

Fl. pollicis longus

Pronator quadratus

TABLE B-3 Muscles Acting on the Wrist and Fingers

Muscle	Insertion	Action	Nerve Supply
Abductor digiti minimi	Pisiform bone TO base of proximal phalanx of little finger	Little finger abduction	Ulnar nerve; C8
Abductor pollicis brevis	Scaphoid; trapezium TO base of proximal phalanx	Thumb abduction	Median nerve; C6, C7
Abductor pollicis longus	Middle of radius TO radial side of base of 1st metacarpal	Thumb abduction	Posterior interosseous branch of radial nerve; C6, C7
Adductor pollicis	Capitate; base of 2nd, 3rd metacarpals TO base of proximal phalanx of thumb	Thumb adduction	Ulnar nerve; C8, T1
Dorsal interossei	Between metacarpals of four fingers TO base of proximal phalanx of 2nd–4th fingers	Index, middle, ring finger abduction; middle finger adduction	Ulnar nerve; C8, T1
Extensor carpi radialis brevis	Lateral epicondyle of humerus TO base of 3rd metacarpal	Hand extension, radial flexion	Radial nerve; C6, C7
Extensor carpi radialis longus	Lateral supracondylar ridge of humerus TO base of 2nd metacarpal	Hand extension, radial flexion	Radial nerve; C6, C7
Extensor carpi ulnaris	Lateral epicondyle of humerus TO base of 5th metacarpal	Hand extension, ulnar flexion	Posterior interosseous branch of radial nerve; C6–C8
Extensor digiti minimi	Tendon of extensor digitorum TO proximal phalanx of little finger	Extension of proximal phalanx of little finger	Posterior interosseous branch of radial nerve; C6–C8
Extensor digitorum	Lateral epicondyle of humerus TO dorsal hoods of four fingers	1st phalanx extension; hand extension	Posterior interosseous branch of radial nerve; C6–C8
Extensor indicis	Lower ulna, interosseous membrane TO dorsal hood of index finger	Extension of proximal phalanx of index finger	Posterior interosseous branch of radial nerve; C6–C8
Extensor pollicis brevis	Middle of radius, ulna TO base of proximal phalanx of thumb	Thumb extension	Posterior interosseous branch of radial nerve; C6, C7
Extensor pollicis longus	Middle third of ulna, interosseous membrane TO base of distal phalanx of thumb	Thumb extension	Posterior interosseous branch of radial nerve; C6–C8
Flexor carpi radialis	Medial epicondyle of humerus TO base of 2nd, 3rd metacarpal	Hand flexion, radial flexion	Median nerve; C6, C7
Flexor carpi ulnaris	Medial epicondyle TO pisiform; hamate; base of 5th metacarpal	Hand flexion, ulnar flexion	Ulnar nerve; C8, T1
Flexor digiti minimi brevis	Hamate bone TO proximal phalanx of little finger	Flexion of little finger	Ulnar nerve; C8
Flexor digitorum profundus	Anterior, medial ulna TO base of distal phalanx of four fingers	Proximal, middle, distal phalanx flexion; hand flexion	Anterior interosseous nerve; C8, T1
Flexor digitorum superficialis	Medial epicondyle TO base of middle phalanx of four fingers	Proximal, middle phalanx flexion; hand flexion	Median nerve; C7, C8, T1
Flexor pollicis brevis	Trapezium; trapezoid; capitate TO base of proximal phalanx of thumb	Thumb flexion	Median nerve; ulnar nerve
Flexor pollicis longus	Middle radius, interosseous membrane TO base of distal phalanx of thumb	Thumb flexion	Anterior interosseous from median nerve; C8, T1
Lumbricales	Tendon of flexor digitorum profundus TO dorsal hoods of four fingers	Proximal phalanx flexion; middle, distal phalanx extension	Median nerve; C6, C7; ulnar nerve; C8
Opponens digiti minimi	Hamate bone TO 5th metacarpal	Opposition of little finger	Ulnar nerve; C8, T1
Opponens pollicis	Trapezium TO 1st metacarpal	Thumb opposition	Median nerve; C6, C7
Palmar interossei	Sides of 2nd, 4th, 5th metacarpal TO base of proximal phalanx of same fingers	Adduction of index, ring, little fingers	Ulnar nerve; C8, T1
Palmaris longus	Medial epicondyle TO palmar aponeurosis	Hand flexion	Median nerve; C6, C7

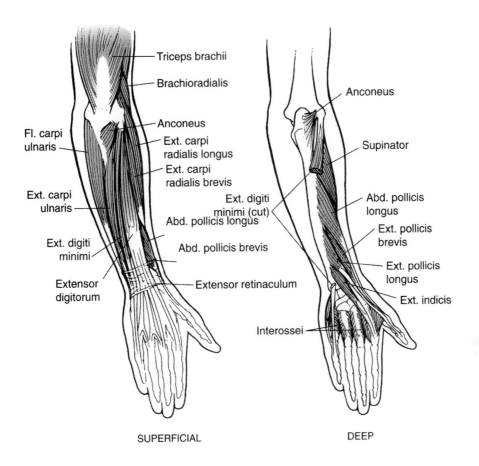

Triceps brachii

Brachioradialis

Fl. carpi ulnaris

Anconeus

Ext. carpi radialis longus

Ext. carpi radialis brevis

Ext. carpi ulnaris

Ext. digiti minimi (cut)

Abd. pollicis longus

Ext. digiti minimi

Abd. pollicis brevis

Extensor digitorum

Extensor retinaculum

SUPERFICIAL

Anconeus

Supinator

Abd. pollicis longus

Ext. pollicis brevis

Ext. pollicis longus

Ext. indicis

Interossei

DEEP

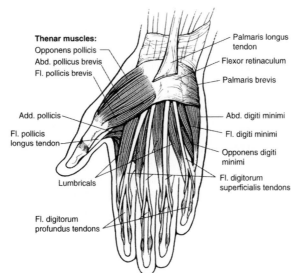

Thenar muscles:
Opponens pollicis
Abd. pollicus brevis
Fl. pollicis brevis

Add. pollicis

Fl. pollicis longus tendon

Lumbricals

Fl. digitorum profundus tendons

Palmaris longus tendon

Flexor retinaculum

Palmaris brevis

Abd. digiti minimi

Fl. digiti minimi

Opponens digiti minimi

Fl. digitorum superficialis tendons

TABLE B-4 Muscles Acting on the Hip Joint

Muscle	Insertion	Action	Nerve Supply
Adductor brevis	Inferior rami of pubis TO upper half of posterior femur	Thigh adduction	Anterior obturator nerve; L3, L4
Adductor longus	Inferior rami of pubis TO middle third of posterior femur	Thigh adduction, internal rotation	Anterior obturator nerve; L3, L4
Adductor magnus	Anterior pubis, ischial tuberosity TO linea aspera on posterior femur, adductor tubercle	Thigh adduction, internal rotation	Posterior obturator, sciatic; L3, L4
Biceps femoris	Ischial tuberosity TO lateral condyle of tibia, head of fubula	Thigh extension; shank flexion, external rotation	Tibial, peroneal portion of sciatic nerve; L5, S1–S3
Gemellus inferior	Ischial tuberosity TO greater trochanter on femur	Thigh external rotation	Sacral plexus; L4, L5, S1 sacral nerve
Gemellus superior	Ischial spine TO greater trochanter	Thigh external rotation	Sacral plexus; L5, S1, S2 sacral nerve
Gluteus maximus	Posterior ilium, sacrum, coccyx TO gluteal tuberosity; iliotibial band	Thigh extension, external rotation	Inferior gluteal nerve; L5 S1, S2
Gluteus medius	Anterior, lateral ilium TO lateral surface of greater trochanter	Thigh abduction, internal rotation	Superior gluteal nerve; L4, L5, S1
Gluteus minimus	Outer, lower ilium TO front of greater trochanter	Thigh abduction, internal rotation	Superior gluteal nerve; L4, L5, S1
Gracilis	Inferior rami of pubis TO medial tibia (pes anserinus)	Thigh adduction, internal rotation; leg flexion, internal rotation	Anterior obturator nerve; L3, L4
Iliacus	Inner surface of ilium, sacrum TO lesser trochanter	Thigh flexion	Femoral nerve; L2, L3
Obturator internus	Sciatic notch, margin of obturator foramen TO greater trochanter	Thigh external rotation	Sacral plexus; L5, S1, S2
Obturator externus	Pubis, ischium, margin of obturator foramen TO upper posterior femur	Thigh external rotation	Obturator nerve; L3, L4
Pectineus	Pectineal line on pubis TO below lesser trochanter	Thigh adduction, flexion	Femoral nerve; L2–L4
Piriformis	Anterior lateral sacrum TO superior greater trochanter	Thigh external rotation, abduction	S1, S2, L5
Psoas	Transverse processes, body of L1–L5, T12 TO lesser trochanter	Thigh flexion; trunk flexion	Femoral nerve; L1–L3
Quadratus femoris	Ischial tuberosity TO greater trochanter	Thigh external rotation	Sacral plexus; L4, L5, S1
Rectus femoris	Anterior inferior iliac spine TO patella, tibial tuberosity	Thigh flexion; leg extension	Femoral nerve; L2, L3, L4
Sartorius	Anterior superior iliac spine TO medial tibia (pes anserinus)	Thigh flexion, external rotation; leg flexion, internal rotation	Femoral nerve; L2, L3
Semimembranosus	Ischial tuberosity TO medial condyle of tibia	Thigh extension, internal rotation; leg flexion, internal rotation	Tibial portion of sciatic nerve; L5, S1, S2
Semitendinosus	Ischial tuberosity TO medial tibia (pes anserinus)	Thigh extension, internal rotation; leg flexion, internal rotation	Tibial portion of sciatic nerve; L5, S1, S2
Tensor fascia latae	Anterior superior iliac spine TO iliotibial tract	Thigh flexion, abduction, internal rotation	Superior gluteal nerve; L4, L5, S1

TABLE B-5 Muscles Acting on the Knee Joint

Muscle	Insertion	Action	Nerve Supply
Biceps femoris	Ischial tuberosity TO lateral condyle of tibia, head of fibula	Thigh extension; leg flexion, external rotation	Tibial, peroneal portion of sciatic nerve; L5, S1–S3
Gastrocnemius	Medial, lateral condyles of femur TO calcaneus	Leg flexion; foot plantarflexion	Tibial nerve; S1, S2
Gracilis	Inferior rami of pubis TO medial tibial (pes anserinus)	Thigh adduction, internal rotation; leg flexion, internal rotation	Anterior obturator nerve; L3, L4
Popliteus	Lateral condyle of femur TO proximal tibia	Leg internal rotation, flexion	Tibial nerve
Rectus femoris	Anterior inferior iliac spine TO patella, tibial tuberosity	Thigh flexion; leg extension	Femoral nerve; L2–L4
Sartorius	Anterior superior iliac spine TO medial tibia (pes anserinus)	Thigh flexion, external rotation; leg flexion, internal rotation	Femoral nerve; L2, L3
Semimembranosus	Ischial tuberosity TO medial condyle of tibia	Thigh extension, internal rotation; leg flexion, internal rotation	Tibial portion of sciatic nerve; L5, S1, S2
Semitendinosus	Ischial tuberosity TO medial tibia (pes anserinus)	Thigh extension, internal rotation; leg flexion, internal rotation	Tibial portion of sciatic nerve; L5, S1, S2
Vastus intermedius	Anterior lateral femur TO patella, tibial tuberosity	Leg extension	Femoral nerve; L2–L4
Vastus lateralis	Intertrochanteric line; linea aspera TO patella, tibial tuberosity	Leg extension	Femoral nerve; L2–L4
Vastus medialis	Linea aspera; trochanteric line TO patella, tibial tuberosity	Leg extension	Femoral nerve; L2–L4

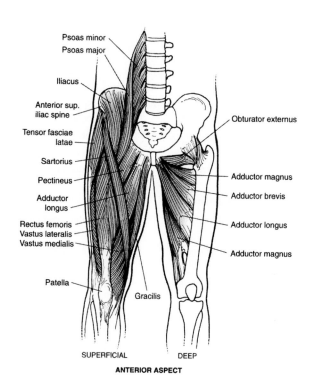

ANTERIOR ASPECT

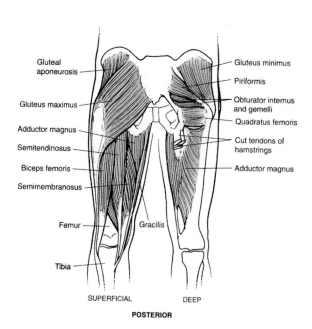

POSTERIOR

TABLE B-6 Muscles Acting on the Ankle and Foot

Muscle	Insertion	Action	Nerve Supply
Abductor digiti minimi	Lateral calcaneus TO base of proximal phalanx of 5th toe	Little toe abduction	Lateral plantar nerve
Abductor hallucis	Medial calcaneus TO medial base of proximal phalanx of 1st toe	Big toe abduction	Medial plantar nerve
Adductor hallucis	2nd, 3rd, 4th metatarsal TO lateral side of proximal phalanx of big toe	Big toe adduction	Lateral plantar nerve
Dorsal interossei	Sides of metatarsals TO lateral side of proximal phalanx	Abduct toes 2–4; adduct 2nd toe; flex proximal phalanx	Lateral plantar nerve
Extensor digitorum brevis	Lateral calcaneus TO proximal phalanx of 1st, 2nd, 3rd toes	Extend toes 1–4	Deep peroneal nerve
Extensor digitorum longus	Lateral condyle of tibia; fibula; interosseous membrane TO dorsal expansion of toes 2–5	Foot dorsiflexion, eversion; toe 2–5 extension	Deep peroneal nerve
Extensor hallucis longus	Anterior fibula; interosseous membrane TO distal phalanx of big toe	Big toe extension; forefoot adduction	Deep peroneal nerve
Flexor digiti minimi brevis	5th metatarsal TO proximal phalanx of little toe	Little toe flexion	Lateral plantar nerve
Flexor digitorum brevis	Medial calcaneus TO middle phalanx of toes 2–5	Toe 2–5 flexion	Medial plantar nerve
Flexor digitorum longus	Posterior tibia TO distal phalanx of toes 2–5	Toe 2–5 flexion; foot plantarflexion	Tibial nerve
Flexor hallucis brevis	Cuboid TO medial side of proximal phalanx of big toe	Big toe flexion	Medial plantar nerve
Flexor hallucis longus	Lower 2–3 of posterior fibula, interosseous membrane	Big toe flexion; forefoot adduction	Tibial nerve
Gastrocnemius	Medial, lateral condyles of femur TO calcaneus	Leg flexion; foot plantarflexion	Tibial nerve; S1, S2
Lumbricals	Tendon of flexor digitorum longus TO base of proximal phalanx of toes 2–5	Proximal phalanx flexion, toes 2–5	Medial, lateral plantar nerve
Peroneus brevis	Lower lateral fibula TO 5th metatarsal	Foot eversion, plantarflexion	Superficial peroneal nerve
Peroneus longus	Lateral condyle of tibia, upper lateral fibula TO 1st cuneiform; lateral 1st metatarsal	Foot eversion, plantarflexion; forefoot abduction	Superficial peroneal nerve
Peroneus tertius	Lower anterior fibula; interosseous membrane TO base of 5th metatarsal	Foot eversion	Deep peroneal nerve
Plantar interossei	Medial side of 3–5 metatarsal TO medial side of proximal phalanx of toes 3–5	Toe 3–5 abduction	Lateral plantar nerve
Plantaris	Linea aspera on femur TO calcaneus	Foot plantarflexion	Tibial nerve
Quadratus plantae	Medial lateral inferior calcaneus TO flexor digitorum tendon	Toe 2–5 flexion	Lateral plantar nerve
Soleus	Upper posterior tibia, fibula, interosseous membrane TO calcaneus	Foot plantarflexion	Tibial nerve
Tibialis anterior	Upper lateral tibia, interosseous membrane TO medial plantar surface of 1st cuneiform	Foot dorsiflexion, inversion	Deep peroneal nerve
Tibialis posterior	Upper posterior tibia, fibula, interosseous membrane TO inferior navicular	Foot inversion, plantarflexion	Tibial nerve

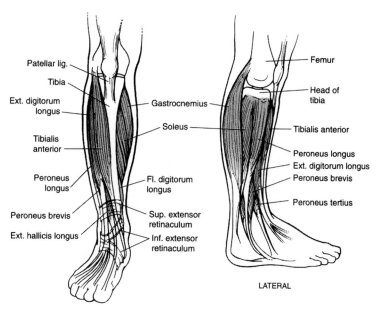

Patellar lig.
Tibia
Ext. digitorum longus
Tibialis anterior
Peroneus longus
Peroneus brevis
Ext. hallicis longus
Gastrocnemius
Soleus
Fl. digitorum longus
Sup. extensor retinaculum
Inf. extensor retinaculum

ANTERIOR

Femur
Head of tibia
Tibialis anterior
Peroneus longus
Ext. digitorum longus
Peroneus brevis
Peroneus tertius

LATERAL

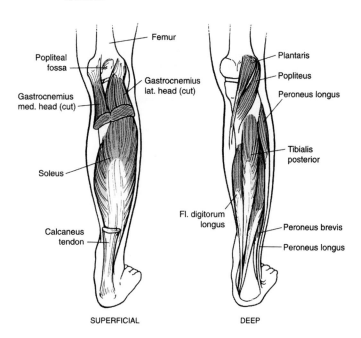

Popliteal fossa
Gastrocnemius med. head (cut)
Soleus
Calcaneus tendon

Femur
Gastrocnemius lat. head (cut)

SUPERFICIAL

Plantaris
Popliteus
Peroneus longus
Tibialis posterior
Fl. digitorum longus
Peroneus brevis
Peroneus longus

DEEP

POSTERIOR ASPECT

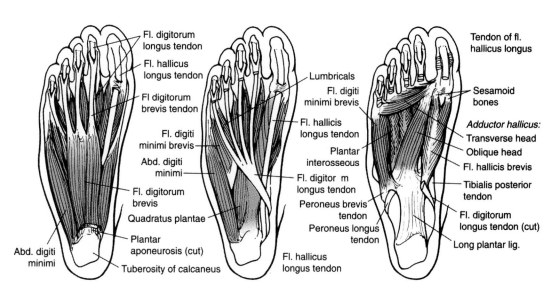

Fl. digitorum longus tendon
Fl. hallicus longus tendon
Fl digitorum brevis tendon
Fl. digiti minimi brevis
Abd. digiti minimi
Fl. digitorum brevis
Quadratus plantae
Plantar aponeurosis (cut)
Tuberosity of calcaneus
Abd. digiti minimi

Lumbricals
Fl. digiti minimi brevis
Fl. hallicis longus tendon
Plantar interosseous
Fl. digitor m longus tendon
Peroneus brevis tendon
Peroneus longus tendon
Fl. hallicus longus tendon

Tendon of fl. hallicus longus
Sesamoid bones
Adductor hallicus:
Transverse head
Oblique head
Fl. hallicis brevis
Tibialis posterior tendon
Fl. digitorum longus tendon (cut)
Long plantar lig.

443

TABLE B-7 Muscles Acting on the Vertebral Column

Muscle	Insertion	Action	Nerve Supply
External oblique (ABD)	9th–12th ribs alternating with l. dorsi, s. ant TO anterior superior spine; pubic tubercle; ant iliac crest	Trunk flexion, lateral flexion, rotation to opposite side	Intercostal nerve; T7–T12
Iliocostalis (ES) lumborum	Sacrum; spinous processes of L1–L5, T11, T12; iliac crest TO lower 6 or 7 ribs	Trunk extension, lateral flexion, rotation to same side	Spinal nerves; dorsal rami
Iliocostalis thoracis	Lower 6 ribs TO upper 6 ribs; transverse process of C7	Trunk extension, lateral flexion, rotation to same side	Spinal nerves; dorsal rami
Iliocostalis cervices	3rd–6th ribs TO transverse processes of C4–C6	Trunk extension, lateral flexion, rotation to same side	Spinal nerves; dorsal rami
Iliopsoas	Bodies of T12, L1–L5; transverse processes of L1–L5; inner surface of ilium, sacrum TO lesser trochanter	Thigh flexion; trunk flexion	Femoral nerve; ventral rami; L1, L3
Internal oblique (ABD)	Iliac crest, lumbar fascia TO ribs 8–10; linea alba	Trunk flexion, lateral flexion, rotation to same side	Intercostal nerves; T7–T12, L1
Interspinales (DP)	Spinous process TO spinous process	Trunk extension, hyperextension	Spinal nerves; dorsal rami
Intertransversarii (DP)	Transverse process TO transverse process	Trunk extension, lateral flexion	Spinal nerves; ventral, dorsal rami
Longissimus (ES) Thoracis	Posterior transverse process of L1–L5; thoracolumbar fascia TO transverse process of T1–T12	Trunk extension, lateral flexion, rotation to same side	Spinal nerves; dorsal rami
Longissimus cervices	Transverse process of T1–T5 TO transverse process of C4–C6	Trunk extension, lateral flexion, rotation to same side	Spinal nerves; dorsal rami
Longissimus capitis	Transverse process of T1–T5, C4–C7 TO mastoid process	Head extension, lateral flexion, rotation	Spinal nerves; dorsal rami
Longus capitis	Transverse process of C3–C6 TO occipital bone	Head, cervical flexion, lateral flexion	Cervical nerves; C1–C3
Longus cervicis, colli	Transverse process of C3–C5; bodies of T1–T2; bodies of C5–C7, T1–T3 TO atlas; transverse process of C5–C6; bodies of C2–C4	Cervical flexion, lateral flexion	Cervical nerves; C2–C7
Multifidus (DP)	Sacrum; iliac spine; transverse processes L5–C4 TO spinous process of next vertebrae side	Trunk extension, lateral flexion, rotation to opposite	Spinal nerves; dorsal rami
Quadratus lumborum	Iliac crest; transverse process of L2–L5 TO transverse process of L1–L2; last rib	Trunk lateral flexion	Thoracic nerves; T12; Lumbar nerves; ventral rami
Rotatores (DP)	Transverse process TO laminae of next vertebrae	Trunk extension, rotation to opposite side	Spinal nerves; dorsal rami
Scaleni	Transverse process of cervical vertebrae TO ribs 1, 2	Cervical lateral flexion, flexion	Cervical nerves
Semispinalis capitis	C4–C6 facets; transverse process of C7 TO base of occipital flexion	Trunk extension, lateral flexion	Cervical nerves; dorsal rami
Semispinalis cervicis	Transverse process of T1–T6 TO spinous process of C1–C5	Trunk extension, lateral flexion, rotation	Cervical nerves; dorsal rami
Semispinalis thoracis	Transverse processes of T6–T10 TO spinous processes of T1–T4, C6, C7	Trunk extension, lateral flexion, rotation	Thoracic nerves; dorsal rami
Spinalis (ES) thoracis	Spinous processes of L1–L2, T11–T12 TO spinous process of T1–T8 ligamentum nuchae	Trunk extension, lateral flexion	Spinal nerves; dorsal rami
Spinalis cervicis	Spinous process of C7 TO spinous process of axis	Trunk extension, lateral flexion	Spinal nerves; dorsal rami
Splenius capitis	Ligamentum nuchae; spinous process of C7, T1–T3 TO mastoid process, occipital bone	Cervical extension, lateral flexion, rotation to same side	Cervical nerves; dorsal rami
Splenius cervicis	Spinous process of T3–T6 TO transverse process of C1–C3	Cervical extension, lateral flexion, rotation to same side	Cervical nerves; dorsal rami

Sternocleidomastoid	Sternum, clavicle TO mastoid process	Head, cervical flexion, lateral flexion, rotation to same side	Accessory nerve; cranial nerve XI
Transverse abdominus (ABD)	Last 6 ribs; iliac crest; inguinal ligament; lumbodorsal fascia TO linea alba; pubic crest	No specific action; increases internal abdominal pressure through compression	Intercostal nerves; T7–T12, L1

ABD, abdominals; ES, Erector Spinae; DP, Deep Posterior muscles.

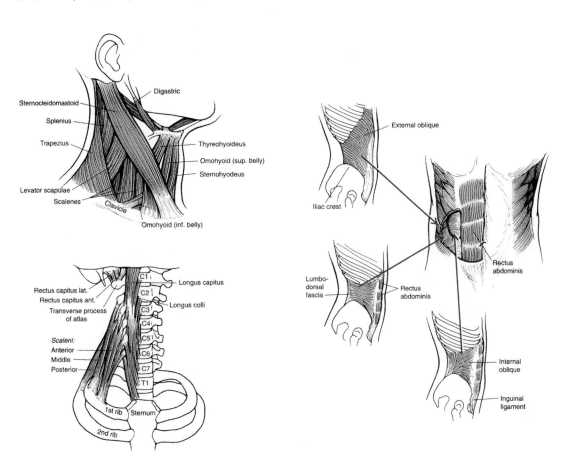

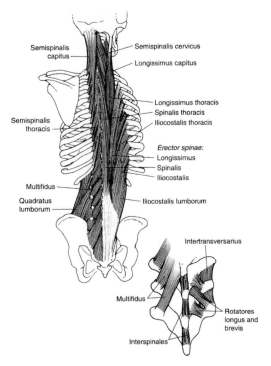

The Metric System and SI Units

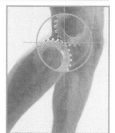

All measurements in the biomechanics literature are expressed in terms of the metric system. This system of measurement uses units that are related to one another by some power of 10. Table C-1 presents the prefixes associated with these powers.

TABLE C-1 Prefixes for the Powers of 10

Prefix	Multiplier	Symbol	Example
Giga	10^9	G	Gigabyte (Gb)
Mega	10^6	M	Megawatt (MW)
Kilo	10^3	k	Kilogram (kg)
centi	10^{-2}	c	centimeter (cm)
milli	10^{-3}	m	milligram (mg)
micro	10^{-6}	μ	microsecond (μs)
nano	10^{-9}	ν	nanosecond (ns)

The standard length in the metric system is the meter. This standard measure was originally indicated by two scratches on a platinum–iridium alloy bar kept at the International Bureau of Weights and Measures in Sèvres, France. Table C-2 illustrates the use of these prefixes in common units of length.

TABLE C-2 Units of Length

Metric Unit	Power	Symbol
Kilometer	10^{-3}	Km
Meter	—	M
Decimeter	10^{-1}	dm
Centimeter	10^{-2}	cm
Millimeter	10^{-3}	mm
Micrometer	10^{-6}	μm

The uniform system for the reporting of numerical values is known as the Système International d'Unites, or SI. This system was developed through international cooperation to standardize the report of scientific information. The base dimensions used in biomechanics are **mass, length, time, temperature, electric current, amount of substance**, and **luminous intensity**. The base units in SI corresponding to the base dimensions are the kilogram, the meter, the second, and the degree kelvin. Table C-3 presents the base units of SI.

TABLE C-3 Base Units of Measurement

Dimension	Unit	Symbol
Mass	Kilogram	kg
Length	Meter	m
Time	Second	s
Temperature	Degree kelvin	K
Electrical current	Ampere	A
Amount of substance	Mole	mol
Luminous intensity	Candela	cd

Other units of measurement that are used in biomechanics are derived. These units are presented in Table C-4.

TABLE C-4 Derived Units of Measurement

Dimension	Unit	Symbol
Acceleration	Meters per second squared	m/s^2
Angle	Radian	rad
Area	Meter squared	m^2
Capacitance	Farad	F
Concentration	Moles per meter cubed	mol/m^3
Density	Mass per unit volume	kg/m^3
Energy	Joule	J
Impulse	Force * time	$N \cdot s$
Luminous flux	Lumen	lm
Moment of inertia	Kilogram-meters squared	kgm^2
Momentum	Kilogram-meters per second	kgm/s
Power	Watts	W
Pressure	Pascal	Pa
Resistance	Ohm	Ω
Speed	Meters per second	M/s
Torque	Newton-meter	Nm
Voltage	Volt	V
Volume	Meter cubed	m^3
Work	Joule	J

TABLE C-5 Common Conversions

Length

1 inch = 25.40 mm	1 inch = 2.54 cm	1 foot = 0.3048 m	1 foot = 30.48 cm
1 yard = 0.9144 m	1 mile = 1609.34 m	1 cm = 0.3937 inches	1 cm = 0.0328 feet
1 m = 39.37 inches	1 m = 3.2808 feet	1 m = 1.0936 yard	1 m = 1.0936 yard
1 km = 0.6214 miles			

Area

1 in = 645.16 mm^2	1 ft^2 = 0.0929 m^2	1 yd^2 = 0.8361 m^2	1 cm^2 = 0.155 in^2
1 m^2 = 10.76 ft^2			

Volume

1 in^3 = 16.387 cm^3	1 ft^3 = 0.0283 m^3	1 yd^3 = 0.7645 m^3	1 yd^3 = 0.7645 m^3
1 cm^3 = 0.061 in^3	1 m^3 = 35.32 ft^3	1 m^3 = 1.308 yd^3	

Mass

1 oz = 28.349 g	1 lb = 0.4536 kg	1 slug = 14.5939 kg	1 slug = 32.2 lb
1 g = 0.0353 oz.	1 kg = 2.2046 lb	1 kg = 0.0685 slug	

Density

1 lb-ft^3 = 16.02 kg/m^3	1 slug-ft^3 = 515.38 kg/m^3

Moment of Inertia

1 slug-ft^2 = 1.36 kgm^2	1 lb-ft^2 = 0.042 kgm^2

Velocity

1 in/s = 24.4 mm/s	1 ft/s = 0.305 m/s	1 mph = 0.447 m/s	1 mph = 1.467 ft/s
1 m/s = 3.60 km/hr	1 m/s = 3.28 ft/s	1 m/s = 2.237 m/hr	1 cm/s = 0.0328 ft/s

Force

1 poundal = 0.1383 N	1 lb-force = 4.448 N	1 kg-force = 9.81 N	1 N = 0.102 kg
1 N = 0.2248 lb			

Pressure

1 poundal/ft^2 = 1.4881 Pa	1 pound-force /ft^2 = 47.889 Pa	1 pound-force/in^2 = 6.8947 Pa
1 mm mercury = 133.322 Pa		

Work and Energy

1 foot poundal = 0.0421 J	1 foot pound-force = 1.3558 J	1 foot pound-force = 0.1383 kgm	1 kgm = 7.2307 ft-lb
1 BTU = 1.0551 kJ	1 kilocalorie = 4.1868 kJ	1 J = 0.7376 ft-lb	1 J = 0.1020 kgm

Power

1 hp (British) = 745.700 W	1 hp (metric) = 735.499 W	1 hp (metric) = 735.499 W	1 ft-lb force/s = 1.3558 W

Torque

1 Nm = 0.74 lb-ft	1 lb-ft = 1.36 Nm	1 kgm = 7.23 lb-ft	1 kg-cm = 0.0723 lb-ft

BTU, British thermal unit.

Trigonometric Functions

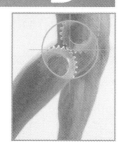

Trigonometry is a branch of mathematics concerned with the measurements of the sides and angles of triangles and their relationships with each other. Many concepts in biomechanics require knowledge of trigonometry. A triangle is composed of three sides and three angles. The sum of the three angles of a triangle equals 180°. A right triangle is a triangle in which one of the angles is a right angle, that is, one of the angles equals 90°. The sum of the remaining angles, therefore, also equals 90°. Consider the triangle with vertices A, B, and C and sides of length AB, AC, and BC in Figure D-1.

The side opposite the right angle, AB, is always the longest side in the right triangle and is referred to as the hypotenuse. The other two sides are named according to which of the other angles is under consideration. If angle A is considered, the side AC is called the adjacent side and the side BC is called the opposite side. If angle B is considered (as in the triangle on the right below), BC is the adjacent side and AC is the opposite side.

Based on the right triangle, trigonometric functions may be defined. A mathematical function is a quantity whose value varies and depends on some other quantity or quantities. Trigonometric functions vary with and depend on the values of the two acute (i.e., less than 90°) angles in a right triangle and the lengths of the sides of the triangle. The trigonometric functions are the ratios of the lengths of the sides of the triangle based on one of the two acute angles in the triangle. There are six such functions: (*a*) sine (abbreviation is sin); (*b*) cosine (abbreviation is cos); (*c*) tangent (abbreviation is tan); (*d*) cosecant; (*e*) secant; and (*f*) cotangent.

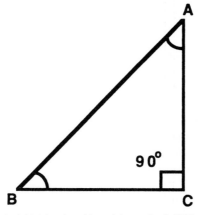

FIGURE D-1 A right triangle with a right angle C (90°) and two acute angles, A and B. A and B sum to 90°.

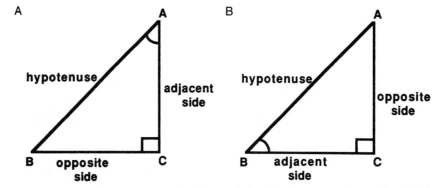

FIGURE D-2 Descriptions of the sides of a right triangle based on the acute angles A (**A**) and B (**B**).

In biomechanics, only the first three of these functions are important. The trigonometric functions are thus defined for angle A (Figure D-2*A*) as:

1. The sine of an angle is the ratio of the side opposite the angle to the hypotenuse.

$$\sin A = \frac{\text{opposite side}}{\text{hypotenuse}} = \frac{BC}{AB}$$

2. The cosine of an angle is the ratio of the side adjacent to the angle to the hypotenuse.

$$\cos A = \frac{\text{adjacent side}}{\text{hypotenuse}} = \frac{AC}{AB}$$

3. The tangent of an angle is the ratio of the side opposite to the angle to the side adjacent to the angle.

$$\tan A = \frac{\text{opposite side}}{\text{adjacent side}} = \frac{BC}{AC}$$

Similarly, the ratios for angle B in Figure D-2*B* may be defined as:

$$\sin B = \frac{\text{opposite side}}{\text{hypotenuse}} = \frac{AC}{AB}$$

$$\cos B = \frac{\text{adjacent side}}{\text{hypotenuse}} = \frac{BC}{AB}$$

$$\tan B = \frac{\text{opposite side}}{\text{adjacent side}} = \frac{AC}{BC}$$

For any angle, the ratios formed by the sides of the right triangle will always be the same. For example, the sine of an angle of 32 will always equal 0.5299 regardless of the size of the sides of the triangle. The same is true for the cosine and tangent of the angle. The values for the sine, cosine, and tangent of angles can be presented in tables. Table D-1 presents these values for angles ranging from 0 to 90°.

The values in this table may also be used to determine the angle when the sides of the triangle are known. Consider the triangle in Figure D-3. The length of the hypotenuse, AC, is 0.05 m and the length of the side opposite angle C is 0.03 m. The ratio of AB to AC is the sine of angle C. Thus:

$$\sin C = \frac{AB}{AC} = \frac{0.03 \text{ m}}{0.05 \text{ m}} = 0.6$$

If the sine values in Table D-1 are examined, it can be determined that the angle whose sine is 0.6 is approximately 37°. This is the arcsin of the angle. Thus:

$$C = \arcsin \frac{AB}{AC}$$

The ratio of the side AB to the hypotenuse AC is the cosine of angle A in Figure D-3. The ratio is still 0.6, and the angle whose cosine is 0.6 is approximately 53. This is referred to as the arccosine of an angle.

Two other useful trigonometric relationships are applicable to all triangles, not only right triangles. The first of these relationships is the law of sines, which states that the ratio of the length of any side to the sine of the angle opposite that side is equal to the ratio of any other side to the angle opposite that side. Consider the triangle in Figure D-4.

For this triangle, the law of sines can be stated as follows:

$$\frac{A}{\sin \alpha} = \frac{B}{\sin \beta} = \frac{C}{\sin \gamma}$$

The other trigonometric relationship that is applicable to any triangle is the *law of cosines*. This relationship states

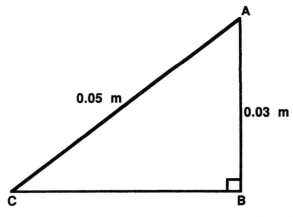

FIGURE D-3 A right triangle with two sides of known lengths and two unknown angles.

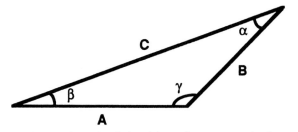

FIGURE D-4 A scalene triangle (no right angle, no two angles the same

that the square of the length of any side of a triangle is equal to the sum of the squares of the other two sides minus twice the product of the lengths of the other two sides and the cosine of the angle opposite the original side. Consider the triangle in Figure D-4. For side A of this triangle, the law of cosines can be stated as follows:

$$A^2 = B^2 + C^2 - 2BC \cos \alpha$$

Similarly, the law of cosines can be stated for sides B and C.

TABLE D-1 Trigonometric Functions

Degrees	Radian	Sine	Cosine	Tangent	Degrees	Radian	Sine	Cosine	Tangent
0	0.000	0.0000	0.0000	0.0000	27	0.471	0.4540	0.8910	0.5095
1	0.017	0.0175	0.9998	0.0175	28	0.489	0.4695	0.8829	0.5317
2	0.035	0.0349	0.9994	0.0349	29	0.506	0.4848	0.8746	0.5543
3	0.052	0.0523	0.9986	0.0524	30	0.524	0.5000	0.8660	0.5774
4	0.070	0.0698	0.9976	0.0699	31	0.541	0.5150	0.8572	0.6009
5	0.087	0.0872	0.9962	0.0875	32	0.559	0.5299	0.8480	0.6249
6	0.105	0.1045	0.9945	0.1051	33	0.576	0.5446	0.8387	0.6494
7	0.122	0.1219	0.9925	0.1228	34	0.593	0.5592	0.8290	0.6745
8	0.140	0.1392	0.9903	0.1405	35	0.611	0.5736	0.8192	0.7002
9	0.157	0.1564	0.9877	0.1584	36	0.628	0.5878	0.8090	0.7265
10	0.175	0.1736	0.9848	0.1763	37	0.646	0.6018	0.7986	0.7536
11	0.192	0.1908	0.9816	0.1944	38	0.663	0.6157	0.7880	0.7813
12	0.209	0.2079	0.9781	0.2126	39	0.681	0.6293	0.7771	0.8098
13	0.227	0.2250	0.9744	0.2309	40	0.698	0.6428	0.7660	0.8391
14	0.244	0.2419	0.9703	0.2493	41	0.716	0.6561	0.7547	0.8693
15	0.262	0.2588	0.9659	0.2679	42	0.733	0.6691	0.7431	0.9004
16	0.279	0.2756	0.9613	0.2867	43	0.750	0.6820	0.7314	0.9325
17	0.297	0.2924	0.9563	0.3057	44	0.768	0.6947	0.7193	0.9657
18	0.314	0.3090	0.9511	0.3249	45	0.785	0.7071	0.7071	1.0000
19	0.332	0.3256	0.9455	0.3443	46	0.803	0.7193	0.6947	1.0355
20	0.349	0.3420	0.9397	0.3640	47	0.820	0.7314	0.6820	1.0724
21	0.367	0.3584	0.9336	0.3839	48	0.838	0.7431	0.6691	1.1106
22	0.384	0.3746	0.9272	0.4040	49	0.855	0.7547	0.6561	1.1504
23	0.401	0.3907	0.9205	0.4245	50	0.873	0.7660	0.6428	1.1918
24	0.419	0.4067	0.9135	0.4452	51	0.890	0.7771	0.6293	1.2349
25	0.436	0.4226	0.9063	0.4663	52	0.908	0.7880	0.6157	1.2799
26	0.454	0.4384	0.8988	0.4877	53	0.925	0.7986	0.6018	1.3270

		Angle					Angle		
Degrees	Radian	Sine	Cosine	Tangent	Degrees	Radian	Sine	Cosine	Tangent
54	0.942	0.8090	0.5878	1.3764	73	1.274	0.9563	0.2924	3.2709
55	0.960	0.8192	0.5736	1.4281	74	1.292	0.9613	0.2756	3.4874
56	0.977	0.8290	0.5592	1.4826	75	1.309	0.9659	0.2588	3.7321
57	0.995	0.8387	0.5446	1.5399	76	1.326	0.9703	0.2419	4.0108
58	1.012	0.8480	0.5299	1.6003	77	1.344	0.9744	0.2250	4.3315
59	1.030	0.8572	0.5150	1.6643	78	1.361	0.9781	0.2079	4.7046
60	1.047	0.8660	0.5000	1.7321	79	1.379	0.9816	0.1908	5.1446
61	1.065	0.8746	0.4848	1.8040	80	1.396	0.9848	0.1736	5.6713
62	1.082	0.8829	0.4695	1.8807	81	1.414	0.9877	0.1564	6.3138
63	1.100	0.8910	0.4540	1.9626	82	1.431	0.9903	0.1392	7.1154
64	1.117	0.8988	0.4384	2.0503	83	1.449	0.9925	0.1219	8.1443
65	1.134	0.9063	0.4226	2.1445	84	1.466	0.9945	0.1045	9.5144
66	1.152	0.9135	0.4067	2.2460	85	1.484	0.9962	0.0872	11.4300
67	1.169	0.9205	0.3907	2.3559	86	1.501	0.9976	0.0698	14.3010
68	1.187	0.9272	0.3746	2.4751	87	1.518	0.9986	0.0523	19.0810
69	1.204	0.9336	0.3584	2.6051	88	1.536	0.9994	0.0349	28.6360
70	1.222	0.9397	0.3420	2.7475	89	1.553	0.9998	0.0175	57.2900
71	1.239	0.9455	0.3256	2.9042	90	1.571	1.0000	0.0000	∞
72	1.257	0.9511	0.3090	3.0777					

Sample Kinematic and Kinetic Data

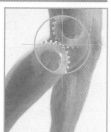

Subject: 50 − kg female

Activity: Walking sampled at 120 Hz; one cycle from right foot touchdown to right foot touchdown

Markers: Head, R shoulder, R elbow, R wrist, R hand, R crest (IC), R greater trochanter (GT), R knee, R ankle, R heel, R fifth metatarsal (met), R toe

Stride events: Right foot touchdown (RTD), left foot touchdown (LTD), right foot toe-off (RTO)

TABLE E-1 Kinematic Data in Millimeters

Frame Number	Head x	Head y	Shoulder x	Shoulder y	Elbow x	Elbow y	Wrist x	Wrist y	Hand x	Hand y	IC x	IC y
−1	−28.000	1458.867	−155.0670	1340.267	−272.4000	1122.533	−337.067	891.2001	−383.333	821.1334	−129.6670	959.4000
0	−16.1104	1460.070	−142.8280	1340.392	−259.5290	1122.318	−323.567	890.5505	−369.112	820.3072	−117.0390	960.8488
1	−5.8344	1460.187	−132.3700	1339.994	−249.0580	1121.832	−313.184	889.9189	−358.828	819.6309	−105.7240	960.9595
2	5.5109	1460.400	−120.8120	1339.625	−237.4180	1121.333	−301.533	889.244	−347.240	818.8842	−93.2708	961.1825
3	17.5563	1460.741	−108.5230	1339.332	−224.9500	1120.857	−288.895	888.5603	−334.605	818.0917	−80.1029	961.5585
4	30.0691	1461.238	−95.7353	1339.154	−211.8550	1120.43	−275.419	887.8932	−321.052	817.2701	−66.4896	962.1211
5	42.8924	1461.910	−82.6015	1339.121	−198.2620	1120.073	−261.185	887.2629	−306.650	816.4315	−52.6116	962.8947
6	55.9139	1462.766	−69.2294	1339.257	−184.2630	1119.802	−246.242	886.6854	−291.434	815.5863	−38.5936	963.8934
7	69.0503	1463.812	−55.6970	1339.575	−169.9210	1119.628	−230.618	886.1729	−275.426	814.7437	−24.5215	965.1221
8	82.2388	1465.042	−42.0612	1340.085	−155.2870	1119.557	−214.338	885.7347	−258.640	813.9131	−10.4521	966.5772
9	95.4311	1466.451	−28.3636	1340.787	−140.4000	1119.594	−197.423	885.3776	−241.090	813.1049	3.5790	968.2484
10	108.5901	1468.027	−14.6346	1341.677	−125.2930	1119.737	−179.898	885.1063	−222.789	812.3306	17.5514	970.1204
11	121.6875	1469.759	−0.8958	1342.746	−109.9920	1119.984	−161.786	884.9250	−203.753	811.6043	31.4545	972.1739
12	134.7022	1471.634	12.8372	1343.984	−94.5150	1120.33	−143.116	884.8385	−184.000	810.9424	45.2829	974.3861
13	147.6191	1473.641	26.5539	1345.378	−78.8790	1120.769	−123.916	884.8523	−163.550	810.3641	59.0335	976.7316
14	160.4287	1475.767	40.2467	1346.915	−63.0930	1121.295	−104.216	884.9739	−142.428	809.8916	72.7026	979.1822
15	173.1259	1478.001	53.9102	1348.583	−47.1645	1121.902	−84.044	885.2129	−120.660	809.5491	86.2856	981.7078
16	185.7099	1480.331	67.5403	1350.371	−31.0984	1122.585	−63.431	885.5804	−98.278	809.3627	99.7773	984.2767
17	198.1837	1482.743	81.1334	1352.268	−14.8980	1123.338	−42.404	886.0891	−75.315	809.3590	113.1725	986.8570
18	210.5535	1485.224	94.6867	1354.265	1.4333	1124.158	−20.994	886.7517	−51.808	809.5640	126.4673	989.4174
19	222.8278	1487.757	108.1977	1356.350	17.8911	1125.040	0.769	887.5803	−27.798	810.0020	139.6598	991.9286
20	235.0169	1490.325	121.6645	1358.513	34.4694	1125.979	22.855	888.5847	−3.327	810.6936	152.7498	994.3636
21	247.1322	1492.907	135.0860	1360.738	51.1596	1126.972	45.232	889.7718	21.557	811.6552	165.7388	996.6990
22	259.1851	1495.481	148.4623	1363.009	67.9504	1128.010	67.868	891.1447	46.811	812.8972	178.6293	998.9143
23	271.1866	1498.022	161.7945	1365.305	84.8281	1129.083	90.730	892.7023	72.384	814.4236	191.4245	1000.9920
24	283.1469	1500.506	175.0846	1367.602	101.7767	1130.179	113.786	894.4395	98.228	816.2318	204.1278	1002.9180
25	295.0749	1502.905	188.3354	1369.872	118.7793	1131.283	137.003	896.3469	124.296	818.3120	216.7429	1004.6800
26	306.9781	1505.195	201.5501	1372.084	135.8182	1132.374	160.351	898.4120	150.543	820.6483	229.2738	1006.2670
27	318.8635	1507.350	214.7321	1374.207	152.8768	1133.433	183.801	900.6194	176.924	823.2191	241.7250	1007.6700
28	330.7369	1509.343	227.8844	1376.207	169.9397	1134.433	207.327	902.9514	203.398	825.9987	254.1017	1008.8810
29	342.6039	1511.150	241.0096	1378.052	186.9933	1135.350	230.903	905.3885	229.928	828.9584	266.4099	1009.8910
30	354.4694	1512.748	254.1096	1379.707	204.0269	1136.158	254.505	907.9105	256.478	832.0680	278.6570	1010.6930
31	366.3380	1514.117	267.1859	1381.145	221.0321	1136.831	278.110	910.4961	283.017	835.2977	290.8521	1011.2800
32	378.2137	1515.238	280.2396	1382.337	238.0038	1137.344	301.699	913.1249	309.516	838.6193	303.0058	1011.6470
33	390.1003	1516.097	293.2721	1383.259	254.9391	1137.677	325.249	915.7772	335.949	842.0071	315.1308	1011.7900
34	402.0008	1516.683	306.2855	1383.893	271.8378	1137.810	348.740	918.4351	362.290	845.4393	327.2408	1011.7050
35	413.9182	1516.986	319.2833	1384.222	288.7014	1137.729	372.151	921.0827	388.514	848.8983	339.3495	1011.3910
36	425.8549	1517.005	332.2706	1384.240	305.5328	1137.424	395.460	923.7070	414.599	852.3707	351.4696	1010.8470
37	437.8128	1516.737	345.2549	1383.941	322.3352	1136.889	418.643	926.2978	440.517	855.8474	363.6112	1010.0730
38	449.7935	1516.188	358.2454	1383.330	339.1115	1136.124	441.675	928.8475	466.242	859.3229	375.7819	1009.0720
39	461.7983	1515.364	371.2537	1382.416	355.8636	1135.134	464.529	931.3510	491.746	862.7949	387.9873	1007.8460
40	473.8288	1514.277	384.2926	1381.215	372.5915	1133.928	487.175	933.8054	516.996	866.2632	400.2315	1006.4040
41	485.8867	1512.942	397.3759	1379.749	389.2927	1132.521	509.583	936.2089	541.957	869.7286	412.5176	1004.7530
42	497.9743	1511.377	410.5173	1378.045	405.9619	1130.932	531.722	938.5610	566.592	873.1921	424.8483	1002.9080
43	510.0948	1509.607	423.7298	1376.137	422.5906	1129.184	553.559	940.8610	590.859	876.6538	437.2262	1000.8850

Frame Number	GT x	GT y	Knee x	Knee y	Ankle x	Ankle y	R Heel x	R Heel y	Met x	Met y	R Toe x	R Toe y	Stride Events
−1	−151.9330	815.6667	60.0000	499.2000	179.6667	122.5333	137.0667	32.5333	318.8667	107.8000	389.6000	174.6000	
0	−138.8750	817.3138	71.2735	500.1740	184.3008	122.2974	139.1965	33.7988	321.1163	101.7447	393.5727	166.1098	RTD
1	−127.3660	817.3990	81.5479	499.6656	188.6009	121.3638	140.9553	35.7224	324.5082	97.1523	399.1105	158.2565	
2	−114.6950	817.6133	92.8275	499.2010	193.2326	120.3715	142.8490	37.7833	328.1142	92.1631	404.9800	149.7856	
3	−101.2980	818.0074	104.7070	498.8362	197.9802	119.3710	144.7892	39.8826	331.7479	86.9928	410.8690	141.0844	
4	−87.4525	818.6227	116.9140	498.6061	202.6871	118.3970	146.7124	41.9504	335.2787	81.8026	416.5578	132.4334	
5	−73.3523	819.4881	129.2452	498.5237	207.2340	117.4741	148.5699	43.9356	338.6140	76.7251	421.8916	124.0495	
6	−59.1365	820.6188	141.5343	498.5822	211.5301	116.6186	150.3248	45.8008	341.6912	71.8718	426.7681	116.1024	
7	−44.9065	822.0160	153.6362	498.7572	215.5108	115.8410	151.9499	47.5205	344.4730	67.3340	431.1295	108.7213	
8	−30.7351	823.6689	165.4220	499.0134	219.1348	115.1469	153.4265	49.0797	346.9431	63.1805	434.9549	101.9964	
9	−16.6723	825.5570	176.7789	499.3102	222.3823	114.5388	154.7436	50.4725	349.1014	59.4569	438.2521	95.9820	
10	−2.7509	827.6524	187.6139	499.6091	225.2517	114.0165	155.8960	51.7004	350.9600	56.1862	441.0497	90.6994	
11	11.0093	829.9228	197.8582	499.8779	227.7565	113.5791	156.8838	52.7708	352.5393	53.3706	443.3898	86.1411	
12	24.5970	832.3331	207.4701	500.0946	229.9220	113.2248	157.7112	53.6945	353.8654	50.9957	445.3221	82.2754	
13	38.0060	834.8476	216.4356	500.2475	231.7811	112.9514	158.3862	54.4842	354.9672	49.0342	446.8991	79.0518	
14	51.2330	837.4310	224.7652	500.3347	233.3704	112.7559	158.9206	55.1539	355.8746	47.4500	448.1728	76.4052	
15	64.2766	840.0502	232.4894	500.3617	234.7272	112.6339	159.3292	55.7181	356.6170	46.2022	449.1921	74.2612	
16	77.1368	842.6746	239.6519	500.3383	235.8862	112.5799	159.6301	56.1915	357.2221	45.2480	450.0017	72.5414	
17	89.8161	845.2775	246.3037	500.2760	236.8787	112.5868	159.8431	56.5886	357.7151	44.5457	450.6412	71.1686	
18	102.3196	847.8358	252.4979	500.1857	237.7323	112.6466	159.9886	56.9235	358.1183	44.0552	451.1447	70.0707	
19	114.6559	850.3299	258.2861	500.0763	238.4710	112.7506	160.0858	57.2092	358.4507	43.7393	451.5414	69.1836	
20	126.8370	852.7439	263.7166	499.9540	239.1157	112.8897	160.1514	57.4574	358.7282	43.5629	451.8558	68.4523	
21	138.8776	855.0646	268.8339	499.8230	239.6849	113.0557	160.1989	57.6785	358.9634	43.4934	452.1079	67.8310	
22	150.7940	857.2812	273.6783	499.6856	240.1949	113.2410	160.2386	57.8810	359.1665	43.5010	452.3141	67.2823	
23	162.6026	859.3842	278.2859	499.5426	240.6593	113.4397	160.2780	58.0722	359.3451	43.5592	452.4875	66.7770	
24	174.3181	861.3651	282.6890	499.3944	241.0892	113.6478	160.3224	58.2579	359.5049	43.6464	452.6383	66.2925	
25	185.9522	863.2155	286.9158	499.2408	241.4929	113.8631	160.3755	58.4427	359.6502	43.7458	452.7746	65.8131	
26	197.5134	864.9266	290.9908	499.0815	241.8764	114.0852	160.4402	58.6309	359.7843	43.8463	452.9024	65.3286	
27	209.0071	866.4890	294.9362	498.9164	242.2435	114.3149	160.5187	58.8257	359.9092	43.9411	453.0261	64.8349	
28	220.4373	867.8925	298.7722	498.7453	242.5968	114.5535	160.6126	59.0307	360.0264	44.0271	453.1489	64.3328	
29	231.8087	869.1266	302.5183	498.5675	242.9386	114.8020	160.7236	59.2494	360.1368	44.1037	453.2730	63.8270	
30	243.1287	870.1817	306.1950	498.3820	243.2710	115.0613	160.8529	59.4857	360.2404	44.1718	453.3998	63.3243	
31	254.4073	871.0497	309.8237	498.1867	243.5966	115.3314	161.0014	59.7442	360.3372	44.2329	453.5304	62.8319	
32	265.6574	871.7253	313.4281	497.9788	243.9186	115.6124	161.1695	60.0295	360.4265	44.2890	453.6651	62.3560	
33	276.8928	872.2063	317.0341	497.7539	244.2404	115.9045	161.3575	60.3465	360.5074	44.3418	453.8039	61.9004	
34	288.1276	872.4932	320.6698	497.5071	244.5661	116.2084	161.5659	60.7002	360.5789	44.3932	453.9465	61.4670	
35	299.3745	872.5881	324.3649	497.2322	244.8999	116.5255	161.7948	61.0952	360.6402	44.4445	454.0924	61.0557	
36	310.6444	872.4946	328.1502	496.9222	245.2467	116.8578	162.0449	61.5363	360.6906	44.4970	454.2406	60.6650	
37	321.9457	872.2165	332.0572	496.5696	245.6118	117.2078	162.3167	62.0285	360.7300	44.5517	454.3904	60.2924	
38	333.2847	871.7587	336.1172	496.1665	246.0014	117.5787	162.6114	62.5774	360.7588	44.6091	454.5409	59.9354	
39	344.6653	871.1267	340.3614	495.7055	246.4221	117.9745	162.9301	63.1895	360.7782	44.6698	454.6915	59.5913	
40	356.0901	870.3273	344.8206	495.1796	246.8816	118.4002	163.2748	63.8730	360.7903	44.7337	454.8418	59.2576	
41	367.5610	869.3682	349.5252	494.5830	247.3890	118.8621	163.6482	64.6386	360.7982	44.8007	454.9916	58.9322	
42	379.0804	868.2585	354.5053	493.9119	247.9545	119.3685	164.0544	65.4995	360.8056	44.8704	455.1414	58.6129	
43	390.6524	867.0091	359.7906	493.1643	248.5902	119.9296	164.4993	66.4728	360.8171	44.9424	455.2919	58.2975	

Frame Number	Head x	Head y	Shoulder x	Shoulder y	Elbow x	Elbow y	Wrist x	Wrist y	Hand x	Hand y	IC x	IC y
44	522.2518	1507.657	437.0246	1374.059	439.1667	1127.303	575.060	943.1083	614.715	880.1120	449.6549	998.70
45	534.4501	1505.557	450.4108	1371.850	455.6750	1125.319	596.194	945.3013	638.117	883.5624	462.1389	996.39
46	546.6946	1503.340	463.8944	1369.549	472.0967	1123.261	616.927	947.4374	661.022	886.9977	474.6841	993.97
47	558.9905	1501.042	477.4785	1367.196	488.4105	1121.160	637.231	949.5129	683.390	890.4071	487.2987	991.48
48	571.3426	1498.698	491.1625	1364.831	504.5930	1119.047	657.077	951.5224	705.182	893.7759	499.993	988.93
49	583.7549	1496.348	504.9425	1362.491	520.6193	1116.949	676.440	953.4589	726.364	897.0853	512.7801	986.37
50	596.2307	1494.029	518.8112	1360.212	536.4642	1114.896	695.298	955.3139	746.906	900.3132	525.6751	983.82
51	608.7714	1491.778	532.7583	1358.027	552.1032	1112.913	713.631	957.0778	766.783	903.4340	538.6957	981.31
52	621.3773	1489.633	546.7705	1355.967	567.5132	1111.025	731.424	958.7397	785.976	906.4198	551.8615	978.88
53	634.0468	1487.627	560.8318	1354.057	582.6737	1109.255	748.666	960.2883	804.471	909.2411	565.1934	976.54
54	646.7767	1485.791	574.9236	1352.324	597.5668	1107.623	765.348	961.7119	822.262	911.8676	578.7122	974.33
55	659.5620	1484.151	589.0253	1350.788	612.1782	1106.150	781.463	962.9990	839.345	914.2688	592.4363	972.28
56	672.3964	1482.731	603.1137	1349.467	626.4967	1104.854	797.011	964.1389	855.722	916.4159	606.3795	970.41
57	685.2723	1481.550	617.1643	1348.376	640.5142	1103.749	811.991	965.1218	871.399	918.2821	620.5474	968.73
58	698.1809	1480.623	631.1516	1347.527	654.2255	1102.850	826.407	965.9398	886.383	919.8438	634.9364	967.27
59	711.1130	1479.962	645.0503	1346.926	667.6275	1102.164	840.264	966.5865	900.683	921.0807	649.5323	966.04
60	724.0594	1479.574	658.8367	1346.579	680.7194	1101.697	853.568	967.0580	914.311	921.9768	664.3104	965.05
61	737.0114	1479.463	672.4901	1346.484	693.5017	1101.452	866.329	967.3524	927.277	922.5203	679.2368	964.29
62	749.9620	1479.627	685.9935	1346.638	705.9764	1101.426	878.554	967.4700	939.592	922.7038	694.2704	963.76
63	762.9059	1480.060	699.3351	1347.032	718.1463	1101.611	890.255	967.4127	951.268	922.5244	709.3649	963.47
64	775.8406	1480.750	712.5073	1347.654	730.0155	1101.999	901.441	967.1836	962.314	921.9839	724.4703	963.38
65	788.7655	1481.681	725.5068	1348.486	741.5892	1102.574	912.121	966.7866	972.741	921.0883	739.5354	963.50
66	801.6824	1482.833	738.3333	1349.510	752.8741	1103.321	922.308	966.2256	982.556	919.8477	754.5085	963.80
67	814.5944	1484.184	750.9880	1350.703	763.8783	1104.220	932.011	965.5046	991.770	918.2762	769.3395	964.25
68	827.5048	1485.710	763.4733	1352.042	774.6117	1105.254	941.240	964.6271	1000.388	916.3914	783.9819	964.85
69	840.4169	1487.389	775.7909	1353.502	785.0856	1106.401	950.004	963.5969	1008.417	914.2144	798.3947	965.57
70	853.3326	1489.199	787.9426	1355.059	795.3122	1107.645	958.312	962.4177	1015.865	911.7689	812.5442	966.39
71	866.2526	1491.119	799.9299	1356.693	805.3045	1108.967	966.174	961.0942	1022.737	909.0815	826.4058	967.30
72	879.1757	1493.128	811.7548	1358.382	815.0755	1110.353	973.597	959.6320	1029.043	906.1808	839.9639	968.30
73	892.0995	1495.209	823.4208	1360.107	824.6380	1111.790	980.589	958.0385	1034.791	903.0973	853.2113	969.39
74	905.0204	1497.344	834.9334	1361.852	834.0043	1113.264	987.157	956.3222	1039.989	899.8622	866.1494	970.55
75	917.9341	1499.516	846.3014	1363.601	843.1862	1114.767	993.311	954.4936	1044.651	896.5072	878.7880	971.81
76	930.8362	1501.708	857.5371	1365.343	852.1953	1116.289	999.058	952.5641	1048.789	893.0635	891.1464	973.16
77	943.7226	1503.906	868.6569	1367.064	861.0429	1117.822	1004.410	950.5459	1052.419	889.5609	903.2537	974.61
78	956.5902	1506.093	879.6808	1368.753	869.7412	1119.360	1009.377	948.4516	1055.557	886.0268	915.1477	976.17
79	969.4370	1508.252	890.6320	1370.400	878.3033	1120.899	1013.972	946.2936	1058.223	882.4857	926.8735	977.83
80	982.2618	1510.366	901.5361	1371.995	886.7441	1122.431	1018.210	944.0840	1060.436	878.9586	938.4812	979.59
81	995.0647	1512.416	912.4197	1373.526	895.0804	1123.954	1022.109	941.8336	1062.220	875.4634	950.0233	981.43
82	1007.8470	1514.380	923.3101	1374.984	903.3311	1125.462	1025.690	939.5526	1063.596	872.0145	961.5525	983.33
83	1020.6090	1516.238	934.2332	1376.355	911.5175	1126.948	1028.974	937.2496	1064.591	868.6240	973.1191	985.28
84	1033.3530	1517.966	945.2139	1377.627	919.6627	1128.403	1031.987	934.9323	1065.230	865.3018	984.7677	987.24
85	1046.0810	1519.540	956.2747	1378.785	927.7914	1129.817	1034.758	932.6072	1065.541	862.0560	996.5345	989.19
86	1058.7940	1520.939	967.4357	1379.812	935.9296	1131.176	1037.315	930.2805	1065.556	858.8937	1008.4450	991.08
87	1071.4940	1522.141	978.7147	1380.693	944.1037	1132.463	1039.691	927.9574	1065.307	855.8212	1020.5140	992.89
88	1084.1810	1523.124	990.1266	1381.411	952.3407	1133.663	1041.920	925.6434	1064.830	852.8441	1032.7460	994.59
89	1096.8570	1523.870	1001.6840	1381.949	960.6672	1134.758	1044.036	923.3441	1064.163	849.9679	1045.1340	996.14
90	1109.5220	1524.363	1013.3960	1382.293	969.1091	1135.730	1046.076	921.0654	1063.349	847.1981	1057.6670	997.52

Frame Number	GT x	GT y	Knee x	Knee y	Ankle x	Ankle y	R Heel x	R Heel y	Met x	Met y	R Toe x	R Toe y	Stride Events
44	402.2833	865.6323	365.4101	492.3406	249.3104	120.5581	164.9916	67.5794	360.8379	45.0161	455.4447	57.9836	
45	413.9826	864.1425	371.3921	491.4435	250.1318	121.2689	165.5426	68.8445	360.8736	45.0907	455.6017	57.6685	
46	425.7624	862.5563	377.7643	490.4779	251.0741	122.0795	166.1676	70.2976	360.9301	45.1652	455.7655	57.3491	
47	437.6376	860.8923	384.5530	489.4505	252.1602	123.0099	166.8858	71.9725	361.0138	45.2383	455.9388	57.0217	
48	449.6248	859.1707	391.7842	488.3699	253.4165	124.0820	167.7211	73.9066	361.1312	45.3084	456.1251	56.6824	
49	461.7424	857.4121	399.4829	487.2455	254.8731	125.3197	168.7025	76.1405	361.2889	45.3743	456.3279	56.3267	
50	474.0093	855.6371	407.6740	486.0878	256.5635	126.7479	169.8648	78.7167	361.4933	45.4355	456.5518	55.9497	
51	486.4451	853.8651	416.3824	484.9072	258.5252	128.3919	171.2490	81.6790	361.7507	45.4938	456.8016	55.5460	
52	499.0691	852.1139	425.6334	483.7140	260.7993	130.2768	172.9024	85.0714	362.0677	45.5543	457.0836	55.1095	
53	511.9001	850.3997	435.4529	482.5174	263.4308	132.4263	174.8798	88.9365	362.4523	45.6266	457.4059	54.6334	
54	524.9558	848.7370	445.8680	481.3257	266.4682	134.8621	177.2433	93.3147	362.9149	45.7260	457.7787	54.1101	
55	538.2520	847.1390	456.9072	480.1456	269.9636	137.6026	180.0630	98.2425	363.4703	45.8735	458.2149	53.5311	
56	551.8018	845.6168	468.6003	478.9818	273.9725	140.6631	183.4173	103.7511	364.1388	46.0956	458.7312	52.8864	
57	565.6142	844.1796	480.9787	477.8369	278.5537	144.0548	187.3924	109.8648	364.9479	46.4237	459.3485	52.1647	
58	579.6932	842.8347	494.0746	476.7118	283.7696	147.7851	192.0818	116.5996	365.9339	46.8940	460.0931	51.3535	
59	594.0364	841.5867	507.9210	475.6049	289.6859	151.8575	197.5852	123.9614	367.1434	47.5465	460.9979	50.4391	LTD
60	608.6337	840.4378	522.5499	474.5135	296.3716	156.2711	204.0059	131.9451	368.6348	48.4256	462.1044	49.4077	
61	623.4672	839.3875	537.9915	473.4333	303.8978	161.0196	211.4477	140.5324	370.4799	49.5791	463.4636	48.2472	
62	638.5101	838.4326	554.2720	472.3594	312.3368	166.0903	220.0112	149.6902	372.7646	51.0562	465.1384	46.9498	
63	653.7275	837.5678	571.4115	471.2875	321.7593	171.4627	229.7893	159.3682	375.5898	52.9052	467.2046	45.5158	
64	669.0768	836.7864	589.4216	470.2143	332.2322	177.1082	240.8623	169.4967	379.0706	55.1688	469.7528	43.9582	
65	684.5092	836.0806	608.3036	469.1397	343.8152	182.9895	253.2933	179.9845	383.3353	57.8796	472.8908	42.3077	
66	699.9719	835.4432	628.0463	468.0684	356.5576	189.0610	267.1239	190.7183	388.5238	61.0557	476.7449	40.6152	
67	715.4105	834.8681	648.6252	467.0117	370.4949	195.2689	282.3695	201.5629	394.7855	64.6967	481.4629	38.9541	
68	730.7715	834.3520	670.0022	465.9895	385.6464	201.5527	299.0160	212.3643	402.2761	68.7818	487.2153	37.4164	
69	746.0055	833.8949	692.1253	465.0319	402.0134	207.8452	317.0172	222.9540	411.1545	73.2680	494.1952	36.1063	
70	761.0693	833.5012	714.9302	464.1787	419.5800	214.0742	336.2964	233.1561	421.5793	78.0903	502.6152	35.1289	
71	775.9278	833.1797	738.3418	463.4794	438.3152	220.1630	356.7498	242.7956	433.7019	83.1627	512.6991	34.5766	
72	790.5556	832.9440	762.2759	462.9903	458.1768	226.0319	378.2556	251.7072	447.6596	88.3795	524.6682	34.5153	
73	804.9377	832.8115	786.6420	462.7713	479.1165	231.5979	400.6838	259.7432	463.5649	93.6183	538.7225	34.9722	
74	819.0697	832.8028	811.3455	462.8813	501.0830	236.7762	423.9086	266.7791	481.4957	98.7442	555.0212	35.9293	
75	832.9578	832.9400	836.2902	463.3738	524.0245	241.4812	447.8179	272.7165	501.4864	103.6165	573.6661	37.3241	
76	846.6178	833.2444	861.3812	464.2920	547.8890	245.6286	472.3199	277.4831	523.5240	108.0956	594.6932	39.0584	RTO
77	860.0739	833.7345	886.5270	465.6647	572.6235	249.1396	497.3450	281.0300	547.5494	112.0514	618.0732	41.0124	
78	873.3571	834.4230	911.6413	467.5040	598.1741	251.9441	522.8448	283.3286	573.4650	115.3715	643.7214	43.0613	
79	886.5038	835.3152	936.6445	469.8040	624.4861	253.9848	548.7892	284.3665	601.1465	117.9675	671.5116	45.0897	
80	899.5530	836.4076	961.4648	472.5408	651.5061	255.2193	575.1624	284.1450	630.4558	119.7792	701.2915	47.0030	
81	912.5449	837.6876	986.0383	475.6746	679.1844	255.6219	601.9611	282.6769	661.2527	120.7769	732.8957	48.7337	
82	925.5189	839.1341	1010.3090	479.1515	707.4776	255.1832	629.1921	279.9857	693.4044	120.9621	766.1557	50.2438	
83	938.5117	840.7193	1034.2300	482.9071	736.3500	253.9097	656.8714	276.1059	726.7898	120.3650	800.9062	51.5241	
84	951.5555	842.4100	1057.7600	486.8694	765.7741	251.8223	685.0226	271.0822	761.3018	119.0424	836.9882	52.5912	
85	964.6761	844.1692	1080.8670	490.9622	795.7294	248.9548	713.6750	264.9703	796.8452	117.0729	874.2502	53.4839	
86	977.8912	845.9573	1103.5240	495.1083	826.2008	245.3527	742.8620	257.8366	833.3345	114.5524	912.5479	54.2587	
87	991.2104	847.7333	1125.7100	499.2321	857.1769	241.0716	772.6188	249.7584	870.6895	111.5892	951.7430	54.9853	
88	1004.6350	849.4551	1147.4090	503.2616	888.6476	236.1757	802.9806	240.8236	908.8328	108.2993	991.7024	55.7423	
89	1018.1610	851.0812	1168.6090	507.1302	920.6024	230.7369	833.9800	231.1305	947.6873	104.8021	1032.2970	56.6135	
90	1031.7800	852.5717	1189.3010	510.7773	953.0286	224.8342	865.6452	220.7872	987.1745	101.2173	1073.4010	57.6847	

Frame Number	Head x	Head y	Shoulder x	Shoulder y	Elbow x	Elbow y	Wrist x	Wrist y	Hand x	Hand y	IC x	IC y
91	1122.1780	1524.589	1025.2720	1382.429	977.6909	1136.564	1048.081	918.8136	1062.432	844.5402	1070.3300	998.7059
92	1134.8250	1524.536	1037.3170	1382.347	986.4352	1137.245	1050.090	916.5961	1061.459	842.0001	1083.1050	999.6655
93	1147.4650	1524.197	1049.5320	1382.041	995.3621	1137.763	1052.148	914.4208	1060.479	839.5836	1095.9770	1000.3870
84	1160.1020	1523.572	1061.9210	1381.507	1004.4890	1138.108	1054.301	912.2968	1059.545	837.2960	1108.9330	1000.8560
95	1172.7400	1522.661	1074.4800	1380.745	1013.8300	1138.275	1056.598	910.2335	1058.710	835.1422	1121.9610	1001.0630
96	1185.3860	1521.474	1087.2070	1379.759	1023.3960	1138.259	1059.087	908.2402	1058.030	833.1259	1135.0540	1000.9990
97	1198.0500	1520.024	1100.0940	1378.556	1033.1920	1138.063	1061.813	906.3257	1057.559	831.2495	1148.2070	1000.6620
98	1210.7410	1518.332	1113.1330	1377.149	1043.2210	1137.688	1064.820	904.4973	1057.355	829.5134	1161.4160	1000.0520
99	1223.4720	1516.420	1126.3120	1375.550	1053.4790	1137.144	1068.144	902.7599	1057.472	827.9161	1174.6800	999.1736
100	1236.2490	1514.314	1139.6170	1373.776	1063.9570	1136.441	1071.818	901.1171	1057.963	826.4537	1187.9990	998.0358
101	1249.0780	1512.043	1153.0310	1371.846	1074.6410	1135.594	1075.871	899.5702	1058.880	825.1201	1201.3720	996.6514
102	1261.9590	1509.631	1166.5340	1369.781	1085.5120	1134.623	1080.325	898.1190	1060.268	823.9072	1214.7950	995.0374
103	1274.8870	1507.109	1180.1040	1367.603	1096.5420	1133.550	1085.200	896.7623	1062.169	822.8048	1228.2650	993.2150
104	1287.8500	1504.502	1193.7160	1365.336	1107.7010	1132.399	1090.508	895.4979	1064.614	821.8015	1241.7710	991.2089
105	1300.8320	1501.839	1207.3390	1363.007	1118.9540	1131.197	1096.251	894.3228	1067.629	820.8849	1255.2970	989.0475
106	1313.8080	1499.151	1220.9350	1360.641	1130.2590	1129.969	1102.426	893.2339	1071.225	820.0424	1268.8180	986.7625
107	1326.7450	1496.467	1234.4590	1358.266	1141.5710	1128.740	1109.012	892.2280	1075.401	819.2618	1282.3000	984.3880
108	1339.5990	1493.820	1247.8540	1355.909	1152.8390	1127.533	1115.977	891.3019	1080.135	818.5322	1295.6950	981.9608
109	1352.3100	1491.240	1261.0510	1353.599	1164.0020	1126.369	1123.268	890.4531	1085.389	817.8444	1308.9420	979.5194
110	1364.8020	1488.760	1273.9640	1351.363	1174.9900	1125.264	1130.814	889.6794	1091.097	817.1916	1321.9620	977.1038
111	1376.9790	1486.412	1286.4910	1349.228	1185.7180	1124.232	1138.519	888.9791	1097.170	816.5699	1334.6530	974.7546
112	1388.7200	1484.224	1298.5100	1347.222	1196.0800	1123.284	1146.261	888.3509	1103.487	815.9788	1346.8920	972.5130
113	1399.8780	1482.223	1309.8780	1345.372	1205.9500	1122.428	1153.894	887.7934	1109.898	815.4207	1358.5280	970.4190
114	1410.2790	1480.435	1320.4330	1343.704	1215.1790	1121.670	1161.243	887.3054	1116.221	814.9016	1369.3830	968.5109
115	1419.7300	1478.880	1329.9900	1342.240	1223.5910	1121.013	1168.110	886.8860	1122.249	814.4294	1379.2550	966.8234
116	1428.0220	1477.574	1338.3540	1341.002	1231.0000	1120.463	1174.283	886.5345	1127.759	814.0141	1387.9280	965.3857
117	1434.9580	1476.527	1345.3370	1340.002	1237.2200	1120.020	1179.554	886.2509	1132.526	813.6654	1395.1920	964.2192
118	1440.3830	1475.740	1350.7930	1339.246	1242.1030	1119.685	1183.750	886.0347	1136.362	813.3915	1400.8820	963.3334
119	1444.2530	1475.199	1354.6820	1338.724	1245.6000	1119.453	1186.789	885.8832	1139.165	813.1953	1404.9460	962.7195
120	1446.7480	1474.865	1357.1890	1338.399	1247.8630	1119.307	1188.778	885.7864	1141.016	813.0679	1407.5700	962.3362
121	1448.4950	1474.645	1358.9430	1338.183	1249.4580	1119.209	1190.200	885.7190	1142.352	812.9777	1409.4110	962.0807
122	1535.0000	1468.600	1446.2670	1331.267	1332.6670	1115.000	1271.000	881.6667	1222.533	807.7334	1503.2670	954.0667

Frame Number	GT x	GT y	Knee x	Knee y	Ankle x	Ankle y	R Heel x	R Heel y	Met x	Met y	R Toe x	R Toe y	Stride Events
91	1045.4800	853.8901	1209.4790	514.1490	985.9099	218.5530	897.9977	209.9099	1027.2140	97.6617	1114.8910	59.0417	
92	1059.2530	855.0042	1229.1370	517.1985	1019.2250	211.9852	931.0504	198.6207	1067.7200	94.2472	1156.6450	60.7684	
93	1073.0900	855.8873	1248.2710	519.8859	1052.9450	205.2283	964.8050	187.0457	1108.6050	91.0794	1198.5420	62.9454	
94	1086.9820	856.5187	1266.8780	522.1782	1087.0360	198.3838	999.2498	175.3125	1149.7730	88.2566	1240.4600	65.6477	
95	1100.9190	856.8826	1284.9580	524.0499	1121.4520	191.5556	1034.3570	163.5488	1191.1220	85.8689	1282.2760	68.9418	
96	1114.8900	856.9678	1302.5100	525.4825	1156.1350	184.8474	1070.0800	151.8817	1232.5400	83.9973	1323.8630	72.8823	
97	1128.8790	856.7668	1319.5380	526.4650	1191.0160	178.3600	1106.3500	140.4368	1273.9020	82.7122	1365.0880	77.5078	
98	1142.8670	856.2758	1336.0510	526.9944	1226.0050	172.1887	1143.0730	129.3379	1315.0730	82.0706	1405.8150	82.8383	
99	1156.8330	855.4942	1352.0600	527.0763	1260.9970	166.4202	1180.1300	118.7044	1355.9030	82.1127	1445.9060	88.8720	
100	1170.7550	854.4260	1367.5830	526.7247	1295.8660	161.1292	1217.3720	108.6481	1396.2270	82.8590	1485.2190	95.5835	
101	1184.6140	853.0799	1382.6470	525.9632	1330.4660	156.3753	1254.6250	99.2689	1435.8710	84.3064	1523.6130	102.9216	
102	1198.3950	851.4703	1397.2810	524.8242	1364.6330	152.1993	1291.6890	90.6500	1474.6500	86.4260	1560.9450	110.8074	
103	1212.0860	849.6176	1411.5220	523.3494	1398.1890	148.6200	1328.3410	82.8528	1512.3730	89.1621	1597.0790	119.1344	
104	1225.6780	847.5482	1425.4110	521.5883	1430.9430	145.6326	1364.3410	75.9138	1548.8460	92.4315	1631.8780	127.7686	
105	1239.1620	845.2944	1438.9880	519.5977	1462.7010	143.2082	1399.4320	69.8418	1583.8800	96.1250	1665.2140	136.5525	
106	1252.5260	842.8939	1452.2900	517.4393	1493.2680	141.2944	1433.3560	64.6175	1617.2900	100.1100	1696.9680	145.3103	
107	1265.7520	840.3885	1465.3500	515.1776	1522.4550	139.8191	1465.8530	60.1938	1648.9040	104.2365	1727.0330	153.8557	
108	1278.8090	837.8237	1478.1860	512.8766	1550.0890	138.6949	1496.6760	56.4992	1678.5610	108.3453	1755.3130	162.0012	
109	1291.6520	835.2469	1490.7990	510.5973	1576.0100	137.8264	1525.5960	53.4431	1706.1190	112.2787	1781.7270	169.5697	
110	1304.2180	832.7062	1503.1670	508.3945	1600.0780	137.1185	1552.4090	50.9230	1731.4590	115.8918	1806.2040	176.4070	
111	1316.4240	830.2491	1515.2380	506.3149	1622.1730	136.4850	1576.9420	48.8343	1754.4840	119.0627	1828.6820	182.3930	
112	1328.1590	827.9207	1526.9250	504.3956	1642.1950	135.8571	1599.0540	47.0793	1775.1250	121.7017	1849.1040	187.4518	
113	1339.2880	825.7624	1538.1000	502.6643	1660.0600	135.1893	1618.6440	45.5762	1793.3400	123.7588	1867.4180	191.5581	
114	1349.6500	823.8110	1548.5950	501.1398	1675.7030	134.4637	1635.6440	44.2660	1809.1160	125.2282	1883.5680	194.7383	
115	1359.0580	822.0975	1558.2070	499.8333	1689.0760	133.6909	1650.0260	43.1152	1822.4670	126.1492	1897.5000	197.0671	
116	1367.3130	820.6466	1566.7050	498.7500	1700.1520	132.9067	1661.8020	42.1148	1833.4310	126.6039	1909.1600	198.6590	
117	1374.2220	819.4747	1573.8630	497.8898	1708.9330	132.1643	1671.0280	41.2741	1842.0700	126.7078	1918.5100	199.6550	
118	1379.6320	818.5875	1579.4960	497.2469	1715.4760	131.5218	1677.8230	40.6102	1848.4840	126.5941	1925.5590	200.2064	
119	1383.4960	817.9734	1583.5340	496.8057	1719.9390	131.0243	1682.4070	40.1330	1852.8560	126.3889	1930.4270	200.4570	
120	1385.9930	817.5894	1586.1500	496.5313	1722.6820	130.6790	1685.1930	39.8256	1855.5500	126.1770	1933.4640	200.5254	
121	1387.7470	817.3316	1587.9920	496.3473	1724.4700	130.4152	1686.9810	39.6145	1857.3240	125.9547	1935.4950	200.4826	RTD
122	1483.7330	808.6667	1679.0000	487.2667	1780.3330	116.5333	1731.2670	38.6666	1917.8670	95.6666	1937.5250	200.4398	

TABLE E-2 Kinetic Data in Newtons

Number	Fx	Fy	Fz	Events	Number	Fx	Fy	Fz	Events
−1	0	0	0		39	−10.7067	−7.1134	275.6521	
0	1.5647	−0.2007	7.04480	RTD	40	−12.2693	−3.5299	285.8246	
1	−1.2618	6.1802	53.34734		41	−12.0855	−2.9519	288.7185	
2	1.7255	9.5325	111.1378		42	−13.0966	−0.4550	303.9773	
3	9.4928	−4.6627	184.3624		43	−13.0047	1.9262	313.3606	
4	21.0518	−22.5572	235.4881		44	−14.2915	5.1167	336.9503	
5	28.9799	−41.3995	289.6832		45	−12.2693	9.0932	351.0691	
6	30.0140	−54.5544	335.5472		46	−13.0966	12.9773	379.3943	
7	26.0155	−66.6458	385.7960		47	−12.4531	18.4103	396.6701	
8	18.2023	−73.6048	427.9769		48	−14.4984	22.5949	428.9415	
9	10.7337	−82.5751	459.7222		49	−14.9120	29.7157	451.6543	
10	6.8501	−85.7424	485.8550		50	−15.9921	34.6401	482.5227	
11	5.7930	−89.8577	499.7984		51	−16.8883	43.2636	508.2171	
12	1.3808	−89.5803	520.2312		52	−18.2211	48.9741	533.8238	
13	−5.6510	−93.1406	529.8775		53	−20.1745	57.4127	558.2904	
14	−14.5903	−92.2852	545.6625		54	−21.4843	63.2157	574.0754	
15	−19.1174	−89.9271	544.9609		55	−23.7823	71.7005	592.9296	
16	−25.3220	−88.2393	555.5719		56	−24.4717	78.2664	600.9098	
17	−26.9306	−82.4133	549.9595		57	−26.5399	85.8033	610.5562	
18	−28.0796	−76.7952	553.0288		58	−24.8624	93.0165	604.5930	
19	−25.8505	−68.7728	540.5762		59	−24.8624	98.9813	604.4176	
20	−24.7705	−62.7387	533.2099		60	−22.2427	104.5069	583.8094	
21	−22.6563	−54.2539	514.1803		61	−20.4043	107.3506	570.0415	
22	−21.1166	−49.3988	496.4661		62	−17.0032	110.4948	535.1392	
23	−19.6229	−42.0237	474.8933		63	−14.2686	110.7029	503.3062	
24	−17.8075	−38.0703	444.9019		64	−9.7185	109.1077	452.5313	
25	−17.2790	−31.8743	428.5030		65	−6.2944	101.1315	404.6502	
26	−16.0840	−28.5682	397.5470		66	−3.8356	91.2132	345.5443	
27	−17.3019	−23.9212	382.2882		67	−3.1002	77.4110	285.2985	
28	−15.6474	−21.3319	356.4184		68	−3.6287	66.4524	228.9111	
29	−16.3138	−19.1818	341.4227		69	−3.0542	51.3323	171.8222	
30	−14.5214	−17.2860	316.2545		70	−4.2952	39.7495	128.9397	
31	−14.2226	−16.3843	310.0282		71	−4.4330	26.8258	88.1619	
32	−11.9476	−14.4423	290.2970		72	−4.6399	18.1560	61.6782	
33	−11.2352	−14.4885	288.2801		73	−2.3648	10.2261	34.0546	
34	−9.9023	−12.8933	275.9152		74	−2.0431	5.3710	25.1975	
35	−9.6495	−13.1014	275.0382		75	0.0480	2.8972	9.3248	
36	−9.5346	−10.3964	269.6889		76	−1.4916	0.9089	10.99105	RTO
37	−9.4657	−11.1593	271.7935						
38	−10.2700	−7.5758	273.8105						

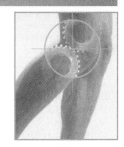

Index

Page numbers in *italics* denote figures; those followed by t denote tables